Leukocyte Typing II

VOLUME 1
Human T Lymphocytes

Leukocyte Typing II

Leukocyte Typing II

VOLUME 1
Human T Lymphocytes

Edited by
Ellis L. Reinherz   Barton F. Haynes
Lee M. Nadler   Irwin D. Bernstein

With 123 Illustrations

Springer-Verlag
New York Berlin Heidelberg Tokyo

Ellis L. Reinherz, M.D., Division of Tumor Immunology, Dana-Farber Cancer Institute, Boston, MA 02115 U.S.A.

Barton F. Haynes, M.D., Department of Medicine, Duke University School of Medicine, Durham, NC 27710 U.S.A.

Lee M. Nadler, M.D., Division of Tumor Immunology, Dana-Farber Cancer Institute, Boston, MA 02115 U.S.A.

Irwin D. Bernstein, M.D., Program in Pediatric Oncology, Fred Hutchinson Cancer Research Center, Seattle, WA 98104 U.S.A.

Library of Congress Cataloging in Publication Data
Main entry under title:
Leukocyte typing II.
    Papers presented at the Second International
Workshop on Human Leukocyte Differentiation Antigens,
held in Boston, Sept. 17–20, 1984.
    Includes bibliographies and indexes.
    Contents: v. 1. Human T lymphocytes—v. 2. Human
B lymphocytes—v. 3. Human myeloid and hematopoietic
cells.
    1. Leucocytes—Classification—Congresses.
2. Histocompatibility testing—Congresses. 3. Tissue
specific antigens—Analysis—Congresses. I. Reinherz,
Ellis L. II. International Workshop on Human
Leukocyte Differentiation Antigens (2nd : 1984 : Boston,
Mass.) III. Title: Leukocyte typing 2. IV. Title:
Leukocyte typing two.
QR185.8.L48L48   1985   616.07′9   85-22229

Typeset by Bi-Comp Inc., York, Pennsylvania.
Printed and bound by Halliday Lithograph, West Hanover, Massachusetts.
Printed in the United States of America.

9 8 7 6 5 4 3 2 1

ISBN 0-387-96175-5 Springer-Verlag New York Berlin Heidelberg Tokyo
ISBN 3-540-96175-5 Springer-Verlag Berlin Heidelberg New York Tokyo

Preface

The Second International Workshop on Human Leukocyte Differentiation Antigens was held in Boston, September 17–20, 1984. More than 350 people interested in leukocyte differentiation agreed to exchange reagents and participate in this joint venture. All in all, in excess of 400 antibodies directed against surface structures on T lymphocytes, B lymphocytes, and myeloid-hematopoietic stem cells were characterized. Because of the enormous quantity of serologic, biochemical, and functional data, *Leukocyte Typing II* has been divided into three volumes.

These books represent the written results of workshop participants. They should be helpful to both researchers and clinicians involved in scientific endeavors dealing with these broad fields of immunobiology. To those who delve into the various sections of the volumes, it will become evident that the work speaks for itself.

I am deeply indebted to the section editors, Barton F. Haynes, *Volume 1, Human T Lymphocytes,* Lee M. Nadler, *Volume 2, Human B Lymphocytes,* and Irwin D. Bernstein, *Volume 3, Human Myeloid and Hematopoietic Cells* for their major contributions in planning, executing, and summarizing the workshop, as well as council members John Hansen, Alain Bernard, Laurence Boumsell, Walter Knapp, Andrew McMichael, Cesar Milstein, and Stuart F. Schlossman. I would also like to thank the National Institutes of Health, World Health Organization, and International Union of Immunological Societies for making this meeting possible. Needless to say, I am most grateful to all of my colleagues who contributed to this effort and helped to accelerate the characterization of human immunobiology through their endeavors.

Ellis L. Reinherz, M.D.

Contents

Contributors

Martine Amiot INSERM U93, Hôpital Saint-Louis, Paris, France

I. Ando ICRF, Human Tumour Immunology Group, School of Medicine, University College London, London WC1E 6JJ, U.K.

R. Andreesen Medizinischen Klinik der Albert-Ludwigs-Universität, Freiburg, F.R.G.

G. Bátory National Institute of Haematology and Blood Transfusion, Egyt Pharmacochemical Works, Budapest, Hungary

Patrick G. Beatty Puget Sound Blood Center, University of Washington, Seattle, Washington 98104, U.S.A.

Alain Bernard Laboratoire d'Immunologie des Tumeurs de l'Enfant, Institut Gustave-Roussy, Villejuif, France

Peter Bettelheim I. Department of Medicine, University of Vienna, Austria

Peter C.L. Beverley ICRF, Human Tumour Immunology Group, School of Medicine, University College London, London WC1E 6JJ, U.K.

A. Bewick Nuffield Department of Surgery, John Radcliffe Hospital, Oxford, U.K.

Robert D. Bigler The Rockefeller University, New York, New York 10021, U.S.A.

Els Blokland Department of Immunohaematology and Bloodbank, University Hospital, 2333 AA Leiden, The Netherlands

Marie-Luise Blue Division of Tumor Immunology, Dana-Farber Cancer Institute, Boston, Massachusetts 02115, U.S.A.

Laurence Boumsell Laboratoire d'Immunologie des Tumeurs de l'Enfant, Institut Gustave-Roussy, Villejuif, France

A.W. Boylston Department of Pathology, St. Mary's Hospital Medical School, London, U.K.

Jean Brochier INSERM U.80, Hôpital E. Herriot, 69374 Lyon Cedex 08, France

K.J. Bross Medizinischen Klinik der Albert-Ludwigs-Universität, Freiburg, F.R.G.

Philippe Brottier Laboratoire d'Immunologie des Tumeurs de l'Enfant, Institut Gustave-Roussy, Villejuif, France

Hans Bruning Department of Immunohaematology and Bloodbank, University Hospital, 2333 AA Leiden, The Netherlands

Bernard Caillou INSERM U93, Hôpital Saint-Louis, Paris, France

N. Carter Nuffield Department of Surgery, John Radcliffe Hospital, Oxford, U.K.

Dominique Charmot Centre d'Immunologie, INSERM-CNRS de Marseille-Luminy, Case 906, 13288 Marseille Cedex 9, France

Nicholas Chiorazzi The Rockefeller University, New York, New York 10021, U.S.A.

Edward A. Clark University of Washington, Seattle, Washington 98104, U.S.A.

Loran T. Clement Cellular Immunobiology Unit, Tumor Institute, University of Alabama in Birmingham, Birmingham, Alabama 35294, U.S.A.

Max D. Cooper Cellular Immunobiology Unit, Tumor Institute, University of Alabama in Birmingham, Birmingham, Alabama 35294, U.S.A.

D.H. Crawford Department of Haematology, School of Medicine, University College London, London WC1E 6HX, U.K.

John F. Daley Division of Tumor Immunology, Dana-Farber Cancer Institute, Boston, Massachusetts 02115, U.S.A.

M. De Felice Dipartimento di Biologia e Patologia Cellulare e Molecolare, II Facoltà di Medicina e Chirurgia, Università di Napoli, Napoli, Italy

L. Del Vecchio Centro Trasfusionale, Ospedale Cardarelli, Napoli, Italy

D.W. Dongworth Nuffield Department of Medicine, John Radcliffe Hospital, Oxford, U.K.

H.G. Drexler Edward J. Hines, Jr. Veterans Administration Hospital, Hines, Illinois 60141, U.S.A.

Patrice Dubreuil Centre d'Immunologie, INSERM-CNRS de Marseille-Luminy, Case 906, 13288 Marseille Cedex 9, France

Bo DuPont Human Immunogenetics Laboratory, Memorial Sloan-Kettering Cancer Center, New York, New York 10021, U.S.A.

Dienne Elferink Department of Immunohaematology and Bloodbank, University Hospital, 2333 AA Leiden, The Netherlands

S. Ellis Nuffield Department of Medicine, John Radcliffe Hospital, Oxford, U.K.

N. Emi First Department of Internal Medicine, Department of Pediatrics, Nagoya University School of Medicine, Nagoya 466, Japan

Alfred C. Feller Abteilung Pathologie, Universität Kiel, Hospitalstrasse 42, D-2300 Kiel, F.R.G.

Hans-Dieter Flad   Forschungsinstitut Borstel, Parkallee 3a, D-2061 Borstel, F.R.G.

Neal Flomenberg   Human Immunogenetics Laboratory, Memorial Sloan-Kettering Cancer Center, New York, New York 10021, U.S.A.

Junichiro Fujimoto   Department of Pathology, Sapporo Medical College, Sapporo 060, Japan

Véronique Gay-Bellile   INSERM U93, Hôpital Saint-Louis, Paris, France

Eric Georget   Laboratoire d'Immunologie des Tumeurs de l'Enfant, Institut Gustave-Roussy, Villejuif, France

S. Gignac   Edward J. Hines, Jr. Veterans Administration Hospital, Hines, Illinois 60141, U.S.A.

Heinz Gisslinger   Department of Medicine, University of Vienna, Vienna, Austria

Gy. Görög   National Institute of Haematology and Blood Transfusion, Egyt Pharmacochemical Works, Budapest, Hungary

F.M. Gotch   Nuffield Department of Medicine, John Radcliffe Hospital, Oxford, U.K.

Els Goulmy   Department of Immunohaematology and Bloodbank, University Hospital, 2333 AA Leiden, The Netherlands

Shizuo Hagiwara   Nichirei Research and Development Institute, Higashimurayama 189, Japan

John A. Hansen   Puget Sound Blood Center, University of Washington, Seattle, Washington 98104, U.S.A.

Elizabeth A. Harden   Department of Medicine, Duke University School of Medicine, Durham, North Carolina 27710, U.S.A.

Barton F. Haynes   Department of Medicine, Duke University School of Medicine, Durham, North Carolina 27710, U.S.A.

Lucinda L. Hensley   Department of Medicine, Division of Rheumatology and Immunology, Duke University Medical Center, Durham, North Carolina 27710, U.S.A.

J. Heyman   Nuffield Department of Medicine, John Radcliffe Hospital, Oxford, U.K.

Winifred Ho   Department of Medicine, Division of Rheumatology and Immunology, Duke University Medical Center, Durham, North Carolina 27710, U.S.A.

Wolfgang Holter   Institute of Immunology, University of Vienna, Vienna, Austria

Thomas H. Hutteroth   I. Med. Klinik u. Poliklinik, Johannes Gutenberg Universität Mainz, F.R.G.

Yoshifumi Ishii   Department of Pathology, Sapporo Medical College, Sapporo 060, Japan

M. Jonker   Primate Center TNO, Rijswijk, The Netherlands

Marrie Kardol Department of Immunohaematology and Bloodbank, University Hospital, 2333 AA Leiden, The Netherlands

Claudine Kieda Centre de Biophysique Moléculaire, Centre National de la Recherche Scientifique, 45045 Orléans Cedex, France

Kokichi Kikuchi Department of Pathology, Sapporo Medical College, Sapporo 060, Japan

Walter Knapp Institute of Immunology, University of Vienna, Vienna, Austria

Robert W. Knowles Human Immunogenetics Laboratory, Memorial Sloan-Kettering Cancer Center, New York, New York 10021, U.S.A.

Ursula Köller Institute of Immunology, University of Vienna, Vienna, Austria

Shinichiro Kon Department of Pathology, Sapporo Medical College, Sapporo 060, Japan

Frits Koning Department of Immunohaematology and Bloodbank, University Hospital, 2333 AA Leiden, The Netherlands

Eugen Kopp Institute for Immunology, University of Munich, Munich, F.R.G.

Jolanta E. Kunicka Memorial Sloan-Kettering Cancer Center, New York, New York 10021, U.S.A.

R. Kurrle Research Laboratories of Behringwerke AG, D-3550 Marburg/L., F.R.G.

J.R. Lamb ICRF Human Tumour Immunology Group, School of Medicine, University College London, London WC1E 6JJ, U.K.

Andrew J. Laster Department of Medicine, Duke University School of Medicine, Durham, North Carolina 27710, U.S.A.

T. Laskay National Institute of Haematology and Blood Transfusion, Egyt Pharmacochemical Works, Budapest, Hungary

Jeffrey A. Ledbetter Department of Medicine, University of Washington, Seattle, Washington 98104, U.S.A.

Virginia Lepage Laboratoire d'Immunologie des Tumeurs de l'Enfant, Institut Gustave-Roussy, Villejuif, France

Norman L. Letvin Division of Tumor Immunology, Dana-Farber Cancer Institute, Boston, Massachusetts 02115, U.S.A.

Herbert Levine Division of Tumor Immunology, Dana-Farber Cancer Institute, Boston, Massachusetts 02115, U.S.A.

David C. Linch Department of Haematology, School of Medicine, University College and Middlesex Hospitals, London, U.K.

Kristof Liszka Institute of Immunology, University of Vienna, Vienna, Austria

David F. Lobach Department of Medicine, Duke University School of Medicine, Durham, North Carolina 27710, U.S.A.

G.W. Löhr Medizinische Klinik der Albert-Ludwigs-Universität, Freiburg, F.R.G.

C. Lo Pardo   Centro Trasfusionale, Ospedale Cardarelli, Napoli, Italy

M. Maio   Dipartimento di Biologia e Patologia Cellulare e Molecolare, Il Facoltà di Medicina e Chirurgia, Università di Napoli, Napoli, Italy

Otto Majdic   Institute of Immunology, University of Vienna, Vienna, Austria

Patrice Mannoni   Department of Pathology, University of Alberta, Edmonton, Alberta, Canada

Paul J. Martin   Fred Hutchinson Cancer Research Center, University of Washington, Seattle, Washington 98104, U.S.A.

T. Maruyama   Laboratory of Chemotherapy and Cell Biology, Aichi Cancer Center Research Institute, Nagoya 464, Japan

Claude Mawas   Centre d'Immunologie, INSERM-CNRS de Marseille-Luminy, Case 906, 13288 Marseille Cedex 9, France

A.J. McMichael   Nuffield Department of Medicine, John Radcliffe Hospital, Oxford, U.K.

P. McShane   Nuffield Department of Surgery, John Radcliffe Hospital, Oxford, U.K.

Cornelis J.M. Melief   Central Laboratory, Netherlands Red Cross, Blood Transfusion Service, Amsterdam, The Netherlands

M. Menon   Edward J. Hines, Jr. Veterans Administration Hospital, Hines, Illinois 60141, U.S.A.

Stefan C. Meuer   I. Med. Klinik u. Poliklinik, Johannes Gutenberg Universität Mainz, F.R.G.

K. H. Meyer zum Büschenfelde   I. Med. Klinik u. Poliklinik, Johannes Gutenberg Universität Mainz, F.R.G.

Frank Miedema   Central Laboratory, Netherlands Red Cross, Blood Transfusion Service, Amsterdam, The Netherlands

Saburo Mimami   First Department of Internal Medicine, Nagoya University, Nagoya, Japan

J. Minowada   Edward J. Hines, Jr. Veterans Administration Hospital, Hines, Illinois 60141, U.S.A.

B. Misra   Edward J. Hines, Jr. Veterans Administration Hospital, Hines, Illinois 60141, U.S.A.

Kanji Miyamoto   First Department of Internal Medicine, Nagoya University, Nagoya, Japan

Shin-ichi Mizuno   First Department of Internal Medicine, Nagoya University, Nagoya, Japan

T. Monnheimer   Medizinische Klinik der Albert-Ludwigs-Universität, Freiburg, F.R.G.

Michel Monsigny   Centre de Biophysique Moléculaire, Centre National de la Recherche Scientifique, 45045 Orléans Cedex, France

Chikao Morimoto   Division of Tumor Immunology, Dana-Farber Cancer Institute, Boston, Massachusetts 02115, U.S.A.

Yasuo Morishima   First Department of Internal Medicine, Nagoya University, Nagoya, Japan

P.J. Morris   Nuffield Department of Surgery, John Radcliffe Hospital, Oxford, U.K.

Simin Naipal-van den Berge   Department of Immunohaematology and Bloodbank, University Hospital, 2333 AA Leiden, The Netherlands

Kazuyuki Naito   Department of Medicine, Duke University School of Medicine, Durham, North Carolina 27710, U.S.A.

K. Nishida   Laboratory of Chemotherapy and Cell Biology, Aichi Cancer Center Research Institute, Nagoya 464, Japan

F.J.M. Nooij   Primate Center TNO, Rijswijk, The Netherlands

Tomoko Noumi   First Department of Internal Medicine, Nagoya University, Nagoya, Japan

Kieran O'Flynn   Department of Haematology, School of Medicine, University College and Middlesex Hospitals, London, U.K.

Ryuzo Ohno   First Department of Internal Medicine, Nagoya University, Nagoya, Japan

Ken-ichi Ohya   First Department of Internal Medicine, Nagoya University, Nagoya, Japan

Masao Okumura   First Department of Internal Medicine, Nagoya University, Nagoya, Japan

Katja Olas   Sandoz Forschungsinstitut, Vienna, Austria

Daniel Olive   Centre d'Immunologie, INSERM-CNRS de Marseille-Luminy, Case 906, 13288 Marseille Cedex 9, France

J. Osterholz   Medizinische Klinik der Albert-Ludwigs-Universität, Freiburg, F.R.G.

K. Ota   Laboratory of Chemotherapy and Cell Biology, Aichi Cancer Center Research Institute, Nagoya 464, Japan

Tom Ottenhoff   Department of Immunohaematology and Bloodbank, University Hospital, 2333 AA Leiden, The Netherlands

E. Pace   Centro Trasfusionale, Ospedale Cardarelli, Napoli, Italy

Thomas J. Palker   Department of Medicine, Division of Rheumatology and Immunology, Duke University Medical Center, Durham, North Carolina 27710, U.S.A.

M. Palmer   Nuffield Department of Medicine, John Radcliffe Hospital, Oxford, U.K.

Christian Peschel   Department of Medicine, University of Innsbruck, Austria

G. Gy. Petrányi   National Institute of Haematology and Blood Transfusion, Egyt Pharmacochemical Works, Budapest, Hungary

Chris D. Platsoucas   Memorial Sloan-Kettering Cancer Center, New York, New York 10021, U.S.A.

Jos Pool   Department of Immunohaematology and Bloodbank, University Hospital, 2333 AA Leiden, The Netherlands

Marguerite Ragueneau   Centre d'Immunologie, INSERM-CNRS de Marseille-Luminy, Case 906, 13288 Marseille Cedex 9, France

Gerti Rank   Institute for Immunology, University of Munich, Munich, F.R.G.

Brigitte Raynal   INSERM U93, Hôpital Saint-Louis, Paris, France

Peter Rieber   Institute for Immunology, University of Munich, Munich, F.R.G.

Gert Riethmüller   Institute for Immunology, University of Munich, Munich, F.R.G.

Kimitaka Sagawa   Department of Immunology, Kurume University School of Medicine, Kurume 830, Japan

Ellen Saltz-Tal   Weizmann Institute of Science, Department of Cell Biology, Rehovot, Israel

Richard M. Scearce   Department of Medicine, Division of Rheumatology and Immunology, Duke University Medical Center, Durham, North Carolina 27710, U.S.A.

Stuart F. Schlossman   Division of Tumor Immunology, Dana-Farber Cancer Institute, Boston, Massachusetts 02115, U.S.A.

Daniel Schmitt   INSERM U.209, Hôpital E. Herriot, 69374 Lyon Cedex 08, France

Wolfgang Scholz   Forschungsinstitut Borstel, Parkallee 3a, D-2061 Borstel, F.R.G.

F.R. Seiler   Research Laboratories of Behringwerke AG, D-3550 Marburg/L., F.R.G.

W. Seyfert   Research Laboratories of Behringwerke AG, D-3550 Marburg/L., F.R.G.

L. Skowron   Edward J. Hines, Jr. Veterans Administration Hospital, Hines, Illinois 60141, U.S.A.

Hannes Stockinger   Institute of Immunology, University of Vienna, Vienna, Austria

T. Takahashi   Laboratory of Chemotherapy and Cell Biology, Aichi Cancer Center Research Institute, Nagoya 464, Japan

S. Takamoto   Laboratory of Chemotherapy and Cell Biology, Aichi Cancer Center Research Institute, Nagoya 464, Japan

Takashi Takei   Department of Pathology, Sapporo Medical College, Sapporo 060, Japan

Thomas F. Tedder   Cellular Immunobiology Unit, Tumor Institute, University of Alabama in Birmingham, Birmingham, Alabama 35294, U.S.A.

Annemarie Termijtelen   Department of Immunohaematology and Bloodbank, University Hospital, 2333 AA Leiden, The Netherlands

Fokke G. Terpstra   Central Laboratory, Netherlands Red Cross, Blood Transfusion Service, Amsterdam, The Netherlands

A. Trautwein   Research Laboratories of Behringwerke AG, D-3550 Marburg/L., F.R.G.

I. Tsuge   First Department of Internal Medicine, Department of Pediatrics, Nagoya University School of Medicine, Nagoya 466, Japan

M.C. Turco Istituto di Scienze Biochimiche, Il Facoltà di Medicina e Chirurgia, Università di Napoli, Napoli, Italy

R. Ueda Laboratory of Chemotherapy and Cell Biology, Aichi Cancer Center Research Institute, Nagoya 464, Japan

Artur J. Ulmer Forschungsinstitut Borstel, Parkallee 3a, D-2061 Borstel, F.R.G.

Tehila Umiel Beilinson Medical Center, Department of Pediatric Hematology/Oncology, Petah Tikva, Israel

K. Utsumi Laboratory of Chemotherapy and Cell Biology, Aichi Cancer Center Research Institute, Nagoya 464, Japan

C. Vacca Centro Trasfusionale, Ospedale Cardarelli, Napoli, Italy

Jan van der Poel Department of Immunohaematology and Bloodbank, University Hospital, 2333 AA Leiden, The Netherlands

S. Venuta Istituto di Scienze Biochimiche, Il Facoltà di Medicina e Chirurgia, Università di Napoli, Napoli, Italy

Nicolas L. von Jeney Sandoz Forschungsinstitut, Vienna, Austria

D.L. Wallace ICRF Human Tumour Immunology Group, School of Medicine, University College London, London WC1E 6JJ, U.K.

Martin Wilhelm Institute for Immunology, University of Munich, Munich, F.R.G.

B. Winkler-Lowen Department of Pathology, University of Alberta, Edmonton, Alberta, Canada

Sybille Wirth Institute for Immunology, University of Munich, Munich, F.R.G.

Kaori Yasuda Department of Immunology, Kurume University School of Medicine, Kurume 830, Japan

Mitchel Mitsuo Yokoyama Department of Immunology, Kurume University School of Medicine, Kurume 830, Japan

S. Zappacosta Dipartimento di Biologia e Patologia Cellulare e Molecolare, Il Facoltà di Medicina e Chirurgia, Università di Napoli, Napoli, Italy

Part I. Introduction

Summary of T Cell Studies Performed during the Second International Workshop and Conference on Human Leukocyte Differentiation Antigens

Barton F. Haynes

T Cell Protocol Areas of Study

For the Second International Workshop and Conference on Human Leukocyte Differentiation Antigens, eight areas of study were chosen (Table 1.1). The results of serologic and cluster analysis will be discussed later in this chapter, while data obtained from functional, biochemical, and phylogeny studies will be presented in individual reports in this volume.

Regarding anti–T cell monoclonal antibodies, the general goals of this workshop were to 1) study a large number of anti–T cell monoclonal antibodies to determine if additional major cluster (CD) groups (1) were yet to be defined, 2) to make available many reagents of a particular specificity for epitope and phylogeny studies, 3) to establish initial clusters of reagents that define antigens of activated T cells, and 4) to identify a large, well-characterized panel of reagents for more select, in-depth studies to be performed at subsequent workshops. The participants in all the serologic and cluster analysis for the T cell section are listed in Appendix 1.

T Cell Antibody Panel

One hundred and fifty-one antibodies were accepted for the T cell section of the Workshop. With eight controls added to the panel the total number of reagents was 159. Because antibodies arriving in the US from certain countries were irradiated prior to redistribution in aliquots to participants, irradiated and nonirradiated positive and negative controls were included. The eight additions to the T cell panel were: A3D8 (anti-p80, pan leukocyte positive control) (2,3); A3D8 irradiated (positive control); P3X63,

Table 1.1. T cell protocol areas of study.

1. Serologic and cluster analysis of reagents in T cell panel
2. Functional studies
3. Biochemical studies
4. Phenotypic characterization of T cell leukemias and lymphomas
5. Phylogenetic studies of T cell antibodies
6. Study of anti–T cell antibodies on frozen tissue sections of human tissue
7. Study of antibodies reactive with antigens of activated T cells
8. Study of T cell leukemia-associated antigens

IgG_1 (negative control) (4); P3X63, IgG_1 irradiated (negative control); PBS-BSA (negative control) × 2; 11G6 (anti-HTLV$_I$ p24), IgG2 (negative control) (5); and $3A1_A$, irradiated (to control for irradiation of an anti–T cell antibody) (6). The final T cell antibody panel is listed in Table 1.2. Each antibody was coded, divided into 100-μl aliquots, and sent to participating laboratories either with or without 0.1% sodium azide.

Based on information provided to the Workshop at the time of antibody submission, the T cell panel was divided into 12 groups (Table 1.3). This was done to facilitate the study of select antigens by laboratories, while maintaining the panel code. As will be seen, not all antibodies originally included in the groupings turned out to be of that specificity.

Methods for Serologic and Cluster Analysis of Monoclonal Antibodies in the T Cell Panel

For participation in this part of the Workshop, the following protocol was adopted. The panel of target cells against which the T cell antibody panel was tested included:

1. Purified peripheral blood (PB) T cells from five donors.
2. Purified PB non-T lymphocytes from five donors.
3. Five target cell suspensions from the following categories: (a) Con A activated T cells, (b) PHA activated T cells, (c) IL-2 dependent T cell lines, (d) MLR activated T cells, (e) thymocytes, or (f) leukemia cells.

On each type of target cell, the following data were provided by the participating laboratories: the percentage of E-rosette positive cells by E-rosette assay or anti–E-rosette monoclonal antibody, percentage of surface immunoglobulin positive B cells, percentage monocytes by anti-monocyte monoclonal antibody or by latex bead ingestion, and viability of suspension at the time of assay. The form used for data entry for each protocol was that designed by Bernard *et al.* for the First Workshop (1).

The mandatory assay for serologic comparison of the T cell antibody panel was immunofluorescence, either using a fluorescent microscope or flow microfluorometry. Since each antibody ascites submitted had a saturation titer of >1 : 1000, the dilution for all reagents in immunofluorescence was 1 : 400. Of 41 laboratories that agreed to participate in serologic analysis of the panel, 24 laboratories submitted completed data (Appendix 1). The number of individual target protocols submitted was 270. Of these, 217 protocols were accepted by the criteria outlined below. Thus, in the serologic comparison of 151 anti–T cell antibodies, 34,503 individual assay results were collected and analyzed.

Table 1.4 shows the target cell types against which the T cell panel of reagents were assayed, and the number of targets of each type assayed by participating laboratories. The criteria for deletion of individual target protocols was as follows:

1. Based on method of study—i.e., if other than microscopy or cytofluorography;
2. If two or more negative controls (panel numbers 1, 2, 35, 157, 158), for targets 1, 3–21 were >10;
3. If two or more negative controls for target 2 were >20; or
4. If positive controls (panel numbers 3, 156) were <60 on all targets except thymocytes and T cell leukemic cells.

As mentioned, using these criteria 217 of 270 submitted protocols were accepted and the data entered for computer analysis.

All data analysis was performed by Dr. Shiangtai Tuan, at the Duke University Computation Center through the Triangle University Computation Center. The computer was an IBM 3081, using the WYLBUR program to edit data and as a utility program and Statistical Analysis System (SAS) programs for actual data analysis (7). The mean, standard deviation, and standard error of the mean were computed for each antibody on each target. Cluster analysis of the 159 antibodies in the T cell panel was performed using an SAS program based on an algorithm using average linkage of variables on squared euclidian distances (8).

Next, criteria were established to assess reproducibility of results submitted by each laboratory. There were four pairs of duplicates in the panel:

1, 157 = P3X63, negative control
39, 40 = $3A1_A$
2, 35 = PBS-BSA, negative control
3, 156 = A3D8, positive control

A reproducibility score was calculated as the sum of absolute differences of each pair divided by the total number of times a pair was run. Thus, the reproducibility score was an average of the absolute difference of values

Table 1.2. Antibody panel for T cell studies of the second international workshop on human leukocyte differentiation antigens—1984.

Antibody group	Code number	Antibody name	Binds SPA	Fixes C	Ig subclass	Lab number	Investigator
Negative control	1	P3X63	No	No	IgG1	105	Haynes
Negative control	2	PBS-BSA	NA	NA	NA	105	Haynes
Positive control	3	A3D8	No	Yes	IgG1	105	Haynes
CD5	4	H65	No	No	IgG1	26	Knowles
	5	6-2	Yes	Yes	IgG2a	28	Naito
	6	SJ10-2H10	NK	NK	IgG1	31	Melvin
	7	L17F12/Leu 1	NK	Yes	IgG2a	47	Warner
	8	MT 61	Yes	NK	IgG2b	61	Rieber
	9	MT 215	No	NK	IgG1	61	Rieber
	10	2H4	NK	No	IgG1	75	Morimoto
	11	XIX102-3	Yes	Yes	IgG2a	96	Bourel
	12	BL-T2	NK	No	IgG2b	116	Ambrosius
CD2	13	9-1	NK	Yes	IgG2b	28	Naito
	14	9-2	NK	Yes	IgM	28	Naito
	15	G19-3.1	No	No	IgG1	36	Ledbetter
	16	S2/Leu 5b	NK	NK	IgG2a	47	Warner
	17	MT 26	No	NK	IgG1	61	Rieber
	18	MT 910	No	NK	IgG1	61	Rieber
	19	MT 1110	No	NK	IgG1	61	Rieber
	20	T11/3Pt2H9	No	No	IgG1	72	Reinherz
	21	T11/ROLD2-1H8	Yes	No	IgG1	72	Reinherz
	22	T11/3T4-8B5	Yes	Yes	IgG2a	72	Reinherz
	23	T11/7T4-7A9	No	Yes	IgM	72	Reinherz
	24	T11/7T4-7E10	Yes	Yes	IgG2b	72	Reinherz
	25	9.6	Yes	Yes	IgG2a	79	Martin
	26	35.1	Yes	Yes	IgG2a	79	Martin
	27	T411B5	NK	Yes	IgG1/G2	88	Girardet
	28	KOLT-2	NK	No	IgG1	71	Sagawa

Group	No.	Antibody			Ig	Ref	Author
CD7	29	9-3	NK	Yes	IgG2b	28	Naito
	30	G3-7	No	No	IgG1	36	Ledbetter
	31	4H9/Leu 9	Yes	NK	IgG2a	47	Warner
	32	BW264/50	No	Yes	IgM	53	Kurrle
	33	BW264/217	No	Yes	IgM	53	Kurrle
	34	BW264/215	No	Yes	IgM	53	Kurrle
	35	PBS-BSA	No	No	NA	105	Haynes
	36	A1	Yes	Yes	IgG2	88	Girardet
	37	4D12.1	NK	MK	IgG1	100	Mawas
	38	8H8.1	Yes	NK	IgG2a	100	Mawas
	39	3A1A	Yes	Yes	IgG1	105	Haynes
	40	3A1$_A$(irrad)	Yes	Yes	IgG1	105	Haynes
	41	3A1$_B$-4G6	Yes	Yes	IgG2	105	Haynes
	42	3A1$_C$-5A12	No	Yes	IgM	105	Haynes
	43	4A	Yes	Yes	IgG2	107, 28	Dupont, Naito
	44	1-3	Yes	Yes	IgG2a	107, 28	Dupont, Naito
	45	I21	Yes	NK	IgG	103	Bernard, Boumsell
CD6	46	T12/3Pt12B8	No	Yes	IgM	72	Reinherz
	47	12.1.5	Yes	Yes	IgG2a	79	Martin
Pan T other or unknown	48	T10B9	NK	Yes	IgM	21	Thompson
	49	T12A10	NK	Yes	IgM	21	Thompson
	50	E9	NK	NK	IgG	27	McMichael
	51	G3-5	No	No	IgG1	36	Ledbetter
	52	G10-2.1	No	No	IgG1	36	Ledbetter
	53	G19-1.2	No	No	IgG1	36	Ledbetter
	54	T55	Yes	Yes	IgG2a	46	Maeda
	55	T56	No	Yes	IgM	46	Maeda
	56	T57	NK	Yes	IgG	46	Maeda
	57	BW239/347	Yes	Yes	IgG	53	Kurrle
	58	MT 211	No	NK	IgG1	61	Rieber
	59	MT 421	No	NK	IgG1	61	Rieber

Table 1.2. *Continued*

Antibody group	Code number	Antibody name	Binds SPA	Fixes C	Ig subclass	Lab number	Investigator
	60	CRIS-3	Yes	Yes	IgG	69	Vilella
	61	CRIS-7	Yes	Yes	IgG	69	Vilella
	62	CRIS-8	Yes	Yes	IgG	69	Viellla
	63	K20	NK	NK	NK	103	Bernard, Boumsell
	64	K50	NK	NK	NK	103	Bernard, Boumsell
	65	G144	No	Yes	IgM	103	Bernard, Boumsell
	66	D47	Yes	Yes	IgG2	103	Bernard, Boumsell
CD4	67	T10C5	NK	Yes	IgM	21	Thompson
	68	G19-2	No	No	IgG1	36	Ledbetter
	69	91d6	Yes	NK	IgG2a	42	Winchester
	70	94b1	Yes	NK	IgG2a	42	Winchester
	71	BW264/123	No	Yes	IgM	53	Kurrle
	72	MT 151	Yes	Yes	IgG2a	61	Rieber
	73	MT 321	No	No	IgG1	61	Rieber
	74	T4/12T4D11	Yes	No	IgG1	72	Reinherz
	75	T4/18T3A9	Yes	No	IgG1	72	Reinherz
	76	MT 310	No	No	IgG1	61	Rieber
	77	T4/19THY5D7	Yes	Yes	IgG2	72	Reinherz
	78	T4/7T4-6C1	No	Yes	IgM	72	Reinherz
	79	66.1	No	Yes	IgM	79	Martin
	80	TII19-4-7	NK	NK	NK	94	Feller
CD8	81	14	NK	NK	IgG1	25	Hogg
	82	M236	No	NK	IgG1	26	Knowles
	83	G10-1.1	Yes	Yes	IgG2a	36	Ledbetter
	84	C12/D3	Yes	Yes	IgG1	43	Petranyi
	85	BW264/162	Yes	Yes	IgG2a	53	Kurrle
	86	BW135/80	Yes	Yes	IgG2a	53	Kurrle

#	Name			Ig		Investigator
87	MT 415	No	No	IgG1	61	Rieber
88	MT 1014	No	Yes	IgM	61	Rieber
89	MT 122	No	No	IgG1	61	Rieber
90	T8/21thy2D3	Yes	No	IgG1	72	Reinherz
91	T8/7Pt3F9	Yes	Yes	IgG2	72	Reinherz
92	T8/2T8-1B5	Yes	Yes	IgG2b	72	Reinherz
93	T8-2T8-1C1	Yes	No	IgG1	72	Reinherz
94	T8/2T8-2A1	Yes	Yes	IgG2b	72	Reinherz
95	T8/2ST8-5H7	NK	NK	NK	72	Reinherz
96	66.2	Yes	Yes	IgG	79	Martin
97	51.1	Yes	Yes	IgG2a	79	Martin
98	T411E1	Yes	Yes	IgG2	88	Girardet
99	T41D8	Yes	No	IgG2	88	Girardet
100	BL-TS1	NK	NK	IgG	116	Ambrosius
101	Withdrawn					
102	D44	Yes	Yes	IgG2b	103	Bernard, Boumsell
103	SK11/Leu 8	Yes	No	IgG2a	47	Warner
104	3AC5	No	NK	IgG1	66	Clark
105	CRIS-4	No	Yes	IgG	69	Vilella
106	CRIS-5	No	Yes	IgM	69	Vilella
107	EDU-2	Yes	Yes	IgG	69	Vilella
108	TQ1/28T17G6	Yes	No	IgG1	72	Reinherz
109	GM1	NK	NK	IgG1	78	Jonker
110	10B4.6	NK	NK	IgG1	100	Mawas
111	8E-1.7	Yes	Yes	IgG2b	100	Mawas
112	6F10.3	NK	NK	IgG1	100	Mawas
113	13B8.2	NK	NK	IgG1	100	Mawas
114	K51	NK	Yes	NK	103	Bernard, Boumsell
115	BL-TS20	NK	NK	IgG	116	Ambrosius
116	BL-TS14	NK	NK	IgG	116	Ambrosius

T cell subset

other

Table 1.2. *Continued*

Antibody group	Code number	Antibody name	Binds SPA	Fixes C	Ig subclass	Lab number	Investigator
CD3	117	G19-4.1	No	No	IgG1	36	Ledbetter
	118	SK7/Leu 4	No	No	IgG1	47	Warner
	119	89b1	NK	NK	NK	42	Winchester
	120	BW264/56	Yes	Yes	IgG2a	53	Kurrle
	121	BW242/55	Yes	No	IgG3	53	Kurrle
	122	T3/2Ad2A2	No	Yes	IgM	72	Reinherz
	123	T3/2T8-2F4	No	No	IgG1	72	Reinherz
	124	T3/RW2-4B6	Yes	Yes	IgG2b	72	Reinherz
	125	T3/RW2-8C8	Yes	No	IgG1	72	Reinherz
	126	X35-3	Yes	Yes	IgG2a	96	Bourel
	127	NU-T1	NK	No	IgG1	71	Sagawa
CD1	128	M-241	No	No	IgG1	26	Knowles
	129	NA1/34	Yes	Yes	IgG2a	27	McMichael
	130	SK9/Leu 6	Yes	Yes	IgG2b	47	Warner
	131	4A76	Yes	Yes	IgG2a	100	Mawas
	132	10D12.2	NK	NK	IgG1	100	Mawas
	133	NU-T2	NK	No	IgG1	71	Sagawa
	134	I-19	NK	Yes	IgG	103	Bernard, Boumsell
T-Activation	135	T1A	NK	Yes	IgG2	9	Morishima
	136	TS145	Yes	NK	IgG1	10	Ueda
	137	100-1A5	NK	NK	NK	69	Vilella
	138	1 MONO 2A6	Yes	Yes	IgG3	72	Reinherz
	139	4EL1C7	Yes	No	IgG1	72	Reinherz
	140	Tac/1HT4-4H3	NK	NK	NK	72	Reinherz

No.	Description	Clone			Isotype	Cluster	Investigator
141		B149.9	Yes	Yes	IgG2a	100	Mawas
142		B1.19.2	Yes	Yes	IgG2a	100	Mawas
143		23A9.3	NK	NK	*NK	100	Mawas
144		39C1.5	NK	NK	*NK	100	Mawas
145		39C6.5	NK	NK	*NK	100	Mawas
146		33B3.1	NK	NK	*NK	100	Mawas
147		33B7.3	NK	NK	*NK	100	Mawas
148		39C8.18	NK	NK	*NK	100	Mawas
149		39H7.3	NK	NK	*NK	100	Mawas
150		41F2.1	NK	NK	*NK	100	Mawas
151		K0LT-1	NK	No	IgG1	71	Sagawa
152	Leukemia associated	6-4	Yes	Yes	IgG2a	28	Naito
153	T-Activation	AA3	NK	NK	IgG1	89	Chiorazzi
154	Leukemia associated	3-40	No	Yes	IgM	107, 28	Dupont, Naito
155	Leukemia associated	3-3	Yes	Yes	IgG2b	107, 28	Dupont, Naito
156	Positive control	A3D8(irrad.)	No	Yes	IgG1	105	Haynes
157	Negative control	P3(irrad.)	No	No	IgG1	105	Haynes
158	Negative control	11G6(HTLV-8 anti-HTLV$_1$ p24)	Yes	Yes	IgG2	105	Haynes
159	T-Activation	Tac	Yes	Yes	IgG2a	106	Waldmann

NK = not known.
NA = not applicable.
* = Rat monoclonal antibody.

Table 1.3. T cell antibody panel groups.

Group (representative antibody)	Number
Controls	8
CD1 (T6)	7
CD2 (T11)	16
CD3 (T3)	11
CD4 (T4)	14
CD5 (T1)	9
CD6 (T12)	2
CD7 (3A1)	15
CD8 (T8)	20
Pan T other or unknown	19
T cell subset other	16
T cell activation	19
Leukemia associated	3
Total	159

Table 1.4. Target cell types in T cell protocol.

Target no.	Type	Number of protocols accepted
1	PB T cells	55
2	PB Non-T cells	33
3	Thymocytes	13
4	Tonsil cells	11
5	Lymph node cells	0
6	Spleen cells	2
7	PHA blasts, 3 days	24
8	Con A blasts, 3 days	1
9	ALL MLC blasts, 6 days	0
10	T-ALL blasts from children (<15 yr)	10
11	T-ALL blasts from adults (>15 yr)	2
12	T lymphoma blasts from children	2
13	T lymphoma blasts from adults	0
14	Cutaneous T cell lymphoma	0
15	T cell chronic lymphocytic leukemia	2
16	T cell clone—TCGF grown	1
17	B cell chronic lymphocytic leukemia	13
18	B lymphoblastoid cell line	4
19	Non-T cell leukemia	12
20	T cell line "spontaneously grown"	17
21	Other	15
	Total	217

for the duplicates run by each laboratory. A high score meant a high average difference between duplicates and a low score meant a low average difference between duplicate samples. Figure 1.1 shows this analysis for 22 of the 24 laboratories participating in serologic analysis. Only 4 of 22 laboratories had considerable variability in their results.

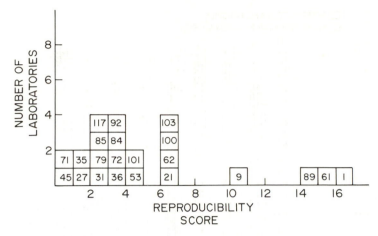

Fig. 1.1. Phenotyping laboratory reproducibility scores for 22 laboratories.

Next, five laboratories were chosen as reference laboratories and the data from the reference laboratories against PB T and non-T cells were analyzed for 13 representative antibodies and compared to the data from the non-reference laboratories. The reference laboratories were numbers 27 (McMichael), 72 (Reinherz), 79 (Martin), 100 (Mawas), and 103 (Bernard and Boumsell). As seen in Fig. 1.2(A), the results on PB T cells of the reference and non-reference laboratories were nearly identical. When the data were plotted with the mean value of the reference labs reported as one value with bars showing ±1SD, and each non-reference laboratory reported as a single point, we saw that each non-reference laboratory except one performed as well or better than the reference laboratories [Fig. 1.2(B), 1.2(C)].

Report of Serologic and Cluster Analysis of Monoclonal Antibodies in the T Cell Panel

Once it was established that the data collected were reproducible and reliable, then cluster analysis was performed (SAS Program, "average" method) (8), for the panel on each target. The clusters for each target were then compared with each other to obtain a combined cluster analysis based on all antibodies assayed on all target cells.

Using SAS cluster analysis, 28 clusters of antibodies in the T cell panel were identified (Tables 1.5 and 1.6). Table 1.5 shows those antibodies that clustered with either the positive or negative controls, or with known antibodies of CD1–8 specificity. Table 1.6 shows those clusters (designated here by a temporary antibody group) that were not defined by known CD1–8 antibodies (1).

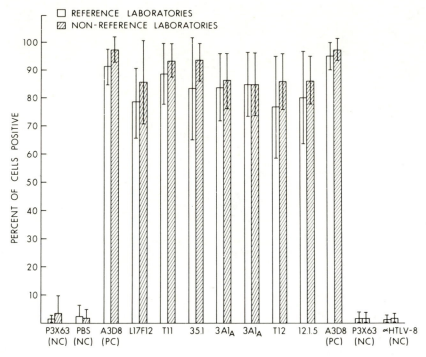

Fig. 1.2A.

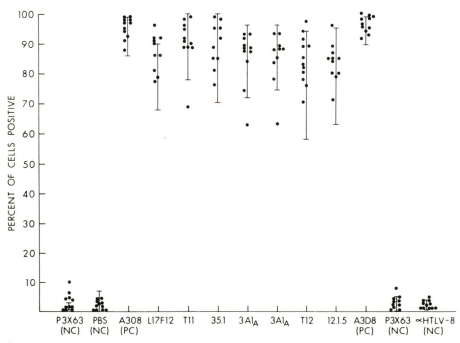

Fig. 1.2B.

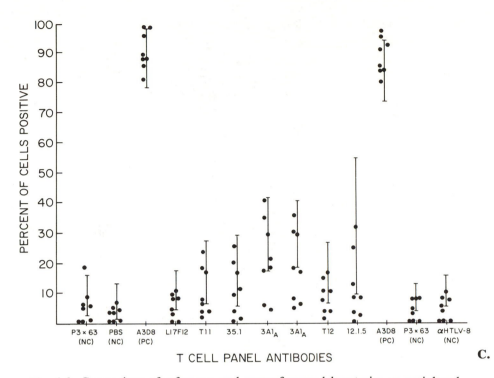

Fig. 1.2. Comparison of reference and non-reference laboratories on peripheral blood T cells (A and B) and on peripheral blood non-T cells (C).

Those antibodies whose specificity for CD group 1–8 have been confirmed by biochemistry or other assays will be listed below (see Table 1.16). Sixteen antibodies that were included in the First Workshop in 1982 (1) were also included in the Second Workshop. To assess the reliability of our cluster analysis, we looked at the results from the First Workshop and compared them with the Second (Table 1.7). In the case of each antibody, the CD designation was the same for both workshops. Tables 1.8–1.13 summarize the data for reactivity of the 28 cluster groups on nonmalignant lymphocytes, malignant cells, and lymphoid and myeloid cell lines.

Antibodies within CD groups 1, 2, 4, 5, 6, 7, and 8 were uniformly tightly grouped and cluster groups were readily apparent. However, known antibodies in the CD3 group to the T3 antigen (9) clustered in three well-defined separate subclusters, arbitrarily designated subclusters A, B, and C (Table 1.8). The only appreciable difference among subclusters CD3 A, B, and C appeared to be in thymocyte reactivity with the mean percent of thymocytes reacting with antibodies within groups A, B, and C, 71%, 51%, and 33% respectively. Reactivity on PB non-T cells was highest (20%) with CD7 antibodies, reflecting CD7 positivity on Fc recep-

Table 1.5. Anti–T cell antibodies clustering within defined cluster groups.

Cluster (no. antibodies)	Antibodies
Negative controls (10)	P3X63, PBS-BSA, BLTS-20, BLTS-1, BLTS-14, 33B7.3, 3-40, 3-3, A-1
Positive control (1)	A3D8
CD1 (9)	D-47, T411E1, M-241, NA1/34, SK9/Leu 6, 4A76, 10D12.2, NU-T2, I-19
CD2 (19)	9-1, MT 1110, S2/Leu 5b, MT 910, 9.6, MT 26, T11/7T4-7E10, T411B5, T11/3Pt2H9, T11/3T4-8B5, T11/ROLD2-1H8, 35.1, T57, 9-2, 89b1, 39C1.5, T11/7T4-7A9, 6F10.3, NU-T1
CD3 (16)	A. SK7/Leu 4, T3/2Ad2A2, BW242/55, 39H7.3, 41F2.1 B. T3/RW2-4B6, T3/RW2-8C8, X35-3, G19-4.1, BW264/56, KOLT-2, T10B9, CRIS-7, BW239/347 C. T10C5, T3/2T8-2F4
CD4 (14)	G19-2, 91d6, 94b1, 13B8.2, T4/12T4D11, T4/18T3A9, MT 310, MT 151, T4/19THY5D7, EDU-2, 66.1, BW264/123, MT 321, T4/7T4-6C1
CD5 (5)	H65, G19-3.1, 6-2, L17F12/Leu 1, MT 61
CD6 (7)	T12/3Pt12B8, 12.1.5, SJ10-2H10, MT421, G3-5, T12A10, MT 211
CD7 (10)	3A1$_A$, 3A1$_B$-4G6, MT 215, G3-7, 4H9/Leu 9, 8H8.1, I21, 4A, 1-3, T55
CD8 (21)	M236, T8/21thy2D3, G10-1.1, C12/D3, MT 415, 4D12.1, 8E-1.7, T8/7Pt3F9, T8-2T8-1C1, T41D8, 66.2, 51.1, MT 122, BW135/80, T8/2T8-2A1, T8/2ST8-5H7, 14, MT 1014, T8/2T8-1B5, BW264/162, 10B4.6

tor-positive large granular lymphocytes in the E-negative fraction of PB mononuclear cells (10).

The reactivity of CD1–8 clusters on fresh malignant target cells (Table 1.9) was similar to data presented by Bernard *et al.* from the First Workshop (1). CD7 reagents were reaffirmed again as the best marker of the T lineage in T ALL, and reacted poorly with HTLV$_I^+$ ATL cells (11). As seen before, CD7-defined p40 antigen was the only T cell lineage antigen found on a small percentage of AML cells (12,13).

CD5 and CD6 reagents both bound B CLL cells in addition to malignant T cells (Table 1.9) (14).

In the 16 remaining temporary cluster groups identified by our com-

Table 1.6. Anti–T cell antibody temporary groups other than defined CD groups.

Temporary antibody group	Number of antibodies	Antibodies
II.	2	3A1$_C$-5A12, K50
IV.	2	BW264/215, SK11/Leu 8
V.	4	D-44, 100-1A5, GM1, K51
VII.	4	T56, 39C8.18, 1MONO2A6, G144
IX.	1	KOLT-1
X. (TACT$_A$)	4	TII19-4-7, TS-145 4EL1C7, B1.19.2
XI. (TACT$_B$)	8	T1A, TAC/1HT4-4H3, TAC, B149.9, 23A9.3, 33B3.1, 39C6.5, AA3
XIII.	3	E9, CRIS-8, CRIS-5
XIV.	2	G10-2.1, G19-1.2
XV.	3	BW264/217, CRIS-3, 6-4
XVII.	1	TQ1/28T17G6
XXI.	1	K-20
XXIV.	1	9-3
XXVI.	2	2H4, CRIS-4
XXVII.	2	BL-T2, 3AC5
XXVIII.	2	XIX102-3, BW264/50

Table 1.7. Antibodies analyzed in both first and second workshops.

Antibody	CD 1st workshop	CD 2nd workshop
9.6	CD2	CD2
T4/12T4D11	CD4	CD4
NA1/34	CD1	CD1
T8/21thy2D3	CD8	CD8
PBS-BSA	NC	NC
A3D8	PC	PC
D47	CD1	CD1
3-40	NC	NC
35.1	CD2	CD2
T11/3Pt2H9	CD2	CD2
12.1	CD6	CD6
3A1	CD7	CD7
4A	CD7	CD7
H65	CD5	CD5
TAC	T-Act	T-Act
T3/2Ad2A2	CD3	CD3

NC = negative control.
PC = positive control.
T Act = antigen of activated T cells.

Table 1.8. Summary of reactivity of clusters CD1–8 on nonmalignant lymphoid target cells.

Antibody group	PB T cells (55)[a]	PB Non-T cells (33)	Thymocytes (13)	Tonsil cells (11)	Spleen cells (2)	PHA blasts (24)	Con A blasts (1)
			Mean % cells positive[b]				
Negative control	4	7	8	3	7	10	9
Positive control (A3D8)	96	90	44	73	85	86	99
CD1	5	6	73	3	7	8	9
CD2	84	11	87	8	23	84	97
CD3 A	69	7	71	5	27	62	44
B	82	7	51	13	20	72	91
C	70	7	33	17	26	50	64
CD4	54	10	73	12	6	46	58
CD5	83	8	68	22	11	79	84
CD6	78	11	31	15	13	63	83
CD7	82	20	64	10	23	84	95
CD8	29	8	66	4	10	36	42

[a] Number in parentheses indicates number of target cells assayed.
[b] Data are mean values for all antibodies within each cluster (see Table 1.5).

puter analysis (Table 1.6), several interesting groups of reagents were identified. The serologic characterization of these groups of reagents are summarized in Tables 1.11, 1.12, and 1.13. Group II contained a known anti-CALLA reagent (K-50). Group VII (consisted of a tight cluster of reagents [T56, 39C8.18, 1 Mono 2A6, and G144 (D-66 cl 2)] that have all been shown by Knowles (this volume, Chapter 22) and Bernard, Boumsell, and coworkers (this volume, Chapter 4) to bind to the CD2 (E-rosette receptor associated) p50 molecule, but, unlike the CD2 cluster of reagents (Table 1.5), which reacted with 84% of resting PB T cells, group VII reagents reacted with only 47%. As noted by Meuer *et al.* (this volume, Chapter 5) and Bernard, Boumsell, and coworkers (this volume, Chapter 4), these reagents are CD2 reagents that bind to epitopes whose expression is increased on activated T cells.

Group IX contains three antibodies (TII19-4-7, TS-145, and 4EL1C7) that define a p120, 200 T cell antigen of activation and was given the preliminary cluster designation of CDw26 (see below).

Group X contains antibodies against the IL-2 receptor and was given the cluster designation CD25 (see below).

Group XIV reagents were against the transferrin receptor, and antibody TQ1/28T17G6 clustered by itself, as did antibodies K-20 and 9-3. Interestingly, antibody TQ1/28T17G6, which has been reported to define functional subsets of T cells (15), was found to immunoprecipitate a p50 CD2-

Table 1.9. Summary of reactivity of clusters CD1–8 on fresh malignant target cells.

Antibody group	T ALL children (10)[a]	T ALL adults (2)	T LL children (2)	T CLL (2)	B CLL (13)	CALLA+ non-TALL (6)	CALLA− non-TALL (1)	Japanese ATL (6)	AML (2)
				Mean % cells positive[b]					
Negative control	9	3	11	6	4	9	5	5	3
Positive control (A3D8)	82	83	92	92	87	76	98	97	74
CD1	15	33	57	2	6	9	5	8	3
CD2	52	35	97	86	9	8	8	88	4
CD3 A	30	14	84	50	8	9	6	49	3
B	23	14	84	94	11	8	7	74	4
C	14	10	43	79	15	8	6	49	4
CD4	24	9	93	91	8	8	10	93	4
CD5	75	34	97	91	63	7	7	82	3
CD6	36	9	47	97	48	9	15	44	3
CD7	91	48	66	68	9	10	11	32	29
CD8	25	23	64	10	6	8	6	8	3

[a] Number in parentheses indicates number of target cells assayed.
[b] Data are mean values for all antibodies within each cluster (see Table 1.5).

Table 1.10. Summary of reactivity of clusters CD1–8 on hematopoietic cell lines.

Antibody group	T cell clone (1)[a]	B lympho- blastoid line (4)	REH (3)	K562 (1)	RPMI-8402 (2)	HPB-ALL (4)	MOLT-4 (5)	CEM (2)	JURKAT (2)	MOLT-3 (1)	HSB-2 (1)	NALM-16 (1)	NALM-1 (1)	KG-1 (1)	MC-1 (1)
Negative control (1)[a]	11	11	6	6	25	16	13	14	9	17	3	19	0	4	0
Positive control (A3D8)	94	76	7	54	84	83	76	97	50	98	99	95	95	88	100
						% of cells positive[b]									
CD1	12	8	6	5	2	55	49	14	11	65	4	7	0	1	0
CD2	98	14	5	5	59	70	35	10	43	18	8	21	0	1	0
CD3 A	95	8	17	5	26	65	26	19	12	NA	NA	8	0	0	0
B	95	14	17	4	14	66	33	37	33	18	13	30	0	0	6
C	80	7	20	4	17	57	34	14	2	NA	NA	10	0	0	0
CD4	42	15	15	4	21	71	55	50	2	66	3	15	5	0	0
CD5	95	13	3	8	96	68	72	95	19	97	78	15	5	0	0
CD6	96	16	4	5	18	46	45	22	13	NA	NA	31	0	4	0
CD7	84	22	7	25	65	53	54	77	88	97	96	21	0	3	3
CD8	80	7	25	5	5	61	59	6	1	9	8	16	0	0	0

NA = Not available.
[a] Number in parentheses indicates number of target cells assayed.
[b] Data are mean values for all antibodies within each cluster (see Table 1.5).

Table 1.11. Summary of reactivity of temporary antibody groups on nonmalignant lymphoid target cells.

Antibody group: temporary group number (representative antibody)	PB T cells (55)[a]	PB non-T cells (33)	Thymocytes (13)	Tonsil cells (11)	Spleen cells (2)	PHA blasts (24)	Con A blasts (1)
			Mean % of cell positive[b]				
II (K-50, CALLA)	8	9	21	6	5	12	8
IV (Leu 8)	52	21	23	14	17	55	5
V (D 44)	22	17	64	8	12	17	8
VII (G144)	43	6	71	3	9	55	91
IX (KOLT-1)	42	5	48	2	12	40	88
X (TACT_A)	23	15	25	5	5	38	56
XI (TACT_B)	4	8	12	4	12	53	82
XIII (CRIS-8)	72	45	75	65	74	73	88
XIV (transferrin receptor)	85	48	57	17	29	78	97
XV (BW264/217)	91	56	75	62	44	84	93
XVII (TQ1)	82	32	83	23	40	76	82
XXI (K-20)	61	51	38	18	35	67	98
XXIV (9.3)	68	12	34	21	19	72	45
XXVI (2H4)	66	47	30	64	86	73	84
XXVII (BL-T2)	65	25	51	29	14	59	33
XXVIII (XIX102-3)	77	22	26	31	31	64	31

[a] Number in parentheses indicates number of target cells assayed.
[b] Data are mean values for all antibodies within each group (see Table 1.6).

like molecule (this volume, Chapter 22) and to block E-rosette formation (this volume, Chapter 4).

Finally, three of the reagents [Leu 8 (no. 103), TQ1 (no. 108), and BW264/215 (no. 34)] did not react with all donors tested. Moreover, when positive, they reacted with a wide range of positivity. While TQ1 clustered alone (temporary group XVII, Table 1.6) antibodies Leu 8 and BW264/215 clustered together (group IV, Table 1.6). These data are summarized in Table 1.14.

Summary of Biochemical Studies Performed

Three laboratories (102, 26, and 105) were the primary contributors of biochemical data on the T cell panel of antibodies (Table 1.15). Their reports are summarized in detail elsewhere in this book (Chapters 4, 22, and 24) and will not be repeated here. In general there was excellent concordance between serologic cluster analysis and biochemical analysis.

Table 1.12. Summary of reactivity of temporary antibody groups on fresh malignant target cells.

Antibody group: temporary group number (representative antibody)	T ALL children (10)[a]	T ALL adults (2)	T LL children (2)	T CLL (2)	B CLL (13)	CALLA+ non-T ALL (6)	CALLA- non-T ALL (1)	Japanese ATL (6)	AML (2)
					% Cells positive[b]				
II (K-50, CALLA)	41	27	40	4	5	47	8	10	3
IV (Leu 8)	14	8	57	15	35	13	7	22	10
V (D44)	80	64	31	15	20	47	25	25	37
VII (G144)	39	19	93	23	6	9	11	23	3
IX (KOLT-1)	16	2	72	54	3	12	5	30	3
X (TACT$_A$)	14	6	28	23	13	14	6	9	3
IX (TACT$_B$)	11	22	17	9	7	24	5	15	3
XIII (CRIS-8)	51	63	93	93	70	56	12	83	17
XIV (transferrin receptor)	86	79	96	93	72	89	89	94	50
XV (BW264/217)	69	32	95	95	31	26	49	72	13
XVII (TQ1)	70	43	94	66	40	11	7	91	18
XXI (K-20)	85	86	53	97	17	85	86	64	59
XXIV (9.3)	36	72	99	80	30	32	9	80	3
XXVI (2H4)	42	7	76	71	48	56	35	45	9
XXVII (BL-T2)	24	24	73	82	49	25	8	59	6
XXVII (XIX102-3)	14	5	79	62	34	7	5	35	3

[a] Number in parentheses indicates number of target cells assayed.
[b] Data are mean values for all antibodies within each group (see Table 1.6).

Table 1.13. Summary of reactivity of temporary antibody groups on hematopoietic cell lines+.

Antibody group: temporary group no. (representative antibody)	T cell clone (1)[a]	B lympho-blastoid line (4)	REH (3)	K562 (1)	RPMI-8402 (2)	HPB-ALL (4)	MOLT-4 (5)	CEM (2)	JURKAT (2)	MOLT-3 (1)	HSB-2 (1)	NALM-16 (1)	NALM-1 (1)	KG-1 (1)	MC-1 (1)
							% Cells positive[b]								
II (K-50, CALLA)	7	25	52	4	63	50	21	24	8	4	3	55	50	0	0
IV (Leu 8)	17	54	4	4	64	22	32	11	22	NA	NA	10	12	0	0
IV (D44)	51	14	6	6	72	71	60	23	57	NA	NA	50	6	10	24
VII (G144)	95	12	3	5	16	57	3	5	18	NA	NA	3	0	0	1
IX (KOLT-1)	32	10	3	4	2	65	8	10	1	67	3	0	0	0	0
X (TACT$_A$)	93	21	4	4	15	12	12	5	1	5	3	25	4	4	11
XI (TACT$_B$)	58	16	3	9	9	5	6	13	7	16	15	25	0	36	8
XIII (CRIS-8)	97	43	49	5	7	58	32	31	43	NA	NA	40	38	32	0
XIV (transferrin receptor)	97	85	63	99	98	75	89	74	76	96	3	100	100		100
XV (BW264/217)	97	65	3	4	36	77	88	89	17	97	65	67	16	62	68
XVII (TQ1)	96	16	3	5	32	76	31	9	42	6	5	0	0	0	0
XXI (K-20)	97	49	38	96	100	64	74	98	99	98	96	100	100	82	100
XXIV (9.3)	41	40	13	4	37	56	22	35	1	98	3	90	39	0	0
XXVI (2H4)	74	65	46	21	3	43	25	32	36	NA	NA	45	51	28	0
XXVII (BL-T2)	41	39	24	6	9	52	42	44	1	34	5	15	0	22	0
XVIII (XIX102-3)	98	72	4	5	33	42	20	7	13	NA	NA	20	45	0	0

NA = No data available.

[a] Number in parentheses indicates number of target cells assayed.

[b] Data are mean values for all antibodies within each group (see Table 6).

Table 1.14. Comparison of reactivities of antibodies leu 8 (103), TQ1 (108), and BW264/215 (34).

Target	Leu 8	BW264/215	TQ1
No. T cell			
donors positive	54/55	54/55	52/55
PB T	49 ± 24	55 ± 36	82 ± 24
Range of positives	(10–96%)	(10–100)	(29–99)
PB non-T	28 ± 26	14 ± 24	31 ± 24
Thymocytes	16 ± 20	29 ± 31	83 ± 16
Tonsil	18 ± 17	10 ± 7	23 ± 18
Spleen	31 ± 43	3 ± 1	40 ± 55
PHA blasts	52 ± 18	59 ± 33	76 ± 18
T ALL children	23 ± 17	6 ± 5	70 ± 32
T ALL adults	8 ± 11	4 ± 3	43 ± 58
TLL children	37 ± 53	76 ± 14	93 ± 5
TCLL	20 ± 12	9 ± 11	66 ± 18
B lymphoblastoid cells	26 ± 21	81 ± 13	15 ± 21
B CLL			
No. donors positive	12/13	7/13	11/13
Range of positives	(13–96)	(21–76)	(14–97)
Mean ± SD of cells positive	44 ± 31	26 ± 29	40 ± 28

Table 1.15. Laboratories that performed evaluations of anti–T cell monoclonal antibodies.

Laboratory number	Investigator(s)	Antibody group studied	Reference in this book
103	Bernard, Boumsell	CD1, CD2	Chapter 4
26	Knowles	Entire T cell panel	Chapter 22
105	Haynes, Palker	CD7	Chapter 24

Final Antibody Clusters and New Cluster Designations

Table 1.16 shows the final anti–T cell antibody cluster groups that were confirmed by biochemical analysis or blocking studies. In addition, two new CD groups, CD25 (anti–IL-2 receptor antibodies) (16) and CDw26 (anti-p120, p200 T cell activation antigen antibodies) were approved by the Workshop Nomenclature Committee and their confirmed antibodies are shown as well in Table 1.16.

The combined analysis of the CD2 and CD3 antibodies deserve particular comment. The official CD designation for each cluster is CD2 and CD3. The subclusters A, B, and C for each cluster are *operational* and have not been approved as final by the Workshop Nomenclature Committee. The significance of these subclusters are as follows:

Table 1.16. Final anti–T cell antibody clusters and approved new CD groups.

Cluster (no. antibodies)	Antibodies
CD1 (8)	D-47, M-241, NA1/34, SK9/Leu 6, 4A76, 10D12.2, NU-T2, I-19
CD2A (18)	9-1, MT 1110, S2/Leu 5b, MT 910, 9.6, MT 26, T11/7T4-7E10, T411B5, T11/3Pt2H9, T11/3T4-8B5, T11/R0LD2-1H8, 35.1, T57, 9-2, 39CL.5, T11/7T4-7A9, 6F10.3, NU-T1
CD2B (4)	T-56, 39C8.18, 1 Mono 2A6, G144(D66c12)
CD2C (2)	39H7.3, 41F2.1
CD3$_A$ (2)	SK7/Leu4, T3/2Ad2A2
CD3$_B$ (6)	T3/RW2-4B6, T3/RW2-8C8, G19-4.1, BW264/56, CRIS-7, BW239/347
CD3$_C$ (1)	T3/2T8/2F4
CD4 (13)	G19-2, 91d6, 94b1, 13B8.2, T4/12T4D11, T4/18T3A9, MT 310, MT 151, T4/19THY5D7, EDU-2, 66.1, MT 321, T4/7T4-6C1
CD5 (4)	H65, 6-2, L17F12/Leu 1, MT 61
CD6 (2)	T12/3P512B8, 12.1.5
CD7 (9)	3A1$_A$, 3A1$_B$-4G6, G3-7, 4H9/Leu9, 8H8.1, I21, 4A, 1-3, T55
CD8 (18)	M236, T8/21thy2D3, G10-1.1, C12/D3, MT 415, 4D12.1, T8/7Pt3F9, T8/2T8-1C1, T41D8, 66.2, 51.1, MT 122, BW135/80, T8/2T8-2A1, T8/2ST8-5H7, 14, MT 1014, T8/2T8-1B5
New CD groups	
CD25[a] (7)	T1A, TAC/1HT4-4H3, TAC, B149.9, 23A9.3 33B3.1, 39C6.5
CDw26[b] (3)	T11119-4-7, TS-145, 4EL1C7

[a] Anti-IL-2 receptor.
[b] Anti-p120, p200 T activation antigen.

CD2A. This subcluster of 18 reagents contains those pan T cell reactive antibodies that react with most PB T cells, immunoprecipitate the p50 E-rosette receptor, and most of which block E-rosette formation (this volume, Chapter 4).

CD2B. These 4 reagents also immunoprecipitate the p50 E-rosette receptor, but in the serologic cluster analysis, clustered together and away from CD2A reagents. This was due to low reactivity with resting PB T cells and high reactivity with activated cells (this volume, Chapter 4).

CD2C. These 2 reagents grouped by computer analysis of serologic data with the CD3A reagents, but by immunoprecipitation and SDS-PAGE analysis (this volume, Chapter 22) immunoprecipitated the CD2 antigen, and by immunofluorescence analysis blocked the binding of OKT11 antibody (this volume, Chapter 4).

CD3 Subclusters A, B, and C. As mentioned, these antibodies fell into 3 distinct subclusters on the basis of their serologic reactivity (Table 1.5). Some antibodies in these three subclusters blocked both OKT3 and BW239/347 (anti-CD3) binding (SK7/Leu 4, T3/RW2-4B6, T3/RW2-8C8, X35-3, G19-4.1, BW264/56) while others (T3/2Ad2A2, T3/2T8-2F4) did not (this volume, Chapter 11). In contrast, antibodies T3/2Ad2A2 and T3/2T8-2F4 blocked the binding of the anti-CD3 reagent UCHT-1, but not OKT3 or BW239/347 (this volume, Chapter 11). Gotch *et al.* in their cluster analysis of Workshop reagents found that T3/2Ad2A2 and T3/2T8-2F4 clustered near to but not with other known CD3 reagents and speculated that these two antibodies may be reactive with antigens similar to but distinct from CD3 (this volume, Chapter 2). Antibodies SK7/Leu4, T3RW2-4B6, G19-4.1, BW264/56, and CRIS-7 were all confirmed biochemically to be against the CD3 antigen (this volume, Chapter 22). Antibody T3/2Ad2A2 was clustered with CD3 reagents in the First Workshop (1) and T3/2T8-2F4 was mitogenic (this volume, Chapter 5), inhibited T cell mediated cytolysis (this volume, Chapter 2), and co-capped with UCHT-1 (this volume, Chapter 2). The possibility exists that some of these CD3 reagents may well be reactive with other molecules associated with the T3 antigen.

Guidelines for Future Study

It is important now to look back over this enormous amount of work and to assess in broad terms what we have learned and where future workshops should focus attention and efforts in the future. From the T cell part of this workshop several major points have been learned. First, we have found that with standard techniques, no new T lineage clusters have emerged, and the CD1–8 clusters defined by A. Bernard and L. Boumsell in the First Workshop define the major T lineage antigens. Whether more T lineage antigens remain to be discovered by novel immunization strategies, such as using primate T cells, remains to be seen. However, for the large part, future workshops can forgo serologic analysis of large numbers of unknown reagents and instead can concentrate on the biology of the antigens defined.

Second, this workshop has identified 97 well-characterized antibodies in the CD1–8, CD25, and CDw26 clusters that now form the reagent panel for the Third Workshop to be held in two years in Oxford, England.

Third, we have learned that many laboratories with well-focused goals can contribute to a coherent big picture. We do not necessarily need high numbers of repetitive observations for clear patterns of monoclonal antibody reactivity to emerge.

Based on data presented to the Second Workshop, a number of areas for future study by the Third Workshop in the T cell area were apparent:

1. Biochemical, serologic, and functional analysis of the CD3 reagents regarding their heterogeneity and the possibility that some members of the CD3 cluster might react with T3-associated molecules.
2. Evaluate subsets of CD1 molecules based on variation in size of the CD1 antigen-bearing chain.
3. Evaluation of possible polymorphisms of the CD7 molecule (see Palker *et al.* this volume, Chapter 24) and search for the function of the CD7 p40 molecule.
4. Evaluate functional correlates of new T cell activation antigen of CDw26 cluster; expand number of antibodies in this cluster.
5. Identification, clustering, and functional significance of T cell-related non-MHC allotypic antigens, e.g., defined by antibodies BW264/215, SK11/Leu 8, and TQ 1 (Table 1.14).
6. Further study of CD2 epitopes defined by the large panel of CD2 reagents.
7. Begin earnest search for antibodies that selectively define early stages of T cell ontogeny and maturation stages. There is a great need for specific markers of T cell precursors.
8. Produce monoclonal antibodies that react with nonpolymorphic regions of the T cell antigen receptor.
9. Produce monoclonal antibodies against functional surface molecules with which T cells interact with intra- and extra-thymic microenvironments for trafficing, information transfer, and activation.

With the powerful set of reagents identified by this Second Workshop, coupled with the functional, biochemical, and other studies presented in the T cell section, the stage is set for the Third Workshop in 1986 to be the focal point for a series of in-depth studies that should aid in further unraveling the role T cells play in modulating the human immune response.

Acknowledgments. The author acknowledges the support of the Duke Workshop Team, Lucinda Hensley, Winifred Ho, Richard Scearce, Joyce Lowery, Linda Powell, and Shiangtai Tuan for their invaluable help during the workshop.

Appendix

Laboratories Participating in the Serologic Analysis of the T Cell Panel

Lab #1 Claudine Kieda
Centre de Biophysique Moléculaire, Centre Nationale de la Recherche Scientifique, 1, rue Haute, 45045 Orléans, France

Lab #9 Yasuo Morishima
Saburo Mimami, Masao Okumura, First Department of Internal Medicine, Nagoya University, 65 Tsurumai-cho, Showa-ku, Nagoya 466, Japan

Lab #10 Ryuzo Ueda
Ikuya Tsuge, Reiko Namikawa, Toshitada Takahashi, Aichi Cancer Center Research Institute, Tashiro-cho, Chikusa-ku, Nagoya 464, Japan

Lab #21 John Thompson
University of Kentucky, Department of Medicine, Room MN62, 800 Rose Street, Lexington, KY 40536

Lab #27 A.J. McMichael*
F.M. Gotch, Nuffield Department of Medicine, John Radcliffe Hospital, Headington, Oxford OX3 9DU, United Kingdom

Lab #31 Stephen Peiper, Susan Melvin
St. Jude Children's Research Hospital, 332 North Lauderdale, P.O. Box 318, Memphis, Tennessee 38101

Lab #35 Loran Clement
224 Tumor Institute, University of Alabama, Birmingham, Alabama 35294

Lab #36 Jeff Ledbetter
Genetic Systems Corporation, 3005 First Avenue, Seattle, Washington 98121

Lab #45 Branislav D. Jankovic
Immunology Research Centre, Vojvode Stepe 458, 11221 Belgrade, Yugoslavia

Lab #53 R. Kurrle
K. Bosslet, H.-U. Schorlemmer, Research Laboratories of Behringwerke AG, P.O. Box 1140, D-3550 Marburg/Lahn, West Germany

Lab #61 Peter Rieber
Gert Reithmüller, Institute for Immunology, University of Munich, Schillerstrasse 42, D-8000 Munich, West Germany

Lab #62 Carlos Izaguirre, M.T. Aye, D. Senger
Department of Medicine, University of Ottawa and Ottawa General Hospital, 451 Smyth Road, Ottawa, Ontario K16 8M5, Canada

Lab #71 Kimitaka Sagawa, Keiji Okubo, Yoshinobu Matsuo, M. Mitsuo Yokoyama
Department of Immunology, Kurume University School of Medicine, 67 Asahimachi, Kurume 830, Japan

Lab #72 Ellis L. Reinherz*
Dana-Farber Cancer Institute, 44 Binney Street, Boston, Massachusetts 02115

Lab #79 Paul Martin*
Fred Hutchinson Cancer Research Center, 1124 Columbia Street, Seattle, Washington 98104

Lab #84 Soren Avnstrom
Finsen Institute, Strandboulevarden 49, DK-2100 Copenhagen, Denmark

Lab #85 C. Boucheix, J.Y. Perrot, M. Mirshahi, C. Rosenfeld, C. Soria, J. Soria
INSERM U253, Hôpital Paul Brousse, 16 bis, av. Paul Vaillant Couturier, 94805 Villejuif, France

Lab #88 Christophe Girardet
Institute of Biochemistry, Chemin des Boveresses, CH-1066 Epalinges, Switzerland

Lab #89 Nicholas Chiorazzi
The Rockefeller University, 1230 York Avenue, New York, New York 10021

Lab #92 Peter Wernet
Medizin. Univ. Klinij, Alfried Miller Strasse 10, D7500 Tubingen, West Germany

Lab #100 Claude Mawas, B. Malissen, D. Olive*
Centre d'Immunologie INSERM-CNRS, Case 906, 13288 Marseille Cedex 9, France

Lab #101 Jerome Ritz
Dana Farber Cancer Institute, 44 Binney Street, Boston, Massachusetts 02115

Lab #103 Alain Bernard*
Institut Gustave-Roussy, Pavillon de Recherche, Rue Camille Desmoulins, 94805 Villejuif Cedex, France

Laurence Boumsell*, INSERM U93, Hôpital Saint-Louis, 75010 Paris, France

Lab #117 Helmet Fiebig
Karl Marx University Leipzig, Section of Biosciences, DDR 7010 Leipzig Tolstr. 33, German Democratic Republic

References

1. Bernard, A., L. Boumsell, and C. Hill. 1984. Joint report of the First International Workshop on Human Leucocyte Differentiation Antigens by the investigators of the participating laboratories. In: *Leucocyte typing,* A. Bernard, L. Boumsell, J. Dausett, C. Milstein, and S.F. Schlossman, eds. Springer-Verlag, Berlin, Heidelberg, 1984, p. 9.

---

* Serologic phenotyping reference laboratory.

2. Telen, M.J., G.S. Eisenbarth, and B.F. Haynes. 1983. Human erythrocyte antigens. Regulation of expression of a novel red cell surface antigen by the inhibitor Lutheran In(Lu) gene. *J. Clin. Invest.* **71**:1878.

3. Telen, M.J., T.J. Palker, and B.F. Haynes. 1984. The In(Lu) gene regulates expression of an antigen on an 80 kilodalton protein of human erythrocytes. *Blood* **64**:599.

4. Haynes, B.F., D.L. Mann, M.E. Hemler, J.A. Schroer, J.A. Shelhamer, G.S. Eisenbarth, C.A. Thomas, H.S. Mostowski, J.L. Strominger, and A.S. Fauci. 1980. Characterization of a monoclonal antibody which defines an immunoregulatory T cell subset for immunoglobulin synthesis in man. *Proc. Natl. Acad. Sci. U.S.A.* **77**:2914.

5. Palker, T.J., R.M. Scearce, S.E. Miller, M. Popovic, D.P. Bolognesi, R.C. Gallo, and B.F. Haynes. 1984. Monoclonal antibodies against human T cell leukemia-lymphoma virus (HTLV) p24 internal core protein: Use as diagnostic probes and cellular localization of HTLV. *J. Exp. Med.* **159**:1117.

6. Haynes, B.F. 1981. Human T cell antigens as defined by monoclonal antibodies. *Immunol. Rev.* **57**:127.

7. *SAS user's guide: Basics.* 1982 Edition. SAS Institute Inc., Cary, NC.

8. *SAS user's guide: Statistics.* 1982 Edition. SAS Institute, Inc., Cary, NC.

9. Reinherz, E.L., and S.F. Schlossman. 1980. The differentiation and function of human T lymphocytes. *Cell* **19**:821.

10. Titus, J.A., B.F. Haynes, C.A. Thomas, A.S. Fauci, and D.M. Segal. 1982. Analysis of Fc (IgG) receptors on human peripheral blood leukocytes by flow microfluorometry. I. Receptor distribution on monocytes, T cells, and cells labeled with 3A1 anti-T cell monoclonal antibody. *Eur. J. Immunol.* **12**:474.

11. Harden, E.A. and B.F. Haynes. 1985. Phenotypic and functional characteristics of human malignant T cells. *Seminars in Hematology* **22**:13–26.

12. Mann, D.L., B.F. Haynes, C. Thomas, D. Cole, A.S. Fauci, and D.G. Poplack. 1983. Heterogeneity of cell surface markers on acute lymphocytic leukemia as detected by monoclonal antibodies. *J. Natl. Cancer Inst.* **71**:11.

13. Sutherland, D.R., C.E. Rudd, and M.F. Greaves. 1984. Isolation and characterization of a human T lymphocyte associated glycoprotein (gp40). *J. Immunol.* **133**:327.

14. Boumsell, L., H. Coppin, D. Rham, B. Raynal, J. Lemerle, J. Dausset, and A. Bernard. 1980. An antigen shared by a human T cell subset and B cell chronic lymphocytic leukemia cells. Distribution on normal and malignant lymphoid cells. *J. Exp. Med.* **152**:229.

15. Reinherz, E.L., C. Morimoto, K.A. Fitzgerald, R.E. Hursey, J.A. Daley, and S.F. Schlossman. 1982. Heterogeneity of human T4+ inducer T cells as defined by a monoclonal antibody that delineates two functionally distinct subpopulations. *J. Immunol.* **128**:463.

16. W.J. Leonard, J.M. Depper, R.J. Robb, T.A. Waldmann, and W.G. Greene. 1983. Characterization of the human receptor for T cell growth factor. *Proc. Natl. Acad. Sci. U.S.A.* **80**:6957.

Part II. Functional Studies

Part II. Functional Studies

CHAPTER 2

Binding and Functional Analysis of the Workshop T Cell Specific Set of Monoclonal Antibodies

Frances M. Gotch, Nigel Carter, Shirley Ellis,
Philip McShane, Josephine Heyman, Mark Palmer,
David W. Dongworth, Amanda Bewick, Peter J. Morris,
and Andrew J. McMichael

Introduction

One hundred and fifty-nine samples were studied in the T cell set of monoclonal antibodies. The first part of this report analyzes the binding data obtained following the protocol of the workshop. The second part describes the use of these antibodies in blocking virus-specific HLA-restricted cytotoxic T lymphocyte activity and natural killer cell-mediated lysis, stimulation of T cell proliferation, co-capping with a standard CD3 specific antibody, and blocking of E-rosette formation. Combining the two types of analysis has allowed most of the antibodies to be placed into known CD clusters. Although no new clusters were clearly defined, a number of individual antibodies gave unusual patterns of reactivity or functional properties.

Methods

Cell Types and Preparation

Peripheral blood sheep red cell (E) receptor positive and tonsil E receptor negative lymphocytes were prepared exactly as described previously (1). Special cells were the T leukemia lines HPB.ALL and MOLT4, thymocytes, Sezary cells (kindly given by Professor I.C. MacLennan, University of Birmingham), a B cell chronic lymphatic leukemia, and PHA blast cells (prepared as described in Ref. 1).

Binding Assay and Cytofluorometric Analysis

The method was as described previously (1) except that 5.0×10^5 cells were labeled in each tube. The second antibody was fluoresceinated goat anti–mouse immunoglobulin (Sigma Laboratories Ltd). Cells were fixed before analysis in 1% fetal calf serum (FCS, Gibco, Biocult), 1% formalin in phosphate buffered saline pH 7.4. Cytofluorography was carried out in an Orthocytofluorograf 50L (Ortho Diagnostics Inc). Dead cells, debris, and large cells, including monocytes, were gated out using forward and 90° scatter measurements. Positively stained cells were identified as those above a fluorescence threshold determined with a relevant negative control. Results were expressed as percent positive.

Inhibition of Virus-Specific CTL Activity

Influenza virus-specific CTLs were prepared by incubating 50×10^6 leukopheresed peripheral blood lymphocytes (PBL) with Influenza A/Hong Kong/68 virus (H3N2) at final dilution of virus of 10^{-3}. After 1 hr in serum-free medium (RPMI 1640) pooled human AB serum or fetal calf serum was added to 10% and the incubation continued for 7 days. Targets were PBL infected with Influenza A virus and labeled with ^{51}chromium (Amersham) 2 or 3 days after stimulation with PHA (2,3). HLA mismatched and target cells infected with Influenza B/Hong Kong virus were specificity controls. Cell mediated lysis was carried out at effector : target ratios ranging from 6 : 1 to 50 : 1 as described previously (2,3). In all experiments CTL activity was HLA Class I antigen restricted and virus type specific.

Epstein–Barr virus-specific CTLs were prepared as described previously (2). PBLs were stimulated for 10 days with autologous irradiated lymphoblastoid cell line cells at a ratio of 40 : 1. Medium, RPMI 1640–10% FCS, was changed at 5 days. Lytic activity was assessed as described previously (2).

In blocking experiments, 10 μl of monoclonal antibody at a dilution of 1 in 20 (at least 20 times saturating concentration) were added to the effector and target cells in 150-μl RPMI–10% FCS. These were at a ratio that gave less than maximal lysis, and antibody was added immediately after they had been mixed together. Antibodies without azide were used wherever possible, although we have shown that sodium azide up to 150 mM has no effect on CTL activity (1).

Inhibition of Natural Killer (NK) Cell Activity

Freshly prepared PBLs were mixed with ^{51}Cr-labeled K562 at ratios of 6 : 1 to 50 : 1. For inhibition experiments a K : T ratio (25 : 1) that gave less than maximal lysis was used; otherwise conditions were as described above for CTL.

Proliferation Assay

Freshly prepared PBLs were suspended at 10^6/ml in RPMI–10% AB serum and 100 μl dispensed into round-bottomed microtiter plates (Sterilin).

Antibodies in 10-μl aliquots at 1 in 20 and 1 in 200 were added to the plate which was incubated for 3 days. Tritiated thymidine was added and 4 hours later the plate was harvested and the incorporated tritiated thymidine counted. Controls were cultures stimulated with PHA, 10% FCS, and 10% AB serum.

Co-capping

HPB.ALL cells, 10^7, were incubated overnight in 2-ml RPMI 1640–10% FCS with 4 μg/ml anti–CD3 antibody, UCHT1 (a kind gift of Dr. P. Beverley, University College, London). After 16 hr at 37°C cells were cooled to 4°C and a binding assay carried out with workshop antibodies as described. HPB.ALL that had not been incubated with UCHT1 were assayed in parallel. Assessment of co-capping was made by comparing fluorescence profiles on the Cytofluorograf and calculating the percent positive cells above a capped control to which no second monoclonal antibody was added. This value was compared with the percent binding above the same gate for the uncapped cells.

Inhibition of E-rosette Formation

This was carried out as previously described (1).

Results

Binding and Cluster Analysis of the T Cell Antibody Set

Each of the antibodies was tested on eight cell types. Each pattern thus obtained was compared with that for each of the other antibodies and correlation coefficients (r) calculated. Clusters were constructed where the r value between each member of the cluster was 0.99 or 1.0. Twenty-five clusters (groups) of two or more identically reacting antibodies were thus generated (Fig. 2.1). The mean binding percentage for each antibody with each cell line in each group was calculated. Correlations between the groups were then calculated and they were reclustered at $r > 0.98$ (Fig. 2.2). This brought together closely related groups into clusters, most of which corresponded with the previously described CD binding patterns. The binding pattern of each cluster is shown in Fig. 2.3. The differences in patterns between the groups in each cluster were very small.

Only one possible new cluster emerged, composed of antibodies 80 and 139. One antibody, 64, bound only to HPB.ALL and is likely to be clonotypic, possibly specific for the receptor; antibody 42 gave a similar pattern though with an r value of only 0.8 when compared with 64. Several antibodies defined activation antigens found only on PHA blasts.

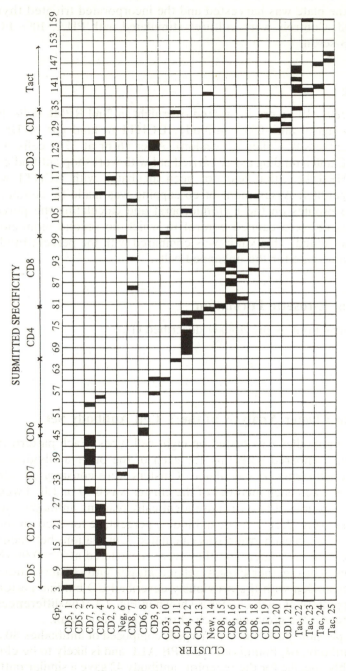

Fig. 2.1. Grouping of identical antibodies. The patterns of binding of each antibody to eight different cell types (see text or legend to Fig. 2.3) were compared and correlation coefficients (*r*) calculated.   Antibodies 1–159 were divided into 25 groups, each with an *r* value of 0.99 or 1.00. The final designation of each group is shown on the extreme left.

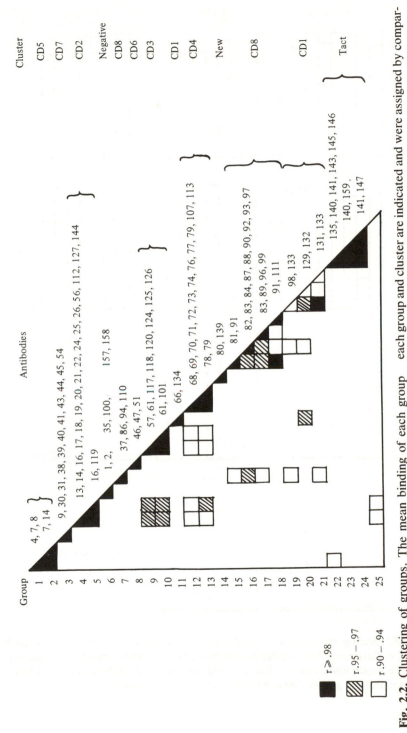

Fig. 2.2. Clustering of groups. The mean binding of each group and cluster are indicated and were assigned by comparison of their binding patterns with Ref. 1. The antibodies in each group were compared and clustered according to r values. The antibodies in

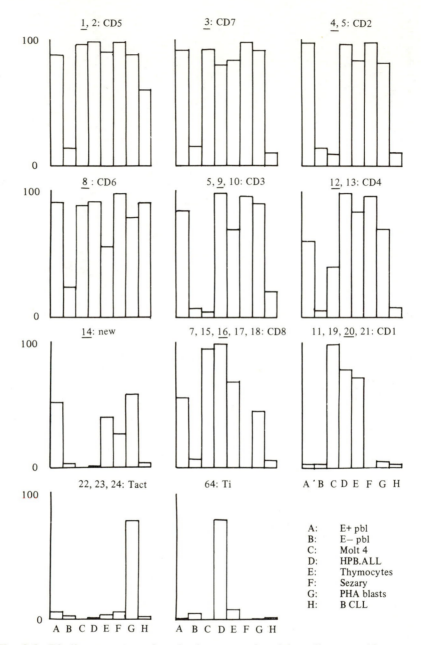

Fig. 2.3. Binding patterns of each cluster on the eight cell types. Above each pattern is shown our final cluster assignation and the component groups (see Fig. 2.1). The group underlined is that contributing the most antibodies to the cluster and its pattern is shown. Binding is shown as % cells positive.

Table 2.1. Unique antibodies: binding and functional studies.

| Antibody | Extent of binding[a] to | | | | | | | | Prolif.[b] | CTL[c] | NK[c] | Cap[d] | E[e] | Nearest Ab | r |
	E+	E−	M4	HPB	Thy	Sez	PHA	BCLL							
6	H	L	L	O	M	H	M	M	nt	nt	nt	nt	−	134 (CD7)	0.84
11	H	M	L	H	M	H	M	H	0.7	0	20	−	−	32	0.91
28	H	O	M	H	M	H	H	O	0.4	16	22	−	++	57 (CD3)	0.94
29	H	L	O	M	L	H	H	H	0.1	0	15	na	−	108	0.77
32	H	M	O	H	M	H	M	H	1.6	0	27	−	−	11	0.91
42	L	O	L	M	O	O	L	L	0.0	0	15	na	−	64	0.80
55	M	O	O	H	H	L	H	L	0.3	18	30	−	−	65	0.99
62	H	H	O	H	H	H	H	H	1.2	0	10	−	−	106	0.77
65	M	O	O	H	M	O	H	O	2.0	27	40	−	−	55	0.99
67	H	L	L	M	M	H	M	M	3.0	22	10	na	−	36	0.95
95	L	O	O	H	M	O	L	O	0.5	43	10	−	−	65	0.84
102	L	O	H	H	M	L	H	O	3.7	12	12	++	−	96 (CD8)	0.93
103	H	L	O	O	M	L	H	H	nt	19	nt	nt	−	142	0.78
108	H	L	O	H	H	O	H	M	0.1	nt	22	−	++	123	0.90
114	M	O	H	H	H	H	L	M	0.0	0	12	−	−	82	0.93
121	H	O	O	H	H	H	H	O	2.5	80	5	−	−	31 (CD7)	0.96
[122	H	L	O	H	H	L	H	M]	nt	72	nt	[++	−	55	0.93
[123	H	L	O	H	H	H	H	H]	2.1	60	12	++]	−	122	0.90
128	O	L	H	H	H	O	O	M	2.9	0	0	na	−	129 (CD1)	0.85
136	M	O	O	O	L	M	M	O	2.9	30	0	na	−	139	0.92
137	H	O	H	H	H	O	L	M	0.0	0	0	−	−	81 (CD8)	0.90
138	H	O	O	H	H	L	H	L	nt	0	nt	nt	−	65	0.96
153	L	L	O	M	L	O	H	L	0.1	1	5	na	−	143 (T-act)	0.75
154	M	L	M	H	L	M	L	M	1.5	6	0	na	nt	65	0.82
155	O	L	H	H	L	O	M	M	0.1	30	0	na	−	128	0.76

[a] H, 67–100%, M, 33–66%, L, 10–32%, 0, 0–9%.

[b] Proliferation assay: Antibodies tested at final dilutions of 2×10^{-2} and 2×10^{-3}; results expressed as cpm $\times 10^{-3}$. [³H]Thymidine taken up by 10^5 PBL on day 3. CD3 antibody 117 gave 21×10^3 cpm and PHA 31×10^3. Background cpm of 0.8×10^3 was subtracted.

[c] Blocking of Influenza-specific CTL and NK lysis, expressed as percent inhibition. Specific lysis by unblocked CTL and NK was 44% and 20%, respectively. nt = not tested.

[d] Co-capping with UCHT1. HPB.ALL cells incubated overnight with UCHT1 and tested with each antibody by direct immunofluorescence and cytofluorography. Results expressed as ++ for >75% reduction, − for <10 and na if binding too weak for assessment.

[e] Inhibition of E-rosette formation: ++, >80% inhibition; −, <10% inhibition.

A number of antibodies that did not appear to belong to any of the clusters are described in Table 2.1, where their nearest relative is also indicated. Some of these probably belong to the above clusters but give anomalous results for reasons such as low affinity or reactivity with epitopes that may be masked on some cell types.

Functional Assays

Blocking of Virus-Specific CTL

Antibodies that gave identical ($r > 0.99$) patterns and which clearly belonged to the well-defined clusters were pooled (Table 2.2) and these pools, representing clusters 1–7, and T cell activation antigens were tested for inhibition of lysis by both EBV- and influenza-specific CTL. As shown in Table 2.2, CD3, CD8, and CD2 pools inhibited lysis confirming previous data (reviewed in Ref. 4). All of them were then tested individually. The CD3 antibodies all inhibited to a marked degree, particularly on influenza-specific CTL (Table 2.3). Similarly, antibodies clustered as CD2 individually inhibited EBV-specific CTL by 45–79% (data not shown). Not all of the CD8 antibodies inhibited: 81, 82, 85, 93, and 99 failed to block influenza-specific CTL at all; 84, 87, 89, 90, 91, 94, 96, and 99 blocked by 15–36%. However, all of these antibodies blocked EBV-specific CTL by 11–14%.

The antibodies shown in Table 2.1 were also tested individually. Three—121, 122, and 123—gave strong inhibition; these antibodies show many characteristics of CD3 and were submitted to the workshop as such. Antibodies 95, 136, and 155 also gave inhibition that was more than background.

We have previously found that EBV cell line-stimulated CTL can lyse NK sensitive cell lines such as K562, after longer periods in culture. The

Table 2.2. Blocking with pooled antibodies.

Pool	Antibodies	% Inhibition	
		Flu CTL	NK
CD1	129, 131, 133, 134	16	22
CD2	13, 16–22, 24, 25	36	15
CD3	117–120, 124–127	96	0
CD4	68–70, 72–74, 76, 77	22	22
CD5	4, 5, 7, 8	10	20
CD6	46, 47	16	—
CD7	31, 38–41, 43–45	22	0
CD8	83, 84, 86, 87, 89–97, 99	88	22
T-act	140, 141, 143, 145, 146, 155, 159	22	25

Table 2.3. Functional studies on the CD3 antibodies.

Antibody	Class	UCHT1 : cap[a] % positive Uncapped	Capped	Proliferation: [³H]thy uptake cpm × 10⁻³	% Inhibition of lysis[b] CTL Flu	EBV	TNK	NK	Correlation coefficient with Leu 4[c]
117	IgG1	94	5.5	12.9	75	28	0		.99
118	IgG1	96	5.2	13.7		38	0		1.00
119	nt	95	95	18.6	20	44	0		.98
120	IgG2a	93	11.1	11.2	75	39	35		.99
121	IgG3	92	87	2.5	80			5	.78
122	IgM	99	8.7	nt	72				.84
123	IgG1	60	8.9	2.1	73			12	.85
124	IgG2b	93	8.3	4.8	60	37	0	0	.99
125	IgG1	94	49	23.0		44	0	0	.99
126	IgG2a	92	4.2	10.2	nt	57	0		.99
127	IgG1			3.2			0		.97
57	IgG	94	61	3.1					.99
61	IgG	96	9.5	5.6					.99
CD3 pool					98	100	7	0	
MHM23 (LFAβ)	IgG1					79	76	65	
MHM24 (LFAα)	IgG1					38	30	5	

[a] HPB.ALL cells were capped by overnight incubation with UCHT1 anti-CD3.
[b] Effectors tested for incubation were Influenza A virus-specific CTL on autologous target cells (25–44% specific lysis), Epstein–Barr virus-specific CTL on autologous B lymphoblastoid cell lines (39% lysis), EBV-stimulated T cells on K562 (33% specific lysis), and NK lysis of K562 (20% specific lysis).
[c] r Values based on binding to cell types shown in Fig. 2.3. Note that antibodies 121, 122, and 123 show significant deviations in binding patterns.
nt = not tested.

effector cells are T cells (2,4) and the Workshop antibody pools were tested for blocking of this form of cytotoxicity (TNK). None inhibited, although the anti–lymphocyte function antigen (LFA) MHM23 (anti–β chain) and MHM24 (anti–α chain), added to the experiment as controls, blocked (Table 2.3). Individually the CD2, CD3, and CD8 reagents were tested (data not shown). Only 13 (29% inhibition), 19 (36%), and 120 (35%) blocked.

Blocking of NK Activity

The pools described above were tested, as well as the set of antibodies shown in Table 2.1 which were tested individually. No antibody blocked NK activity, although the positive control anti–LFA-β chain MHM23 (5) did inhibit by 65% (Table 2.3).

Proliferation Assay

None of the pools stimulated proliferation, including that representing CD3. The CD2 pool and individual CD2 reagents were also tested at 7 days and again failed to stimulate proliferation. The antibodies belonging to the CD3 cluster were tested individually and most, but not all, were mitogenic at 3 days (Table 2.3). The reagents shown in Table 2.1 were also tested individually and poor but positive proliferative responses were obtained only with numbers 65, 67, 121, 123, and 128.

Co-capping with UCHT1 (Anti-CD3)

When the pools (see Table 3.2 for their composition) were tested none of the antigens clearly co-capped with UCHT1. When the CD3 antibodies were tested individually, it was found that 119 did not cap at all, and 125 only partially co-capped (Table 2.3); all of the other CD3 antibodies co-capped. Of the antibodies shown in Table 2.1, 102, 122, and 123 co-capped and the others, including 121, did not. 121, 122, and 123 were submitted as anti-CD3 reagents and show strong similarities to the CD3 cluster in their functional properties. Unfortunately the putative anti–T cell receptor reagent gave relatively weak fluorescence on uncapped HPB.ALL cells and it could not be determined whether the antigen co-capped with CD3.

Blocking of E-rosette Formation

All of the antibodies submitted as CD2 or subsequently shown as belonging to the cluster (Fig. 2.3) and the unique antibodies (Table 2.1) were tested individually. All of the CD2 antibodies except 13 blocked. Antibodies 28 and 108 also blocked.

Discussion

Clustering of antibodies by binding reactivities with cells and cell lines clearly depends on the target cells used in analysis. Each of the special cells used in this study was chosen because it was known to discriminate between one of the defined CD types, e.g., B CLL for CD5 or Sezary cells for CD4/CD8. This method therefore has limitations and there may be leukemic or normal cells which can further split the clusters defined here. The method of analysis should not be considered in isolation, although it was capable of distinguishing CD5, CD6, and CD7 in the last workshop (1,6). Biochemical analysis of the nature of the antigens identified by particular monoclonal antibodies is an essential part of the full characterization and the results described here should be compared with other studies where immunoprecipitations have been carried out. Similarly the effects of adding antibodies to functional assays can support groupings and define further splits.

Antibodies in the well-defined CD1–7 clusters for the most part behaved as expected in functional assays (see Ref. 6 for review). In particular, the CD3, 8, and 2 reagents inhibited virus-specific CTL activity. Most CD3 antibodies stimulated mitogenic responses (7) and co-capped (8) with a known CD3 reagent UCHT1. Most CD2 reagents blocked E-rosette formation.

In these clusters, however, there were exceptions. The CD3 cluster and the related antibodies 121, 122, and 123 (which were submitted as CD3) are particularly interesting. The CD3 antibodies 119 and 121 did not co-cap with UCHT1 and 125 and 57 capped poorly. 121, 123, 124, 127, 57, and 61 stimulated proliferation only weakly. 121, 122, and 123 gave anomalous binding data, e.g., 121 bound to MOLT4 which, according to the other antibodies does not bear the CD3 antigen. Yet all of these antibodies blocked CTL function. The fact that the CD3 antigen is complex with some of the reagents binding to different chains may account for some of these findings. Further study is indicated.

A similar problem arose in the CD2 group when antibody 13 repeatedly failed to inhibit E-rosette formation, possibly simply because it binds to a different epitope. Two of the antibodies in Table 2.1—28 and 108—blocked E-rosette formation but differed markedly in their binding patterns from each other and CD2.

In the CD8 cluster there were five component groups (Figs. 2.1 and 2.3) with slightly different binding patterns. Not all of the antibodies inhibited influenza-specific CTL equally well. These results suggest heterogeneity in the antigen and more detailed analysis would be worthwhile.

In the unique group of reagents a few stand out as interesting. 121, 122, and 123 are probably related to CD3. 102 gave a very unusual binding pattern yet co-capped with UCHT1; in other respects it looked more like a CD8 or activation antigen. 28 and 108 may be related to CD2. Biochemical analysis will help to determine whether these reagents identify new functionally important antigens.

In this and the previous workshop about 200 anti–T cell monoclonal antibodies have been tested for their effects on these T cell functions. Although the aberrant data discussed above could be explained by new differentiation antigens, the evidence is inconclusive and it is more likely that most of the anomalous binding patterns and functional effects represent antibodies binding to different epitopes of the known antigens with different activities. Thus most of the T cell antigens involved in T cell function have probably already been defined. However there are possibilities that some could have been missed. As an example, the antibodies to the lymphocyte function antigen were excluded from the T cell set because of their broader reactivity, yet they clearly have profound effects on T cell function (5,9). It is possible that other reagents which do not fit into simple patterns of binding, i.e., primarily to T cells, may similarly affect T cell function. Also antigens which are expressed in very low amounts may have effects on T cell function, and attention may have to be directed to reagents which have greater effects on function in proportion to their binding. One important antigen/epitope still to be found is the constant part of the T cell receptor. This may be present in low amounts on resting T cells and, by analogy with immunoglobulin, antibodies to this part of the molecule might not affect binding, although it would be expected to co-cap with CD3 (8). Of the antibodies analyzed here only 102 seems to be a candidate but a definitive answer awaits biochemical characterization.

Acknowledgments. This work was supported by grants from the Medical Research Council to A.J. McM and PJM. We thank Mrs. R. Bryan for preparing the manuscript.

Note added in proof. It is now clear that Antibody 64 binds to CD9.

References

1. Gotch, F.M., P.D.K. Hildreth, N.P. Carter, P. McShane, D.W. Dongworth, and A.J. McMichael. 1984. Analysis of the T cell specific sets of monoclonal antibodies. In: *Leucocyte typing,* A. Bernard, L. Boumsell, J. Dausset, C. Milstein, and S.F. Schlossman, eds. Springer-Verlag, Berlin, Heidelberg, pp. 224–230.
2. Dongworth, D.W., F.M. Gotch, N.P. Carter, P.D.K. Hildreth, and A.J. McMichael. 1984. Inhibition of virus specific HLA restricted T cell mediated lysis by monoclonal anti T cell antibodies. In: *Leucocyte typing,* A. Bernard, L. Boumsell, J. Dausset, C. Milstein, and S.F. Schlossman, eds. Springer-Verlag, Berlin, Heidelberg, pp. 320–328.
3. McMichael, A.J., and B.A. Askonas. 1978. Influenza virus specific cytotoxic T cells in man: induction properties of the cytotoxic cell. *Eur. J. Immunol.* **8**:705.
4. Dongworth, D.W., and A.J. McMichael. 1984. Inhibition of human T lymphocyte function. *Brit. Med. Bull.* **40**:254.
5. Hildreth, J.E.K., F.M. Gotch, P.D.K. Hildreth, and A.J. McMichael. 1983. A human lymphocyte-associated antigen involved in cell mediated lympholysis. *Eur. J. Immunol.* **13**:202.
6. Bernard, A., L. Boumsell, J. Dausset, C. Milstein, and S.F. Schlossman, eds. 1984. *Leucocyte typing.* Springer-Verlag, Berlin, Heidelberg.
7. Van Wauwe, J.P., J.R. De Mey, and J.G. Goussens. 1980. OKT3: A monoclonal anti human T lymphocyte antibody with potent mitogenic properties. *J. Immunol.* **124**:2708.
8. Reinherz, E.L., S.C. Meuer, K.A. Fitzgerald, R.E. Hussey, H. Levine, and S.F. Schlossman. 1982. Antigen recognition by human T lymphocytes is linked to surface expression of the T3 molecular complex. *Cell* **30**:735.
9. Sanchez-Madrid, F., A.M. Krensky, C. F. Ware, E. Robbins, J.L. Strominger, S.J. Burakoff, and T.A. Springer. 1982. Three distinct antigens associated with human T-lymphocyte-mediated cytolysis: LFA-1, LFA-2, and LFA-3. *Proc. Natl. Acad. Sci. U.S.A.* **79**:7489.

CHAPTER 3

Functional Studies Performed with the Second International Workshop T Cell Panel of Monoclonal Antibodies

Dominique Charmot, Daniel Olive, Patrice Dubreuil, Marguerite Ragueneau, and Claude Mawas

The primary mixed lymphocyte reaction (MLR), anti–class I cytotoxic T lymphocyte (CTL) clones as well as population cell-mediated lympholysis (CML), and the interleukin-2 (IL-2)-dependent growth of T cell lines were studied using the complete set of the monoclonal antibodies (mAbs) submitted. Anti–class II CML and natural killer (NK) lysis on K562 were studied using a selection of the mAbs provided. In some experiments local mAbs either submitted or not submitted to the Workshop were studied in parallel.

Materials and Methods

The *in vitro* assays used were routinely performed. mAbs from the functional set were always used at the final dilution 1/400 except when otherwise stated. mAbs were considered inhibitory (or stimulatory) when MLR was modified ±50%, CML ±30%, and IL-2-dependent growth ±75% of their relevant control (1). The clusters of differentiation (CD) were those ascribed by the organizers to the mAbs before the distribution of the mAbs to the laboratories.

Results and Discussion

The results of the studies undertaken on the complete panel of mAbs are displayed in Table 3.1 and described in the following.

Table 3.1. Summary of the functional studies with T cell panel mAbs.

CD	Effect of mAb on					
	MLR		IL2		CMLI	
	↗	↗	↗	↗	↗	↗
CD5	7,9	6,8,10	4		None	
CD2	All but 15,26,28		None		14,23	
CD7	29		36		None	31
CD6	47		None		46	
Pan T other	56,59,60		All but 49,50,51,52,60,61,62		61	
CD4	All but 67,73,78,80		All but 79		None	
CD8	86,87,88,89,96	82,83,90	All but 86,95,97,98,100		All but 81,84,85,91,98,100	
T cell subset	101,107,113	104,108,110 111	All but 108,111,114		101,102,106	
CD3	117,118,119,124,125,127		119,120,123,124	118	117,118,119,120,122,123,125	
CD1	130,133		129,133		None	
T-activation	144,145,146,148,149,151,159	140,150	135,139,140,144,146,151,159		136,144,150	138

Primary Mixed Lymphocyte Reaction

CD5

mAbs 7 and 9 gave concordant inhibition in repeats. mAb 7 was later announced to contain azide! Discordant results in repeats were seen with mAbs 6, 8, and 10.

CD2

All mAbs submitted were strongly inhibitory (mean inhibition > 75%) except mAbs 15 (G19-3.1), 26 (35.1), and 28 (KOLT-2).

CD7

None of the mAbs were found inhibitory except mAb 29 (9-3).

CD6

Only mAb 47 (12.1.5) was inhibitory.

Group Pan T, Other, or Unknown

Three mAbs were inhibitory—56 (T57), 59 (MT 421), and 60 (CRIS-3).

CD4

All mAbs were strongly inhibitory except mAbs 67 (T10C5), 73 (MT 321), 78 (T4/7T4-6C1), and 80 (TII19-4-7). Except for mAb 67, the three others gave inhibition around 30%.

CD8

Five mAbs gave strong inhibitions: 86 (BW135/80), 87 (MT 415), 88 (MT 1014), 89 (MT 122), and 96 (66.2). mAbs 82, 83, 90 gave inhibitions between 30 and 45%. Data with mAb 97 (51.1) are questionable since the values are so low that azide is suspected.

T Cell Subset, Other

Strong inhibitions were seen with mAbs 101 (BRC-T1), 107 (EDU-2), 113 (13B8.2); 101 contains azide. Strong stimulation is seen with mAb 111 (8E 1.7). mAbs 104 (3AC5), 108 (TQ1/28T17G6), and 110 (10B4.6) (an anti-T8 mAb) gave inhibitions between 30 and 45%.

CD3

mAbs 117 (G19-4.1), 118 (SK7/Leu 4), 119 (89bl), 124 (T3/RW2-4B6), 125 (T3/RW2-8C8), and 127 (NU-T1) were strongly inhibitory; 118 contains azide.

CD1

mAbs 130 (SK9/Leu 6) and 133 (NU-T2) were inhibitory but 130 contains azide.

T Activation

mAbs 144 (39C1.5), 145 (39C6.5), 146 (33B3.1), 148 (39C8.18), 149 (39H7.3), and 151 (KOLT-1) were strongly inhibitory. However, 39C1.5, 39C8.18 and 39H7.3 are not anti-Il-2 receptor mAbs. mAb 159 (TAC) was also strongly inhibitory.

mAbs 140 (Tac/1HT4-4H3) and 150 (41F2.1) gave inhibition between 30–45%; 150 is an anti–E-rosette receptor mAb.

Cell-mediated Lympholysis

Population CML and anti–class I CTL clones.

CD5

No mAb found inhibitory (at the dilution used for the Workshop).

CD2

Only mAb 14 (9-2) and 23 (T11/7T4-7A9), both IgM, were inhibitory at the dilution used in this Workshop screening. All were inhibitory at higher concentration.

CD7

No mAb was found inhibitory; mAb 31 (4H9/Leu 9) enhanced the cytolysis, a fact already noticed with some local mAbs.

CD6

mAb 46 (T12/3Pt12B8), IgM, was strongly inhibitory.

Pan T, Others and Unknown

mAb 61 (CRIS-7) was inhibitory.

CD4

None was found inhibitory of anti–class I CTL clones or population CML. The assay on anti–class II CTL was a technical failure.

CD8

All mAbs blocked anti–class I CTL clones and population CML except 6: mAbs 81 (14), 84 (C12/D3), 85 (BW246/162), 91 (T8/7Pt3F9), 98 (T411E1), and 100 (BL-TS1).

T Cell Subset, Others

Three mAbs were blocking: mAbs 101 (BRC-T1), 102 (D44), and 106 (CRIS-5).

CD3

7 out of 11 were strong inhibitors of anti–class I CML: 117 (G19-4.1), 118 (SK7/Leu 4), 119 (89b1), 120 (BW264/56), 122 (T3/2Ad2A2), 123 (T3/2T8-2F4), and 125 (T3/RW2-8C8).

T Activation

Three mAbs in this group blocked anti–class I CML: 136 (TS145), 144 (39C1.5), and 150 (41F2.1). mAb 138 (1 MONO 2A6) enhanced anti–class I CML (> 50% of control).

IL-2-dependent Growth of an IL-2-dependent T Cell Line

Analysis of the data was based on taking into account all inhibition >75% concordant in two independent experiments without duplicates.

In these experiments, TAC gave 75% inhibition; control 1 gave no inhibition but control 2 gave 55% inhibition (!).

CD5

mAb 4 (H65) was an inhibitor.

CD2

No mAb inhibitor.

CD7

Only mAb 36 (A1) was an inhibitor.

CD6

None.

Pan T, Others and Unknown

12 out of 19 were strong inhibitors: the seven nonblocking are the mAbs 49, 50, 51, 52, 60, 61, and 62.

CD4

All mAbs were inhibitors except mAb 79 (66.1).

CD8

All mAbs were inhibitors except 86 (BW135/80), 95 (T8/2ST8-5H7), 97 (51.1), 98 (T411E1), and 100 (BL-TS1).

T Cell Subset, Other

Only mAb 108 (TQ1/28T17G6), 111 (8E-1.7) and 114 (K51) were not inhibitory.

CD3

The following mAbs were found inhibitory: 119 (89b1), 120 (BW264/56), 123 (T3/2T8-2F4), 124 (T3/RW2-4B6). An inhibition between 50–75% was seen with mAb 118 (SK7/Leu 4).

CD1

mAb 129 (NA1/34) and 133 (NU-T2) were strongly inhibitory.

T Activation

mAbs 135 (T1A), 139 (4EL1C7), 140 (Tac/1HT4-4H3), 144 (39C1.5), 146 (33B3.1), 151 (KOLT-1), and 159 (TAC) are strongly inhibitory.

   Unfortunately, the two negative controls 157 and 158 are also inhibitory!

Special Functional Studies

CD2 Selected MAbs

In the screening of the T cell panel, in functional assays, with the standard dilution of 1/400 final, we were surprised to see that although most CD2s were inhibitory of the primary MLR, the vast majority, except two IgM mAbs, were unable to block CML or NK lysis. This was not so if the mAb final concentration was 1/40 in these assays as can be seen in Table 3.2. mAbs T144, T150, T149, and T148 were strong inhibitors of anti–class I and anti–class II CTL clones as well of NK effectors (tested on K562).

Table 3.2. Special studies on a selection of anti-E-rosette and IL-2 receptor mAbs.

mAbs added	Anti-class I CTL clones		Anti-class II CTL clones	NK effectors
	PHA blasts	EBV targets	EBV targets	K562
None	55	45	52	86
Controls				
H8-109.14 (irrelevant)	55	52	55	85
25.3 (LFA-1)	*24 (56)*	*13 (71)*	*20 (62)*	*56 (35)*
T110 10B4.6 (CD8)	*23 (58)*	18 (60)	61	85
BL.4 (CD2)	60	NT	*33 (37)*	82
T141 B149.9 (IL-2 receptor)	46 (16)	40	50	70 (19)
Anti-IL-2 receptors				
18E6.4	53	NT	NT	*56 (35)*
27E4.6	46 (16)	33 (27)	51	*54 (37)*
T146 33B3.1	44 (20)	NT	55	71 (17)
T145 39C6.5	51	NT	48	70 (19)
22D611	45 (17)	NT	NT	64 (26)
T147 33B7.3	54	NT	NT	70 (19)
E-rosette receptor				
5B64	*39 (29)*	*29 (36)*	NT	*57 (34)*
19E36	*46 (16)*	NT	NT	*64 (26)*
T144 39C1.5	*42 (24)*	*28 (38)*	*19 (63)*	*59 (31)*
T150 41F2.1	*43 (22)*	*32 (29)*	51	NT
T149 39H7.3	*46 (16)*	*27 (40)*	*24 (54)*	*50 (42)*
T148 39C8.18	48	*20 (56)*	*21 (60)*	*60 (30)*

Anti–IL-2 Receptor MAbs

While screening these mAbs on anti–class I and anti–class II CTL clones as well as on NK effectors (population) we found strong NK inhibition by mAbs T143 and 27E4.6 (not submitted) and weak inhibitions by mAbs T141, T146, T145, and T147 (Table 3.2).

Conclusions

Many mAbs belonging to the various clusters of differentiation have been found to interfere with *in vitro* assays (1). MLR is a very sensitive assay: most mAbs belonging to CD3, CD4, CD8, CD2, or directed against the IL-2 receptor were found inhibitory. In the other groups, individual mAbs are often found inhibitory. Equally sensitive is the IL-2-dependent growth assay: here again, most mAbs belonging to CD3, CD4, and CD8 are inhibitory as well as many of those directed against the IL-2 receptor. However, most CD2 mAbs are not inhibitory in contrast to a majority of pan T mAbs not classified in a given cluster or mAbs belonging to the T cell subset group.

Against anti–class I CTL clones, as expected mAbs belonging to CD3 and CD8 block effectively while those belonging to CD5, CD7, and CD4 are ineffective. CD2 mAbs are effective blockers of CML against class I and II as well as of NK lysis.

Finally, NK lysis is inhibited reproducibly to various degree by most mAbs directed against the IL-2 receptor.

In these studies, we have not looked extensively for stimulatory effects. However we have noticed one mAb (111) strongly enhancing the primary MLR and two the CML (CD7:31; T-activation:138).

Although this functional mass screening might be affected by technical errors, the data look coherent and allow these results to be confirmed and expanded in more controlled experiments.

Acknowledgments. This work was supported in part by INSERM and CNRS.

Reference

1. Olive, D., D. Charmot, P. Dubreuil, A. Tounkara, M. Ragueneau, C. Mawas, and P. Mannoni. 1985. Human lymphocyte functional antigens. In: *Human T cell clones: A new approach to immune regulation. 19th Leucocyte culture conference,* A. Mitchison and M. Feldman, eds. Humana Press, Cambridge, England (in press).

CHAPTER 4

The Epitopic Dissection of the CD2 Defined Molecule: Relationship of the Second Workshop Antibodies in Terms of Reactivities with Leukocytes, Rosette Blocking Properties, Induction of Positive Modulation of the Molecule, and Triggering T Cell Activation

Alain Bernard, Philippe Brottier, Eric Georget, Virginia Lepage, and Laurence Boumsell

Before the era of monoclonal antibodies (mAbs), several reports indicated that the T cell surface molecule responsible for rosette formation with sheep erythrocytes (E) is a 50-Kd molecule (1,2). This was confirmed and extended by obtention of mAbs directed against this molecule (3–5) and the First International Workshop on Human Leucocyte Differentiation Antigens could define the typical clusters of differentiation as CD2 [T, gp50] with mAbs 9.6, 35.1, and T11$_1$ (6). We have also described another mAb, termed D66, reactive with the same molecule, but to a distinct epitope, since we observed no cross-blocking between the binding of D66 and the binding of 9.6/T11$_1$ antibodies. Several of our observations indicated that remarkable features characterize this epitope (4): the density of D66 is high on immature and activated T cells, whereas T-PBLs display only a low density of D66 epitopes; the low density of D66 on T-PBL can be explained, to a large extent, by their coverage with sialic acid residues (as such, D66 could not be classified, strictly speaking, as a CD2 mAb since the definition of CD by the First Workshop relied both on tissue distribution and M.W. determinations). In addition, D66 would not block T cell rosettes with E pretreated with AET or neuraminidase while it would efficiently block rosettes with untreated E, either at 4 or at 37°C. Moreover we observed a cell metabolism-independent positive modulation phenomenon of the CD2 defined molecule through the D66 epitope: binding of a second Ab, even an Fab fragment, on D66 mAb can totally reverse inhibition of E-rosette formation, and evidence that this is due to emergence of initially hidden D66 epitopes was provided by cytofluorometric studies.

Quite recently, Meuer *et al.* (7) have obtained a series of mAbs permitting them to define, on the CD2 molecules, three distinct epitopes (which they termed $T11_1$, $T11_2$, and $T11_3$) and showed that co-binding of mAb $T11_2$ and $T11_3$ on the molecule triggers T cell activation. In addition, they also observed a positive modulation phenomenon, since they reported that $T11_3$ is not displayed on resting T-PBLs but appears on these cells after binding of $T11_2$ mAb under cell metabolism-independent conditions.

The present work was undertaken with the T cell panel of the Second Workshop, in order to relate the various effects of binding mAb to the CD2 defined molecule.

Materials and Methods

Cells and Reagents Used and Their Preparation

PBLs were obtained after Ficoll–Hypaque centrifugation, activated T cells were recovered on day 3 after stimulation with optimal doses of phytohemagglutinin (PHA), and thymocytes were obtained from children undergoing cardiac surgery and were kept frozen as previously described (8). In addition to the T cell panel of the Second Workshop, other mAbs were used in the present study: D66 clones 1 and 2 have been previously described (4,9) (D66 clone 2 is included in the Second Workshop panel— also termed G144—and coded XT65); FITC–OKT11 was kindly provided by Ortho Diagnostic Co. (Raritan, NJ, USA) and was previously described (5); finally, mAb L129 was obtained in our laboratory and is under further study and mAb Och was obtained by Drs. Jacques Colombani and Virginia Lepage (INSERM U93, Hôpital Saint-Louis, Paris). These reagents were used as dilutions of ascites having a titer of maximum reactivity in IF greater than 10^{-3}.

Immunofluorescence Assays and mAb Binding Studies

Indirect immunofluorescence assays were performed using a FITC-anti–mouse Ig from Meloy Laboratories (Springfield, VA, USA) and the batch used was the same as used for common studies of the T cell protocol. Fluorescence was measured using cytofluorometry (Ortho System 50H, Ortho Diagnostic Co., Westwood, MA, USA). For cross-blocking studies, antibodies from the T cell battery were used at 1:50 dilutions and other antibodies at saturating amounts determined by preliminary experiments. Biotinylation of mAbs D66 clone 2 and Och have been performed using a technique previously described (4).

Rosette Formation

Rosette formation with untreated sheep E or AET-pretreated[1] E was performed as previously described (4). mAbs were added at a final dilution of 1 : 20 in PBS without sodium azide and no washing was performed between the co-incubation of T cells with mAbs and the addition of sheep E.

Assays for Mitogenicity of mAbs

PBLs ($5 \times 10^4/200$ μl) were incubated with combinations of mAbs, and preliminary experiments had shown that optimal tritiated thymidine incorporation occurs after 80 hours of culture. This was observed both for the D66 + 9.6/T11$_1$ combination and the XT23 + XT138 combination, for instance. The optimal dilution for these two mAbs was found to be 1 : 500, and therefore the other mAbs were screened after dilution at 1 : 500. They were dialyzed when their preparation included sodium azide.

Results

Systematic Search for mAbs Blocking E-rosettes in the T Cell Battery. Are There Molecules Other Than CD2 Involved in the Process of Rosette Formation?

The ideal strategy to search for mAbs directed against the CD2 defined molecule would be to select mAbs reacting with a 50-Kd protein from the T cell surface, and to confirm the identity of the protein by sequential immunoprecipitation with a CD2 reference antibody. This is underway in our laboratory. Another approach was to systematically search for mAbs that blocked E-rosettes. This was done, using thymocytes and T-PBL, and rosetting with either untreated sheep E at 4 and 37°C or with E pretreated with AET. As indicated in Table 4.2, four different patterns of rosette blockings were observed. Antibody no. 138, giving no rosette inhibitions, could be related to the CD2 molecule because, as will be described below, another screening procedure was followed, namely to systematically search for antibodies inducing T cell proliferation with CD2 reference antibodies. It is clear, however, that this screening strategy might have missed other mAbs directed against the CD2 molecule and giving no rosette inhibition nor inducing mitogenicity in the combinations tested. The list of mAbs selected and investigated here is given in Table 4.1.

---

[1] AET = 2-amino-ethylisothiouronium bromide.

Table 4.1. List of antibodies used in the present study.

Code number	Antibody name	Code number	Antibody name
13	9-1	25	9.6
14	9-2	26	35.1
16	S2/Leu 5b	27	T411B5
17	MT 26	55	T56
18	MT 910	56	T57
19	MT 1110	65	G144 (D66 clone 2)
20	T11/3Pt2H9	108	TQ1/28T17G6
21	T11/ROLD2-1H8	144	39C1.5
22	T11/3T4-8B5	148	39C8.18
23	T11/7T4-7A9	149	39H7.3
24	T11/7T4-7E10	150	41F2.1
—	Och[a]	—	L129[a]

[a] The two antibodies Och and L129 were not in the T cell battery.

On another hand we have, surprisingly, observed strong inhibitions with mAbs that reacted with antigens that could not be affiliated to the CD2 molecule, like mAb no. 108 (TQ1) (10) or a mAb of our own, also reacting with non–T cells, and termed L129. Thus the stable interaction between T cells and sheep E may require molecules other than CD2. This is further supporting by co-capping studies, which showed independent movements of the CD2 molecule and L129-defined antigen (11).

Correspondence Between the Pattern of Rosette Inhibition and Reactivities with Leukocytes

Table 4.2 also shows the reactivities of the anti–T cell MAbs we could affiliate to the CD2 molecule or found to inhibit E-rosette formation. The panel of cells we used to screen all reagents from the T cell protocol included three different preparations of thymocytes, T-PBLs, and activated T cells. In addition, it included the malignant cells from one case of leukemia, known to be CD2 unreactive; the malignant cells of one case of lymphoblastic lymphoma, known to be CD2 reactive; and the cells from one case of B cell chronic lymphocytic leukemia (B CLL) (CD2 unreactive). From the results of the First Workshop (6) and by comparison with appropriate controls a typical pattern of reactivities with CD2 reagents could be defined based both on the percent of reactive cells and the stage of fluorescence histograms, clearly distinct from other defined CDs or other pan-T reagents. In Table 4.1, it can be seen that a clear correspondence emerged from the comparison between the patterns of rosette inhibition and leukocyte reactivities of the selected antibodies. Namely, all antibodies but one (no. 28) which had a typical CD2 pattern of reactivity could inhibit rosette formation under all circumstances. On the other

Table 4.2. mAbs found to block E-rosettes within the T Cell battery and leukocyte reactivities of antibodies found to be useful to investigate the CD2 defined molecule.

Rosette inhibition[a]									T cell reactivities[b]					Reference antibodies	List of Workshop mAbs[c]
Thymocytes			T-PBL			T-PHA			Thy	T-PBL	T-PHA	T-ALL	T-LL		
E4°C	E37°C	EAET	E4°C	E37°C	EAET	E4°C	E37°C	EAET							
C	C	C	C	C	C	C	C	C	9/H	8/H	5/VH	–	+	9.6/T11$_1$	14,16,17,18,19 20,21,22,24,25 26,27,56,144
C	C	C	C	C	C	C	C	C	9/H	6-8/L	5/VH	–	+		23,149,150
C	C	C	C	C	C	C	C	C	9/H	2/VL	5/VH	–	+		148
C	C	N	C	C	N	C	C	N	9/H	6-8/VL	5/VH	–	+	D66	55,65,Och*
P	P	N	P	P	N	P	N	N	9/H	8/M	5/VH	–	+		13
M	N	N	N	N	N	M	N	N	8/M	2/N	5/VH	–	+		138
C	C	C	C	C	C	C	C	C	Most T-cells + monocytes			–	+		108
P	C	C	C	NT	C	P	NT	C	Most T-cells + monocytes			–	+		L129*

[a] E4°C and E37°C when rosette assays were performed at 4° or at 37°C, respectively, with untreated sheep E. EAET when rosette assays were performed with AET-pretreated sheep E. C for complete blocking (percentage of rosette inhibition >80); P for partial inhibition (inhibition between 30 and 80%); N for no inhibition; NT for not tested.

[b] Three different samples of thymocytes (thy), T-PBL, and T-PHA were investigated. T-ALL: T-cell acute leukemia known to be CD2 unreactive; T-LL: T-cell lymphoblastic lymphoma known to be CD2 reactive. In addition, these antibodies were tested on cells from one case of B-CLL cells and found to be unreactive. The number is the percent of positive cells $\times 10^{-1}$; H for high density; VH for very high density; L for low density; VL for very low density; M for intermediate density; N for null density. Tissue distribution of antibody nos. 108 and L129 showed differences.

[c] The sign * indicates two mAbs that were not included in the Second Workshop battery. Among the mAbs listed in CD2, results dealing with two mAbs (nos. 15 and 28) are not reported here, since they were not found to inhibit rosette formation. No. 28, however, had a leukocyte reactivity typical of CD2.

hand, among the four antibodies (nos. 13, 55, 65, and Och—this last antibody was not included in the Workshop battery but introduced in our study for characterization) that gave a peculiar pattern of rosette inhibition, three gave a faint reactivity with most T-PBLs, while no. 13 gave a level of fluorescence density intermediate between D66 and $9.6/T11_1$.

Competitive Binding Studies

These studies were performed on thymocytes. Two mAbs, representative of critical epitopes could be used, FITC–OKT11 and biotinylated D66 (D66 clone 2 = G144 = XT65). In addition, we could prepare biotinylated Och. As indicated in Table 4.3, and from comparisons with results displayed in Table 4.2, it can be seen that most mAbs able to block EAET rosette formation could totally inhibit the binding of OKT11 but not the binding of D66. Conversely, all mAbs unable to block rosettes with EAET, but able to block rosettes with untreated E, did block D66 binding but not OKT11 binding. However some noticeable exceptions were ob-

Table 4.3. Competitive binding studies.[a]

Second labeled mAb[b]	Binding inhibition induced by first mAb[c]		
	Total	Partial	Null
OKT11	$9.6/T11_1$		D66
	14,16,18,19	26	13,55,65,Och*
	24,25,56,148		
	149	144,150	27
		17	23
			138
			108,L129*
D66	D66		$9.6/T11_1$
	13,55,65,Och*	24	25,56,148,149
		26	16,18,19,20
			144,150
			17,23
			138
			108,L129*
Och	D66		$9.6/T11_1$
	Och*		20,24
			26
			144,150
			17,23
			108,L129*

[a] These studies were performed on thymocytes.
[b] OKT11A was directly conjugated with fluorescein; D66 and Och were biotinylated and revealed with FITC–avidin; readings were performed by cytofluorometry.
[c] All mAbs of the series listed in Table 4.2 could not be investigated here for lack of materials.

served. mAb 26 could partially block the binding of both OKT11 and D66. mAbs 23 and 138 blocked neither OKT11 nor D66 binding and mAb 17 only partially blocked OKT11 binding. mAbs 144 and 150 induced a partial blocking of OKT11 fixation, and, finally, mAbs 108 and L129* induced no blocking. It can also be seen that the pattern of blocking of biotinylated Och is similar to that of biotinylated D66.

Ability of Various Combinations of mAbs to Trigger T Cell Activation

Since Meuer *et al.* (7) have recently shown that combination of mAbs $T11_3$ with mAb $T11_1$ and $T11_2$ could induce T cell activation, and that $T11_3$ antibodies produce no rosette inhibition, a systematic search for mAbs inducing T cell activation with $T11_1$ was performed ($T11_1$ was a generous gift from Dr. E. Reinherz). Only one mAb not able to block E-rosette formation but able to induce mitogenicity was found: antibody no. XT138 (results not shown). As indicated in Table 4.2, we found the antigen defined by XT138 to be present on most thymocytes, lacking on T-PBLs, and present in very high density on activated T cells. Guided by the preceding results, a series of combinations of mAbs were assayed two by two for their ability to induce T-PBL proliferation. The results are depicted in a summarized form in Fig. 4.1. All combinations of mAbs affiliated to the $9.6/T11_1$ epitope were not mitogenic; similarly all combinations of antibodies affiliated to the D66 epitope were not mitogenic. However, all combinations of one antibody affiliated to the $9.6/T11_1$ epitope and any antibody affiliated to the D66 epitope (with the exception of three antibodies: 27, 144, and 150) were strongly mitogenic, and so on as indicated by the arrows in Fig. 4.1. The combinations inducing no activation should be emphasized: all antibodies affiliated to the D66 epitope and antibody no. 138, and all antibodies affiliated to the $9.6/T11_1$ epitope and either antibody no. 17 or no. 23.

These results clearly indicate that activation of T cells through the CD2 defined molecule arises by "touching" the molecule at combinations of selective areas, rather than solely from intrinsic properties of some mAbs against the CD2 molecule.

Studies of Modulations of the CD2 Defined Molecule

Since two types of "positive modulations" of the molecule have been demonstrated, we decided to investigate, with selected mAbs, the possible relationships between both types of modulations. As recalled in the introduction section, the first type is the reappearance of free D66 epitopes after binding of a second antibody on saturating amounts of anti-D66, producing a reversal of rosette inhibition. As shown in Table 4.4, this was investigated with a selection of antibodies affiliated to the 9.6/T11

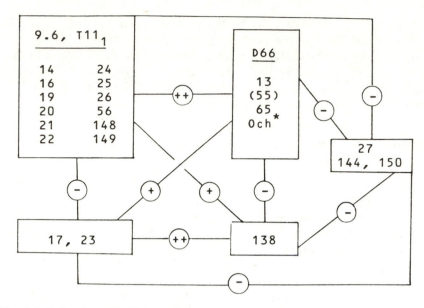

Fig. 4.1. Induction of T-PBL proliferation by combinations of pairs of mAbs from the T cell battery selected for reactivity with the CD2 defined molecule. Tritiated thymidine incorporation was measured at day 4, which was found to be the optimal period for typical combinations (D66 + 9.6/T11$_1$; D66 + 23; 23 + 138; T11$_1$ + 23). Combinations listed + gave 25,000 to 75,000 cpm; combinations listed ++ usually gave more than 150,000 cpm. Controls ranged from 500–5000 cpm. Combinations of antibodies in the same box led to no T cell proliferation. In addition, antibody nos. 108 and L129 were not found to be mitogenic in all combinations tested.

Table 4.4. Positive modulation typical of D66 epitope[a] investigated with the second workshop battery.

| mAbs sensitizing T cells | Rosette inhibition[b] | | | | | |
| | Without Fab anti–mouse Ig | | | After adding Fab anti–mouse Ig | | |
	E4°C	E37°C	EAET	E4°C	E37°C	EAET
9.6/T11	+	+	+	+	+	+
D66	+	+	−	−	−	−
55,65,Och	+	+	−	−	−	−
13	±	−	−	+	+	±
23	+	+	+	+	+	±
17,20,24,25,26 144,150	+	+	+	+	+	+

[a] In these experiments, as indicated in Materials and Methods, thymocytes were incubated with an amount of mAbs known to inhibit rosette formation. Next the sheep E were added without intermediate washings.
[b] Rosette inhibition is indicated + when inhibition was greater than 80% of the number of rosettes occurring as compared to the positive control; −, when less than 20% inhibition occurred; ± when 20–80% inhibition was observed.

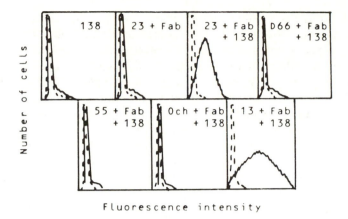

Fig. 4.2. Fluorescence histograms showing induction of 138 (T11$_3$) epitopes after incubations with mAbs able to induce positive modulation of D66 epitopes.

epitopes, with all the antibodies affiliated to the D66 epitopes, and with antibody nos. 17 and 23. As can be seen from Table 4.4, the positive modulation phenomenon was observed with none of the antibodies affiliated to 9.6/T11$_1$ epitopes, nor with antibody no. 17. Three out of the four antibodies affiliated to D66 epitopes gave rise to reversal of rosette inhibition, upon binding of a second antibody; surprisingly, antibody no. 23 also could produce such a phenomenon but with EAET only. Finally no. 13 gave a very peculiar phenomenon after binding of a second antibody, since the blockage of rosettes with E4°C was drasticaly increased, while it did appear with E37°C and EAET rosettes.

Next, it was of interest to check whether these antibodies could induce appearance of 138 epitopes on T-PBLs. In these experiments, T-PBLs were first incubated with the antibody to be tested; in a second step an Fab fragment of anti–mouse Ig was added under saturating conditions so that no fluorescence by a developing reagent could be accounted for by the first antibody (see controls, Fig. 4.2). In a third step, antibody no. 138 was added followed by a fluorescent reagent. Figure 4.2 displays the fluorescence histograms given by cytofluorometry. While antibody no. 23 did induce appearance of 138 epitopes, antibodies 65, 55, and Och did not. Surprisingly, antibody no. 13, which showed a peculiar pattern of modulation of rosette inhibition, could induce 138 epitopes in even higher densities than antibody no. 23.

Discussion

The CD2 [T, gp50] defined molecule displays remarkable features and the discovery of its functional role(s) and mode of action will certainly bring much to our understanding of T cell physiology. A summary of the conclusions from the present study, where we took advantage of the exchange of reagents during the time course of the Second Workshop blind studies, appears in Fig. 4.3. Several epitopes can be defined on the CD2 molecules, and the availability of several mAbs against a single epitope—or epitope group—has permitted us to show that the various effects of mAb binding on the properties displayed by the molecule are due to the touching of critical regions, and not so much to the intrinsic properties of a given mAb. In addition, attempts can be made to relate some of the various properties displayed by the molecule. Indeed, the scheme depicted in Fig. 4.3 has no topological pretension, but it might provide useful guidelines when a detailed biochemical analysis of the molecule will be accomplished.

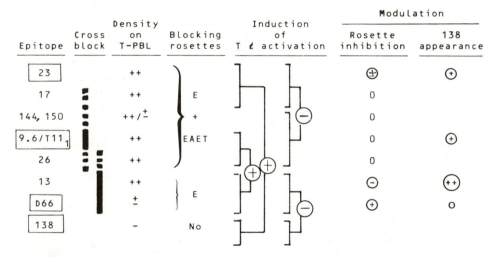

Fig. 4.3. Epitopic dissection of the CD2 defined molecule: a recapitulation. Four major epitopic groups could be defined. One represented by antibody no. 23, the second by antibodies 9.6 and $T11_1$, the third by antibody D66, and the fourth by antibody no. 138. Of note, antibody no. 17, which shares many features in common with no. 23, could partially block the binding of an antibody representative of the $9.6/T11_1$ epitope. No. 26 could partially block the binding of antibodies representative of both the $9.6/T11_1$ epitope and the D66 epitope. A clear correlation appears between the density of these epitopes—always found high on thymocytes and very high on activated T cells—on the T-PBL surface, and their ability to block E-rosettes: Most mAbs able to block rosettes with AET-pretreated E were found in high densities on T-PBL, whereas all the antibodies which can only block rosettes with untreated E were found to be in low density on T-PBL. Finally antibody no. 138, unable to block E-rosettes, cannot be detected on T-PBL. These data can be accounted for by a model of rosette formation we have previously proposed (4). The induction of T cell activation by pairs of mAbs against the CD2 molecule can solely occur by combinations of antibodies selective of given epitopes. Similarly, the two types of cell metabolism-independent modulation phenomena of the CD2 molecule are epitope dependent.

The tight correspondence, in the mAb groups that could be delineated here, between their pattern of E-rosette inhibition, tissue distribution—particularly the epitope density on the T-PBL surface, and their ability to induce modulation of the molecule and to trigger T cell activation, gives rise to some conclusions and useful speculations. Thus, the epitopic dissection of the CD2 molecule allows a deeper insight into the mechanism of E-rosette formation. This is certainly a complex phenomenon which is highly dependent on certain requisites of the procedure used, and the T cell populations marked by E-rosetting critically depend upon the conditions followed during the assay. Thus, pretreatment of sheep E with AET or neuraminidase permits the detection of the largest population of T cells. The observation we made (4,9) that binding mAbs to a region (D66) which is present in low density of T-PBL—to a large extent because it is masked by sialic acid residues—does not induce rosette blocking with EAET but block rosettes with untreated E while mAbs directed against another region ($9.6/T11_1$), which is always exposed on the T cell surface do block rosette formation, sheds light on reasons why certain populations of T cells, particularly according to their stage of maturation, do or do not form rosettes depending upon the technical conditions. As to the mechanism of rosette formation, we have proposed a model involving interaction of E with two different regions of the CD2 molecule, which can account for the known properties of the phenomenon (4,9); yet a single interacting region could be allosterically influenced, and the results obtained in the present work are still compatible with both possibilities. However, the finding that two different mAbs—one included in the Workshop panel (no. T108 = TQ1), the other from our own laboratory (L129), both reacting with monocytes in addition to T cells, and able to inhibit rosette formation, indicate that either a variant of the CD2 molecule would exist on monocytes, or that molecule other than CD2 would be necessary for stable rosette formation. Although definitive conclusions on this require biochemical characterization of the molecules recognized by these mAbs both on T-cells and monocytes; it is clear that the CD2 molecule remains the major T cell surface component in determining the conditions of rosette formation. As we also showed (9) that rosette formation between T cells and erythrocytes from numerous species also depend on the CD2 molecule, it is tempting to speculate on the relationships between this property of the molecule and its physiological role.

Another astonishing feature of the molecule are the events called here "epitope modulation" (4,7). The present work shows that the appearance of further D66 epitopes after binding a second antibody on mAbs directed against D66 epitope on the one hand, and appearance of $T11_3$ epitope after binding of mAb against $T11_2$ epitope on the other, are not experimental translations of the same phenomenon, although both indicate remarkable mobility or/and plasticity of the molecule on the cell surface and are therefore probably related. This is also indicated by the results observed

here with antibody no. 13, which gave rise to an increase in rosette inhibition after binding of a second antibody and appeared also to be very
efficient in inducing the appearance of $T11_3$ epitopes; both effects are
opposite to what we observed for the other antibodies belonging to the
D66 epitopic group.

It is also tempting to speculate on the possible relationships between
modulation phenomena and activation of T cells by selective combinations of antibodies. It is quite probable that T cell activation which occurs
after touching both the $T11_2$ and $T11_3$ epitopes and after touching both the
$T11_1$ and D66 epitopes follows the same process since they have identical
kinetics and IL-2 requirements (12), even though the initial interactions
occurring at the level of the CD2 molecule are clearly not the same. Here
also it must be recalled that several reports have shown that binding a
single antibody on the $9.6/T11_1$ groups leads to inhibition of many T cell
functions (13,14). We have also shown that binding antibody on the D66
epitope leads to inhibition of many T cell functions. Yet some discrimina-
tions in the functions inhibited have been described with antibody no. 26
(35.1) (15), a finding which fits the observations made here of the particular pattern of this antibody. It thus appears that the types of interactions
exerted on definite regions of the CD2 defined molecule do have exquisite
effect on T cell activation, either triggering or preventing it, a way through
which a fine tuning of T cell activities might be exerted.

Summary

The anti–T cell battery of mAbs for the Second Workshop was systematically screened for reagents against the CD2 [T, gp50] defined molecule. In
order to ensure the sorting of reagents of putative interest to investigate
the properties of the molecule, two screening procedures were used on
the whole T cell battery: blocking E-rosette formation, and induction of T
cell proliferation in conjunction with reference antibodies. The selected
mAbs were systematically investigated for competitive inhibition studies,
and results of their reactivities with leukocyte populations were compared
to their pattern of blocking E-rosettes, to induce a cell metabolism-independent mechanism of modulation and to induce in combinations T-cell
proliferation. As summarized in Fig. 4.3, at least four different epitopic
groups could be defined which are characterized by remarkable properties. It appears that selectively "touching" the CD2 defined molecule at
definite regions produces events which can control T cell activation.

Acknowledgments. We thank Catherine Simon for secretarial assistance;
Ortho Diagnostic Co. for providing FITC OKT11; Dr. E. Reinherz for
providing $T11_1$ and Dr. J. Colombani for providing Och. In addition, we
are very grateful to the teams of Dr. Langlois (Hôpital Bichat, Paris) and

Dr. Neveu (Hôpital Laënnec, Paris) for providing us with thymus specimens. This work was supported by l'Association pour la Recherche sur le Cancer, Villejuif 94800, France.

References

1. Gurtler, L.G. 1981. Glycolipid and p40 are the binding sites in the sheep erythrocyte and T-lymphocyte membrane responsible for rosette formation. *Immunobiol.* **158**:426.
2. Gross, N., and C. Bron. 1980. Identification and partial characterization of surface antigens specific for human normal and leukemic T-cells. *Eur. J. Immunol.* **10**:417.
3. Kamoun, M., P.J. Martin, J.A. Hansen, M.A. Brown, A.W. Siadak, and R.C. Nowinski. 1981. Identification of a human T-lymphocyte surface protein associated with the E-rosette receptor. *J. Exp. Med.* **153**:207.
4. Bernard, A., C. Gelin, B. Raynal, D. Pham, C. Gosse, and L. Boumsell. 1982. Phenomenon of human T-cells rosetting with sheep erythrocytes analyzed with monoclonal antibodies. "Modulation" of a partially hidden epitope determining the conditions of interaction between T-cells and erythrocytes. *J. Exp. Med.* **155**:1317.
5. Verbi, W., M.F. Greaves, C. Schneider, K. Koubek, G. Janossy, H. Stein, P. Kung, and G. Goldstein. 1982. Monoclonal antibodies OKT11 and OKT11A have pan-T reactivity and block sheep erythrocyte "receptors". *Eur. J. Immunol.* **12**:81.
6. Bernard, A., L. Boumsell, J. Dausset, C. Milstein, and S.F. Schlossman, eds. 1984. *Leucocyte typing,* Springer-Verlag, Berlin, Heidelberg.
7. Meuer, S.C., R.E. Hussey, M. Fabbi, D. Fox, O. Acuto, K.A. Fitzgerald, J.C. Hodgdon, J.P. Protentis, S.F. Schlossman, and E.L. Reinherz. 1984. An alternative pathway of T-cell activation: a functional role for the 50 Kd T11 sheep erythrocyte receptor protein. *Cell* **36**:897.
8. Boumsell, L., and A. Bernard. 1980. High efficiency of Biozzi's high responder mouse strain in the generation of antibody secreting hybridomas. *J. Immunol. Methods* **38**:225.
9. Amiot, M., A. Bernard, C. Gelin, B. Raynal, and L. Boumsell. 1984. Phenomenon of rosette formation of human T-cells analyzed with monoclonal antibodies. The same mechanism of interaction accounts for rosette formation with erythrocytes from many species, including autologous erythrocytes. In: *Leucocyte typing,* A. Bernard, L. Boumsell, J. Dausset, C. Milstein, and S.F. Schlossman, eds. Springer-Verlag, Berlin, Heidelberg, pp. 281–293.
10. Reinherz, E.L., C. Morimoto, K.A. Fitzgerald, R.E. Hussey, J.F. Daley, and S.F. Schlossman. 1982. Heterogeneity of human T4$^+$ inducer T-cells defined by a monoclonal antibody that delineates two functional subpopulations. *J. Immunol.* **128**:463.
11. Bernard, A., and L. Boumsell, manuscript a preparation.
12. Brother, P., A. Bernard, and L. Boumsell, submitted for publication.
13. Hansen, J.A., P.J. Martin, P.G. Beatty, E.A. Clark, and J.A. Ledbetter. 1984. Human T lymphocyte cell surface molecules defined by the Workshop monoclonal antibodies ("T Cell Protocol"). In: *Leucocyte typing,* A. Bernard, L.

Boumsell, J. Dausset, C. Milstein, and S.F. Schlossman, eds. Springer-Verlag, Berlin, Heidelberg, pp. 195–212.

14. Palacios, R., and O. Martinez-Maza. 1982. Is the E receptor on human T lymphocytes a "negative signal receptor"? *J. Immunol.* **129:**2479.

15. Martin, P.J., G. Longton, J.A. Ledbetter, W. Newman, M.P. Braun, P.A. Beatty, and J.A. Hansen. 1983. Identification and functional characterization of two distinct epitopes on the human T cell surface protein T, p. 50. *J. Immunol.* **131:**180.

CHAPTER 5

Monoclonal Antibodies as Probes to Define Critical Surface Structures Involved in T Cell Activation

Stefan C. Meuer, Thomas H. Hutteroth, and
K.H. Meyer zum Büschenfelde

Introduction

The production of monoclonal antibodies directed against surface structures of human T lymphocytes has provided unique probes to define discrete stages of T cell differentiation as well as individual T cell subpopulations that are programmed to perform regulatory and effector functions in the immune response (1–3). Importantly, besides their usefulness for phenotypic characterization of normal and malignant cells of the T lineage, these reagents have also been employed to characterize the physiologic role of their respective membrane molecules. For example, it was possible to identify by monoclonal antibodies the transferrin receptor (4), the receptor for interleukin-2 (5), and, more recently, the T cell antigen receptor (6). Moreover, on the basis of functional antibody effects *in vitro,* it was suggested that the subset restricted glycoproteins, T4 and T8, are themselves involved as associative recognition structures for constant portions of, respectively, class II or class I MHC gene products in effector–target cell interaction (7). This view originated from studies in which antibodies were utilized to block *in vitro* responses such as cytotoxicity or/and proliferation (8,9,10).

In contrast, the finding that certain monoclonal antibodies deliver positive signals such as induction of T cell activation (11) is believed to be due to their capacity to replace natural ligands involved in this process. This notion is supported by experiments in which monoclonal antibodies to the T cell antigen receptor (i.e., anti-T3, anti-Ti) in appropriate form were demonstrated to mediate identical effects to those of the natural ligand of this molecular complex, namely specific antigen itself. Thus, IL-2 receptor expression, proliferation, mediator release, and regulatory function were inducible as a consequence of antireceptor-antibody binding to the T cell surface (12,13).

Most recently, a T cell receptor independent "alternative" pathway of activation was discovered which can be triggered by monoclonal antibodies directed at the T lineage-restricted 50-Kd T11 glycoprotein (14). Particularly, in this case, the potential of monoclonal antibodies for functional studies is underlined by the fact that a natural ligand that could engage this mode of T cell activation remains yet to be identified.

In the present studies, monoclonal antibodies were investigated for their capacity to induce T cell proliferation *in vitro* via the T3–Ti antigen receptor or, alternatively, the T11 pathway of T cell activation. The data to be presented below demonstrate how functional tests can help to identify individual antibody specificity and to define critical structures involved in physiologic cell function.

Materials and Methods

Derivation of Lymphocyte Populations

Lymphocytes were obtained by Ficoll–Hypaque density centrifugation of heparinized blood from healthy donors. A T cell-enriched fraction was prepared by rosetting with sheep erythrocytes. Subsequently the E^+ population was plated onto sterile glass petri dishes for 2 hr at 37°C and the nonadherent fraction treated with two cycles of monoclonal antibodies anti-I1 (15) and anti-Mo1 (16) (kindly provided by Drs. L.M. Nadler and R.F. Todd, respectively, DFCI, Boston) and rabbit complement. This population is referred to as "purified resting T lymphocytes."

Monoclonal Antibodies

An azide-free panel of monoclonal antibodies as submitted to the Second Intl. Workshop on Human Leukocyte Differentiation Antigens was employed. In general, antibodies were investigated at final dilutions 1:300, 1:900, and 1:2700 of ascites in culture medium (RPMI 1640 + 10% fetal bovine serum, supplemented with 1% penicillin–streptomycin). All other monoclonal antibodies were provided by Dr. E.L. Reinherz (DFCI, Boston).

Proliferative Assays

Proliferation of T lymphocytes to monoclonal antibodies was determined by culturing 1×10^5 cells/0.2 ml total volume in 96-well round-bottomed microtiter plates (Coster, Cambridge, MA). Cultures were pulsed individually after 3 days with 1 µCi of [^{3}H]thymidine (NEN, Dreieich, FRG) and harvested 18 hours later on a Skatron Cell Harvester. ^{3}H-TdR incorporation was measured in a Packard Scintillation Spectrometer (Packard Instruments, Downers Grove, ILL). Background ^{3}H-TdR uptake was determined by substituting media for monoclonal antibodies. Each value represents the mean of triplicate cultures. Standard deviations were <15%. Each experiment demonstrated is representative for at least three individual experiments performed.

Determination of E-rosette Formation

Peripheral blood mononuclear cells (1×10^6 in 0.2 ml of culture medium) were incubated with monoclonal antibody ($1:500$ final concentration) at 4°C for 1 hr and then washed once. Pellets were re-suspended in 0.2 ml of culture medium followed by addition of 30 μl of a 5% sheep red blood cell suspension in medium. Subsequently, samples were centrifuged for 10 min at 600 rpm, incubated for 1 hr at room temperature, and then pellets were gently re-suspended. E-rosettes were evaluated by microscopic examination.

Results

Monoclonal Antibodies Which Activate T Lymphocytes via the T3–Ti Antigen Receptor Complex

Although the majority of monoclonal antibodies designated as anti-T3 appear to be directed at the glycosylated 20-Kd subunit (Fig. 5.1), it is possible that others with a similar reactivity pattern among cells of the T lineage might bind to different molecules and/or epitopes contained

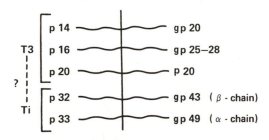

Fig. 5.1. Schematic view of the Ti–T3 molecular complex. Five individual components of the T cell antigen receptor complex have been identified. Whereas the alpha and beta chains are known to be disulfide linked, the association of Ti with T3 as well as the relationship between the various T3 components are unknown (left: M.W. of polypeptide chains; right: M.W. of glycosylated complete subunits).

within the T3–Ti complex. Given the previously described mitogenic effects of anti-T3 antibodies (11) it was necessary to investigate monoclonal reagents of the pan-T cell group as well as those listed under CD3 of the Second Intl. Workshop on Human Leukocyte Differentiation Antigens for their capacity to activate resting T lymphocytes. A comparison of their individual mitogenic activities in combination with biochemical analyses could potentially be useful to provide information on the functional role of some of the T3–Ti subunits. Moreover, additional surface structures which might mediate T cell activation could be identified by such experiments.

Therefore, monoclonal antibodies were individually added to purified resting T lymphocytes in the presence or absence of accessory cells and mitogenic activity was measured by means of ^{3}H-TdR uptake following incubation *in vitro* for 3 days. It was found that none of these antibodies exhibited mitogenic activity in the absence of accessory cells. In contrast, when 5% autologous monocytes were added to the *in vitro* culture, T cell proliferation could be detected. As shown in Table 5.1, the mitogenic effect of antibodies contained within the CD3 group demonstrated a considerable heterogeneity. Thus, whereas antibody nos. 120, 121, 122, and 126 induced stimulation indices (SI) >15, all others were only moderately mitogenic (SI < 10). In line with results published in the literature (20,22), these four antibodies markedly enhanced the responsiveness of T cell blasts (allogeneic T cell lines) to interleukin-2 (not shown). In addition, antibodies nos. 49, 57, 60, 61, and 62 of the pan-T cell panel displayed mitogenic activity, indicating that they might be directed at epitopes contained within the T3–Ti molecular complex (data not shown). Because we investigated all monoclonal antibodies at different dilutions (1:300; 1:900; 1:2700) with consistent results, it is unlikely that the observed quantitative differences in their functional activities were due to differential antibody concentrations. Moreover, our results do not support the view that mitogenic activity of anti-T3 monoclonals correlates with one or another serological antibody subclass.

Table 5.1. Mitogenic activity of monoclonal antibodies contained within the CD3 group.

Antibody no.	SI[a]	Antibody no.	SI
117	4	123	3
118	8	124	8, 5
119	6	125	4
120	21	126	18
121	20	127	6, 5
122	22	PHA	35

[a] SI: stimulation index.

Table 5.2. Epitopes of the T11 glycoprotein as defined by monoclonal antibodies.

	Epitopes		
	$T11_1$	$T11_2$	$T11_3$
Expression			
Thymocytes	+	+	−
Resting T cells	+	+	−
Activated T cells	++	++	++
E-rosette formation	+	−	−
Molecule	50 kd	50 kd	50 kd

Although the affinity of the Ag binding portion of an individual antibody molecule might be responsible for its functional activity, an alternative possibility is that these antibodies could be directed at different epitopes and/or molecules contained within the Ti–T3 molecular complex. Biochemical analysis as well as cross-blocking studies should help to resolve this open question.

Monoclonal Antibodies Triggering the Alternative Pathway of T Cell Activation

Our present studies were aimed at identifying within the anti-T11 (CD2) and anti–pan-T cell antibody groups reagents that are directed at the various epitopes of the 50-Kd T11 glycoprotein (Table 5.2). To this end, in a first set of experiments we investigated all monoclonal antibodies for their capacity to inhibit the formation of E-rosettes by T lymphocytes. As demonstrated in Table 5.3, 13 out of 16 antibodies of the CD2 group and

Table 5.3. Monoclonal antibodies[a] directed at the 50-Kd T11 glycoprotein.

Mitogenic (SI > 3)	Not mitogenic (SI < 3)	
19, 20, 21, 22, 23, 24, 25, 65	14, 15, 16, 17, 18, 27, 56	Inhibition of E-rosette formation
Anti-T11₂[b]	13, 15, 28	No inhibition of E-rosette formation
Anti-T11₃/138 (expressed upon T cell activation)		

[a] Numbers in the table are those assigned to monoclonal antibodies submitted to the Workshop.
[b] Not submitted to the Workshop.

two additional monoclonals of the pan-T cell panel (no. 56 and no. 65) blocked E-rosetting, whereas antibodies 13, 15, 18, and all other pan-T cell antibodies did not. Thus, on the basis of these experiments two groups of anti-T11 antibodies could be defined (Table 5.3).

Since it was previously demonstrated that certain anti-T11 antibodies, particularly the E-rosette receptor-unrelated anti-T11$_2$ (see Discussion), were capable of inducing a proliferative T cell response when added in concert with anti-T11$_3$ (14), it was necessary to investigate whether the CD2 or pan T antibodies submitted to the Workshop would exhibit mitogenic activity by themselves or in combination with anti-T11$_3$.

Moreover, since alternative pathway activation is known to occur independent of accessory cells (14), purified resting T lymphocytes were employed as responder population and proliferation determined by means of [^{3}H]thymidine uptake following a 3-day incubation period. None of the CD2 or pan T antibodies was found to be mitogenic by itself under these experimental conditions. In contrast, when the same reagents were investigated in the presence of saturating concentrations of anti-T11$_3$ antibodies nos. 19–25 and 65 induced T cell proliferation (SI > 3). It should be noted, however, that from a quantitative point of view, these reagents were much weaker mitogens than the previously described anti-T11$_2$ (Table 5.4).

Thus, based on both mitogenicity and influence on E-rosette formation, it is possible to define at least four individual groups of anti-T11 antibodies which could correspond to different epitopes of the 50-Kd glycoprotein (Table 5.3). It should be noted that anti-T11$_2$, which had not been submitted to the Workshop, is unique so far, since all other mitogenic antibodies inhibit E-rosetting whereas anti-T11$_2$ clearly does not. Given that some

Table 5.4. Monoclonal antibodies activating T lymphocytes via the T11 pathway[a].

Antibody no.	SI[b]	Antibody no.	SI
Anti-T11$_{1A}$	4.5	20	4
Anti-T11$_2$	16	21	5
Anti-T11$_3$	1	22	3.8
13	1	23	4.1
14	1	24	3.2
15	1	25	3.3
16	1	27	1
17	2	28	1
18	1.5	56	1
19	3	65	8.4

[a] All monoclonal antibodies were tested in the presence of anti-T11$_3$. None of the antibodies was mitogenic by itself.
[b] SI: stimulation index.

monoclonal antibodies directed at the $T11_1$ epitope were already demonstrated to exhibit weak mitogenic activity in the presence of anti-$T11_3$ (14), one might conclude that the mitogenic, E-rosette-blocking antibodies (nos. 19–25, 65) are directed at the previously defined $T11_1$ epitope. Whether their nonmitogenic counterparts (14–18; 27; 56) bind to a different site than the former remains to be determined. Nevertheless, the capacity of the latter to inhibit E-rosette formation as well suggests that these two epitopes, if they exist, have to be located very close to each other.

Table 5.3 also indicates that one can clearly identify one or more novel epitope(s) of T11, namely the one(s) identified by antibodies No. 13/15/28 which do not block E-rosette formation. As opposed to anti-$T11_2$, they do not induce T cell activation together with anti-$T11_3$. Sequential immunoprecipitation and cross-blocking studies will be necessary to prove that the above three antibodies in fact react with the T11 molecule and, in addition, all define the same determinant.

As demonstrated earlier, the $T11_3$ epitope is only present on activated T cells. Moreover, the capacity of other anti-T11 antibodies (i.e., anti-$T11_1$ or anti-$T11_2$) to produce T cell activation via the alternative pathway appears to be related to their ability to induce expression of this "activation antigen" and thus allow binding of the anti-$T11_3$ monoclonal to the T cell surface. Particularly, anti-$T11_2$ was found to be very potent with regard to this activity (14). In order to identify within the group of monoclonal antibodies directed at "activation antigens" those with anti-$T11_3$-like activity, all reagents contained in this panel were individually added to purified resting T lymphocytes in the presence of anti-$T11_2$ and proliferation determined by means of ^{3}H-TdR uptake in the standard 3 days *in vitro* system. Only one antibody, namely no. 138, was found to produce a strong proliferative signal under these conditions, whereas all others had no effect. A side-by-side comparison of anti-$T11_3$ and no. 138 indicated that they were functionally identical.

Discussion

A number of lineage-specific antigens have been defined on human T lymphocytes by monoclonal antibodies (1). In the case of the 20/25-Kd T3 molecule, both its appearance in late intra-thymic ontogeny at the time of acquisition of immunologic competence and its critical role in T cell function suggested that T3 was closely linked to an important recognition receptor or cell–cell interaction molecule (17,18,19). Antibodies directed against T3 were unique in the ability to block antigen-specific T cell responses (18–20) and were mitogenic for resting T lymphocytes (11). The latter activity was critically dependent on the presence of accessory cells (21). More recent studies have shed some light on the function of the T3 molecule. There it was demonstrated that this 20/25-Kd glycoprotein forms a molecular complex with a 90-Kd heterodimer, termed Ti, which bears clone-specific determinants and serves as receptor for antigen on T cells. Moreover, human T lymphocytes, independent of their subset derivation, specificity, or regulatory function, employ an analogous T3–Ti molecular complex for antigen recognition (6,23).

When tested on human T cell clones, monoclonal antibodies to T3 or Ti produced identical functional effects:

1. Anti-T3 or anti-Ti antibodies, respectively, blocked antigen-specific functions at the level of antigen recognition and/or binding. However, whereas anti-T3 was able to inhibit all T lymphocytes, anti-Ti activity proved to be restricted to individual clones (20,22).
2. Incubation of T cell clones or resting T cells with anti-T3 led to reversible modulation and loss of T3 from the cell surface and co-modulation of Ti (and vice versa) through external shedding, without affecting viability or expression of other known surface structures.
3. This temporary decrease in antigen receptor density following treatment with monoclonal antibodies was accompanied by rapid expression of cellular receptors for interleukin-2. However, this did not lead to endogenous IL-2 production and, consequently, did not result in T cell proliferation (13,22,23).
4. When anti-T3 or anti-Ti were individually coupled to the surface of a solid support, they were themselves capable of triggering clonal T cell proliferation through an IL-2-dependent autocrine pathway, analogous to antigen itself (12,13). This finding suggested that multimeric surface attachment and cross-linking of antigen receptors represents an important signal in T cell activation.

Recent biochemical studies on the components of the T3–Ti antigen receptor indicated that this molecular complex consists of at least 5 individual subunits (Fig. 5.1). Thus, besides the disulfide linked 49–53-Kd alpha chain and the 41–43 beta chain which form the Ti molecule, a 20-Kd glycoprotein, a 20-Kd nonglycosylated polypeptide, and a 25-Kd glycoprotein have been identified (24). However, the precise association of the latter three molecular species with Ti and their functional role in effective antigen recognition and T cell activation are not known at the present time.

In addition, the basis of the mitogenic effect of anti-T3 antibodies, particularly in the case of resting T lymphocytes, requires further investigation. Previous studies have suggested that one of the functional contributions of accessory cells which are required to induce T cell proliferation in this experimental system is to present—via binding of antibody to their Fc receptors—anti-T3 in multimeric form to the responding T lymphocyte and thereby mediate T cell receptor cross-linking (21). That such a mechanism serves as an important signal in T cell activation is supported by recent studies in which purified anti-T3 (or anti-Ti), covalently coupled to the surface of a solid support, was demonstrated to trigger proliferation of T cell clones (12,13). However, for resting T cells additional signals, i.e., lymphokines, provided by accessory cells might be required for T cell activation.

Nevertheless, a critical signal naturally produced by physical interaction of antigen-presenting cells with T lymphocytes can be replaced by a monoclonal antibody (anti-T3). This now provides a potent system to precisely define the requirements for activation of individual functional T cell populations such as helper, suppressor, or cytotoxic cells.

Human T lymphocytes were first identified when it was observed that all thymus-derived cells spontaneously formed E-rosettes with sheep erythrocytes (25,26). This E-rosetting capacity appeared during thymic ontogeny and was maintained on all peripheral T lymphocytes. Subsequently, with the advent of monoclonal antibodies, the receptor for sheep erythrocytes has been identified to be part of a 50-Kd glycoprotein structure (27) which appears at the earliest level of T cell ontogeny (2). Moreover, this structure demonstrates a remarkable antigenic conservation on T lymphocytes in primates (28,29). However, until recently, nothing was known about the physiologic role of this surface molecule.

Recently, a series of monoclonal antibodies against this 50-Kd structure was produced in order to define the function of T11. As a result, three distinct epitopes have been delineated so far on this molecule (Table 5.2). Two of these, termed $T11_1$ and $T11_2$, are expressed on resting T lymphocytes as well as thymocytes, whereas a third epitope, termed $T11_3$, was found exclusively on activated T cells. Moreover, only antibodies directed at $T11_1$ were able to inhibit E-rosette formation.

Perhaps more importantly, it was shown that anti-$T11_2$ and anti-$T11_3$ in concert could activate T lymphocytes to express their individual functional programs. Thus, activation via T11 results in proliferation and release of mediators as well. Moreover, this alternative T cell pathway is not associated with the antigen receptor complex and is independent of accessory cell signals or antigen (14). The expression of T11 on virtually all thymocytes and its presence on all members of the peripheral T cell compartment supports the view that this 50-Kd glycoprotein may be critical in mediating thymocyte growth and differentiation.

Presumably, there is a natural ligand that can engage the alternative pathway of T cell activation. However, its identity as well as the functional significance of an antigen-independent mode of T cell triggering are unknown at present. In striking contrast to ligands of the Ti–T3 antigen receptor (i.e., antigen, anti-T3, or anti-Ti) which activate T lymphocytes only when presented to the responding cell in multimeric form on cellular or artificial surfaces (12,13), anti-T11 antibodies if coupled to a solid support lose their mitogenic capacity. Therefore, the finding that anti-$T11_2$ and anti-$T11_3$ induce T cell proliferation only when employed in soluble form (14) might suggest that their natural counterpart, if it exists, could be a soluble mediator.

Acknowledgments. The authors wish to thank Ms. Martina Hauer and Ms. Gabriele Rasch for their excellent technical assistance and Dr. D.A. Cooper for his critical comments. This work was supported by a grant from the Deutsche Forschungsgemeinschaft (DFG-Me-693/3-1).

References

1. Reinherz, E.L., and S.F. Schlossman. 1980. The differentiation and function of human T lymphocytes: A review. *Cell* **19**:821.
2. Reinherz, E.L., P.C. Kung, G. Goldstein, R. Levey, and S.F. Schlossman. 1980. Discrete stages of human intrathymic differentiation: analysis of normal thymocyte and leukemic lymphoblasts of T lineage. *Proc. Natl. Acad. Sci. U.S.A.* **77**:1588.
3. Reinherz, E.L., P.C. Kung, G. Goldstein, and S.F. Schlossman. 1979. Separation of functional subsets of human T cells by a monoclonal antibody. *Proc. Natl. Acad. Sci. U.S.A.* **76**:4061.
4. Trowbridge, I.A., and M.B. Omary. 1981. Human cell surface glycoprotein related to cell proliferation is the receptor for transferrin. *Proc. Natl. Acad. Sci. U.S.A.* **78**:3039.
5. Leonard, W.J., J.M. Depper, T. Uchiyama, K.A. Smith, T.A. Waldmann, and W.C. Greene. 1982. A monoclonal antibody that appears to recognize the receptor for human T cell growth factor: partial characterization of the receptor. *Nature* **300**:267.
6. Meuer, S.C., O. Acuto, R.E. Hussey, J.C. Hodgdon, K.A. Fitzgerald, S.F. Schlossman, and E.L. Reinherz. 1983. Evidence for the T3 associated 90KD heterodimer as the T cell antigen receptor. *Nature* **303**:808.
7. Meuer, S.C., S.F. Schlossman, and E.L. Reinherz. 1982. Clonal analysis of human cytotoxic T lymphocytes: T4 and T8 effector T cells recognize products of different major histocompatibility regions. *Proc. Natl. Acad. Sci. U.S.A.* **79**:4395.
8. Meuer, S.C., R.E. Hussey, J.C. Hodgdon, T. Hercend, S.F. Schlossman, and E.L. Reinherz. 1982. Surface structures involved in target recognition by human cytotoxic T lymphocytes. *Science* **218**:471.
9. Biddison, W.E., P.E. Rao, M.A. Talle, G. Goldstein, and S. Shaw. 1982. Possible involvement of the OKT4 molecule in T cell recognition of class II HLA antigens. Evidence from studies of cytotoxic T lymphocytes specific for SB antigens. *J. Exp. Med.* **156**:1065.
10. Malissen, B., N. Rebai, A. Liebeuf, and C. Mawas. 1982. Human cytotoxic T cell structures associated with expression of cytolysis. I. Analysis at the clonal cell level of the cytolysis-inhibiting effect of 7 monoclonal antibodies. *Eur. J. Immunol.* **12**:739.
11. Van Wauve, F.P., J.R. De Mey, and J.G. Goossens. 1980. OKT3: A monoclonal anti-human T lymphocyte antibody with potent mitogenic properties. *J. Immunol.* **124**:2708.

12. Meuer, S.C., J.C. Hodgdon, R.E. Hussey, J.P. Protentis, S.F. Schlossman, and E.L. Reinherz. 1983. Antigen-like effects of monoclonal antibodies directed at receptors on human T cell clones. *J. Exp. Med.* **158**:988.

13. Meuer, S.C., R.E. Hussey, D.A. Cantrell, J.C. Hodgdon, S.F. Schlossman, K.A. Smith, and E.L. Reinherz. 1984. Triggering of the T3–Ti antigen receptor complex results in clonal T cell proliferation via an interleukin 2 dependent autocrine pathway. *Proc. Natl. Acad. Sci. U.S.A.* **81**:1509.

14. Meuer, S.C., R.E. Hussey, M. Fabbi, D. Fox, O. Acuto, K.A. Fitzgerald, J.C. Hodgdon, J.P. Protentis, S.F. Schlossman, and E.L. Reinherz. 1984. An alternative pathway of T-cell activation: A functional role for the 50 KD T11 sheep erythrocyte receptor protein. *Cell* **36**:897.

15. Nadler, L.M., P. Stashenko, R. Hardy, J.M. Pesando, E.J. Yunis, and S.F. Schlossman. 1981. Monoclonal antibodies defining serologically distinct HLA-D/DR related Ia-like antigens in man. *Hum. Immunol.* **1**:77.

16. Todd, R.F., L.M. Nadler, and S.F. Schlossman. 1981. Antigens on human monocytes identified by monoclonal antibodies. *J. Immunol.* **126**:1435.

17. Reinherz, E.L., P.C. Kung, G. Goldstein, and S.F. Schlossman. 1979. A monoclonal antibody with selective reactivity with functionally mature thymocytes and all peripheral human T cells. *J. Immunol.* **123**:1312.

18. Reinherz, E.L., E.L. Hussey, and S.F. Schlossman. 1980. A monoclonal antibody blocking human T cell function. *Eur. J. Immunol.* **10**:758.

19. Chang, T.W., P.C. Kung, S.P. Gingras, and G. Goldstein. 1981. Does OKT3 monoclonal antibody react with an antigen recognition structure on human T cells? *Proc. Nat. Sci. U.S.A.* **78**:1895.

20. Reinherz, E.L., S.C. Meuer, K.A. Fitzgerald, R.E. Hussey, H. Levine, and S.F. Schlossman. 1982. Antigen recognition by human T lymphocytes is linked to surface expression of the T3 molecular complex. *Cell* **30**:735.

21. Kaneoka, H., G. Perez-Rojas, T. Sasasuki, C.J. Benike, and E.G. Engleman. 1983. Human T lymphocyte proliferation induced by a Pan-T monoclonal antibody (anti-Leu 4): Heterogeneity of response is a function of monocytes. *J. Immunol.* **131**:158.

22. Meuer, S.C., K.A. Fitzgerald, R.E. Hussey, J.C. Hodgdon, S.F. Schlossman, and E.L. Reinherz. 1983. Clonotypic structures involved in antigen specific human T cell function: Relationship to the T3 molecular complex. *J. Exp. Med.* **157**:705.

23. Meuer, S.C., D.A. Cooper, J.C. Hodgdon, R.E. Hussey, K.A. Fitzgerald, S.F. Schlossman, and E.L. Reinherz. 1983. Identification of the antigen/MHC-receptor on human inducer T lymphocytes. *Science* **222**:1239.

24. Borst, J., S. Alexander, J. Elder, and C. Terhost. 1983. The T3 complex on human T lymphocytes involves four structurally distinct glycoproteins. *J. Biol. Chem.* **8**:5135.

25. Brain, P., J. Gordon, and W.A. Willetts. 1970. Rosette formation by peripheral lymphocytes. *Clin. Exp. Immunol.* **6**:681.

26. Coombs, R.R.A., B.W. Gurner, A.B. Wilson, G. Holm, and B. Lindgren. 1970. Rosette-formation between human lymphocytes and sheep red blood cells not involving immunoglobulin receptors. *Int. Arch. Allergy App. Immunol.* **39**:658.

27. Howard, F.D., J.A. Ledbetter, J. Wong, C.P. Bieber, E.B. Stinson, and L.A.

Herzenberg. 1981. A human T lymphocyte differentiation marker defined by monoclonal antibodies that blocks E rosette formation. *J. Immunol.* **126**:2117.
28. Haynes, B.F., B.L. Dowell, L.L. Hensley, F. Gore, and R.S. Metzgar. 1982. Human T cell antigen expression by primate T cells. *Science* **215**:298.
29. Letvin, N.L., N.W. King, E.L. Reinherz, R.D. Hunt, H. Lanes, and S.F. Schlossman. 1983. T lymphocyte surface antigens in primates. *Eur. J. Immunol.* **13**:345.

CHAPTER 6

The Development of Monoclonal Antibodies against Human Immunoregulatory T Cell Subsets: The Isolation of Human Suppressor Inducer T Cell Subset

Chikao Morimoto, Norman L. Letvin, and
Stuart F. Schlossman

It is now well established that T cells are involved in a complex series of interactions which regulate the immune response (1,2). Considerable impetus to the dissection of T cell heterogeneity came with development of monoclonal antibodies capable of dividing T cells into functionally distinct T4 and T8 populations which also show preferential recognition of class II and I antigens, respectively (3–8).

Moreover, within these two major populations of T lymphocytes, numerous studies have now shown that there exists both functional and phenotypic heterogeneity (5,9–12). A number of monoclonal and auto-antibodies have permitted the dissection of these cells into distinct subsets. For example, antibody to Ia has allowed for the division of $T4^+$ cells into two subsets following activation. Both the $T4^+Ia^+$ and $T4^+Ia^-$ lymphocyte subsets are required to induce optimal Ig secretion by B cells (12). Naturally occurring anti–T cell antibodies found in some patients with active juvenile rheumatoid arthritis (JRA) have been used to subdivide $T4^+$ cells into a helper population ($T4^+JRA^-$) and an inducer of suppressor population ($T4^+JRA^+$) for PWM- and antigen-driven immunoglobulin production (9,10). Using a monoclonal antibody it was shown that the major inducer of help was $T4^+JRA^-TQ1^-$ (13). While these studies have provided an initial phenotypic definition of the heterogeneity within the major populations of T cells, the precise relationship of individual subsets with one another has been more difficult to define because of the small size of the populations and the less than optimal available serologic reagents.

We and others have shown a substantial conservation of antigenic determinants on the surface of lymphocytes of a wide array of primate species (14,15). Since some of the conserved antigens between man and phylogenetically lower primate species may be more immunodominant on lymphocytes of the lower primate species, we reasoned that immunization of mice with lymphocytes from lower primates might prove a useful strategy for developing monoclonal antibodies which recognize functionally important structures on human lymphocytes.

We have now produced a monoclonal antibody using splenocytes from mice immunized with lower primate lymphocytes which is reactive with a subset of human T4$^+$ cells. Functional studies indicate that this antibody, anti-2H4, defines the human suppressor inducer subset of lymphocytes previously described as T4$^+$JRA$^+$.

Materials and Methods

Isolation of Lymphoid Populations

Human peripheral blood mononuclear cells were isolated from healthy volunteer donors by Ficoll–Hypaque density gradient centrifugation (Pharmacia Fine Chemicals, Piscataway, NJ). Unfractionated mononuclear cells were first depleted of macrophages by adherence to plastic as previously described (16). The adherent cells were recovered and used as a macrophage-enriched population. The macrophage-depleted mononuclear cells were separated into erythrocyte rosette (E-rosette) positive (E$^+$) and E-rosette-negative (E$^-$) populations with 5% sheep erythrocytes (Microbiological Associates, Bethesda, MD) as previously described (9,10). The T cell population thus obtained was 95% E$^+$ and 94% reactive with the monoclonal antibody anti-T3 (17). The E-population was further fractionated into B and null cell populations by complement-mediated lysis with anti-Mol and anti-B1, respectively (18,19). Reanalysis of antibody and complement-lysed subpopulations of E$^-$ cells demonstrated less than 5% residual antibody-reactive cells in either population. Suspensions of human thymocytes were made from fragments of thymus obtained at cardiac surgery from infants (age 2 mo to 4 yr).

Production and Characterization of Monoclonal Antibodies

The monoclonal antibody anti-2H4 was produced by standard techniques after immunization of a BALB/c J mouse (Jackson Laboratories, Bar Harbor, ME) with cells of a T lymphocyte line derived from *Aotus trivirgatus*. The hybridoma antibody described here, anti-2H4, was shown to be of the IgG1 subclass by the specificity of the staining with fluorescein-labeled goat anti–mouse IgGl (Meloy Laboratories, Springfield, VA) and its failure to be stained by fluorescein-labeled antibodies directed against other subclasses of mouse immunoglobulin. Two T cell-specific monoclonal antibodies, anti-T4 and anti-T8, reacted with nonoverlapping reciprocal populations of human peripheral T cells comprising approximately 60 and 30% of the circulating E^+ population. These antibodies of the IgG_2 subclass have been described elsewhere (20,21) and are available through Coulter Immunology, Hialeah, FL.

Human Cell Lines

Epstein–Barr virus-transformed B lymphoid lines (Laz 461, Laz 509, Laz 388, and Laz 156), Burkitt's lines (Raji and Daudi), T cell lines (HSB, CEM, JM and Molt 4), the myeloblastoid line KG1, and histiocytic line U937, and the erythroleukemia line K562 were used in this study.

Complement-dependent Lysis of Lymphocytes with Monoclonal Antibodies

E^+ lymphocytes were treated with anti-T4 or anti-T8 monoclonal antibodies and rabbit C (Pel-Freeze Biologicals) as previously described (21,22,23). After lysis of cells with anti-T4 and C, greater than 90% of the residual cells were $T8^+$ and less than 5% were $T4^+$. After lysis with anti-T8 and C, greater than 90% of the remaining cells were $T4^+$ and less than 5% were $T8^+$. These two populations will be referred to as $T8^+$ and $T4^+$ cells, respectively.

Analysis and Separation of Lymphocyte Populations with a Fluorescence-activated Cell Sorter

Cytofluorographic analysis of cell populations and cell separation was performed by means of indirect immunofluorescence with fluorescein-conjugated $F(ab')_2$ goat anti–mouse $F(ab')_2$ on an Epics V cell sorter (Coulter Electronics) or a FACS I (Becton-Dickinson) as previously described (13).

Detection of *in vitro* Secretion of IgG

Unfractionated and separated populations of lymphocytes were cultured in round-bottomed microtiter culture plates (Falcon) at 37°C in a humidified atmosphere with 5% CO_2 for 7 days in RPMI 1640 supplemented with 20% heat-inactivated fetal calf serum (Microbiological Associates), 0.5% sodium bicarbonate, 200 mM L-glutamine, 25 mM HEPES, and 1% penicillin–streptomycin in the presence of PWM. Macrophages were added to all populations at a 5% final concentration at the initiation of *in vitro* cultures. In some experiments, various numbers of T8 cells were added to a mixture containing 2×10^4 cells of a subpopulation of $T4^+$ cells and 5×10^4 B cells with PWM. On day 7, cultures were terminated, supernatants were harvested, and IgG secretion into the supernatant was determined by solid-phase radioimmunoassay (RIA) as previously described (9,22).

Results

Reactivity of Anti-2H4 with Human Lymphoid Cells and Cell Lines

In an effort to generate monoclonal antibodies against non-human primate cells which may prove useful in dissecting the heterogeneity of T4+ and T8+ cells, Balb/c mice were immunized with peripheral blood lymphocyte lines derived from *A. trivirgatus*. Hybridoma cells, the supernatants of which were found to be reactive with a subset of human T lymphocytes, were developed for further characterization. One clone of interest secreted the monoclonal antibody termed anti-2H4. Figure 6.1 shows a representative cytofluorographic pattern of cells stained with this antibody. Anti-2H4 was reactive with 42 ± 4% of peripheral blood human T lymphocytes, with 41 ± 5% of T4+ lymphocytes and 54 ± 4% (n = 15) of T8+ lymphocytes. Thus, 2H4+ T cells were found in both T4+ and T8+ subpopulations of cells. Anti-2H4 was not reactive with human thymocytes, did not react with the immature human T cell lines tested, and reacted only slightly with the more mature human T cell line JM. Its reactivity was not restricted to the T lineage: it reacted with all 6 B cell lines tested and 2 of 3 human hematopoietic lines, as well as subsets of human peripheral blood B cells and null cells.

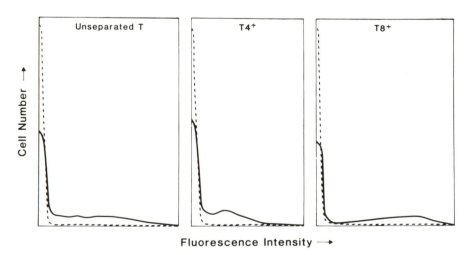

Fig. 6.1. Cytofluorographic analysis of unfractionated T, T4, and T8 cells with anti-2H4 antibody.

Only T4+2H4− Lymphocytes Have Helper Inducer Function for B Cell Ig Synthesis

We sought to determine whether T cell help for B cell immunoglobulin production was restricted to the T4+2H4− or T4+2H4− cell population. T4+2H4+ and T4+2H4− cells were mixed with B lymphocytes, stimulated with PWM *in vitro,* and total IgG production was measured after 7 days in culture. As shown in Fig. 6.2, the addition of T4+2H4+ cells to B cells resulted in virtually no augmentation in IgG synthesis when compared with IgG synthesis by B cells alone. T4+2H4− cells, however, provided significant helper function for this IgG synthesis. In repeated experiments the addition of increasing numbers of T4+2H4− cells resulted in increasing IgG synthesis by B cells. Thus, the majority of helper activity for antibody production in response to PWM by B cells resides in the T4+2H4− subset of cells.

T4+2H4+ Cells Are Required for Suppression of PWM-stimulated IgG Secretion

Previous studies have shown that a subset of T4+ cells is required for the generation of suppressor function (9,19,22). We, therefore, sought to determine whether the T4+2H4+ or T4+2H4− cells are required for this function. As shown in Table 6.1, graded numbers of T8+ cells were added to either B cells + T4+2H4+ or B cells + T4+2H4− cells. These populations were then stimulated with PWM and IgG synthesis was measured.

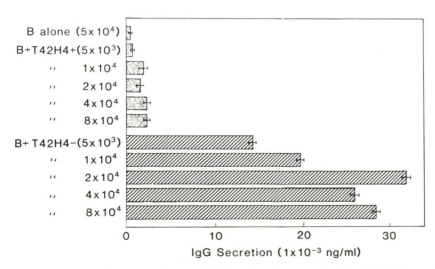

Fig. 6.2. Quantitative comparison of helper function provided by T4+2H4+ and T4+2H4− cells for PWM-stimulated IgG synthesis.

Table 6.1. T4$^+$2H4$^+$ are required for suppression of PWM-stimulated IgG secretion.

Cell combinations[a]	T8 cells added	IgG (ng/ml)	
		Exp 1	Exp 2
A. B (5 × 10⁴) + T4$^+$2H4$^+$ (2 × 10⁴)	0	3000[b]	4200
	1 × 10⁴	560(81)[c]	2480(41)
	2 × 10⁴	280(91)	500(88)
	4 × 10⁴	5(100)	140(97)
B. B (5 × 10⁴) + T4$^+$2H4$^-$ (2 × 10⁴)	0	15400	26000
	1 × 10⁴	21600(0)	36000(0)
	2 × 10⁴	15600(0)	13600(40)
	4 × 10⁴	8000(47)	5600(78)

[a] Varying numbers of T8$^+$ T cells were added to a constant number of B cells (5 × 10⁴), and to this were added fractionated T4$^+$2H4$^+$ or T4$^+$2H4$^-$T cells (2 × 10⁴) in the presence of PWM. Total IgG production was measured after 7 days.
[b] Values are expressed as mean ng/ml of triplicate samples. SEM was always less than 10%.
[c] Number in parentheses equals % suppression calculated by the following formula:

$$\frac{\text{Control IgG} - \text{IgG observed by the addition of T8 cells}}{\text{Control IgG production}} \times 100$$

While the addition of increasing numbers of T8$^+$ cells did not result in increasing suppression of IgG synthesis by the B + T4$^+$2H4$^-$ cell populations, marked suppression of IgG synthesis did occur when T8$^+$ cells were added to the B + T4$^+$2H4$^+$ cells. It should be noted that when excess numbers of T8$^+$ cells (4 × 10⁴) were added to T4$^+$2H4$^-$ and B cells, a moderate amount of suppression of IgG production was seen.

T4$^+$2H4$^+$ Cells Induce Suppressor Effector Function

To demonstrate directly that T4$^+$2H4$^+$ cells are necessary for the induction of suppression, varying numbers of T4$^+$2H4$^+$ or T4$^+$2H4$^-$ cells were added to a constant number of B cells and T4$^+$2H4$^-$ or T4$^+$2H4$^+$ cells and T8 cells in the presence of PWM.

As shown in Fig. 6.3, the addition of increasing numbers of T4$^+$2H4$^+$ cells to a cell combination of B cells + T4$^+$2H4$^-$ cells + T8 cells resulted in a cell number-dependent suppression of IgG synthesis. In contrast, the addition of increasing numbers of T4$^+$2H4$^-$ cells resulted in an augmentation of IgG production. To rule out the possibility that T4$^+$2H4$^+$ cells are themselves suppressor effector cells, varying numbers of T4$^+$2H4$^+$ or T4$^+$2H4$^-$ cells were added to a constant number of B cells (5 × 10⁴) and T4$^+$2H4$^+$ or T4$^+$2H4$^-$ cells (2 × 10⁴) in the presence or absence of T8$^+$ cells (1 × 10⁴) with PWM. When increasing numbers of T4$^+$2H4$^+$ T cells were added to the mixture of B cells and T4$^+$2H4$^-$ T cells, no suppression was observed. However, when increasing numbers of T4$^+$2H4$^+$ cells were added to the mixture of B cells and T4$^+$2H4$^-$ cells including T8 cells, marked suppression was seen as previously shown in Fig. 6.3 (data not shown). Thus, T4$^+$2H4$^+$ cells were not themselves effectors of suppres-

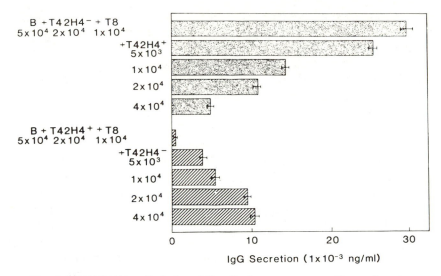

Fig. 6.3. T4⁺2H4⁺ cells induce T8 cells for suppressor effector function.

sion; rather they induced or activated T8⁺ cells to suppress the immune response.

Discussion

In these studies, we have shown that the monoclonal antibody anti-2H4 subdivides peripheral blood T4⁺ cells into two functionally distinct populations: one provides poor help to B cells for PWM-induced Ig synthesis (T4⁺2H4⁺); the other provides a good helper signal for PWM-induced Ig synthesis (T4⁺2H4⁻). Moreover, this monoclonal antibody defines the subset of T4⁺ cells which is the inducer of T8⁺ suppressor cells.

The strategy employed in creating this monoclonal antibody was based on our previous studies demonstrating the conservation of various T lymphocyte-specific surface antigens in all primate species (14). We reasoned that the production of new monoclonal antibodies which might be useful in further subdividing T cell populations into functionally distinct subpopulations may have been difficult up until now because of a lack of immunodominance of such important surface structures on human T cells. Such structures may be conserved on simian lymphocytes and be expressed in a more highly antigenic configuration than they are on human cells.

This monoclonal antibody defines with a new level of precision a cell population which has been studied in murine and human systems. Eardley *et al.* (23) and Cantor *et al.* (24) showed that the murine Lyt-1⁺ subset of cells is heterogeneous and that the maintenance of immunologic homeostasis is governed by the Qa1 feedback inhibitory circuit. In their studies, a cell with the Lyt-1 Qal$^+$ phenotype was required to induce Lyt123$^+$ Qal$^+$ T cells to exert feedback suppressor activity (23,24). Other studies have also indicated that this Lyt-1 suppressor inducer cell may express the I-J determinant (25). The Lyt-1$^+$ IJ$^-$ cell provides a helper signal for B cells. Thus, it would appear that the T4$^+$2H4$^+$ lymphocyte subset is functionally analogous to the Lyt1$^+$ Qal$^+$ IJ$^+$ subset, whereas the T4$^+$2H4$^-$ subset is comparable to the Lyt1$^+$ IJ$^-$ subset in mice (25).

Our previous studies demonstrated that the T4$^+$ subset of cells defined by naturally occurring anti–T cell antibodies found in some patients with active JRA (T4$^+$JRA$^+$) is responsible for the induction of T8$^+$ suppressor activity and that the T4$^+$JRA$^-$ subset of cells accounts for most of the help for antibody synthesis by B cells (9,10,22). Thus, the subset of T4$^+$ cells defined by anti-2H4 is functionally similar to that defined by naturally occurring JRA anti-T cell antibodies. The present studies directly demonstrate that the T4$^+$2H4$^+$ subset of lymphocytes is an important suppressor inducer population and may play a central role in maintaining normal immune homeostasis. Further studies are needed to determine the role of this cell population in human disease states.

Summary

Immunization of mice with lower lymphoid cells has provided a useful strategy for raising monoclonal antibodies against functionally important surface determinants on human T lymphocytes. We have developed a monoclonal antibody, anti-2H4, which defines a functionally important human T cell subset. Anti-2H4 was reactive with approximately 42% of unfractionated T cells, 41% of T4$^+$ inducer cells and 54% of T8$^+$ cytotoxic/suppressor cells. Anti-2H4 was not reactive with human thymocytes but reacted with subsets of peripheral blood B cells and null cells. This antibody subdivided peripheral blood T4$^+$ cells into two functionally distinct populations. T4$^+$2H4$^+$ lymphocytes provide poor help to B cells for PWM-induced immunoglobulin synthesis; T4$^+$2H4$^-$ cells provide a good helper signal for PWM-induced Ig synthesis. Moreover, this antibody defines the subset of T4$^+$ cells which is the inducer of T8$^+$ suppressor cells. These results suggest that anti-2H4 defines the human suppressor inducer subset of lymphocytes previously described as T4$^+$JRA$^+$. Lastly, these results reemphasize the previously documented remarkable structural conservation of certain T cell specific determinants on lymphocytes of phylogenetically distant primate species.

Acknowledgment. This work was supported by NIH grants AI12069, AI20729, and CA19589.

References

1. Reinherz, E.L. and S.F. Schlossman. 1980. Regulation of the immune response: inducer and suppressor T lymphocyte subsets in man. *New England J. Med.* **303**:370.
2. Germain, R.N. and B. Benacerraf. 1980. Helper and suppressor factors. *Springer Semin. Immunopathol.* **3**:93.
3. Reinherz, E.L., P.C. Kung, G. Goldstein, and S.F. Schlossman. 1979. Separation of functional subsets of human T cells by a monoclonal antibody. *Proc. Natl. Acad. Sci. U.S.A.* **76**:4061.
4. Reinherz, E.L., P.C. Kung, G. Goldstein, and S.F. Schlossman. 1980. A monoclonal antibody reactive with the human cytotoxic/suppressor T cell subset previously defined by heteroantiserum termed TH_2. *J. Immunol.* **124**:1301.
5. Thomas, Y., J. Sosman, O. Irigoyen, S. J. Friedman, P.C. Kung, G. Goldstein, and L. Chess. 1980. Functional analysis of human T cell subsets defined by monoclonal antibodies. I. Collaborative T-T interactions in the immunoregulation of B cell differentiation. *J. Immunol.* **125**:2402.
6. Ledbetter, J., R.L. Evans, M. Lipinski, C. Cunningham-Rundels, R.R. Good, and L.A. Herzenberg. 1981. Evolutionary conservation of surface molecules that distinguish T lymphocyte inducer and cytotoxic/suppressor subpopulations in mouse and man. *J. Exp. Med.* **153**:310.
7. Meuer, S.C., S.F. Schlossman, and E.L. Reinherz. 1982. Clonal analysis of human cytotoxic T lymphocyte: T4 and T8 effector T cells recognize products of different major histocompatibility regions. *Proc. Natl. Acad. Sci. U.S.A.* **79**:4395.
8. Krensky, A.M., C. Clayberger, C.S. Reiss, J.L. Strominger, and S.J. Burakoff. 1982. Specificity of $OKT4^+$ cytotoxic T lymphocyte clones. *J. Immunol.* **129**:2001.
9. Morimoto, C., E.L. Reinherz, Y. Borel, E. Mantzouranis, A.D. Steinberg, and S.F. Schlossman. 1981. Autoantibody to an immunoregulatory inducer population in patients with juvenile rheumatoid arthritis. *J. Clin. Invest.* **67**:753.
10. Morimoto, C., J. Distaso, Y. Borel, S.F. Schlossman, and E. L. Reinherz. 1982. Communicative interactions between subpopulations of human T lymphocytes required for generation of suppressor effector function in a primary antibody response. *J. Immunol.* **128**:1645.
11. Gatenby, P.A., B.L. Kotzin, G.S. Kansas, and E.G. Engelman. 1982. Immunoglobulin secretion in human autologous mixed leukocyte reaction. Definition of a suppressor amplifier circuit using monoclonal antibodies. *J. Exp. Med.* **156**:55.
12. Reinherz, E.L., C. Morimoto, A.C. Penta, and S.F. Schlossman. 1981. Subpopulation of the $T4^+$ inducer T cell subset in man. Evidence for an amplifier population preferentially expressing Ia antigen upon activation. *J. Immunol.* **126**:67.
13. Reinherz, E.L., C. Morimoto, K.A. Fitzgerald, R.E. Hussey, J.A. Daley, and S.F. Schlossman. 1982. Heterogeneity of human $T4^+$ inducer T cells as defined by a monoclonal antibody that delineates two functionally subpopulations. *J. Immunol.* **128**:463.

14. Letvin, N.L., N.W. King, E.L. Reinherz, R.D. Hunt, H. Lane, and S.F. Schlossman. 1983. T lymphocyte surface antigens in primates. *Eur. J. Immunol.* **13:**345.
15. Haynes, B.F., B.L. Dowell, L.L. Hensley, I. Gore, and R.S. Metzgar. 1982. Human T cell antigen expression by primate T cells. *Science* **215:**298.
16. Morimoto, C., R.F. Todd, J.A. Distaso, and S.F. Schlossman. 1981. The role of the macrophage in *in vitro* primary anti-DNP antibody production in man. *J. Immunol.* **127:**1137.
17. Reinherz, E.L., P.C. Kung, G. Goldstein, and S.F. Schlossman. 1979. A monoclonal antibody with selective reactivity with functionally mature human thymocytes and all peripheral human T cells. *J. Immunol.* **123:**1312.
18. Todd, R.F., L.M. Nadler, and S.F. Schlossman. 1981. Antigens on human monocytes identified by monoclonal antibodies. *J. Immunol.* **126:**1435.
19. Nadler, L.M., J. Ritz, R. Hardy, J.M. Pesando, and S.F. Schlossman. 1981. A unique cell surface antigen identifying lymphoid malignancies of B cell origin. *J. Clin. Invest.* **67:**134.
20. Reinherz, E.L., S.C. Meuer, K.A. Fitzgerald, R.E. Hussey, H. Levine, and S.F. Schlossman. 1982. Antigen recognition by human T lymphocytes is linked to surface expression of the T3 molecular complex. *Cell* **30:**735.
21. Meuer, S.C., D.A. Cooper, J.C. Hodgdon, R.E. Hussey, C. Morimoto, S.F. Schlossman, and E.L. Reinherz. 1983. Immunoregulatory human T lymphocytes triggered as a consequence of viral infection: Clonal analysis of helper, suppressor inducer and suppressor effector cell populations. *J. Immunol.* **131:**1167.
22. Morimoto, C., E.L. Reinherz, Y. Borel, and S.F. Schlossman. 1983. Direct demonstration of the human suppressor inducer subset by anti-T cell antibodies. *J. Immunol.* **130:**157.
23. Eardley, D.D., J. Hugenberger, L. McVay-Boudreau, F.W. Shen, R.K. Gershon, and H. Cantor. 1978. Immunoregulatory circuits among T cell sets. II. T helper cells induce other T cell sets to exert feedback inhibition. *J. Exp. Med.* **147:**1106.
24. Cantor, H., J. Hugenberger, L. McVay-Boudreau, D.D. Eardley, J. Kemp, F.W. Shen, and R.K. Gershon. 1978. Immunoregulatory circuits among T cell sets: Identification of a subpopulation of T inducer cells that activates feedback inhibition. *J. Exp. Med.* **148:**871.
25. Eardley, D.D., D.B. Murphy, J.D. Kemp, F.W. Shen, H. Cantor, and R.K. Gershon. 1980. Lyt-1 inducer and Lyt 1,2 acceptor T cells in the feedback suppression circuit bear an I-J subregion controlled determinant. *Immunogen.* **11:**549.

CHAPTER 7

Lectin Activation Induces T4, T8 Coexpression on Peripheral Blood T Cells

Marie-Luise Blue, John F. Daley, Herbert Levine, and Stuart F. Schlossman

Recent studies from this and other laboratories have indicated that the T4 and T8 glycoproteins preferentially interact with class II and class I MHC molecules, respectively (1–3). Although the precise mechanism of interaction between T4, T8, and MHC antigens is not known, it has been proposed that T4 and T8 molecules bind to nonpolymorphic regions of MHC antigens (2,4). In this report, using the sensitive technique of two-color fluorescence flow cytometry, we demonstrate the existence of small numbers of T4$^+$T8$^+$ cells in freshly isolated T cell populations and that lectins can induce the coexpression of T4 and T8 on a fraction of peripheral blood T cells. Our results suggest that T4, T8 coexpression occurs on an activated blast-like peripheral blood T cell. Since lymphocyte cell surface phenotype and function appear to be closely linked, the T4$^+$T8$^+$ cell may prove to have an important role in either regulation or differentiation.

Materials and Methods

Cell Preparations

Mononuclear leukocytes were isolated from blood by Ficoll–Hypaque (Pharmacia) gradient centrifugation; E$^+$ (T cells) were isolated by the formation of E-rosettes with sheep red blood cells (SRBC). Isolation of T4$^+$T8$^-$ and T8$^+$T4$^-$ cells, as well as T4$^+$T8$^+$ subfractions, was performed using an Epics V cell sorter (Coulter Corporation) with the appropriate monoclonal antibodies.

Monoclonal Antibodies

Conjugated monoclonal antibodies to stain T4 and T8 antigens included anti-T4 biotin, anti-T8A–FITC, anti-T4–FITC, and anti-T8A biotin (Coulter Immunology, Hialeah, FL 33010). Monoclonal anti-B1 FITC, anti-Mo$_2$ biotin, mouse IgG–FITC, and mouse IgG biotin also were from Coulter Immunology. Other monoclonal antibodies such as anti-T4, anti-T8, anti-T6, anti-T9, anti-T10 (5,6), and anti-N901 (against NK cells, Ref. 7) have been described previously. Another monoclonal antibody, anti-IL-2R (1HT4-4H3) was raised against the IL-2 receptor (8).

TCGF Preparation

IL-2 containing supernatant (TCGF) was produced by alloreaction stimulation between whole peripheral blood mononuclear cells from two different donors (1 : 1 cell ratio) in the presence of phytohemagglutinin (2 μg/ml) and phorbol myristate acetate (5 $\times$ 10^{-9} M) (Sigma) at a cell density of 3.5 $\times$ 10^6 cells/ml. After a 4-hr incubation period, cells were washed and incubated in 1% human serum and RPMI 1640 (Gibco) for 40 hr. The supernatant was harvested and assayed using an IL-2 dependent cell line.

Two-color Fluorescence Flow Cytometry

1 $\times$ 10^6 cells were incubated for 30 min on ice with a biotin-conjugated monoclonal antibody against one surface antigen and another monoclonal, directly conjugated to FITC, directed against the second antigen. Following incubation, the cells were washed twice and incubated with Texas Red avidin. Texas Red avidin was prepared by conjugating avidin (Sigma) with Texas Red (Molecular Probes, Junction City, OR). After three additional washes, cells were fixed in a 1% paraformaldehyde/0.15 M PBS solution, pH 7.2 (9) and stored until analysis time. Cells were analyzed on the Epics V cell sorter (Coulter Electronics) equipped with a dual laser, argon wavelength 488 nm (FITC), krypton wavelength 568 nm (Texas Red). Light scatter and fluorescent signals (both red and green) were passed through log amplifiers, processed and integrated in a Multiple Data Acquisition and Display Unit (MDADS, Coulter Electronics) to generate dual fluorescent contour displays and histograms.

Mitogen Activation

2.5 to 10 $\times$ 10^5 cells/well were assayed in microculture for proliferation to Con A (62.5 μg/ml) (Calbiochem, San Diego), PHA (0.5 μg/ml) (Burrow-Welcome Co., Research Triangle Park, NC), PWM (50 μg/ml) (Grand Island Biological, Grand Island, NY) $\pm$ TCGF (10–12%) in 10% heat-inactivated human AB serum RPMI 1640 (Gibco) media supplemented with pen-strep and glutamine (Microbiological Associates, Bethesda, MD). Final concentration of cells was 0.5 $\times$ 10^6 cells/ml. Cells were labeled with 0.2 μCi of ^{3}H-TdR tritiated thymidine (Schwarz-Mann, Div.

of Becton Dickinson, Orangeburg, NY). After 18 hours cells were harvested on a Mash II apparatus (Microbiological Associates) and ^{3}H-TdR incorporation was measured in a Packard Scintillation Counter (Packard Instruments, Downer's Grove, IL).

Mitogen activation for phenotypic analyses was carried out in tissue culture flasks at the same concentration of cells and mitogen used in the microculture proliferation assays described above.

Results

T4$^+$T8$^+$ Cells in Normal Peripheral Blood

Peripheral blood lymphocytes were isolated from various healthy donors and T cells were obtained by E-rosetting as described (Materials and Methods). T cells were analyzed by two-color fluorescence for the presence of T4$^+$T8$^+$ cells using monoclonal anti-T4 biotin with Texas Red avidin and monoclonal anti-T8 conjugated to fluorescein isothiocyanate (FITC). Reversing the reagents and using T8 biotin with Texas Red avidin and T4 directly conjugated to FITC gave identical results. Analysis of T cells from 19 normal volunteers showed that 3.0 ± 0.5% (S.E.M.) cells coexpressed T4 and T8; the range of T4$^+$T8$^+$ percentages was 0.5–8. Figure 7.1(A) shows a typical two-color profile of normal T cells. Dually labeled cells in Fig. 7.1(A) are seen as a small cluster in the center of the plane and represent 2% of the total E$^+$ population. When T cells were cultured in media alone for several days or more, the percentage of T4$^+$T8$^+$ cells increased slightly. Monocyte contamination in these T cell preparations was less than 1% as determined by log 90° light-scatter analysis or labeling with anti-Mo$_2$, a monocyte specific antibody.

T4$^+$T8$^+$ Cells in Mitogen-Activated Cultures

The number of T4$^+$T8$^+$ cells increased dramatically when T cells were cultured with Con A or PHA with or without TCGF (see Materials and Methods). In some cell samples after 4 or 5 days of lectin stimulation, the proportion of T4$^+$T8$^+$ cells was greater than 50%. The coexpression of T4 and T8 in lectin-stimulated cultures did not depend on the addition of TCGF, but TCGF increased the proliferation in these cultures (Fig. 7.2). Figure 7.1(C) represents the same cells shown in Fig. 7.1(A), following 5 days *in vitro* culture with Con A and TCGF. The T4$^+$T8$^+$ fraction in Fig. 7.1(C) comprises 36%.

To rule out the generation of an artifact by the mechanics of dual laser analysis, 50% of a T cell sample was stained with anti-T4 biotin and Texas Red and 50% with anti-T8 conjugated to FITC, and subsequently the two

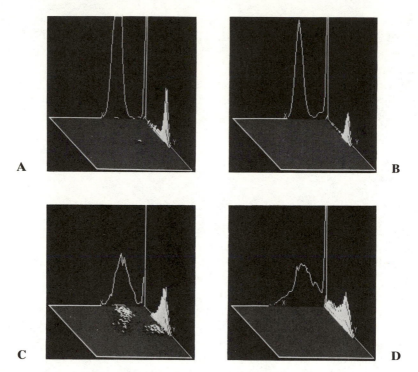

Fig. 7.1. Two-color analysis of T4 and T8 antigens on resting mitogen-treated cells. Cells were stained with anti-T4 biotin/Texas Red and anti-T8 FITC. Log red fluorescence is shown along the *x*-axis and log green fluorescence along the *y*-axis. Cell number is represented on the vertical axis. Panel A: unstimulated peripheral blood T cells; Panel B: the same cells as in panel A, but stained with anti-T4 biotin and Texas Red alone or anti-T8 FITC alone. Cells were mixed (1:1) prior to analysis; Panel C: cells were activated with Con A/TCGF for 5 days prior to staining as in panel A; Panel D: activated cells as in C but stained and mixed as in panel B.

samples were mixed and analyzed. Unstimulated T cells, shown dually labeled in Fig. 7.1(A), when stained and mixed as described gave the histogram shown in Fig. 7.1(B). The same cells following Con A activation, shown dually labeled in Fig. 7.1(C), gave the results represented in Fig. 7.1(D) following single antibody labeling and mixing. Analyses shown in Fig. 7.1(A) and 1(B), and 1(C) and 1(D), were performed at identical fluorescence settings.

Antibody binding to Con A on T cells was not a factor in determining staining patterns. Washing T cells with 0.1 *M* α-methylmannoside prior to staining did not have any significant effect on two-color histogram profiles.

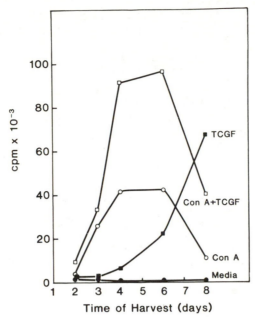

Fig. 7.2. Proliferation of T cells in response to Con A and/or TCGF. Cells were activated with Con A and/or TCGF for various lengths of time (see Materials and Methods).

Correlation of T4, T8 Coexpression and Cell Size

T cells, following 4 or 5 days of activation with Con A, with or without TCGF, contained 50–95% of cells that were clearly larger in size than unstimulated T cells as measured by forward-angle light scattering and/or 90° light scatter. Figure 7.3 shows the forward-angle light-scattering profiles of T cells at various times after Con A/TCGF treatment. During early states of lectin stimulation, up to day 3, a substantial number of small cells are still present (Fig. 7.3). When small and large cells from 3-day lectin-stimulated cultures were analyzed for T4, T8 coexpression, it was found that a high proportion of the large cells (>35%) coexpressed T4 and T8, while small cells were minimally labeled with T4 and T8. Since even unstimulated T cells contain some large cells, we decided to look at T4, T8 coexpression in untreated cultures. Figure 7.4(A) represents a forward-angle light-scattering profile of T cells cultured *in vitro* for 3 days. Large cells, shown from the vertical line to the right, represent about 5% of total T cells. Using identical fluorescence settings, Fig. 7.4(B) shows T4+T8+ cells in the small cell population, while Fig. 7.4(C) shows T4+T8+ cells in the large population. Background readings at the same settings show a higher background for the large cells. However, even after sub-

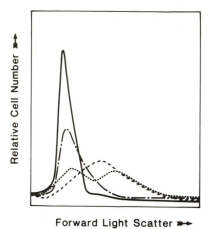

Fig. 7.3. Forward-angle light-scattering profiles of cells activated with Con A/ TCGF for various lengths of time. (——) = 0 time, (–·–) = 2 days, (---) = 3 days, (■■■) = 4 days.

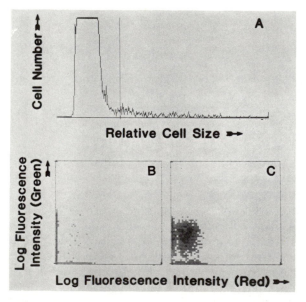

Fig. 7.4. Prevalence of T4⁺T8⁺ cells among small- and large-sized unstimulated cells. Panel A: forward-angle light-scattering profile of total T cell population. Two-color fluorescence contour histogram of small cells (panel B) and large cells (panel C) stained with T4 biotin/Texas Red and anti-T8 FITC.

traction of background, at least 30% of the large cells coexpress T4 and T8, a 27-fold increase over the proportion of $T4^+T8^+$ cells in the small population. Monocytes make up only 2–3% of these large cells as determined by staining with anti-MO_2 antibody.

Correlation with Activation Antigens

To further define the cell that coexpresses T4 and T8, we looked at activation antigens in lectin-stimulated cultures that contained both small and large cells (Table 7.1). Although activation antigens can be detected already on cells treated with Con A/TCGF for 2 days, these cultures contain mostly small cells, while cultures stimulated for 3 days with Con A/TCGF contain nearly equal numbers of small and large cells (Fig. 7.3). Clearly, IL-2 receptors defined by the anti-Tac antibody and anti-T9 and anti-T10, known activation antigens also found on thymocytes (6), are found on both small and large cells. However, the number of cells expressing these activation antigens are two times greater for the large-sized population, where virtually all cells express IL-2R and T9. In addition, the number of antigenic sites recognized on the large cells by anti-IL-2R, anti-T9, and anti-T10 is at least two fold greater (data not shown). The small cells expressed a wide range of fluorescence intensities with these antibodies, while the large cells exhibited a nearly homogeneous fluorescence intensity. Therefore, these activation antigens are already elicited on small cells by lectin treatment, but become fully expressed only on large cells.

The results from Table 7.1 indicate that most or all of the T4, T8 dually labeled cells clearly coexpress the activation antigens, but there are other large cells that exhibit activation antigens but lack detectable T4, T8 coexpression. Another antibody, originally raised against chronic

Table 7.1. Expression of activation antigens on small and large cells.

Antibody	Percent positive cells[a]	
	Small cells	Large cells
Anti-T4 and anti-T8[b]	17	39
Anti-IL-2R	47	87
Anti-T9	47	89
Anti-T10	29	64
Anti-N901[c]	6	5

[a] Values given are after subtraction of background levels. Background levels for small and large cells were determined separately.
[b] Cells were labeled simultaneously with anti-T4 biotin, Texas Red avidin, and anti-T8 FITC. Percentages represent dually labeled cells.
[c] Anti-N901 is a monoclonal antibody against natural killer cells (Ref. 7).

myeloid leukemia cells and found to be specific for natural killer cells (7), did not label large cells more frequently than small cells.

Stability of the T4+T8 Phenotype

After 5 days, viability of cells in Con A or Con A/TCGF cultures usually decreases. We do not know if this is due primarily to an increase in cell density or Con A toxicity. However, if cells following 5 days of Con A/TCGF activation are placed in media containing TCGF or Con A/TCGF at a lower cell density (0.5×10^6 cells/ml), cell viability remains high. Figure 7.5(A) shows a two-color fluorescence contour histogram of T cells after 5 days of exposure to Con A/TCGF. When the same cells are cultured for an additional 3 days in media with TCGF, the number of dually labeled cells decreases [Fig. 7.5(B)]. If, in addition, the media contain Con A, there is no substantial decrease in colabeled cells [Fig. 7.5(C)]. Figure 7.5(B) and quantitation of positively labeled cells (Table 7.2) suggest that large numbers of T4+T8+ may have reverted to T4+T8− and T8+T4− cells. More support for this conclusion was obtained when the T4+T8+ cell fraction (80% pure) was sorted from a T cell population which had been activated for 5 days with Con A/TCGF. Again, there was a substantial increase in T4+T8− and T8+T4− cells when this fraction was cultured in media supplemented with TCGF. On the other hand, incubation of T cells in fresh Con A/TCGF media seemed to block the appearance of T4+T8− and T8+T4− cells (Fig. 7.5(C), Table 7.2). The number of dually labeled cells in Fig. 7.5(A) and 7.5(C) are comparable (Table 7.2), but there appears to be a significant shift to higher fluorescence intensities in Fig. 5(C).

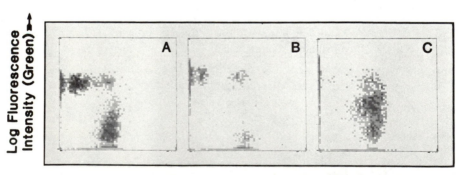

Fig. 7.5. Effect of culture conditions on Con A/TCGF activated T cells. Panel A: T cells were activated for 5 days with Con A/TCGF and stained with anti-T4 biotin/Texas Red and anti-T8 FITC. The 5-day activated cells were cultured either in media with TCGF (panel B) or fresh Con A/TCGF (panel C) for 3 days and stained as in panel A.

Table 7.2. Stability of T4$^+$T8$^+$ phenotype.

Cell treatment	Phenotype (% positive cells)			
	T4$^+$T8$^+$	T4$^+$T8$^-$	T8$^+$T4$^-$	T4$^-$T8$^-$
5 days Con A/TCGF	61	26	11	1
5 days Con A/TCGF and				
3 days media/TCGF	26	45	28	1
5 days Con A/TCGF and				
3 days fresh Con A/TCGF	58	20	19	2

Discussion

We have demonstrated using the sensitive technique of two-color fluorescence flow cytometry the existence of small numbers of T4$^+$T8$^+$ cells in peripheral blood. The majority of normal peripheral blood T lymphocytes, as has been shown previously, express either T4 or T8, but not both. On the other hand, coexpression of T4 and T8 surface antigens on immature cells such as thymocytes or on incompletely differentiated cells found in lymphoblastic lymphomas or cell lines derived from these lymphomas has been well documented (10,11,12).

Since coexpression of T4 and T8 occurred predominantly on large blast-like cells in normal peripheral blood, we examined the ability of various lectins to induce coexpression. Con A at optimal concentrations was most effective but PHA and PWM also induced the T4$^+$T8$^+$ phenotype. In each case, the T4$^+$T8$^+$ phenotype was almost exclusively found on the large cells of the mitogen-activated cultures.

The T4$^+$T8$^+$ cell was partially characterized. It is a large blast-like cell and expresses several activation antigens: T9, T10, and IL-2R. It is a cell highly responsive to TCGF. It bears no detectable amounts of T6, an antigen found on the majority of T4$^+$T8$^+$ thymocytes. This result suggests that the peripheral T4$^+$T8$^+$ cell differs from the majority of T4$^+$T8$^+$ thymocytes and represents a more mature cell type. The T4$^+$T8$^+$ cell also is probably unrelated to a NK cell since lectin-activated T cells are not labeled more frequently with anti-N901, an antibody directed against a NK cell specific antigen, than unstimulated T cells.

Preliminary results suggest that the increased presence of cells coexpressing T4 and T8 in lectin-activated cultures is not due to the selective expansion of a minor population of T4$^+$T8$^+$ cells. Instead, the T4$^+$T8$^+$ cell arises from either a T4$^+$T8$^-$ or T8$^+$T4$^-$ or both cell types. Preliminary experiments with highly purified, sorted T4$^+$T8$^-$ and T8$^+$T4$^-$ cell populations have indicated that the T4$^+$T8$^+$ cells can arise from cells expressing detectable amounts of only one of these antigens. However, the generation of cells coexpressing T4 and T8 may require the presence of cell products from both T4$^+$T8$^-$ and T8$^+$T4$^-$ cell types. The T4$^+$T8$^+$ phenotype appears to revert to the T4$^+$T8$^-$ and T8$^+$T4$^-$ phenotype, within the limits of detection by fluorocytometric techniques upon removal of lectin (Fig. 7.5). Whether cells can alter their surface antigens such that a $T4^+T8^-$ cell becomes a $T8^+T4^-$ cell or vice versa remains to be determined and is currently under investigation.

Both T4 and T8 surface antigens appear to play a crucial role in MHC antigen recognition (1,2,13). Thus, the induction or loss of either T4 or T8 may be decisive in immune regulation or differentiation.

Summary

Using two-color fluorescence flow cytometry, we were able to detect the presence of small numbers of $T4^+T8^+$ cells (about 3%) in freshly isolated peripheral T cell populations derived from normal healthy donors. Coexpression of T4 and T8 was predominantly found on large blast-like cells and appeared to be related to activation. Stimulation of peripheral T cells with Con A for 5 days resulted in the generation of up to 60% of $T4^+T8^+$ cells. Coexpression was accompanied by a two fold increase in the number of T8 antigenic sites/cell. The $T4^+T8^+$ cells in lectin stimulated cultures expressed high levels of the activation antigens T9, T10, and the IL-2 receptor, but lacked T6, an antigen found on a majority of stage II thymocytes. Coexpression of T4 and T8 appeared to be a transitory process since prolonged culture of T cells in the absence of lectin resulted in the loss of the $T4^+T8^+$ phenotype. Since T4 and T8 molecules may directly interact with MHC antigens, coexpression of these molecules may have an important role in immune function.

References

1. Meuer, S.C., S.F. Schlossman, and E.L. Reinherz. 1982. Clonal analysis of human cytotoxic T lymphocytes: $T4^+$ and $T8^+$ effector T cells recognize products of different major histocompatibility complex regions. *Proc. Natl. Acad. Sci. U.S.A.* **79**:4395.
2. Biddison, W.E., P.E. Rao, M.A. Talle, G. Goldstein, and S. Shaw. 1982. Possible involvement of the OKT4 molecule in T cell recognition of class II HLA antigens. *J. Exp. Med.* **156**:1065.
3. Engleman, E.G., C.J. Benike, E. Glickman, and R.L. Evans. 1981. Antibodies to membrane structures that distinguish suppressor/cytotoxic and helper T lymphocyte subpopulations block the mixed leukocyte reaction in man. *J. Exp. Med.* **154**:193.
4. Reinherz, E.L., S.C. Meuer, and S.F. Schlossman. 1983. The delineation of antigen receptors on human T lymphocytes. *Immunol. Today* **1983**(4):5.
5. Reinherz, E.L., P.C. Kung, G. Goldstein, and S.F. Schlossman. 1979. Further characterization of the human inducer T cell subset defined by monoclonal antibody. *J. Immunol.* **123**:2894.

6. Terhorst, C., A. van Agthoven, K. Leclair, P. Snow, E.L. Reinherz, and S.F. Schlossman. 1981. Biochemical studies of the human thymic differentiation antigen T6, T9 and T10. *Cell* **23**:771.

7. Griffin, J.D., T. Hercend, R. Beveridge, and S.F. Schlossman. 1983. Characterization of an antigen expressed by human natural killer cells. *J. Immunol.* **130**:2947.

8. Fox, D.A., R.E. Hussey, K.A. Fitzgerald, A. Bensussan, J.F. Daley, S.F. Schlossman, and E.L. Reinherz. Activation of human thymocytes via the 50 KD T11 sheep erythrocyte binding protein induces the expression of interleukin 2 receptors on both T3$^+$ and T3$^-$ populations. 1984. *J. Immunol.* (in press).

9. Lanier, L.L. and N.L. Warner. 1981. Paraformadehyde fixation of hematopoietic cells for quantitative flow cytometry (FACS) analysis. *J. Immunol. Methods* **47**:25.

10. Reinherz, E.L. and S.F. Schlossman. 1980. The differentiation and function of human T lymphocytes: A review. *Cell* **19**:821.

11. Reinherz, E.L., P.C. Kung, G. Goldstein, R.H. Levey, and S.F. Schlossman. 1980. Discrete stages of human intrathymic differentiation: Analysis of normal thymocytes and leukemic lymphoblasts of T lineage. *Proc. Natl. Acad. Sci. U.S.A.* **77**:1588.

12. Bernard, A., L. Boumsell, E.L. Reinherz, L.M. Nadler, J. Ritz, H. Coppin, Y. Richard, F. Valensi, J. Dausset, G. Flandrin, J. Lemerle, and S.F. Schlossman. 1981. Cell surface characterization of malignant T cells from lymphoblastic lymphomas using monoclonal antibodies: Evidence for phenotypic differences between malignant T cells from patients with acute lymphoblastic leukemia and lymphoblastic lymphoma. *Blood* **57**:1105.

13. Acuto, O., R.E. Hussey, K.A. Fitzgerald, J.P. Protentis, S.C. Meuer, S.F. Schlossman, and E.L. Reinherz. 1983. The human T cell receptor: Appearance in ontogeny and biochemical relationship of α and β subunits on IL-2 dependent clones and T cell tumors. *Cell* **34**:717.

CHAPTER 8

Analysis of the Ontogeny and Function of Human Helper T Cell Subpopulations

Loran T. Clement, Max D. Cooper, and Thomas F. Tedder

Introduction

One characteristic feature of lymphoid cell differentiation is the generation of functionally distinct populations of lymphocytes. This functional
diversification is often accompanied by changes in the expression of cell
surface molecules. While the functional consequences of the acquisition
or loss of a particular membrane component are not always apparent,
these changes may nonetheless serve as useful markers for discriminating
cells with different functions, lineage, or relative maturation.

The advent of monoclonal antibody technology has provided a particularly powerful tool for identifying differentiation antigens which are expressed by functionally distinct subpopulations of human T lymphocytes
(1–3). We have recently produced two monoclonal antibodies, termed
HB-10 and HB-11, which have an unusual pattern of tissue reactivity. In
addition to lymphocytes of B and NK cell lineage, these antibodies react
with a subpopulation of T cells present in adult blood and lymphoid tissues. In this report, we describe studies investigating the ontogeny of T
lineage cells expressing the antigens recognized by the HB-10 and HB-11
antibodies. In addition, the functional capabilities of the subpopulations
of Leu-3$^+$ T helper (T_H) cells defined by these antibodies have been determined.

Materials and Methods

Cell Preparations

Peripheral blood mononuclear cells (MNC) and neutrophils were isolated
by Ficoll–Hypaque density gradient centrifugation (4). Monocytes were
isolated by adherence to plastic at 37°C, then harvested by scraping. Cells

forming rosettes with sheep erythrocytes (E^+ MNC) were separated from non-rosetting (E^-) cells by density gradient centrifugation (5).

Spleen, lymph node, and thymus tissue samples were obtained during surgical procedures or postmortem from individuals without identifiable hematologic disorders, and single cell suspensions were prepared. Informed consent was obtained according to protocols approved by the Human Use Committee of the University of Alabama in Birmingham.

Immunofluorescence Analysis

Methods employed for the analysis of cells by one- or two-color indirect immunofluorescent staining have previously been described in detail (6). Fluorescein (FITC)- or tetramethylrhodamine (RITC)-conjugated goat antibodies specific for the appropriate murine heavy chain isotypes were used as secondary antibodies. Reactivity was assessed by flow cytometry with a fluorescence-activated cell sorter (FACS) or by two-color fluorescence microscopy (6).

Monoclonal Antibody Production

The HB-10 and HB-11 monoclonal antibodies were produced by fusing spleen cells from mice immunized with the human B cell line SB with Ag8.653 myeloma cells (7). Tissue culture supernatants were screened for antibodies reactive with SB cells and blood MNC by indirect immunofluorescence. The hybridomas producing the HB-10 and HB-11 monoclonal antibodies were subcloned twice by limiting dilution, then grown in ascitic form in pristane-primed mice. Each antibody was purified by Na_2SO_4 precipitation and ion exchange chromatography for use in the experiments described herein.

The heavy chain isotypes of the HB-10 and HB-11 antibodies were determined (by immunofluorescence analysis) to be IgM and IgG1, respectively.

FACS Purification of B and T Cell Subpopulations

For purification of Leu-3$^+$ subpopulations, E^+ cells were stained with Leu-2 and Leu-15 antibodies and FITC-conjugated goat anti–mouse immunoglobulin (Ig). Unstained cells, which were >97% Leu-3$^+$, were then isolated with the FACS. These negatively selected Leu-3$^+$ cells were then stained with HB-11 and FITC-goat anti–mouse Ig antibodies, and the Leu 3$^+$/HB-11$^+$ and Leu 3$^+$/HB-11$^-$ subpopulations were FACS-purified.

Small and large IgM$^+$ B cells were purified with the FACS as previously described, using forward-angle light scatter and fluorescence intensity as the selection parameters (8).

Lymphocyte Function Assays

The proliferative responses of T cells to phytohemagglutinin (PHA), pokeweed mitogen (PWM), OKT3 (10 ng/ml), or soluble tetanus toxoid antigen were assessed as previously described (9). Briefly, T cells (1 × 10^5/well) supplemented with 10% monocytes were cultured for 3d (OKT3), 4d (mitogens), or 6d (tetanus antigen) in triplicate microtiter wells. Cells were pulsed with [^{3}H]thymidine (^{3}H-TdR; 1 μCi/well) during the final 16–18 hr of culture, harvested, and ^{3}H-TdR uptake estimated by scintillation counting.

Small and large B cell proliferation was determined by culturing FACS-purified B cells (7.5 × 10^4/well) with mitomycin C-treated Leu-3$^+$ cells (7.5 × 10^4/well) and PHA or PWM for 3 days, as previously described (8). ^{3}H-TdR uptake was determined as described above.

B cell differentiation was assessed by culturing E$^-$ cells (7.5 × 10^4/well) with an equal number of Leu-3$^+$ cells (or Leu-3$^+$ subpopulations) and PWM for 7 days. Plasma cell formation was determined by immunofluorescent staining for cytoplasmic IgM and IgG, as previously described (10).

Results

Tissue Reactivity of HB-10 and HB-11 Antibodies

The reactivity of the HB-10 and HB-11 antibodies with different leukocyte populations present in adult blood was assessed in two-color immunofluorescence staining experiments. As shown in Table 8.1, the HB-10 and HB-11 antibodies had virtually identical patterns of reactivity. Both antibodies reacted with all IgM$^+$ B cells and the vast majority of Leu-11$^+$ (or Leu-7$^+$) NK cells. Approximately 60% of Leu-4$^+$ T cells in adult blood were HB-10$^+$ and 11$^+$, while monocytes and neutrophils did not express either antigen.

Table 8.1. Reactivity of HB-10 and HB-11 with adult blood leukocytes.

Cell type	HB-10$^+$	HB-11$^+$
B cells (IgM$^+$)	99 ± 1[a]	99 ± 2
T cells (Leu-4$^+$)	64 ± 8	63 ± 4
NK cells (Leu-11$^+$)	96 ± 5	96 ± 6
Monocytes (Leu-M1$^+$)	N.D.	1 ± 1
Neutrophils	<1	<1

[a] Percent ± 1SD of each cell type coexpressing the HB-10 or HB-11 antigens, as determined by two-color indirect immunofluorescent staining.

Table 8.2. Tissue distribution of T cell subpopulations expressing the HB-10 reactive antigen.

Cell source	% HB-10[+] cells among:[a]		
	Total T (Leu-4[+])	T_H (Leu-3[+])	T_s (Leu-2[+])
Thymus	11 ± 3[b]		
Blood			
Newborns	92 ± 3	86 ± 10	93 ± 5
Adults	64 ± 8	54 ± 2	74 ± 7
Spleen or tonsils	27 ± 6	14 ± 10	39 ± 21

[a] Percent ± 1SD of Leu-4[+], Leu-3[+], or Leu-2[+] cells from each tissue coexpressing the HB-10 reactive antigen.
[b] Percent ± 1SD of total thymocytes which were HB-10[+]. All T6[+] thymocytes were HB-10[-], whereas 20–40% of Leu-4[+] thymocytes were HB-10[+].

Similar studies were performed to analyze the expression of the HB-10 and HB-11 antigens on T lineage cells as a function of their maturation, membrane antigen phenotype, and tissue distribution. Only a small percentage (9–11%) of thymocytes were reactive with the HB-10 (and HB-11) antibodies (Table 8.2). In two-color immunofluorescence staining experiments, the HB-10 antigen was expressed by 20–40% of OKT3/Leu-4[+] thymocytes but was not detected on the less mature cells reactive with the OKT6 antibody. Virtually all circulating T cells in newborn blood coexpressed the HB-10 (and HB-11) antigen. In adults, however, only 64% of Leu-4[+] cells in blood and 27% in spleen or tonsils were reactive with HB-10. In all instances, the cells reactive with HB-10 were also recognized by HB-11. Although the percentage of Leu-3[+] and Leu-2[+] cells which coexpressed the HB-10 and HB-11 antigens generally paralleled that observed for the total Leu-4[+] population, the coexpression frequency was consistently somewhat higher for the Leu 2[+] subset. Comparable results were obtained using HB-11 and OKT3, OKT4, and OKT8 antibodies.

Functional Capabilities of Leu 3[+]/HB-11[+] and Leu 3[+]/HB-11[-] Helper T Cell Subpopulations

The subpopulations of Leu-3[+] cells defined by the presence or absence of the HB-11 reactive antigen were purified by sequential negative- and positive-selection techniques with the FACS, and their functional capabilities were determined in a variety of *in vitro* assays. Both the Leu 3[+]/HB-11[+] and Leu 3[+]/HB-11[-] subsets proliferated in response to PHA and PWM (Table 8.3). Cross-linkage of T3 antigens with the OKT3 monoclonal antibody was also mitogenic for cells within each subpopulation. In contrast, only the Leu-3[+]/HB-11[-] subpopulation had a recall proliferative response to the soluble tetanus toxoid antigen.

Table 8.3. Proliferative responses of T helper cell subpopulations to mitogens or soluble antigen.

Stimulus	^{3}H-TdR uptake (cpm)[a]		
	Total Leu-3$^+$	Leu-3$^+$/HB-11$^-$	Leu-3$^+$/HB-11$^+$
None	788	843	758
PWM	42,745	30,073	37,882
PHA	120,547	101,958	61,405
OKT3	36,649	18,530	23,857
Tetanus toxoid	9,045	15,063	1,093

[a] Leu-3 cells (1 × 10^5/well) were cultured with 10% adherent cells and the indicated stimulus for 4d (mitogen) or 6d (tetanus toxoid). ^{3}H-TdR uptake during the final 16–18 hr of culture was determined.

The ability of these two T helper subpopulations to induce B cell proliferation was also determined. As shown in Table 8.4, mitomycin C-treated HB-11$^+$ and HB-11$^-$ helper T cells stimulated with PHA could both induce proliferative responses in FACS-purified small B cells. Similarly, mitogen-activated cells in each subpopulation could induce large B cells to proliferate. When culture supernatants from PWM-activated Leu 3$^+$/HB-11$^+$ or Leu 3$^+$/HB-11$^-$ T cells were analyzed for their ability to induce large B cells to proliferate, each contained soluble growth factors promoting proliferation of these B cells (data not shown). Hence, both the Leu 3$^+$/HB-11$^+$ and Leu 3$^+$/HB-11$^-$ helper subsets were capable of inducing B cell proliferation.

Experiments assessing the ability of these helper T cell subpopulations to induce B cell differentiation into antibody-producing plasma cells provided contrasting results. When Leu 3$^+$/HB-11$^+$ cells were cultured with

Table 8.4. Induction of B cell proliferation by mitogen-stimulated T helper subpopulations.

Cells in culture		Mitogen	^{3}H-TdR uptake (cpm)[a]
B	T		
Small B	—	PHA	121
Small B	Leu-3$^+$	PHA	28,405
Small B	Leu-3$^+$/HB-11$^+$	PHA	28,417
Small B	Leu-3$^+$/HB-11$^-$	PHA	39,334
Large B	—	PWM	600
Large B	Leu-3$^+$	PWM	12,029
Large B	Leu-3$^+$/HB-11$^+$	PWM	11,963
Large B	Leu-3$^+$/HB-11$^-$	PWM	19,242

[a] Small and large IgM$^+$ B cells were isolated with the FACS and cultured with mitomycin C-treated Leu-3$^+$ cells (or subpopulations thereof) and the indicated mitogen for 72 hr. ^{3}H-TdR uptake during the final 16 hr of culture was assessed. The ^{3}H-TdR uptake by mitogen-stimulated, mitomycin C-treated T cells alone was <1000 cpm.

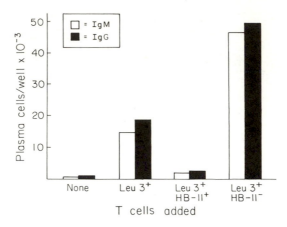

Fig. 8.1. Induction of B cell differentiation by Leu-3$^+$ subpopulations. The Leu 3$^+$/HB-11$^-$ T cell subpopulation contains all helper T cells capable of inducing IgM$^+$ and IgG$^+$ plasma cell formation.

B cells and PWM, no plasma cell formation was induced (Fig. 8.1). In contrast, the Leu 3$^+$/HB-11$^-$ subpopulation stimulated IgM$^+$ and IgG$^+$ plasma cell formation which was correspondingly increased over that observed with the total Leu-3$^+$ population. Quantitative measurements (by radioimmunoassay) of the IgM and IgG secreted in these cultures similarly indicated that only the Leu-3$^+$/HB-11$^-$ cells induced B cell differentiation into antibody-producing cells (data not shown).

Discussion

Two monoclonal antibodies, termed HB-10 and HB-11, have been used to characterize the ontogeny and functional capabilities of two subpopulations of human Leu-3$^+$ helper T cells. The antigens recognized by these two antibodies were not expressed solely by T lineage cells but were also present on virtually all B and NK cells. Neither antigen was detectable on monocytes, neutrophils, or other hemopoietic-derived cells, however. Hence, it appears that these two antigenic determinants are differentiation antigens which mark cells of lymphoid origin, a finding that is consistent with and supports the hypothesis that T, B, and NK lymphocytes are all derived from a common lymphoid stem cell (11).

Among cells differentiating along the T lymphocyte pathway, the HB-10 and HB-11 antigens were expressed first by a small subpopulation of thymocytes. These cells did not express the T6 "common thymocyte" antigen. However, 20–40% of the Leu-4$^+$ thymocytes did coexpress the HB-10 and HB-11 antigens, suggesting that determinants appear late during the intra-thymic phase of T cell differentiation. In newborn blood, virtually all T cells were HB-10$^+$ and HB-11$^+$. With increasing age (and environmental exposure), only 60% of circulating Leu-4$^+$ T cells (and Leu-3$^+$ helper T cells) expressed these antigens, and cells from secondary lymphoid tissues were only 20% HB-10$^+$/HB-11$^+$. These data suggest that the expression of the membrane determinants recognized by these antibodies may be lost as a consequence of T cell activation. This notion is supported by the observation that only Leu 3$^+$/HB-11$^-$ cells have a recall proliferative response to the soluble tetanus toxoid antigen. If this interpretation is correct, our data would indicate that the ability of helper T cells to produce soluble B cell differentiation factors is also dependent on prior exposure to antigen or some other activation stimulus. In contrast, production of B cell growth factors would not appear to require a previous encounter with antigen, since both the "virgin" and "memory" T$_H$ subsets had this capability. We cannot presently exclude the possibility, however, that HB-10/11$^+$ and HB-10/11$^-$ cells derive from separate sublineages which undergo postnatal contraction and expansion, respectively.

Functionally distinct subpopulations of Leu-3/T4$^+$ helper T cells have also been identified with other monoclonal antibodies (12–14). For example, the TQ1 and Leu-8 antibodies have been shown to react with approximately 60–80% of Leu-3/T4$^+$ T cells in peripheral blood (13,14). Functional analyses of the T helper subsets defined with these antibodies demonstrated that many, but not all, of the Leu-3/T4$^+$ helper cells capable of secreting B cell differentiation factors were TQ1$^-$ and Leu-8$^-$. Although these data suggest that there may be considerable overlap of Leu-3$^+$ T cell subsets which do not express the HB-10, HB-11, TQ1, or Leu-8 antigens, two-color immunofluorescence studies using these antibodies have established that the overlap is inexact and that the molecules bearing the TQ1 or Leu-8 determinants are dissimilar from those recognized by the HB-10 and HB-11 antibodies (data not shown). Therefore, it is possible that the mechanisms determining expression of the HB-10 and HB-11 antigens may apply to other T$_H$ membrane differentiation antigens as well.

Summary

We have studied the ontogeny and functional abilities of subpopulations of human Leu-3$^+$ helper cells identified by two monoclonal antibodies, HB-10 and HB-11. The antigens recognized by these antibodies are present on B and NK lineage cells as well as subpopulations of both Leu-2$^+$ and Leu-3$^+$ T cells. Both antigens are expressed by a subset of relatively mature T3$^+$ thymocytes and virtually all circulating T cells in newborns. In adults, however, only 64% of Leu-3$^+$ cells in blood and 27% in lymphoid tissues express these antigens. Functional analysis of the purified Leu-3$^+$ subpopulations defined by HB-10 and HB-11 showed that both subsets responded to mitogens and produced growth factors that supported B cell proliferation. However, the Leu-3$^+$/HB11$^+$ cells were unable to induce B cell differentiation while the Leu-3$^+$/HB-11$^-$ cells were efficient in this regard. Similarly, only Leu-3$^+$/HB-11$^-$ cells had a recall proliferative response to soluble antigen. These results suggest that the HB-10 and HB-11 antigens identify a subpopulation of "virgin" Leu-3$^+$ helper cells that can produce B cell growth factors but are deficient in their ability to produce B cell differentiation factors.

Acknowledgments. This work was supported in part by grants CA 16673, CA 13148, awarded by the National Institutes of Health, and 1-608, awarded by the March of Dimes Birth Defects Foundation.

References

1. Reinherz, E.L., P.C. Kung, G. Goldstein, and S.F. Schlossman. 1979. Further characterization of human inducer T cell subsets defined by monoclonal antibody. *J. Immunol.* **123**:2894.
2. Ledbetter, J.A., R.L. Evans, M. Lipinski, L. Cunningham-Rundles, R.A. Good, and L.A. Herzenberg. 1981. Evolutionary conservation of surface molecules that distinguish T lymphocyte helper/inducer and cytotoxic/suppressor subpopulations in mouse and man. *J. Exp. Med.* **153**:310.
3. Reinherz, E.L., P.C. Kung, G. Goldstein, and S.F. Schlossman. 1980. A monoclonal antibody reactive with the human cytotoxic/suppressor T cell subset previously defined by a heteroantiserum termed TH$_2$. *J. Immunol.* **124**:1301.
4. Boyum, A. 1968. Isolation of mononuclear cells and granulocytes from human blood. *Scand. J. Clin. Lab. Invest.* **21**(Suppl. 97):77.
5. Pellegrino, M.A., S. Ferrone, M.P. Dierich, and R.A. Reisfield. 1975. Enhancement of sheep red blood cell–human lymphocyte rosette formation by the sulfhydryl compound 2-aminoethylisothiouronium bromide. *Clin. Immunol. Immunopathol.* **7**:804.
6. Tedder, T.F., L.T. Clement, and M.D. Cooper. 1984. Expression of C3d receptors during human B cell differentiation: Immunofluorescent analysis with the HB-5 monoclonal antibody. *J. Immunol.* **133**:678.
7. Hammerling, G.J., U. Hammerling, and J.F. Kearney. 1981. *Monoclonal antibodies and T cell hybridomas*. Elsevier/North Holland, New York, p. 563.
8. Clement, L.T., M.K. Dagg, and G.L. Gartland. 1984. Small, resting B cells can be induced to proliferate by direct signals from activated helper T cells. *J. Immunol.* **132**:740.
9. Landay, A., G.L. Gartland, and L.T. Clement. 1983. Characterization of a phenotypically distinct subpopulation of Leu 2$^+$ cells which suppresses T cell proliferative responses. *J. Immunol.* **131**:2757.
10. Gathings, W.E., A.R. Lawton, and M.D. Cooper. 1977. Immunofluorescent studies of the development of pre-B cells, B lymphocytes and immunoglobulin isotype diversity in humans. *Eur. J. Immunol.* **7**:804.

11. Metcalf, D., and M.A.S. Moore. 1971. *Haemopoietic cells*. North-Holland Publishing, Amsterdam.
12. Corte, G., M.C. Mingari, A. Moretta, G. Damiani, L. Moretta, and A. Bargellesi. 1982. Human T cell subpopulations defined by a monoclonal antibody. I. A small subset is responsible for proliferation to allogeneic cells or to soluble antigen and for helper activity for B cell differentiation. *J. Immunol.* **128:**16.
13. Reinherz, E.L., C. Morimoto, K.A. Fitzgerald, R.E. Hussey, J.F. Daley, and S.F. Schlossman. 1982. Heterogeneity of human T4$^+$ inducer T cells defined by a monoclonal antibody that delineates two functional subpopulations. *J. Immunol.* **128:**463.
14. Gatenby, P.A., G.S. Kansas, C.Y. Xian, R.L. Evans, and E.G. Engleman. 1982. Dissection of immunoregulatory subpopulations of T lymphocytes within the helper and suppressor sublineages in man. *J. Immunol.* **129:**1997.

CHAPTER 9

Effects of Workshop Monoclonal Antibodies on the Cytolytic Activity of Alloreactive CD4-Positive T Cell Clones

Neal Flomenberg, Bo Dupont, and Robert W. Knowles

The development of techniques for the production of monoclonal antibodies (mAbs) and for the *in vitro* propagation of T lymphocytes has contributed considerable information to present concepts of T cell function. Studies of T cell-mediated cytotoxicity have successfully utilized mAbs as highly specific probes to identify which of the cell surface molecules play functional roles during the cytolytic process. Antibodies to the CD2, CD3, CD4, CD8, and LFA-1 antigens are capable of blocking T cell-mediated cytotoxicity, while, in contrast, antibodies to the CD5, CD6, and CD7 antigens have not produced similar effects (1–11). In the course of this work, it has been suggested by several investigators that monoclonal antibodies recognizing these functional T cell surface molecules are heterogeneous in their ability to disrupt the cytolytic process (10,12,13). Moreover, T lymphocyte clones also appear heterogeneous in their sensitivity to inhibition by mAbs (12,14–16).

The present studies were performed utilizing workshop mAbs to address three issues. First, we wished to assess the degree of functional heterogeneity of antibodies recognizing the CD2, CD3, CD4, and LFA-1 antigens, by analyzing a larger panel of antibodies than would otherwise be available to a single laboratory. Second, we wished to determine whether uncommon antibodies binding to the CD5, CD6, or CD7 molecules could be identified which were indeed capable of disrupting the cytolytic process. Last, we hoped to identify additional, yet uncharacterized, T cell surface molecules which might play functional roles in T cell-mediated cytotoxicity.

Materials and Methods

Biochemical and functional analyses were performed on each antibody grouped as CD2, CD3, CD4, CD5, CD6, CD7, "activated T cell," "Pan T cell unknown," and "T cell subset unknown" in this workshop. Antibodies in the myelomonocytic workshop which recognized T cells, B cells, but not the erythroleukemia cell line K562 were selected as potentially recognizing the LFA-1 antigen. These antibodies were also included in this analysis.

Functional analyses were performed utilizing four CD4 positive allocytotoxic T lymphocyte clones K1D, K1G, K1I, and K1L. K1I recognizes the HLA-DR7 allospecificity, while K1G recognizes HLA-DP4(SB4). K1L recognizes a subset of HLA-DQ2(MB2) positive cell lines. K1D recognizes a private specificity expressed by DP molecules on a limited number of HLA-DR7 haplotypes. All clones were derived by limiting dilution and propagated by weekly restimulation and culture in Interleukin-2 (IL-2) containing conditioned medium (17).

Clones K1D and K1G were surface-labeled with ^{125}I using lactoperoxidase and lysed with NP-40. Immunoprecipitation and SDS gel electrophoresis were performed utilizing each of the mAbs. Each antibody was scored as positive (+), weak (w), or negative based on a comparison of the amount of radiolabeled material precipitated relative to the other antibodies recognizing the same molecular family (18).

Cell-mediated cytotoxicity assays were carried out utilizing mAbs at a final dilution of 1 : 80 in the test wells. Antibody was preincubated with the effector T cell clones for 0.5 hr prior to addition of ^{51}Cr-labeled target cells. Percent specific cytolysis was measured in a 4-hr chromium release assay. Triplicate determinations were performed for each clone. The percent inhibition by each antibody was calculated as the ratio of the percent specific cytolysis observed in the presence and absence of antibody (17). Antibodies producing 51–100% inhibition were scored as positive (+). Those producing 0–20% inhibition were scored as negative (−), while those producing 21–50% inhibition were scored as weak(w).

Results

One hundred and fifty-two antibodies were tested for their ability to block the cytolytic reactivity of CD4 positive alloreactive T cell clones. The results of these studies are shown in Tables 9.1–9.4. Antibodies are listed in three groups in the tables. The first group includes the antibodies originally designated as falling within the specified CD cluster at the time of initial distribution. The second group consists of additional antibodies biochemically identified as part of the cluster. The final group consists of those antibodies which were serologically included in the cluster.

Antibodies Recognizing CD2 (Table 9.1)

Fifteen of the sixteen antibodies initially grouped as CD2 were confirmed to recognize this antigen by immunoprecipitation. The sixteenth did not

Table 9.1. Blocking effects of mAbs recognizing the CD2, CD3, and CD4 antigens.

Antibody no.	Biochem. ID	Serologic cluster	Blocking activity	Antibody no.	Biochem. ID	Serologic cluster	Blocking activity
mAbs recognizing CD2				mAbs recognizing CD3			
13	CD2	CD2	−	117	CD3	CD3-B	+
14	CD2	CD2	+	118	CD3	CD3-A	+
15	CD2w+CD4w	CD5	−	119	CD4+CD3w	CD2	+
16	CD2	CD2	+	120	CD3	CD3-B	+
17	CD2	CD2	+	121	—	CD3-A	+
18	CD2	CD2	+	122	—	CD3-A	+
19	CD2	CD2	+	123	—	CD3-C	+
20	CD2	CD2	+	124	CD3w	CD3-B	+
21	CD2w	CD2	+	125	—	CD3-B	+
22	CD2	CD2	+	126	—	CD3-B	+
23	CD2w	CD2	+	127	CD2	CD2	+
24	CD2	CD2	+				
25	CD2	CD2	+	61	CD3	CD3-B	+
26	CD2	CD2	+	101	CD3	?	+
27	CD2w	CD2	+				
28	—	CD3-B	−	28	—	CD3-B	−
				48	—	CD3-B	+
56	CD2	CD2	+	57	—	CD3-B	+
78	CD2w	CD4	−	67	—	CD3-C	−
108	CD2	XVII	+	149	CD2	CD3-A	+
112	CD2	CD2	−	150	CD2	CD3-A	+
127	CD2	CD2	+				
138	CD2	VII	−	mAbs recognizing CD4			
144	CD2	CD2	+	67	—	CD3-C	−
148	CD2	VII	+	68	CD4	CD4	w
149	CD2	CD3-A	+	69	CD4	CD4	+
150	CD2	CD3-A	+	70	CD4	CD4	+
				71	CD4	CD4	+
55	CD2w	VII	+	72	CD4	CD4	w
65	—	VII	+	73	CD4	CD4	w
119	CD4+CD3w	CD2	+	74	CD4	CD4	+
				75	CD4	CD4	+
				76	CD4	CD4	w
				77	CD4	CD4	+
				78	—	CD4	−
				79	—	CD4	w
				80	p120, 200	X	−
				107	CD4	CD4	+
				113	CD4	CD4	−
				119	CD4+CD3w	CD2	+

yield a detectable precipitate. Eleven additional antibodies capable of immunoprecipitating the CD2 antigen were identified in other workshop groups, although not all of these clustered with the CD2 group serologically. Three of these antibodies were grouped in cluster VII and recognize predominantly activated T cells, although they precipitate a CD2 determinant. One additional antibody (T65) serologically clustered with VII, but did not yield a detectable precipitate, and one antibody (T119) was clustered with CD2 but biochemically appeared as a mixture of CD4 and CD3.

Twenty-one of the twenty-six antibodies which precipitated the CD2 antigen produced strong blocking of cell-mediated cytotoxicity, while five antibodies biochemically confirmed as CD2 did not produce effective blocking. It should be noted that the ability to block cytotoxicity did not show an absolute correlation with the immunoprecipitation data. T13, for example, was among the strongest antibodies in immunoprecipitation, yet produced relatively little blocking effect. In contrast, T14 and T21, which immunoprecipitated much less radiolabeled antigen, produced virtually complete inhibition. The immunoglobulin subclass of the antibodies also did not show clear correlation with the presence or absence of blocking effect.

Antibodies Recognizing CD3 (Table 9.1)

Of the eleven antibodies originally grouped as CD3, only four yielded detectable immunoprecipitates of the CD3 complex. Two of the eleven antibodies appeared to precipitate other T cell surface antigens, while five produced no detectable precipitate. Two additional antibodies recognizing the CD3 antigen were detected in other workshop groups, and six additional antibodies clustered serologically with CD3, although two of these immunoprecipitated the CD2 molecule.

All biochemically confirmed CD3 mAbs produced strong blocking effects. It is noteworthy that seven of nine antibodies which did not produce detectable precipitates nevertheless produced strong blocking effects. The CD3 antibodies were, as a group, the most potent of all mAbs capable of blocking cytolytic activity.

Antibodies Recognizing CD4 (Table 9.1)

Ten of the fourteen antibodies initially grouped as CD4 were confirmed biochemically to recognize this antigen. Two mAbs recognized other T cell surface antigens and two failed to yield precipitates. Three additional CD4 antibodies were identified in other groups, although T119 also precipitated CD3 molecules as previously described. Of the twelve confirmed CD4 antibodies, eleven produced blocking effects. The degree of blocking was frequently quantitatively less than that seen with either the CD2 or CD3 antibodies. Like the CD2 antibodies, the degree of blocking could not be clearly related to the amount of radiolabeled material which was precipitated by the antibody nor to the immunoglobulin subclass.

Antibodies Recognizing CD5, CD6, and CD7 (Table 9.2)

None of the antibodies recognizing these T cell differentiation antigens demonstrated strong blocking in cell-mediated cytotoxicity assays. This included analysis of five antibodies serologically grouped as CD5 (four positive in immunoprecipitation), and eleven antibodies serologically grouped as CD7 (10 confirmed biochemically). In the CD6 cluster, neither of the two biochemically confirmed antibodies produced blocking effects. Of the five additional antibodies in this group, two demonstrated blocking effects, but these were weak and variable from clone to clone.

Antibodies to LFA-1 (Table 9.3)

MAb T60 immunoprecipitated the p90,160 complex characteristic of LFA-1. Seven antibodies from the myelomonocytic workshop (M11, M55, M56, M72, M73, M75, and M89) were identified as potentially recognizing LFA-1 based on their pattern of serologic reactivity. M11 did not

Table 9.2. Blocking effects of mAbs recognizing the CD5, CD6, and CD7 antigens.

Antibody no.	Biochem. ID	Serologic cluster	Blocking activity	Antibody no.	Biochem. ID	Serologic cluster	Blocking activity
mAbs recognizing CD5				mAbs recognizing CD7			
4	CD5	CD5	–	30	CD7	CD7	–
5	CD5	CD5	–	31	CD7w	CD7	–
6	—	CD6	–	32	—	XXVIII	–
7	CD5	CD5	–	33	—	XV	–
8	CD5	CD5	–	34	—	IV	–
9	—	CD7	–	35	—	–	–
10	—	XXVI	–	36	—	–	–
11	—	XXVIII	–	37	CD8	CD8	–
12	—	XXVII	–	38	CD7	CD7	–
				39	CD7	CD7	–
15	CD2w+CD4w	CD5	–	40	CD7	CD7	–
				41	CD7	CD7	–
mAbs recognizing CD6				42	—	II	–
46	CD6	CD6	–	43	CD7	CD7	–
47	CD6	CD6	–	44	CD7	CD7	–
				45	CD7	CD7	–
6	—	CD6	–				
49	—	CD6	w/–	54	CD7	CD7	–
51	—	CD6	w/–				
58	—	CD6	–	9	—	CD7	–
59	—	CD6	–				

Table 9.3. Blocking effects of mAbs recognizing the LFA-1 antigen.

Antibody no.	Biochem. ID	Serologic cluster	Blocking activity
mAbs recognizing LFA-1			
M11	ND	CP28	−
M55	90, 160	CDw18	w
M56	90, 160	CDw18	+/w
M72	90, 160	—	+
M73	90, 160w	CDw18	+
M75	90, 160	CDw18	+
M89	90, 160	CDw18	+
T60	90, 160	XV	+/−

yield a detectable immunoprecipitate despite the fact that it exhibited a high titer in binding assays. It failed to demonstrate any blocking activity, and was not clustered with the LFA-1 group in the workshop serologic analysis (Bernstein, I., elsewhere this volume). The other six antibodies did precipitate the p90,160 complex. While T60 and M56 could be distinguished from the other antibodies in this cluster based on their precipitation pattern using ^{125}I-labeled granulocytes, they were identical to the other antibodies in their reactivity with the labeled T lymphocytes. The LFA-1 antibodies showed a broad range of blocking effects ranging from quite weak to very strong. They also showed more variation from clone to clone than CD2, CD3, or CD4 antibodies which exhibited blocking effects. Their blocking activity could not be correlated with titer, Ig subclass, or with the amount of radiolabeled material immunoprecipitated. A more detailed report of the serologic, biochemical, and functional heterogeneity of these antibodies is presented elsewhere in this volume (Flomenberg, Kernan, et al., Volume 3, Chapter 7).

Other Workshop mAbs (Table 9.4)

Several additional T cell surface antigens were biochemically identified in the "activated T cell" and "unknown" workshop groups. Seven antibodies recognized the p55 molecule which has been associated with the IL-2 receptor. None of these were capable of blocking T cell-mediated cytotoxicity. In addition, five additional antigens were detected by eight antibodies in these various workshop groups. None of these antibodies, which are listed in Table 9.4, produced blocking effects. There were in addition, twenty-five antibodies in the "activated T-cell" and "unknown" groups which failed to produce detectable immunoprecipitates. Four of these antibodies produced weak blocking effects (T49, T50, T51,

Table 9.4. Blocking effect of other workshop mAbs.

Antibody no.	Biochem. ID	Serologic cluster	Blocking activity	Antibody no.	Biochem. ID	Serologic cluster	Blocking activity
mAbs recognizing activated T cell antigens				mAbs recognizing unknown pan-T antigens			
135	TAC	XI	−	48	—	C3-B	+
136	p120, 200	X	−	49	—	CD6	w/−
137	—	V	−	50	—	XIII	w/−
138	CD2	VII	−	51	—	CD6	w/−
139	p120, 200	X	−	52	p90	XIV	−
140	TAC	XI	−	53	p90	XIV	−
141	TAC	XI	−	54	CD7	CD7	−
142	p250	X	−	55	CD2w	VII	+
143	TAC	XI	−	56	CD2	CD2	+
144	CD2	CD2	+	57	—	CD3-B	+
145	TAC	XI	−	58	—	CD6	−
146	TAC	XI	−	59	—	CD6	−
147	—	—	−	60	p90, 160	XV	+
148	CD2	VII	+	61	CD3	CD3-B	+
149	CD2	CD3-A	+	62	—	XIII	w/−
150	CD2	CD3-A	+	63	p120, 130, 200	XXI	−
151	CD4/TAC	IX	w	64	—	II	−
153	—	XI	−	65	—	VII	+
159	TAC	XI	−	66	—	CDI	−
mAbs recognizing unknown T subset antigens				mAbs recognizing other T cell antigens			
101	CD3	?	+	29	p48	XXIV	−
102	—	V	−				
103	—	IV	−	63	p120, 130, 200	XXI	−
104	—	XXVIII	−				
105	—	XXVI	−	80	p120, 200	X	−
106	—	XIII	−	136	p120, 200	X	−
107	CD4	CD4	+	139	p120, 200	X	−
108	CD2	XVII	+				
109	—	V	−	142	p250	X	−
110	—	CD8	−				
111	—	CD8	−	52	p90	XIV	−
112	CD2	CD2	−	53	p90	XIV	−
113	CD4	CD4	w				
114	—	V	−				
115	—	—	−				
116	—	—	−				

and T62). Two of these (T49 and T51) were serologically clustered with CD6, as described above. The remaining two antibodies (T50 and T62) produced partial blocking of two of the four clones on which they were tested. These antibodies were clustered serologically as XIII along with T106, which produced no blocking effects.

Discussion

A variety of T cell surface molecules have been identified which appear to play a role in the cytolytic process. Of these, the CD3 molecules appear to be noncovalently associated with the T cell antigen receptor on the cell surface, while the rest appear to represent "accessory" binding molecules (5,6,19). It is therefore not surprising that antibodies to the CD3 complex were the most consistent of all the mAbs studied in their blocking effects. This was true for all of the serological subclusters of CD3 (this volume, Chapter 1). All biochemically confirmed CD3 antibodies produced strong blocking. Moreover, seven of nine antibodies, which were serologically clustered as CD3 but failed to yield immunoprecipitates, also produced strong blocking effects.

Antibodies to the CD2 antigen cluster have been shown to be heterogeneous with regard to their abilities to block sheep red blood cell rosette formation and activate T lymphocytes (10). Moreover, a group of antibodies which immunoprecipitate CD2 molecules bind preferentially to activated T cells and have been separately clustered as VII in this workshop (this volume, Chapter 1). These antibodies also exhibit heterogeneity in their ability to block T cell-mediated cytotoxicity. Twenty-three of twenty-eight antibodies included in this cluster on the basis of their biochemical or serological reactivity produced strong blocking. Only three antibodies which both immunoprecipitated CD2 molecules and clustered serologically as either CD2 (T13 and T122) or VII (T138) failed to produce blocking effects. It should be noted that the inability of these three antibodies to block T cell-mediated cytotoxicity has been independently confirmed (this volume, Chapter 16). Moreover, T13 and T138 also produce less blocking of sheep red blood cell rosette formation than the majority of CD2 antibodies (this volume, Chapters 4 and 5). These findings do not merely reflect a lower affinity of these antibodies for the CD2 molecules. T13 was one of the most potent of the CD2 antibodies in immunoprecipitation, yet it is quite atypical in these other assay systems, suggesting that it recognizes a distinct epitope. It should be reemphasized, however, that the vast majority of antibodies to the CD2 complex (including the VII cluster) exhibit strong blocking effects.

The CD4 molecule is present on the vast majority of HLA-class II specific CTL and absent from the majority of HLA-class I specific CTL. This and other evidence have suggested that this molecule functions as an accessory binding molecule to the constant portions of HLA-class II molecules (5-7,20-22). Only one antibody biochemically and serologically grouped with CD4 failed to produce blocking. However, this group of antibodies was also heterogeneous in the range of blocking activity observed. While the CD2 and CD3 antibodies produced strong (>50%) blocking effects, many of the CD4 antibodies produced weak (20–50%) blocking when studied in the same experiments utilizing the same clones.

Unlike CD2, CD3, and CD4, the LFA-1 antigen is present on a broad variety of bone marrow-derived cells. LFA-1 appears to play a functional role in many of these cell populations, suggesting it may play a role in cell attachment or adherence (9,10,13). This group of antibodies exhibited more variation from clone to clone than that seen for the CD2, CD3, or CD4 antibodies (see Flomenberg et al., Volume 3, Chapter 7).

The other goal of these studies was to identify additional antibodies capable of disrupting T cell-mediated cytolysis. For this purpose, we screened the antibodies recognizing CD5, CD6, or CD7 as well as the unclustered antibodies in the workshop. None of the CD5 or CD7 antibodies demonstrated any functional effect in this assay system. Two antibodies serologically clustered with CD6 (T49 and T51), but which did not yield immunoprecipitates, produced low levels of inhibition. These inhibitory effects, in addition to being weak, were variable from clone to clone. There were two additional antibodies (T50 and T62) which also produced weak blocking effects. These antibodies also produced variable effects from clone to clone. Interestingly, these two antibodies were clustered together serologically in group XIII. In view of the weak nature and variability of the observed inhibition of these four antibodies, the ultimate significance of these findings will require further study.

In summary, this study of 152 workshop antibodies has demonstrated that:

1. Antibodies to CD2 are heterogeneous in their functional effects. While most of these antibodies produce strong inhibition of T-cell mediated cytotoxicity, other strongly binding antibodies are completely without effect.
2. The CD3 mAbs appear to be the most potent and least heterogeneous in their ability to block cytotoxicity.
3. Most mAbs recognizing CD4 are also capable of blocking T cell-mediated cytotoxicity. However, the degree of inhibition is generally less than that seen with CD2 or CD3.
4. Antibodies to the LFA-1 antigens showed more variation from one T cell clone to the next than did other mAbs capable of blocking cytotoxicity.
5. Four additional weakly blocking antibodies were identified through this analysis. However, no antibody was identified in the workshop outside of the CD2, CD3, CD4, and LFA-1 groups which was capable of strong inhibition of CD-4 positive allocytotoxic T cell clones.

Acknowledgments. We thank Donna Williams, Jackie Chin-Louie, Debbie Moshief, Michael Moon, and Bernadette Kienzle for excellent technical assistance and Louise Rozos for help in preparing the manuscript. This work was supported by grants from the U.S. Public Health Services, National Institutes of Health, NCI-CA-22507, CA-08748, CA-19267, CA-23766, CA-33050, and a grant from the Xoma Corporation.

References

1. Evans, R.L., D.W. Wall, C.D. Platsoucas, F.P. Siegal, S.M. Fikrig, and C.M. Testa. 1981. Good RA: Thymus-dependent membrane antigens in man: Inhibition of cell-mediated lympholysis by monoclonal antibodies to TH2 antigen. *Proc. Natl. Acad. Sci. U.S.A.* **78**:544.

2. Reinherz, E.L., E. Hussey, K. Fitzgerald, P. Snow, C. Terhorst, and S.F. Schlossman. 1981. Antibody directed at a surface structure inhibits cytolytic but not suppressor function of human T lymphocytes. *Nature* **294**:168.

3. Chang, T.W., P.C. Kung, S.P. Gingras, and G. Goldstein. 1981. Does OKT3 monoclonal antibody react with an antigen recognition structure on human T cells? *Proc. Natl. Acad. U.S.A.* **78**:1805.

4. Landegren, U., U. Ramstedt, I. Axberg, M. Ullberg, M. Jondal, and H. Wigzell. 1982. Selective inhibition of human T cell cytotoxicity at levels of target recognition or initiation of lysis by monoclonal OKT3 and Leu-2a antibodies. *J. Exp. Med.* **155**:1579.

5. Reinherz, E.L., S. Meuer, K.A. Fitzgerald, R.E. Hussey, H. Levine, and S.F. Schlossman. 1982. Antigen recognition by human T lymphocyte is linked to surface expression of the T3 molecular complex. *Cell* **30**:735.

6. Meuer, S.C., R.E. Hussey, J.C. Hodgdon, T. Hercend, S.F. Schlossman, and E.L. Reinherz. 1982. Surface structures involved in target recognition by human cytotoxic T lymphocytes. *Science* **218**:471.

7. Spits, H., J. Borst, C. Terhorst, and J.E. de Vries. 1982. The role of T cell differentiation markers in antigen-specific and lectin-dependent cellular cytotoxicity mediated by T8$^+$ and T4$^+$ human cytotoxic T cell clones directed at class I and class II MHC antigens. *J. Immunol.* **129**:1563.

8. Spits, H., H. Ijssel, C. Terhorst, and J.E. de Vries. 1982. Establishment of human T lymphocyte clones highly cytotoxic for an EBV-transformed B cell line in serum-free medium: Isolation of clones that differ in phenotype and specificity. *J. Immunol.* **128**:95.

9. Sanchez-Madrid, F., A.M. Krensky, C.F. Ware, E. Robbins, J.L. Strominger, S.J. Burakoff, and T.A. Springer. 1982. Three distinct antigens associated with human T-lymphocyte-mediated cytolysis: LFA-1, LFA-2, and LFA-3. *Proc. Natl. Acad. Sci. U.S.A.* **79**:7489.

10. Krensky, A.M., F. Sanchez-Madrid, E. Robbins, J. Nagy, T.A. Springer, and S.J. Burakoff. 1983. The functional significance, distribution, and structure of LFA-1, LFA-2, and LFA-3: Cell surface antigens associated with CTL–target interactions. *J. Immunol.* **131**:611–616.

11. Fast, L.D., J.A. Hansen, and W. Newman. 1981. Evidence for T-cell nature and heterogeneity with natural killer (NK) and antibody-dependent cellular cytotoxicity (ADCC) effectors: a comparison with cytolytic T lymphocytes. *J. Immunol.* **127**:448.

12. Malissen, B., N. Rebai, A. Liabeuf, and C. Mawas. 1982. Human cytotoxic T cell structures associated with expression of cytolysis. I. Analysis at the clonal level of the cytolysis-inhibiting effect of 7 monoclonal antibodies. *Eur. J. Immunol.* **12**:739.

13. Ware, C.F., F. Sanchez-Madrid, S.J. Burakoff, J.L. Strominger, and T.A. Springer. 1983. Human lymphocyte function associated antigen-1 (LFA-1): Identification of multiple antigenic epitopes and their relationship to CTL mediated cytotoxicity. *J. Immunol.* **131**:1182.

14. MacDonald, H.R., A.L. Glasebrook, and J.C. Cerottini. 1982. Clonal hetero-
    geneity in the functional requirement for Lyt 2/3 molecules on cytolytic T
    lymphocytes: Analysis by antibody blocking and selective trypsinization. *J.
    Exp. Med.* **156:**1711.
15. MacDonald, H.R., N. Thiernesse, and J.C. Cerottini. 1981. Inhibition of T
    cell mediated cytolysis by monoclonal antibodies directed against Lyt-2: Het-
    erogeneity of inhibition at the clonal level. *J. Immunol.* **126:**1671.
16. Moretta, A., G. Pantaleo, M.C. Mingari, L. Moretta, and J.C. Cerottini. 1984.
    Clonal heterogeneity in the requirement for T3, T4, and T8 molecules in
    human cytolytic T lymphocyte function. *J. Exp. Med.* **159:**921.
17. Flomenberg, N., K. Naito, E. Duffy, R.W. Knowles, R.L. Evans, and B.
    Dupont. 1983. Allocytotoxic T cell clones: Both Leu 2^+3^- and Leu 2^-3^+ T
    cells recognize class I histocompatibility antigens. *Eur. J. Immunol.* **13:**905.
18. Knowles, R.W., and W.F. Bodmer. 1982. A monoclonal antibody recognizing
    a humun thymus leukemia-like antigen associated with beta-2 microglobulin.
    Eur. J. Immunol. **12:**676.
19. Meuer, S.C., K.A. Fitzgerald, R.E. Hussey, J.G. Hodgdon, S.F. Schloss-
    man, and E.L. Reinherz. 1983. Clonotypic structures involved in antigen-
    specific human T cell function—Relationship to the T3 molecular complex. *J.
    Exp. Med.* **157:**705.
20. Engleman, E.G., C.J. Benike, C. Grumet, and R.L. Evans. 1981. Activation
    of human T lymphocyte subsets: Helper and suppressor/cytotoxic cell recog-
    nize and respond to distinct histocompatibility antigens. *J. Immunol.*
    127:2124.
21. Meuer, S.C., S.F. Schlossman, and E.L. Reinherz. 1982. Clonal analysis of
    human cytotoxic T lymphocytes: $T4^+$ and $T8^+$ effector cells recognize prod-
    ucts of different major histocompatibility complex regions. *Proc. Natl. Acad.
    Sci. U.S.A.* **79:**4395.
22. Biddison, W.E., P.E. Rao, M.A. Talle, G. Goldstein, and S. Shaw. 1982.
    Possible involvement of the OKT4 molecule in T cell recognition of class II
    HLA antigens. *J. Exp. Med.* **156:**1065.

CHAPTER 10

Effects of the Workshop Anti–T Cell Monoclonal Antibodies on Lymphocyte Proliferative and Cytotoxic Functions

György Görög, Gabriella Bátory, Tamás Laskay, and
Gyözö G. Petrányi

Introduction

Evaluation of the functional effects of anti-lymphocyte monoclonal antibodies is important in basic research and in therapy as well. The investigation of molecules involved in lymphocyte functions may contribute to a
better understanding of how these cells work. On the other hand, when
monoclonal antibodies are given to patients, "peaceful" (non-killing)
actions may lead to main or side effects that must be reckoned with.

Monoclonal antibodies to differentiation antigens on human T lymphocytes often affect different functions when added without complement.
Thus, for example, some CD3 antibodies have been known to induce
proliferation but inhibit antigen- or mitogen-stimulated cell division (1).
Also, CD4 and CD8 antibodies have been shown to block cytotoxic T
lymphocyte (CTL) action (2,3) and the mixed lymphocyte reaction (MLR)
(4). Antibodies against the sheep red-cell receptor diminish natural killer
(NK) cytotoxicity (5) and proliferative responses that require the activation of Ca^{2+} influx (6).

However, as most of the previous studies have employed only a few
(2–5) different antibodies to particular antigens, it could seldom be resolved whether the differences in the effects observed would depend on
antibody subclass, fine epitope specificity, affinity, or other factors. The
present workshop has provided an excellent opportunity to analyze the
role of these factors, since large numbers of antibodies to one particular
molecule could be examined at the same time. Also, a reliable comparison
of antibodies of different CD could be achieved.

In this study, the whole panel of anti–T cell antibodies was analyzed in
a range of proliferative and cytotoxic assays. The influence of antibodies
on lymphokine production as well as indirect antigen modulation were
also investigated.

Methodological Considerations

The methods used have previously been described in detail. On each experimental day, the whole panel was run in a single experiment, using one person's peripheral mononuclear cells (PMC). Variations between different individuals were small. End dilution of antibodies varied between 200 and 500. Usually, triplicates were set up which showed little variability. Evaluations were based on the mean values.

Proliferative assays (7) were carried out in 96-well plates with 10^5 PMC in RPMI 1640 + 5% AB serum. Cells were cultured with suboptimal doses of phytohemagglutinin (PHA), concanavalin A (Con A), or pokeweed mitogen (PWM), or with no mitogen, in the presence of antibodies for 3 days. For the MLR, equal numbers of two unrelated persons' PMC were cultured together for 5 days. Effects on IL-2-dependent proliferation were evaluated by adding antibodies and IL-2 for 24 hr to cells from an MLR on day 10. Lymphokines were determined from the supernatants of the proliferative assays. Interleukin-2 (IL-2) content was judged using a 1-day culture of an IL-2-dependent rat T cell clone. At the end of assays, [³H]thymidine incorporation was measured.

Cytotoxic assays used ^{51}Cr release as a sign of target-cell death. Natural killer (NK) activity was measured against K-562 cells as in Ref. 8. Lectin-dependent cytotoxicity (LDCC) to Raji cells was investigated in the presence of PHA (9). For a selected set of antibodies, NK activity against Raji cells was also measured.

Antiviral activity—putative gamma-interferon content—was assessed on FL5 cells challenged with vesicular stomatitis virus. Modulation of antigens was observed following incubation of the cells in the cold with monoclonal antibody and a FITC-labeled second layer. Capping and endocytosis were allowed to take place at 37°C for 30 and 120 min.

For evaluation using CLINSTAT on an Apple II, the crude results of the particular experiments were treated as a distribution (see Fig. 10.2). Antibodies were grouped according to clear-cut group limits, if any, and standard deviation values of the usually normally distributed data. Thus, groups of strong and weak inhibitors and enhancers (with a body of neutral antibodies in-between) were distinguished whenever possible. Correlations among different assays and donors were computed. Workshop and lab controls fell into the "no effect" group in all cases.

Results

Results will first be discussed according to observations made in the different experimental systems. Next, the findings for the different CD groups are given.

Proliferation Assays and Lymphokine Production

There were remarkable correlations among PHA-, Con A-, and PWM-induced proliferations (Fig. 10.1). Thus, these will generally be referred to as mitogen responses. Inspecting the distribution of, say, PHA values (Fig. 10.2), a group of strong inhibitors could be distinguished. When grouping antibodies according to standard deviation values, inhibition was exerted by 13 of the 15 CD2s [except: G19-3.1 (clustered as CD5) and KOLT-2 (clustered as CD3); 35.1 not tested] and 10 of the 11 CD3s (except: X35-3). In the case of the latter, inhibition was apparent after subtracting cpm values of the cultures with antibody only. The following antibodies[1] showed an inhibitory effect: of the unidentified pan-Ts, T10B9 (CD3), T57 (CD2), BW239/347 (CD3), MT 421 (clustered CD6, but see later), CRIS-3 (not clustered), CRIS-7 (CD3), and CRIS-8 (not clustered); of the antibodies against activated T cells 39C1.5 (CD2), 39C8.18 (not clustered), 39H7.3 (CD3), and 41F2.1 (CD3); from other groups, MT 415 (clustered CD8, but see later) and BRC-T1.[2] Generally, strong inhibitors of mitogen responses blocked MLR as well, as shown in Fig. 10.3. However, some antibodies blocked MLR only (some CD4 and CD8—see Fig. 10.10—and five additional antibodies) and enhancers of these kinds of proliferation were separate antibodies.

When the proliferation mediated by antibodies was studied, some reagents were mitogenic (Fig. 10.4). They mostly belonged to CD3 with 7 other antibodies (some finally clustered CD3). Subtracting thymidine incorporation caused by them from cpm values of antibody + mitogen cultures revealed that mitogenic effects attributable to PHA and Con A were negligible in most of the cases. All antibodies inducing proliferation on day 3 were inhibitory in MLR (day 5).

The IL-2-dependent division of MLR memory cells was also enhanced by a number of CD3s and some other antibodies[3] (Fig. 10.5). Eight of the 19 antibodies to activated T cells diminished this "secondary" proliferation selectively (with no effect on "primary" mitogen responses and MLR)[4] (Fig. 10.6), resulting in a negative correlation between the effects on these two types of proliferation. However, IL-2-dependent proliferation was blocked by some antibodies which inhibited "primary" proliferation as well. In the 24-hr supernatants of lymphocytes incubated with these and a few other antibodies, antiviral activity was found (Table 10.1). Nevertheless, putative gamma-interferon induction does not seem char-

---

[1] Final cluster group given in parentheses.
[2] Removed from study.
[3] 2 clustered CD3, 2 clustered CD5.
[4] Some clustered Tac.

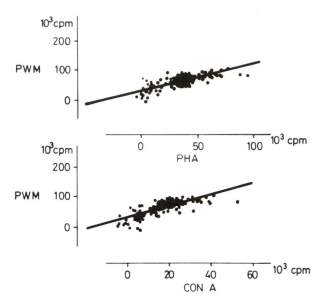

Fig. 10.1. Correlations among antibody effects on PHA-, Con A-, and PWM-induced proliferation.

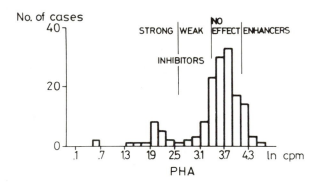

Fig. 10.2. Grouping of antibodies according to their effects on PHA stimulation.

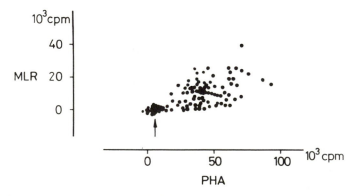

Fig. 10.3. Antibody effects on PHA-induced stimulation and MLR. Note the population of strong inhibitors of both responses (arrow).

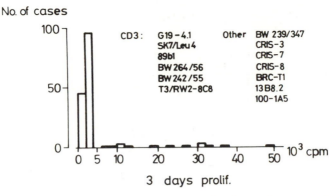

Fig. 10.4. Thymidine incorporation values in day-3 lymphocyte cultures with antibody. Mitogenic antibodies listed.

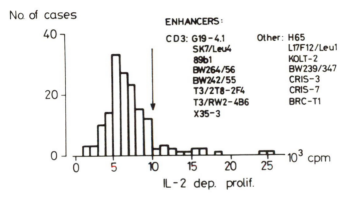

Fig. 10.5. Thymidine incorporation values of day-10 MLR memory cells in culture with antibodies.

Table 10.1. List and effects of monoclonal antibodies causing release of antiviral activity.

| | Proliferation | | | | | |
| | Mitogen induced | | | | | |
IFN inducers	PHA	Con A	PWM	MLR	IL-2 dep.	PWM-IL-2
MT 215 ±	N	N	R	R	N	N
MT 26	R	R	R	R	R	R
MT 910	R	R	R	R	R	R
MT 421	R	R	R	R	R	N-R
MT 151	N-R	R	R	R	R	N-R
MT 310	R	R	R	R	R	R
MT 415	R	R	R	R	R	N
MT 1014	R	N	N-R	R	N	N
MT 122	R	N	R	R	N	N

N = normal; R = reduced.
In tests not indicated all of these antibodies were indifferent.

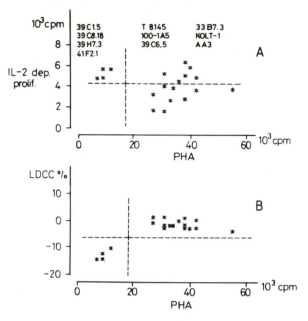

Fig. 10.6. Effects of antibodies to activated T cells on "primary" and "secondary" proliferation and LDCC.

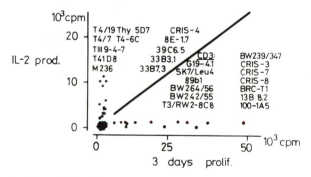

Fig. 10.7. Lack of correlation between 3-day proliferation and IL-2 production on day 1. Respective enhancers listed.

acteristic of any particular antibody group but rather of the MT designation (9 out of 13).[5]

IL-2 release by lymphocytes incubated with antibody only and mitogenicity were clearly attributable to separate antibodies (Fig. 10.7). Similarly, effects on PWM-induced proliferation and IL-2 release were also

---

[5] May be due to mycoplasma contamination (P. Rieber, personal communication).

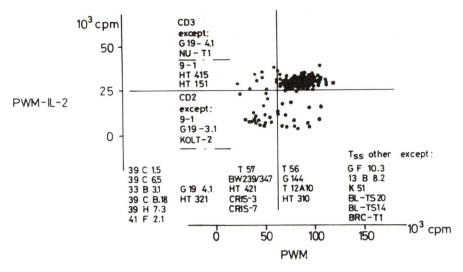

Fig. 10.8. Antibody effects on PWM-induced proliferation and IL-2 production.

separable in a number of cases (Fig. 10.8). Most CD3s inhibited proliferation but not IL-2 release. Eleven out of the 19 antibodies in the "T cell subset other" group exerted a reverse effect. CD2s and some reagents to activated T cells blocked both responses.

Cytotoxic Assays

NK activity against K-562 cells was mostly inhibited by CD2s and 3 other antibodies (Fig. 10.9). Two of these, T57 and 39C1.5 (both clustered CD2), showed CD2-like effects in other tests as well. While monoclonal

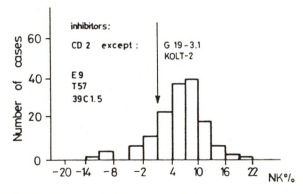

Fig. 10.9. Antibody effects on NK against K-562 cells. Cytotoxicity % with controls subtracted.

antibody 35.1 did not reach us in this panel, it had been proved, too, to block NK in previous experiments (É. Pócsik and G.Gy. Petrányi, unpublished).

LDCC to Raji cells in the presence of PHA (a function of more matured T cells) was lowered by CD2, too, as well as by a group of antibodies to activated T cells (clustered CD2 or CD3) that blocked "primary" proliferative responses (Fig. 10.6). There was some cytotoxic activity against Raji cells without adding PHA. Of the LDCC-blocking antibodies, all but one (9.1) inhibited this NK- like cytotoxicity as well. However, decrease in LDCC exceeded NK blocking so that a specific inhibition of LDCC could be concluded.

Indirect Modulation of Antigens

Modulation of antigens was tested in an indirect assay. There were only minor differences in the time course of capping and endocytosis caused by such cross-linked monoclonal antibodies.

Characterization of the CD Groups

Among pan-T reagents, both CD2 and CD3 tended to inhibit mitogen responses and MLR. They could, however, be distinguished in other tests. CD2 blocked PWM-induced IL-2 production and, more clearly, both cytotoxic reactions while CD3 usually did not. CD3 antibodies stimulated thymidine uptake on day 3 and/or secondary proliferation of MLR memory cells. This effect was not observed with CD2 reagents. Some antibodies included in these groups (CD2: G19-3.1[7] and KOLT-2;[8] CD3: NU-T1[8]) showed no effect in these tests. On the other hand, some reagents provided as "pan T other" or "T cell subset other" exerted clearly CD2 (T57,[9] MT 421) or CD3 (CRIS-3,[10] CRIS-7,[8] CRIS-8,[10] BW239/37[8]) - like effects.

CD5 and CD7 antibodies had no major effect in these tests except for three IgM-type CD7s (BW264/50, BW264/217, BW264/215) that seemed to enhance mitogen responses.

Turning to antibodies reacting with T cell subpopulations, CD4 and CD8 antibodies showed no uniform effects. MLR was more often blocked by CD4[11] (Fig. 10.10). Three antibodies (CD4: MT 151, MT 310 and CD8: MT 415) (see above) inhibited all kinds of proliferative responses and caused release of antiviral activity in the supernatants of lymphocyte cultures (Table 10.1).

---

[7] Clustered CD5.
[8] Clustered CD3.
[9] Clustered CD2.
[10] Not clustered.
[11] One of the exceptions (T10C5) clustered CD3C IgM!

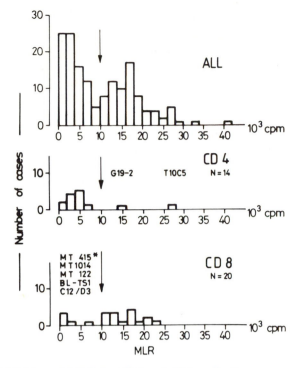

Fig. 10.10. Inhibition of MLR by CD4 and CD8 antibodies.

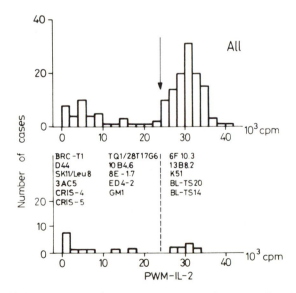

Fig. 10.11. Inhibition of PWM-induced IL-2 production by antibodies to "other T cell subsets."

Sixteen antibodies to other T cell subsets were included in this workshop. Of these, 11 blocked PWM-induced IL-2 production (Fig. 10.11)[12] but, unlike CD2, did not affect proliferative responses.

Antibodies to activated T cells could be divided into three groups according to their functional effects. Eight antibodies including characterized reagents against the IL-2 receptor lowered IL-2-dependent proliferation but not "primary" proliferations or cytotoxicity (Fig. 10.6). Four other antibodies had clearly reverse effects as they blocked all "primary" stimulations (MLR and mitogen responses) with no effect on IL-2-dependent division. These reagents also blocked LDCC (Fig. 10.6) and one of them (39C1.5)[9] blocked NK, too. The remaining 7 antibodies showed no effect in these assays.

Discussion

In this series of experiments, we looked at functional effects of anti–T cell monoclonal antibodies. The relatively high number of antibodies to particular antigens and the completeness of the antibody panel (all well-characterized antigens included) as well as the reliability of the assays used allowed some conclusions to be drawn.

Proliferation could be induced by CD3 with some other antibodies. This may point to a unique role among pan-T antigens of this molecule [see the well-known connection of CD3 to the T cell antigen receptor (2)]. All these antibodies were inhibitory in a day-5 MLR, possibly exhausting the "proliferative capacity" of the cells. To see whether these reagents inhibited mitogen responses, the thymidine incorporation values measured in the control (antibody only) cultures were subtracted from the cpms seen in mitogen-stimulated cultures. As mitogen stimulations employed suboptimal amounts of mitogens, a (roughly) additional effect of antibody and mitogen could have been observed if the antibodies had failed to block mitogen action.

While T cell proliferation is mostly supposed to be mediated by IL-2, there was no correlation between thymidine incorporation on day 3 and IL-2 release into the supernatants of the same cultures on day 1 in two tests (antibody alone and with PWM), although some reagents, including most of the CD2s, blocked both responses. This might allow alternative or additional mechanisms of proliferation inhibition/induction by some anti–T cell monoclonal antibodies. An independent inhibition of IL-2 synthesis and cell proliferation in murine MLR was seen by Macphail and Stutman (10) in the case of some anti–Ia monoclonal antibodies. As found earlier by Palacios and Martinez-Maza (6) for monoclonal antibody T11A, inhibition of "primary" proliferations and IL-2-dependent "secondary"

---

[12] No consequent clustering.

cell growth were separable effects. In the case of T11A, this difference was attributed to blocking of the Ca^{2+} influx required for initiation of cell activation. In our case, CD3 and four antibodies to activated T cells (clustered CD2 or CD3) showed a similar pattern while some other antibodies lowered IL-2-dependent proliferation selectively. As an explanation involving the very early steps of activation seems unlikely for the latter (as these antigens are supposed to appear only later), the mechanism of inhibition of proliferative responses by these monoclonal antibodies remains to be studied further.

NK and LDCC were blocked by CD2 and LDCC was inhibited by the four antibodies to activated T cells that diminished primary proliferations (clustered CD2 or CD3). Further testing of these antibodies showed that, despite their ability to decrease NK to Raji cells, they inhibited LDCC as well. This selective inhibition supports the concept of different effector populations for K-562-NK and Raji-LDCC (11).

NK cells share with cytotoxic T cells the expression of CD8 (12). Neither NK nor LDCC were inhibited by CD8s that are known to affect allogeneic or virus-specific CTL (2). This indicates a basic difference between NK and LDCC on one hand and the specific cytotoxicity on the other, possibly due to different effector populations and/or recognition mechanisms.

The rather uniform behavior of the different T cell antigens with respect to capping and endocytosis with two antibody layers coupled to them may have its significance when patients develop anti–mouse Ig antibodies.

As to the characterization of CD groups, antibodies included into particular pan-T CDs displayed rather uniform activity patterns. This questions the role of factors like subclass,[13] affinity, and epitope specificity. The only case when the role of antibody subclass could be suspected was that of three IgM-type CD7s that slightly enhanced mitogen responses in contrast to other CD7s with no effect.

Pan-T molecules formed two groups as antibodies to CD5 and CD7 had no major effects in any of the functional tests applied while CD2 and CD3 were inhibitory in mitogen-induced proliferation and MLR. However, these latter two could be distinguished by their activity in other reactions. Nonetheless, some antibodies of a given suspected specificity showed different activity patterns in several reactions, while some reagents of the "pan T other" or other groups had CD2- or CD3-like effects. It remains to be seen whether this kind of grouping will be supported by biochemical and tissue section work.[14]

T cell subpopulation specific antibodies failed to show any activity characteristic for the particular CDs. Most CD4s and some CD8s exerted

---

[13] For CD3, our individuals seem to be responders to IgG. Only one IgM CD3 was included and two reclustered and neither was mitogenic.

[14] Mostly confirmed by Workshop clustering.

selective inhibition of MLR with a few reagents from other groups. In the case of these functionally heterogeneous groups, and of antibodies of suspected CD2 or CD3 specificity that did not display functional effects characteristic for their CD, epitope specificity differences remain a possible explanation.

It will be a biochemical task to see whether antibodies to "T cell subset other" that decreased PWM-induced IL-2 release are directed to the same or similar cell surface structure(s).[15]

At least two kinds of antigens could be distinguished on activated T cells. One kind of molecule(s) including that recognized by Tac seems to be involved in IL-2-dependent proliferation. Surface markers other than the IL-2 receptor have been verified to participate in IL-2-driven proliferation by blocking proliferation by monoclonal antibodies to these structures (13). Nonspecific inhibition by monoclonal antibody via suppressor factor release from IL-2-dependent cells was also described (14). The other group may play a role in "primary" stimulations and some sorts of cytotoxicity.[16]

References

1. Van Wauwe, J.P., J.R. De Mey, and J.G. Goossens. 1980. OKT3: a monoclonal anti-human T lymphocyte antibody with potent mitogenic properties. *J. Immunol.* **124**:2708.
2. Reinherz, E.L., S.C. Meuer, S.F. Schlossman. 1983. The human T cell receptor: analysis with cytotoxic T cell clones. *Immunol. Rev.* **74**:83.
3. Dongworth, D.W., F.M. Gotch, N.P. Carter, P.D.K. Hildreth, and A.J. McMichael. 1984. Inhibition of virus-specific, HLA-restricted, T cell-mediated lysis by monoclonal anti-T cell antibodies. In: *Leucocyte typing,* A. Bernard, L. Boumsell, J. Dausset, C. Milstein, and S.F. Schlossman, eds. Springer-Verlag, Berlin, Heidelberg, pp. 316–320.
4. Engelman, E.G., C.J. Benike, E. Glickman, and R.L. Evans. 1981. Antibodies to membrane structures that distinguish between suppressor/cytotoxic and helper T lymphocyte subpopulations block the mixed lymphocyte culture in man. *J. Exp. Med.* **154**:193.
5. Martin, P.J., G. Longton, J. Ledbetter, W. Newman, M.P. Braun, P.G. Beatty, and J.A. Hansen. 1983. Identification and functional characterization of two distinct epitopes on the human T cell surface protein Tp50. *J. Immunol.* **131**:180.
6. Palacios, R., and O. Martinez-Maza. 1982. Is the E receptor on human T lymphocytes a "negative signal receptor"? *J. Immunol.* **129**:2479.
7. Onody, C., G. Batory, and G.Gy. Petranyi. 1980. Age-dependent responsiveness of T lymphocytes to allogeneic and PHA stimulation. *Thymus* **1**:205.
8. Batory, G., M. Benczur, M. Varga, T. Garam, C. Onody, and G.Gy. Petranyi. 1981. Increased killer cell activity in aged humans. *Immunobiol.* **158**:393.

---

[15] Not clustered.
[16] Clustered CD2 or CD3.

9. Bonavida, B., A. Robins, and A. Saxon. 1977. Lectin-dependent cellular cytotoxicity in man. *Transplantation* **23**:261.
10. Macphail, St., and O. Stutman. 1984. Independent inhibition of IL2 synthesis and cell proliferation by anti-Ia antibodies in mixed lymphocyte responses to Mls. *Eur. J. Immunol.* **14**:318.
11. Bonavida, B., and T.P. Bradley. 1983. Relationship between natural killer (NK) cells and both lectin-dependent cellular cytotoxicity (LDCC) and antibody-dependent cellular cytotoxicity (ADCC) measured by the two target conjugate single cell assay. In: *Intercellular communication in leucocyte function,* J.W. Parker, and R.L.O. O'Brien, eds., John Wiley & Sons Ltd, New York, pp. 569–574.
12. Perussia, B., V. Fanning, and G. Trinchieri. 1983. A human NK and K cell subset shares with cytotoxic T cells expression of the antigen recognized by antibody OKT8. *J. Immunol.* **131**:223.
13. Malek, T.R., and E.M. Shevach. 1984. Interleukin 2-driven lymphocyte proliferation is dependent upon a surface antigen distinct from the interleukin 2 receptor: Requirements for inhibition of T cell proliferation by monoclonal antibody 5C3. *Cell Immunol.* **84**:85.
14. Burns, G.F., T. Trigila, and G.A. Varigos. 1984. Mouse monoclonal antibodies can nonspecifically inhibit the proliferation of human T cell growth factor dependent T cells. *Cell Immunol.* **B2**:426.

CHAPTER 11

T Cell Activation by CD3 Antibodies

Roland Kurrle, Waltraud Seyfert, Armin Trautwein, and
Friedrich Robert Seiler

Monoclonal antibodies which recognize the T3 antigen on human T
cells have turned out to be excellent tools for analyzing T cell activation.
The T3 antigen complex seems to be involved in specific immune functions, either as a receptor or as molecules functionally or physically
associated with the receptor (1–3). In contrast to T cell activation by
mitogens, the activation via anti-T3 antibodies seems to reflect
antigen-specific lymphocyte stimulation. It is well established that mere
binding of different anti-T3 antibodies triggers mitogenesis (4,5), induces
the production of immune mediators like interferon (γ-IFN) and inter-
leukin-2 (IL-2) (6–8), and blocks cytotoxic effector functions and antigen-
specific proliferative responses (9). However, to date all studies of the
activation of human T cells via the T3 antigen complex have been carried
out with monoclonal antibodies of the IgG2a isotype (OKT3) or the IgG1
isotype (Leu-4, UCHT1). From the functional point of view the isotypes
of anti-T3 antibodies seem to play a critical role in the efficiency and the
mechanism of T cell activation. Whereas anti-T3 antibodies of the IgG2a
isotype are highly effective in activating T cells from all donors by an IL-
2-dependent mechanism (8,10), for anti-T3 antibodies of IgG1 isotype
nonresponsiveness caused by polymorphism in the accessory cell function has been described (11). Based on blocking experiments with Fc
fragments of normal IgG (12,13) and analysis of different ethnic groups,
the cause of nonresponsiveness seems to be genetic variations of the Fc-γ
receptor of accessory cells (11,14). This study therefore compares the
ability of anti-T3 antibodies of the IgG2b and IgG3 isotypes to activate T
cells with that of IgG2a and IgG1 antibodies. The therapeutic use of
OKT3 (IgG2a) for treatment of patients undergoing an acute allograft
rejection after kidney transplantations and for purging of mature T cells
from donor marrows to prevent acute graft-versus-host diseases (GvHD)
in allogeneic bone transplantations is reported to be highly effective (15–
18). However, the activation of the immune system via T3^{+} cells has to be

considered as therapy-limiting, due to antigenic modulation (19,20) and development of anti-Ig antibodies. The implications resulting from this study for the therapeutic use of anti-T3 antibodies shall be discussed.

Materials and Methods

Monoclonal Antibodies

Monoclonal antibodies which were said to recognize the T3 antigen complex (CD3 group), as well as two antibodies of the IgG2b isotype (BW 239/347; BW 242/412) established previously to react with the T3 antigen, were analyzed (21). To eliminate contamination by sodium azide all antibody samples were dialyzed extensively before being used in functional assays.

Cytofluorometric Assays

Cells were analyzed by an Ortho Cytofluorograph 50H/2150 Computer System, modified for single-step analysis of whole blood (22). The percentage of fluorescein-positive cells was calculated by a modified version of the Ortho Software. Labeling of cells with different antibodies was carried out at +4°C (30 min). After extensive washing, cells were stained with a fluoresceinated rabbit anti–mouse Ig–F(ab)$_2$ (2.Ab–FITC). For cytofluorometric blocking assays, cells were coated with an excess of non-fluoresceinated antibodies. After removing unbound antibodies by washing three times, cells were stained with directly fluoresceinated antibodies (OKT3–FITC; BW 264/56–F(ab)$_2$–FITC). Blocking was defined as a decrease of fluorescence intensity, relative to background values. To measure antigenic modulation, Ficoll-separated lymphocytes (+ accessory cells) were labeled at +4°C (30 min) with the respective antibodies alone or with antibodies + rabbit anti–mouse Ig–FITC. After washing three times, the cells were then incubated for 24 hr at 37°C. Restaining of those cells was carried out at +4°C with the antibody combinations given in the results. The extent of antigenic modulation was determined by comparing the median fluorescence channel of experimental groups versus control groups.

Assays for Proliferative Activity and *In Vitro* IgM Synthesis

To measure the mitogenic properties of anti-T3 antibodies, Ficoll-separated human peripheral blood lymphocytes (+ accessory cells) (1.5×10^5 cells/well) were cultivated for 66 hr in the presence of appropriate amounts of different anti-T3 antibodies (antibody dilution 1 : 200–1 : 10^5) or mitogen (PHA, 10 μg/ml). After 48 hr, the cells were pulsed with [^{14}C]thymidine (0.075 μCi/well; NEN, Dreieich, FRG). Proliferation was assessed by [^{14}C]thymidine uptake. The given results represent the mean cpm incorporation obtained from 6 individual values. *In vitro* IgM synthesis was induced by culturing 1.5×10^5 PBLs in U-shaped microtiter plates in the presence of appropriate amounts of different anti-T3 antibodies (antibody dilution: $1:10^3–1:10^7$). In contrast to all cell culture systems described above where Dulbecco's medium + 15% fetal calf serum was used, cells for IgM synthesis were cultured in serum-free Iscove's medium. On day 10 the culture supernatant was harvested and the IgM content determined in an ELISA system for human IgM (BEHRINGWERKE, Marburg).

Results

Eleven monoclonal antibodies which were said to recognize the T3 antigen complex as well as two antibodies of the IgG2b isotype (BW 239/347, BW242/412) established previously to react with the T3 antigen (21) were analyzed in different functional systems for their ability to activate mature peripheral T cells. With the exception of BW 242/412 all antibodies were included in the serological analysis of the T cell workshop protocol (Section I studies). The percentages of labeled E$^+$ cells, summarized in Table 11.1, indicate that from serological analysis studies only antibody NU-T1

Table 11.1. Reactivity patterns of anti-T3 mAbs.

Antibody name	Ig subclass	E$^+$-cells[a]	mAb + OKT3–FITC	mAb + BW 264/56– F(ab)$_2$–FITC	Blocking capacity
				% Fluorescence-positive human lymphocytes	
G19-4.1	IgG1	89.8 ± 2.3	1.3	0.3	+
SK7/Leu 4	IgG1	89.6 ± 1.3	1.1	2.9	+
T3/2T8-2F4	IgG1	93.0 ± 1.3	78.6	67.2	–
T3/RW2-8C8	IgG1	89.8 ± 2.0	4.3	12.3	+[c]
NU-T1	IgG1	98.2 ± 1.0	80.4	66.0	–
89b1	NK	90.2 ± 1.0	5.9	13.8	+[c]
BW 264/56	IgG2a	90.8 ± 2.0	0.2	1.2	+
X35-3	IgG2a	90.4 ± 2.6	6.0	(65.9)	+[c]
OKT3	IgG2a	n.d.[b]	0.3	1.4	+
BW 239/347	IgG2b	85.2 ± 4.5	4.5	3.8	+[c]
BW 242/412	IgG2b	n.d.[b]	2.1	4.0	+[c]
T3/RW2-4B6	IgG2b	91.6 ± 2.2	5.3	8.2	+[c]
BW 242/55	IgG3	93.2 ± 3.7	6.2	n.d.	+[c]
T3/2Ad2A2	IgM	91.6 ± 1.6	79.1	69.6	–
Medium control	PBS-BSA	2.2 ± 1.2	78.3	65.9	

[a] Test carried out according to the Workshop protocol.
[b] Not done (within these experiments).
[c] Partial (steric) blocking.

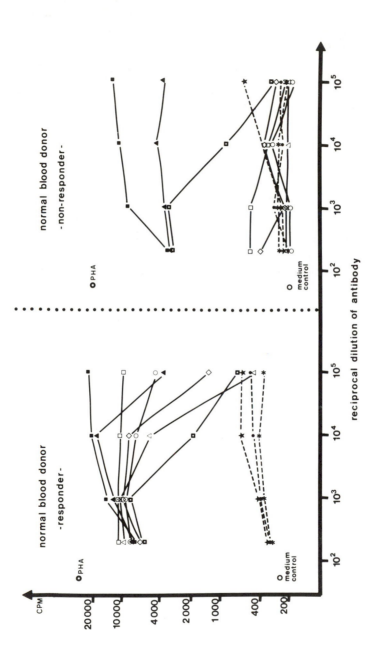

Fig. 11.1. Proliferation of human lymphocytes from normal blood donors incubated for 3 days with appropriate amounts of different anti-T3 antibodies or mitogen (PHA). Proliferation was assessed by [^{14}C]thymidine uptake. Anti-T3 antibodies: IgG1 (□ G19-4.1; ◇ SK7/Leu 4; ○ T3/RW2-8C8; △ 89b1); IgG2a (■ BW264/56; ▲ ×35-3); IgG2b (✳ BW 239/347; ● BW 242/412; ★ T3/RW2-4B6); IgG3 (◨ BW 242/55).

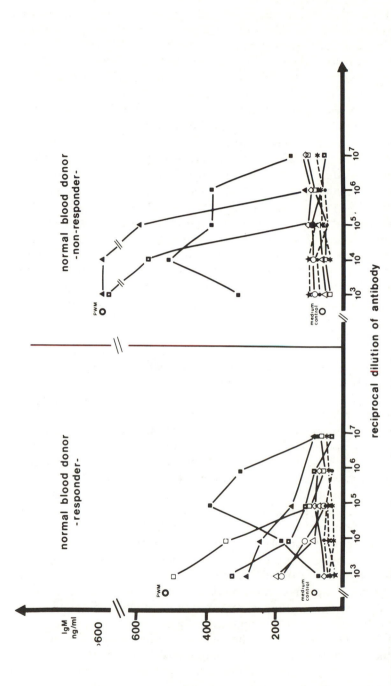

Fig. 11.2. IgM content of human lymphocytes from normal blood donors cultivated for 10 days in serum-free Iscove's medium in the presence of appropriate amounts of different anti-T3 antibodies or mitogen (PWM). The IgM content of the culture supernatant was measured with an ELISA assay for human IgM. For antibody symbols see Fig. 11.1.

does not fit in the reactivity pattern measured. To confirm that all antibodies used for further testing recognize the T3 antigen complex, blocking studies were carried out. For this purpose lymphocytes were preincubated with the respective monoclonal antibody and afterwards stained either with OKT3–FITC or BW 264/56–F(ab)$_2$–FITC. The results listed in Table 11.1 show that only antibodies T3/2Ad2A2, T3/2T8-2F4, and NU-T1 were unable to block the binding of directly labeled anti-T3 antibodies. As these antibodies yielded negative results in all other functional experiments, they were excluded from all further consideration. Interestingly, of the remaining antibodies only a few were able to cause complete blocking, whereas most of them brought about only partial (steric) blocking. This indicates that different epitopes were recognized. To test the mitogenic capacity of the anti-T3 antibodies PBLs from normal blood donors were cultured in the presence of the respective antibody. After 3 days [^{14}C]thymidine uptake was measured. Figure 11.1 shows a sample of all experimental results. The blood donors were previously selected to be a responder (donor L.B.) and a nonresponder (donor W.S.) for Leu-4 (IgG1) respectively. In this experiment it was demonstrated that all IgG1 antibodies only failed to induce DNA synthesis in the nonresponder situation, whereas antibodies of the IgG2b isotype were unable to induce T cell proliferation in all cases tested.

As mentioned above T cell activation via OKT3 results not only in T cell proliferation but also in the induction of γ-IFN production (6). Recently we confirmed these results with the mitogenic antibodies BW 264/56 (IgG2a) and BW 242/55 (IgG3) (data not shown).

On the other hand, cloned murine γ-IFN is reported to act synergistically with other helper factors in the stimulation of B cell antibody responses (23,24). From these data we suggested that T cell-derived lymphokines produced after stimulation with anti-T3 antibodies might be able to induce Ig synthesis *in vitro*. In analogy to the proliferation experiment described above, PBLs from a responder to IgG1 (donor W.L.) and a nonresponder (donor W.S.) were cultured in serum-free Iscove's medium with various dilutions ($1:10^3$–$1:10^7$) of anti-T3 antibodies. After 10 days the culture supernatant was harvested and the IgM content determined in an ELISA system for human IgM. In Fig. 11.2 the results of one of three identical experiments are presented. Although the absolute amount of IgM produced by cells from different individuals varies considerably, the message from all experiments is identical. Under conditions where IgG1 antibodies are mitogenic, they were able to induce IgM synthesis *in vitro*, whereas in the nonresponder situation no IgM could be measured. Antibodies of the IgG2a isotype and the IgG3 antibody are potent inducers of IgM synthesis, correlating with their capability to induce the production of γ-IFN. Under the given conditions IgG2b antibodies failed, in parallel with the lack of mitogenicity, to induce IgM synthesis. However, from a large number of subjects Tax and coworkers (25) found two related per-

Table 11.2. Antigen modulation by anti-T3 mAbs.[a]

| Lymphocytes incubated overnight with | Blood donor L.B. | | | Blood donors W.S. | |
| | Cells labeled with | | | Cells | |
	2.Ab–FITC*	BW 264/56–F(ab)₂–FITC	Starting values	labeled with 2.Ab–FITC	Starting values
Medium	2.0	78.8	3.0	4.2	2.2
G19-4.1	3.0	0.2	82.9	78.3	75.2
SK7/Leu 4	4.3	0.3	81.4	77.4	73.4
T3/RW2-8C8	2.5	3.3	81.3	77.0	74.4
89b1	39.6	2.6	81.3	75.4	70.7
BW 264/56	5.9	3.8	80.5	7.3	73.6
X35-3	5.1	6.4	81.2	14.1	73.8
OKT3	8.2	3.1	79.4	13.9	75.1
BW 239/347	69.2	n.d.	78.0	65.8	69.6
BW 242/412	71.8	15.0	82.7	64.5	69.2
T3/RW2-4B6	73.0	5.6	77.5	68.3	70.1
BW 242/55	9.4	16.2	85.9	n.d.	n.d.

[a] Lymphocytes were incubated overnight at 37°C with the respective anti-T3 antibody. After washing, the cells were labeled at +4°C with 2.Ab–FITC or BW 264/56–F(ab)₂–FITC. As control the cells were kept overnight at +4°C and were then labeled with 2.Ab–FITC (starting values). 2.Ab–FITC = rabbit anti-mouse Ig–F(ab)₂–FITC. Data represent percent of cells fluorescent positive.

sons able to respond with one anti-T3 antibody of IgG2b isotype (SPV-T3a). These results indicate that there might exist, with very low frequency, a polymorphism of Fc-γ2b receptors similar to that of Fc-γ1 receptors (25). Previously we could demonstrate with a few anti-T3 antibodies that under conditions where T cell proliferation could be induced, T3 antigen modulation occurs in parallel. We now designed experiments using the whole panel of anti-T3 antibodies. In experimental approaches constructed in analogy to the proliferation and IgM synthesis experiments, the data listed in Table 11.2 clearly show that antigenic modulation occurs only under conditions where an effective T cell activation is possible.

Discussion

In the present study monoclonal antibodies which recognize the T3 antigen complex were analyzed for their ability to activate mature human T cells. The specificity of the antibodies tested was confirmed by serological analysis with separated lymphocyte populations according to the T cell workshop protocol. Additionally specificity was confirmed by blocking assays and nonblocking antibodies were excluded from further consideration. In summary, all types of experiments designed to study T cell activation gave consistent results. Whenever antigenic modulation was allowed to occur after binding of anti-T3 antibodies, the binding of such antibodies resulted in the induction of DNA and IgM synthesis. Recent studies indicate that the nonresponsiveness of T cells from distinct blood donors to anti-T3 antibodies of the IgG1 isotype is caused by a polymorphism of the Fc-γ-receptor on accessory cells. The data of this study are in accordance with this hypothesis, although the isotype of antibody 89B1 is not known. For the Fc-γ2b receptor a polymorphism may also exist (25); however, in screening more than 20 blood donors with BW 242/412 (Ig2b) we failed to induce T cell activation with this antibody by mere co-cultivation with human leukocytes. However, under artificial conditions, when BW 242/412 was cross-linked with a second antibody (rabbit anti–mouse-Ig) T3 antigenic modulation did occur (21). The same type of experiment was carried out by Tax and coworkers (25) who coupled SPV-T3a (IgG2b) to Sepharose beads. They were able to demonstrate that this antibody, provided it is coupled to Sepharose, is able to activate purified T cells. Taken together, these experiments indicate that the function of accessory cells within T cell activation via anti-T3 antibodies is restricted to their cross-linking, obviously the prerequisite for antigenic modulation. Within this concept, modulation of the T3 antigen complex, without further signals, e.g., lymphokines from accessory cells, seems to play a critical role as trigger signal during T cell activation.

Antigenic modulation of the T3 complex occurs not only under *in vitro* conditions, but is also described for *in vivo* situations after therapeutic application of OKT3 for treatment of patients undergoing acute allograft rejection upon kidney transplantation. Although this treatment seems to be a beneficial approach, in the light of this study it must be taken into consideration that obviously under conditions where antigenic modulation can occur, this is associated with T cell proliferation, induction of immune mediators like IL-2 and γ-IFN, and the activation of B cells. At least for cloned murine γ-IFN it is reported that this mediator induces enhanced expression of Ia and H-2 antigens (26,27). In turn, an enhanced expression of class I and class II major histocompatibility complex antigens may by themselves result in an activation of the host immune system. However, only clinical trials with modulating and nonmodulating anti-T3 antibodies will be able to decide if these *in vitro* results are of relevance in the patient situation.

Acknowledgments. The skillful technical assistance of K. Müller and K. Thomas and the excellent secretarial assistance of C. Walldorf are gratefully acknowledged.

References

1. Chang, T.W., P.C. Kung, S.P. Gingras, and G. Goldstein. 1981. Does OKT3 monoclonal antibody react with an antigen-recognition structure on human T cells? *Proc. Natl. Acad. Sci. U.S.A.* **78:**1805.

2. Reinherz, E.L., S. Meuer, K.A. Fitzgerald, R.E. Hussey, H. Levine, and S.F. Schlossman. 1982. Antigen recognition by human T lymphocytes is linked to surface expression of the T3 molecular complex. *Cell* **30**:735.

3. Meuer, S.C., K.A. Fitzgerald, R.E. Hussey, J.C. Hodgdon, S.F. Schlossman, and E.L. Reinherz. 1983. Clonotypic structures involved in antigen-specific human T cell function. *J. Exp. Med.* **157**:705.

4. Van Wauwe, J.P., J.R. De Mey, and J.G. Goossens. 1980. OKT3: a monoclonal anti–human T lymphocyte antibody with potent mitogenic properties. *J. Immunol.* **124**:2708.

5. Musiani, P., N. Maggiano, F.B. Aiello, L. Lauriola, F.O. Ranelletti, and M. Piantelli. 1984. Ia- and IgG-Fc receptor-positive accessory cell sustains peripheral T lymphocyte but not thymocyte mitogenesis induced by OKT3 monoclonal antibody. *Cell. Immunol.* **84**:333.

6. Pang, R.H.L., Y.K. Yip, and J. Vilcek. 1981. Immune interferon induction by a monoclonal antibody specific for human T cells. *Cell. Immunol.* **64**:304.

7. Welte, K., E. Platzer, C.Y. Wang, E.A. Rinnooy Kan, M.A.S. Moore, and R. Mertelsmann. 1983. OKT8 antibody inhibits OKT3-induced IL2 production and proliferation in OKT8$^+$ cells. *J. Immunol.* **131**:2356.

8. Van Wauwe, J.P., J.G. Goossens, and P.C.L. Beverley. 1984. Human T lymphocyte activation by monoclonal antibodies; OKT3, but not UCHT1, triggers mitogenesis via an interleukin 2-dependent mechanism. *J. Immunol.* **133**:129.

9. Van Wauwe, J.P., J.G. Goossens, and G. Van Nyen. 1984. Inhibition of lymphocyte proliferation by monoclonal antibody directed against the T3 antigen on human T cells. *Cell. Immunol.* **86**:525.

10. Meuer, S.C., R.E. Hussey, D.A. Cantrell, J.C. Hodgdon, S.F. Schlossmann, K.A. Smith, and E.L. Reinherz. 1984. Triggering of the T3-Ti antigen-receptor complex results in clonal T-cell proliferation through an interleukin-2 dependent autocrine pathway. *Proc. Natl. Acad. Sci. U.S.A.* **81**:1509.

11. Tax, W.J.M., H.W. Willems, P.P.M. Reekers, P.J.A. Capel, and R.A.P. Koene. 1983. Polymorphism in mitogenic effect of IgG1 monoclonal antibodies against T3 antigen on human T cells. *Nature* **304**:445.

12. Looney, R.J., and G.N. Abraham. 1984. The Fc portion of intact IgG blocks stimulation of human PBMC by anti-T3. *J. Immunol.* **133**:154.

13. Landegren, U., J. Andersson, and H. Wigzell. 1984. Mechanism of T lymphocyte activation by OKT-3 antibodies. A general model for T cell induction. *Eur. J. Immunol.* **14**:325.

14. Abo, T., A.B. Tilden, C.M. Balch, K. Kumagai, G.M. Troup, and M.D. Cooper. 1984. Ethnic differences in the lymphocyte proliferative response induced by a murine IgG1 antibody, Leu4, to the T3 molecule. *J. Exp. Med.* **160**:303.

15. Russell, P.S., R.B. Colvin, and A.B. Cosini. 1984. Monoclonal antibodies for the diagnosis and treatment of transplant rejection. *Ann. Rev. Med.* **35**:63.

16. Cosimi, A.B., R.C. Burton, R.B. Colvin, G. Goldstein, F.L. Delmonico, M.P. La Quaglia, N. Tolkoff-Rubin, R.H. Rubin, J.T. Herrin, and P.S. Russell. 1981. Treatment of acute renal allograft rejection with OKT3 monoclonal antibody. *Transplantation* **32**:535.

17. Prentice, H.G., G. Janossy, D. Skeggs, H.A. Blacklock, K.F. Bradstock, G. Goldstein, and A.V. Hoffbrand. 1982. Use of anti-T-cell monoclonal antibody

OKT3 to prevent acute Graft-Versus-Host disease in allogeneic bone-marrow transplantation for acute leukemia. *Lancet* **27**:700.

18. Blacklock, H.A., H.G. Prentice, M.J.M.L. Gilmore, E. Price-Jones, S. Schey, N. Tidman, D.D.F. Ma, G. Goldstein, G. Janossy, and A.V. Hoffbrand. 1983. Attempts at T cell depletion using OKT3 and rabbit complement to prevent acute Graft-Versus-Host disease in allogeneic bone marrow transplantation. *Exp. Hematol.* **11**:37.

19. Estabrook, A., C.L. Berger, R. Mittler, P. LoGerfo, M. Hardy, and R.L. Edelson. 1983. Antigenic modulation of human T lymphocytes by monoclonal antibodies. *Transplant. Proc.* **XV**:651.

20. Chatenoud, L., M.F. Baudrihaye, H. Kreis, G. Goldstein, J. Schindler, and J.F. Bach. 1982. Human in vivo antigenic modulation induced by the anti-T cell OKT3 monoclonal antibody. *Eur. J. Immunol.* **12**:979.

21. Kurrle, R., W. Seyfert, A. Trautwein, and F.R. Seiler. 1985. Cellular mechanisms of T-cell activation by modulation of the T3-antigen complex. *Transplant. Proc.* **XVII**:880.

22. Hoffman, R.A., P.C. Kung, W.P. Hansen, and G. Goldstein. 1980. Simple and rapid measurement of human T lymphocytes and their subclasses in peripheral blood. *Proc. Natl. Acad. Sci. U.S.A.* **77**:4914.

23. Leibson, H.J., M. Gefter, A. Zlotnik, P. Marrak, and J.W. Kappler. 1984. Role of γ-interferon in antibody-producing responses. *Nature* **309**:799.

24. Sidman, C.L., J.D. Marshall, L.D. Shultz, P.W. Gray, and H.M. Johnson. 1984. γ-Interferon is one of several direct B cell-maturing lymphokines. *Nature* **309**:801.

25. Tax, W.J.M., H. Spits, H.F.M. Hermes, H.W. Willems, P.J. Capel, and R.A.P. Koene. 1984. Polymorphism of human Fc. *J. Immunol.* (in press).

26. Wong, G.H.W., J. Clark-Lewis, J.L. Mckimm-Breschkin, A.W. Harris, and J.W. Schrader. 1983. Interferon-γ induces enhanced expression of Ia and H-2 antigens on B-lymphoid, macrophage, and myeloid cell lines. *J. Immunol.* **131**:788.

27. King, D.P. and P.P. Jones. 1983. Induction of Ia and H-2 antigens on a macrophage cell line by immune interferon. *J. Immunol.* **131**:315.

CHAPTER 12

Studies of T Cell Proliferation Induced by Monoclonal Antibodies of the Second International Workshop

Paul J. Martin, Jeffrey A. Ledbetter, Patrick G. Beatty, Edward A. Clark, and John A. Hansen

Monoclonal antibodies have proved useful as probes for identifying and studying molecules that mediate or regulate cell function. For example, certain CD3 antibodies are known to activate T cells and cause T cell proliferation (1). These antibodies bind to a noncovalently associated complex of polypeptides with molecular weights between 19,000–28,000 daltons (2–4). The CD3 complex in turn is noncovalently associated with other cell surface molecules that function as antigen receptors for T lymphocytes (5–6). The cross-linking of CD3/T cell antigen receptor complexes by CD3 antibodies is now understood to trigger T cell activation and proliferation in a way that mimics triggering by specific antigen (7). Binding of CD3 antibodies and cross-linking of CD3 on the cell surface can lead to expression of interleukin-2 (IL-2) receptors and secretion of IL-2 into the medium (8).

Other molecules on T cells may also influence T cell activation. For example, it is well recognized that antibodies which react with CD2 or with the IL-2 receptor can inhibit the proliferative response of T cells to stimulation with phytohemagglutinin, conconavalin A, allogeneic cells, or soluble antigen (9–12). Antibody binding to other surface molecules can facilitate activation. For example, we have found that antibody 9.3, which recognizes a homodimeric 90,000-dalton polypeptide expressed on 70% of E-rosette-forming cells, is capable of enhancing the proliferative effect of CD3 antibodies. With this in mind, we screened the Workshop T cell antibody panel in order to answer three questions about T cell activation. First, we tested whether any of the Workshop antibodies could increase or decrease the response of T cells stimulated by an anti-CD3 antibody. Second, we sought to identify non-CD3 antibodies that were mitogenic. Third, we screened for antibodies that could induce IL-2 receptor expression without causing IL-2 secretion.

Methods

Peripheral blood mononuclear cells (PBL) were isolated by density gradient centrifugation over Ficoll–Hypaque (S.G. 1.077). Antibodies of the Workshop panel were distributed individually in round-bottomed wells of microtiter plates. Cells (5×10^4) were cultured for three days (unless indicated otherwise) in 50 ul RPMI 1640–12% fetal calf serum containing antibodies at a final dilution of 1 : 200 (unless indicated otherwise). Proliferation was assessed by [^{3}H]thymidine incorporation. Purified human IL-2 was purchased from Genzyme Corp. (Boston, MA) and its activity was verified by testing its ability to stimulate proliferation of an IL-2-dependent continuously cultured human T cell line.

Fluorescein isothiocyanate (FITC) conjugates of anti-CD3 antibodies 38.1 (IgM) and 64.1 (IgG2a) were prepared according to a modification of the method described by Goding (13) with the use of antibodies purified from ascites fluid by protein A-sepharose column chromatography (14) or euglobulin fractionation. Cross-blocking studies were carried out as described previously (15). Cells stained by direct or indirect immunofluorescence were analyzed by flow microfluorimetry with the use of a FACS IV (Beckton-Dickinson, Mountain View, CA).

Results

We tested the Workshop T cell antibody panel to determine whether any antibodies could enhance or diminish the proliferative response of T cells stimulated by antibody 64.1. The histogram depicted in Fig. 12.1 shows a slight but significant decrease in the proliferation of cells co-stimulated with antibody 64.1 and antibodies of the Workshop anti-T cell panel. There were no outliers on the low end, indicative of complete blocking. Furthermore, the lowest responses were not associated with any particular antibody specificity. When the identity of the individual antibodies was revealed, there was no evidence in this experiment that anti-CD2 antibodies or anti–IL-2 receptor antibodies diminished significantly the proliferative response to stimulation with antibody 64.1.

In contrast, there was one antibody that appeared as an outlier on the high end and gave approximately twice the expected proliferative response. This antibody, designated KOLT-2, was examined in greater detail. The fluorescence histogram of PBL stained with this antibody had a profile identical to the profile of PBL stained with antibody 9.3 (data not shown). Moreover, the antigen immunoprecipitated by the KOLT-2 antibody had a molecular weight of 44,000 daltons under reducing conditions (not shown), similar to what has been described for the antigen immunoprecipitated by antibody 9.3 (4). Finally, it was demonstrated that antibody KOLT-2 could completely block the binding of antibody 9.3 on PBL

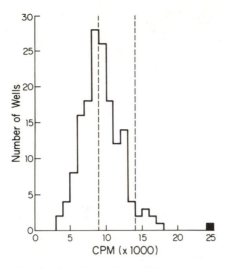

Fig. 12.1. Frequency distribution of T cell proliferation induced by co-stimulation of human PBL with antibodies of the Workshop T cell panel (final dilution 1 : 200) and antibody 64.1 (final dilution 1 : 250). The vertical dotted lines indicate 2 SD above and below the $\bar{X}$ of 12 microcultures stimulated with antibody 64.1 alone.

(not shown). Collectively, these results indicate that antibodies KOLT-2 and 9.3 recognize the same cell surface molecule.

In order to identify mitogenic antibodies, blood mononuclear cells were cultured for three days in microwells containing individual antibodies of the T cell panel and then pulse labeled with [³H]thymidine. There were 17 antibodies that appeared to be mitogenic in the first two screenings (Table 12.1). In a third screen, mitogen-free, purified IL-2 (5 units/ml) was added to each well. There were no antibodies identified that were mitogenic only in the presence of IL-2. All antibodies that were mitogenic in the presence of IL-2 were also mitogenic in the absence of IL-2. These results indicate that the Workshop T cell panel did not contain antibodies capable of inducing IL-2 receptor expression without IL-2 secretion. In further studies, it was found that 10 of the 17 mitogenic antibodies could be demonstrated to have anti-CD3 specificity by cross-blocking studies with FITC-conjugated anti-CD3 antibodies 64.1 and 38.1.

It was possible that some of the non-cross-blocking antibodies recognized CD3, but the concentration or avidity of the antibody was not sufficient to inhibit binding of 64.1 or 38.1. Alternatively, some of these antibodies might recognize novel epitopes of CD3. To test for this, we compared the fluorescence histograms of the CD3 non-cross-blocking antibodies on CD3-modulated cells and unmodulated cells. The fluorescent histogram of PBL incubated overnight in medium and stained by indirect immunofluorescence with antibody T121 showed a bimodal distribution,

Table 12.1. Characteristics of mitogenic antibodies.

Workshop antibody number	Screen (cpm)[a]			Cross-blocking[b]	
	Exp. A	Exp. B	Exp. C (IL-2)	FITC–64.1	FITC–38.1
T57	16,400	41,955	6278	−	+
T60	13,617	29,983	12,975	−	−
T61	5391	4211	5377	−	+
T62	21,834	5232	12,153	−	−
T94	9818	597	7353	−	−
T101	19,647	48,886	10,176	+	+
T105	11,119	807	6711	−	−
T117	16,730	38,601	11,545	+	+
T118	11,483	39,501	8044	+	+
T119	10,917	36,106	13,195	+	+
T120	8520	16,979	9464	+	+
T121	17,396	19,374	9620	−	−
T124	4990	18,460	1701	+	+
T125	13,821	37,612	6628	+	+
T126	7921	24,546	8384	+	−
T128	9434	839	10,034	−	−
T137	8774	4587	8465	−	−
Background	<1000	<2500	<1700		

[a] Human PBL (5×10^4) were incubated in microcultures (50 µl) for three days with individual antibodies of the Workshop T cell panel (final dilution, 1 : 200). Numbers in the table indicate cpm [³H]thymidine incorporation during the last four hours of culture. "A", "B" and "C" represent three independent screening experiments. Experiment "C" was carried out with the addition of lectin-free, purified IL-2 (5 U/ml) to the microculture wells.

[b] Cells were preincubated with the mitogenic antibodies of the Workshop T cell panel and then stained with FITC-conjugated antibodies 64.1 and 38.1 which are known to have CD3 specificity. "+" indicates that preincubation of cells with the Workshop antibody caused a measurable decrease in the intensity of staining by FITC-labeled antibody compared to cells preincubated in medium or irrelevant antibody. "−" indicates that preincubation of cells with the Workshop antibody did not decrease the intensity of staining by FITC-labeled antibody.

suggesting two distinct positive populations (Fig. 12.2). When PBL were incubated overnight with antibody 38.1, all CD3 antigen was modulated, as shown by the negative control curve. The staining pattern of antibody T121 on CD3-modulated cells was distinctly different from the staining of unmodulated cells. The staining of one of the originally positive populations was lost after modulation of the CD3 antigen and the new fluorescence histogram that emerged was suggestive of the characteristic profile seen after staining with anti-CD8 antibody. Thus, it is likely that antibody T121 is a mixture of two antibodies: one which recognizes CD3 and another which recognizes CD8. If this hypothesis is correct, we can conclude that it was the anti-CD3 antibody that caused T cell proliferation (Table 12.1). Two other antibodies, T60 and T137, also showed decreased staining on CD3-modulated cells (not shown), indicating the possible presence of a CD3 antibody.

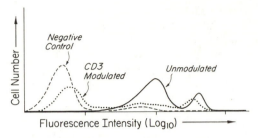

Fig. 12.2. Fluorescence histograms of unmodulated PBL (——) and CD3-modulated PBL (····) stained with antibody T121. The negative control (----) represents staining of CD3-modulated cells with an affinity-purified FITC-conjugated goat anti–mouse immunoglobulin antiserum. This histogram was equivalent to the histogram of unmodulated cells stained by indirect immunofluorescence with an irrelevant (nonbinding) control murine monoclonal antibody (not shown).

In separate studies we have found that the CD3 antibody 64.1 can cause significant mitogenesis at less than ¹/₁₀ of the minimum concentration required to produce threshold staining detectable by indirect immunofluorescence. Thus, the mitogenesis associated with the CD3 non-cross-blocking antibodies could be caused by CD3 antibodies present in concentrations too low to be detected by immunofluorescence methods. All of the CD3 non-cross-blocking mitogenic antibodies except T128 could bind to cells from baboons. If it is this cross-reacting antibody species that causes proliferation of human cells, it should also cause proliferation of baboon cells. If, on the other hand, the mitogenic effect of the antibody were caused by anti-CD3 contamination, then it should not cause baboon cells to proliferate, unless the contaminating CD3 antibody also reacted with a CD3-like molecule on baboon cells. This is unlikely because none of the anti-human CD3 antibodies tested in the previous Workshop or in the present Workshop reacts with cells from lower primates. One of the six CD3 non-cross-blocking mitogenic antibodies, T94, was also mitogenic for baboon cells (Table 12.2). The fluorescence histogram of PBL stained with antibody T94 had a characteristic CD8 profile on both human and baboon cells (not shown).

A kinetic study was carried out in order to determine whether the proliferation induced by antibody T94 could be caused by anti-CD3 contamination. The proliferation induced by the anti-CD3 control (64.1) reached a plateau after two days of culture and remained essentially unchanged on days three and four (Table 12.3). In contrast, the proliferation induced by antibody T94 showed exponential kinetics and did not reach a peak until day five. Culture of PBL in medium containing the anti-CD8 antibody 51.1 (4,15) did not cause proliferation. These data support the conclusion that the proliferative activity of antibody T94 was not caused by a CD3 antibody.

Table 12.2. Studies with cells from non-human primates.

Workshop antibody number	Binding to baboon cells[a]	[³H]Thymidine incorporation[b]
T60	Yes	1137 ± 410
T62	Yes[c]	671 ± 94
T94	Yes	6586 ± 267
T105	Yes[c]	308 ± 45
T128	No	221 ± 10
T137	Yes	513 ± 25

[a] Binding was determined by indirect immunofluorescence and flow microfluorimetry.
[b] Baboon PBL (5×10^4) were incubated in triplicate microcultures (50 μl) for three days with the indicated antibodies of the Workshop T cell panel. Numbers indicate cpm [³H]thymidine incorporation ($\bar{X} \pm$ SEM) during the last four hours of culture. The incorporation by cells cultured in medium was 193 ± 35 cpm.
[c] Decreased fluorescence intensity compared to human cells.

Antibodies 64.1 and T94 had different binding characteristics and different dose–response profiles in proliferative assays. The level of proliferation induced by antibody 64.1 remained constant over a wide range of antibody concentration down to 5 ng/ml, a concentration at which antibody binding was no longer detectable by indirect immunofluorescence (not shown). These data indicate that T cells are exquisitely sensitive to ligand–receptor interaction involving anti-CD3 antibodies and CD3 molecules and that binding to a very low number of receptors is sufficient to initiate the proliferative response. In contrast, the level of proliferation induced by antibody T94 was critically dependent on its concentration. Peak proliferation occurred at the highest concentration tested (1 : 200 dilution) and declined to reach background levels at a dilution of 1 : 50,000. At this dilution, antibody binding was readily detectable by

Table 12.3. Kinetics of proliferation.[a]

	Antibody			
Day	64.1	T94	51.1	Medium
1	115 ± 9	120 ± 10	158 ± 8	146 ± 3
2	10,233 ± 176	2884 ± 335	287 ± 38	304 ± 72
3	10,673 ± 1708	12,811 ± 1315	711 ± 94	396 ± 129
4	12,633 ± 1558	56,921 ± 2153	1887 ± 584	1809 ± 356
5	6299 ± 648	64,636 ± 3248	2413 ± 551	2803 ± 198

[a] Human PBL (5×10^4) were incubated in triplicate microcultures (100 μl) with anti-CD3 (64.1) or anti-CD8 (T94 and 51.1) antibodies or with medium for various periods of time. Numbers in the table indicate cpm [³H]thymidine incorporation ($\bar{X} \pm$ SEM) during the last four hours of culture.

Table 12.4. Proliferation of isolated subsets.

	Antibody T94	Phytohemagglutinin	Medium
PBL	6491 ± 227	79,647 ± 1398	609 ± 31
CD8⁺	738 ± 50	36,587 ± 8500	439 ± 45
CD4⁺	17,379 ± 1142	97,864 ± 1147	884 ± 423

Cells (5×10^4) were incubated in triplicate microcultures (100 μl) for three days with antibody T94 (diluted 1 : 400), phytohemagglutinin (2.5 μg/ml), or with medium. Numbers indicate cpm [³H]thymidine incorporation ($\bar{X} \pm$ SEM) during the last four hours of culture.

indirect immunofluorescence, with approximately 70% saturation of the binding sites (not shown). These data could suggest that a high degree of antigenic occupancy is required for the induction of optimal proliferative responses by this antibody.

The disparity between antibody binding and functional activity detected by titration suggested that the binding of antibody T94 might not be responsible for inducing cell proliferation. The effect of antibody T94 was therefore tested on CD8⁺ and CD4⁺ cells isolated by panning (16). If binding of the antibody were the cause of the proliferation, then it would be expected that CD8⁺ cells would respond and that CD4⁺ cells would not. The data in Table 12.4 shows to the contrary that antibody T94 triggered proliferation of CD4⁺ cells but not CD8⁺ cells. These findings indicate that the proliferation was unrelated to the binding of antibody T94. This observation, together with the finding that the peak response occurred on day five, suggests that the proliferation induced by this ascites fluid represented a soluble antigen response.

Discussion

The data reported here describe our findings concerning the ability of Workshop T cell antibodies to activate T cells or to enhance or block the ability of anti–T cell antibodies to activate T cells. This was accomplished by developing screening strategies that focused efficiently on a relatively small number of candidate antibodies. Further testing was then directed towards determining whether the observed functional effect was specific or whether it represented an artifact caused by contamination with a second antibody or other substance present in the ascites fluid.

We sought to identify antibodies that could modulate the mitogenic effect of an IgG2a anti-CD3 antibody. Tax *et al.* (17) have recently reported that IgG1 antibodies against CD2, CD8, and HLA-A,B,C, antigens could block the mitogenic effect of IgG1 anti-CD3 antibodies but not IgG2a anti-CD3 antibodies. IgG2a antibodies that recognize the CD2, CD8, and HLA-A,B,C blocked the mitogenic effect of both IgG1 and

IgG2a anti-CD3 antibodies. It was suggested that the inhibition by IgG1 antibodies might occur if certain soluble antibody–antigen complexes compete successfully for binding to monocyte Fc receptors, since Fc cross-linking is required for the mitogenic effect of anti-CD3 antibody binding (1,17–21). It was speculated that Ig class nonspecific inhibition could be caused by the interaction of immune complexes with monocyte Fc receptors for IgG2a, inducing the release of products such as prostaglandin E which can suppress lymphocyte proliferation.

Our results did not confirm the notion that the antigenic specificity was a major factor in determining whether an antibody could inhibit anti-CD3 induced proliferation even when only IgG2a antibodies were considered. Instead, it appeared that as a group, the Workshop antibodies caused a unimodal decrease in antibody 64.1-induced proliferation, suggesting that the effect was nonspecific. The magnitude of the inhibition was not as great as that described by other investigators. It is possible that more striking effects could have been overlooked in our experiments since each antibody was tested only as a single replicate at a final dilution of 1 : 200. Alternatively, the proliferation induced by antibody 64.1 may be intrinsically less susceptible to inhibition than the proliferation induced by other anti-CD3 antibodies.

One antibody designated KOLT-2 was capable of enhancing the mitogenic effect of antibody 64.1. Antibody 9.3, which was included in the First Workshop (4), has a similar effect on anti-CD3-induced proliferation. Thus, it was not entirely unexpected to find by immunofluorescence, immune precipitation, and competitive inhibition experiments that the KOLT-2 and 9.3 antibodies appear to recognize similar antigenic specificities. In other experiments, we have found that antibody 9.3 enhances the mitogenic effect of antibody 64.1 both by inducing increased IL-2 receptor expression and by increasing the secretion of IL-2.

Our strategy for identifying mitogenic non-CD3 antibodies involved several screening steps. The ability to induce proliferation of PBL after three days culture in the continuous presence of each antibody was first tested. Subsequent evaluation was carried out in order to determine whether the mitogenic antibody contained an anti-CD3 specificity. This was accomplished by competitive inhibition experiments with known anti-CD3 antibodies and by comparing the fluorescence histograms on CD3-modulated and unmodulated cells. Four of the 17 mitogenic antibodies, T62, T105, T94, and T128, appeared not to contain an anti-CD3 specificity by these criteria.

Further experiments were carried out with the use of cells from non-human primates. Although five of the six antibodies tested could bind to baboon PBL, only one had a mitogenic effect on these cells. The binding of antibodies T62 and T105 on baboon PBL was considerably decreased compared to the binding on human PBL. The mitogenic effect of these antibodies may require more surface binding than can be accommodated on baboon cells. Antibody T128, which was included in the CD1 group, did not bind to either human or baboon cells. It has not been tested whether this antibody can cause proliferation of human thymocytes. Antibody T94 did have a mitogenic effect on baboon cells, but further studies with human cells suggested that the proliferation was the result of triggering by soluble antigen. Studies with purified antibody might determine whether the soluble antigen was the antibody itself or something else present in the ascites fluid.

Summary

Mitogenic antibodies that recognize specificities other than CD3 and antibodies capable of inducing IL-2 receptor expression without IL-2 secretion were not identified among the Workshop T cell panel. The antibodies were also tested for their ability to modulate anti-CD3-induced T cell proliferation. Specific inhibition was not demonstrated, but antibody KOLT-2 enhanced the response. It was demonstrated by indirect immunofluorescence, immunoprecipitation, and cross-blocking that the antigen recognized by antibody KOLT-2 is similar to the one recognized by antibody 9.3, which was included in the first Workshop.

Acknowledgments. We thank Elizabeth Conger, Don Ellingsen, Ingrid Jennings, Gary Longton, and Gloria McDowell for technical assistance and Pauline Marsden for help in the preparation of the manuscript. This work was supported by U.S. Public Health Service grants CA29548 and CA18029 from the National Institutes of Health.

References

1. Van Wauwe, J.P., J.R. De Mey, and J.G. Goossens. 1980. OKT3: a monoclonal anti-human T lymphocyte antibody with potent mitogenic properties. *J. Immunol.* **124**:2708.
2. Van Agthoven, A., C. Terhorst, E. Reinherz, and S. Schlossman. 1981. Characterization of T cell surface glycoproteins T1 and T3 present on all human peripheral T lymphocytes and functionally mature thymocytes. *Eur. J. Immunol.* **11**:18.
3. Borst, J., M.A. Prendiville, and C. Terhorst. 1982. Complexity of the human T lymphocyte-specific cell surface antigen T3. *J. Immunol.* **128**:1560.
4. Hansen, J.A., P.J. Martin, P.G. Beatty, E.A. Clark, and J.A. Ledbetter. 1984. Human T lymphocyte cell surface molecules defined by the workshop monoclonal antibodies ("T cell protocol"). In: *Leucocyte typing,* A. Bernard, L. Boumsell, J. Dausset, C. Milstein, and S.F. Schlossman, eds. Springer-Verlag, Berlin, Heidelberg, pp. 195–212.
5. Meuer, S.C., O. Acuto, R.E. Hussey, J.C. Hodgdon, K.A. Fitzgerald, S.F. Schlossman, and E.L. Reinherz. 1983. Evidence for the T3-associated 90KD heterodimer as the T cell antigen receptor. *Nature* **303**:808.
6. Meuer, S.C., K.A. Fitzgerald, R.E. Hussey, J.C. Hodgdon, S.F. Schloss-

man, and E.L. Reinherz. 1983. Clonotypic structures involved in antigen specific human T cell function: Relationship to the T3 molecular complex. *J. Exp. Med.* **157**:705.

7. Meuer, S.C., O. Acuto, T. Hercend, S.F. Schlossman, and E.L. Reinherz. 1984. The human T-cell receptor. *Annu. Rev. Immunol.* **2**:23.

8. Van Wauwe, J.P., J.G. Goossens, and P.C.L. Beverley. 1984. Human T lymphocyte activation by monoclonal antibodies; OKT3, but not UCHT1, triggers mitogenesis via an interleukin 2-dependent mechanism. *J. Immunol.* **133**:129.

9. Van Wauwe, J.P., J. Goossens, W. Decock, P. Kung, and G. Goldstein. 1981. Suppression of human T-cell mitogenesis and E-rosette formation by the monoclonal antibody OKT11A. *Immunology* **44**:865.

10. Martin P.J., G. Longton, J.A. Ledbetter, W. Newman, M.P. Braun, P.G. Beatty, and J.A. Hansen. 1983. Identification and functional characterization of two distinct epitopes on the human T cell surface protein Tp50. *J. Immunol.* **131**:180.

11. Miyakawa, T., A. Yachie, N. Uwadana, S. Ohzeki, T. Nagaoki, and N. Taniguchi. 1982. Functional significance of Tac antigen expressed on activated human T lymphocyte: Tac antigen interacts with T cell growth factor in cellular proliferation. *J. Immunol.* **129**:2474.

12. Depper, J.M., W.J. Leonard, R.J. Robb, T.A. Waldmann, and W.C. Greene. 1983. Blockade of the interleukin 2 receptor by anti-Tac antibody: inhibition of human lymphocyte activation. *J. Immunol.* **131**:690.

13. Goding, J.W. 1976. Conjugation of antibodies with fluorochromes: modifications to the standard methods. *J. Immunol. Methods* **13**:215.

14. Ey, P.L., S.J. Prowse, and C.R. Jenkin. 1978. Isolation of pure IgG_1, IgG_{2a}, and IgG_{2b} immunoglobulins from mouse serum using protein A-Sepharose. *Immunochem.* **15**:429.

15. Martin, P.J., J.A. Ledbetter, E.A. Clark, P.G. Beatty, and J.A. Hansen. 1984. Epitope mapping of the human surface suppressor/cytotoxic T cell molecule Tp32. *J. Immunol.* **132**:759.

16. Wysocki, L.J., and V.L. Sato. 1978. Panning for lymphocytes. A method of cell separation. *Proc. Natl. Acad. Sci. U.S.A.* **75**:2844.

17. Tax, W.J.M., F.F.M. Hermes, R.W. Willems, P.J.A. Capel, and R.A.P. Koene. 1984. Fc receptors for mouse IgG1 on human monocytes: polymorphism and role in antibody-induced T cell proliferation. *J. Immunol.* **133**:1185.

18. Van Wauwe, J.P., and J.G. Goossens. 1981. Mitogenic actions of Orthoclone OKT3 on human peripheral blood lymphocytes: effects of monocytes and serum components. *Int. J. Immunopharmacol.* **3**:203.

19. Tax, W.J.M., H.W. Willems, P.P.M. Reekers, P.J.A. Capel, and R.A.P. Koene. 1983. Polymorphism in mitogenic effect of IgG1 monoclonal antibodies against T3 antigen on human T cells. *Nature* **304**:445.

20. Kaneoka, H., G. Perez-Rojas, T. Sasasuki, C.J. Benike, and E.G. Engleman. 1983. Human T lymphocyte proliferation induced by a pan-T monoclonal antibody (anti-Leu-4): heterogeneity of response is a function of monocytes. *J. Immunol.* **131**:158.

21. Van Wauwe, J.P., and J. Goossens. 1983. The mitogenic activity of OKT3 and anti-Leu-4 monoclonal antibodies: a comparative study. *Cell. Immunol.* **77**:23.

CHAPTER 13

Phorbol Ester Induces Changes in the Pattern of Cell Surface Molecules Involved in CTL–Target Cell Interaction

Istvan Ando, Dorothy H. Crawford, and
Peter C.L. Beverley

Introduction

Antigen recognition by cytotoxic T lymphocytes (CTLs) is mediated via cell surface molecules (1,2). These involve the T3 molecular complex and the T4, T8, and T11 antigens. Phorbol esters induce a variety of phenotypic changes in lymphocytes, e.g., increased expression of the receptor for interleukin-2 (IL-2) and temporary down-modulation of the T3 receptor complex (3). These phenotypic changes are paralleled by an increased sensitivity to IL-2 and a temporary unresponsiveness to antigen (3). To further characterize the functional changes which accompany the alterations in phenotype we monitored the phorbol ester-induced antigenic changes of cytotoxic T cells defined by monoclonal antibodies to the T11, T8, and T3 molecules and correlated them with the functional changes which occur after phorbol ester stimulation. It was found that after treatment with this most potent tumor promoter—phorbol ester, 12-O-tetradecanoylphorbol-13-acetate (TPA)—the amount of T3, T4, and T8 molecules decreased on the cell surface while T11 increased. These phenotypic changes are paralleled by temporary loss of cytotoxic activity.

Materials and Methods

Materials

TPA and fluorescein-conjugated anti–mouse immunoglobulin were purchased from Sigma, ^{51}Cr was obtained from Amersham International. RPMI 1640 tissue culture medium and fetal calf serum were obtained from Gibco.

Culture Conditions

Cytotoxic T cells were generated with slight modifications of the method described by Moss *et al.* (4). Briefly, 10^6 E$^+$ cells from a healthy donor were cultured in the presence of 4000R irradiated autologous Epstein–Barr virus transformed lymphoblastoid B cell lines (EBV lines) in RPMI 1640 tissue culture medium supplemented with 10% fetal calf serum, glutamine penicillin, and streptomycin. Ten days later the E$^+$ cells were rosetted and restimulated with irradiated EBV line as above in the presence of 20% TCGF from which the phytohemagglutinin was removed and restimulated four times with antigen and TCGF at 10-day intervals. After this the T cells were cloned at 0.3 cell per well density in round-bottomed microtiter plates in the presence of 5×10^4 irradiated EBV cells and 20% TCGF in 200-μl final volume. Growing colonies were expanded in 24-well Costar wells tested for cytotoxic activity and for expression of T cell antigens. Clone C2a is a T3$^+$T8$^+$T4$^-$ MHC class I antigen (HLA-A2) restricted cytotoxic cell line.

Cytotoxic Assay

Cytotoxic activity of the cells was determined in a 4-hr ^{51}Cr release assay using 5×10^3 target cells per well. The spontaneous isotope release was usually <15%.

Stimulation of the Cells with TPA

Cells were seeded at a density of 5×10^5/ml in 24-well Costar plates and TPA (dissolved at 1 mg/ml concentration in DMSO) was added to the cultures at 10 ng/ml concentration. An equal amount of DMSO was used in control cultures.

Antiserum Treatment of the Cells

Cytotoxic T cells (5×10^4/well) were seeded into the wells of U-bottomed microtiter plates in 50-μl complete RPMI 1640 medium and 50-μl antiserum diluted to 1 : 100 was added. The cells were incubated with the antisera for 1 hr at 37°C. Target cells were added in 100-μl volume.

Indirect Immunofluorescence

Cells (5×10^5) were incubated with antibodies (1 : 100) for 1 hr at +4°C, washed three times, and after addition of fluorescein-labeled anti–mouse Ig at appropriate dilution, incubated for 1 hr at +4°C on ice. After three further washes cells were analyzed on a FACS I equipment for fluorescence intensity using a linear amplifier.

Results

Effect of Monoclonal Antibodies on CTL Activity

Antibodies, of CD2, CD8, and CD3 groups, were analyzed for the capacity to block CTL activity of clone C2a. Table 13.1 shows the antibodies which caused more than 50% reduction of CTL activity.

Effect of TPA Treatment on CTL Activity and Phenotype

Cytotoxic T cells were incubated in RPMI 1640 medium in the presence of 20% TCGF. TPA was added to the cultures and the cytotoxic activity of the cells was determined after 12 and 24 hr (Table 13.2). The 12-hr TPA treatment abrogated the cytotoxic activity of the cells. When the cell surface antigens of the cells were analyzed (Table 13.3) an increased level of T11 antigen and a reduced amount of T3 and T8 antigen were seen. In order to study the recovery of cytotoxic activity from TPA treatment, the cells were washed free of TPA after a 12-hr incubation period and seeded into the wells of 24-well Costar plates (5×10^5/ml). Samples of cells were

Table 13.1. The CD2, CD8, and CD3 antibodies which inhibit cell-mediated lympholysis by clone C2a(T3$^+$T8$^+$T4$^-$).

Antibody group	Antibody name	Antibody group	Antibody name
CD2	OKT11	CD3	*Leu 4*
	G19-3.1		*89B1*
	S2/Leu 5b		BW264/56
	MT 26		BW242/55
	MT 910		T3/2Ad2A2
	MT 1110		T3/2T8-2F4
	T11/3Pt2H9		T3/RW2-4B6
	T11/ROLD2-1H8		T3/RW2-8C8
	T11/3T4-8B5		X35-3
	T11/7T4-7E10		NU-T1
	9.6		
	T4IIB5		
CD8	UCHT-4		
	M236		
	G10-1.1		
	C12/D3		
	BW135/80		
	MT 415		
	MT 1014		
	MT 122		
	T8/21thy2D3		
	T8/2T8-2A1		
	T8/2T8-1B5		
	66.2		
	51.1		

Table 13.2. The effect of TPA treatment on the CML activity of clone C2a.

Treatment of effector cells	Percent reduction of CML activity by TPA at E : T		
	1 : 1	0.5 : 1	0.25 : 1
TPA for 12 hours	88	92	100
TPA for 24 hours	84	92	99
12 hours[a]	75	81	85
24 hours[a]	71	80	82
48 hours[a]	43	47	48
72 hours[a]	2	5	3

[a] Cells were treated with TPA for 12 hours, washed, and incubated for the times indicated.

harvested 12, 24, and 72 hr after removal of TPA and the cytotoxic activity and the phenotype of the cells were determined by indirect immunofluorescence (Tables 13.2 and 13.3). It was found that the full cytotoxic activity of the cells returned to normal 48–72 hr after removal of TPA as did T11, T3, and T8 antigens.

Discussion

Tumor promoter phorbol esters induce a variety of phenotypic changes in T lymphocytes, T cell tumors, and cloned T cell lines (5,6). In previous studies we have demonstrated that treatment of cloned T lymphocyte lines with phorbol esters results in a marked increase in the density of IL-2 receptor and loss of the T3 receptor complex from the cell surface (3).

Table 13.3. Fluorescence intensity of TPA treated and control C2a cells stained with OKT11, UCHT4, and Leu 4 monoclonal antibodies.

Treatment of cells	Cells stained with			
	Nonstain	OKT11	UCHT4	Leu 4
None	29	46	81	75
TPA for 12 hours	24	89	34	35
TPA for 24 hours	22	134	37	31
12 hours[b]	22	159	31	34
24 hours[b]	31	171	37	39
48 hours[b]	28	115	57	49
72 hours[b]	25	59	96	83

[a] Figures in the tables are fluorescence peak channel number which is an index of the overall fluorescence intensity of the cell population.
[b] Cells were treated with TPA for 12 hours washed and incubated for the times indicated.

These phenotypic changes are paralleled by increased sensitivity to IL-2 and temporary inability to proliferate in response to specific antigen. From the data presented here it can be seen that CD2, CD8, and CD3 group antibodies reduce the cytotoxic capacity of a T8$^+$ T cell clone. This confirms the previous findings that T11, T8, and T3 molecules are involved in effector–target cell interactions. After phorbol ester treatment the density of these antigens changes dramatically. The amount of the T11 antigen increases while the cytotoxic cells lose T3, T8, and T4 (unpublished results) antigens. These changes are paralleled by an inability to lyse specific target cells.

Several mechanisms can be considered to explain this phenomenon. Firstly, TPA temporarily inactivates the lytic apparatus of cytotoxic T lymphocytes. Secondly, phorbol esters down-regulate the expression of cell surface molecules which are involved in attacker–target cell interactions. At present we cannot distinguish between these two mechanisms but the down-regulation of the antigen-specific receptor complex and the T8 or T4 antigens could be a part of this process.

Summary

After tumor promoter phorbol ester treatment of a T8$^+$ MHC class I antigen restricted cloned cytotoxic T cell line, the capacity of the line to lyse autologous Epstein–Barr virus transformed lymphoblastoid B cell lines is abrogated. At the same time the pattern of the cell surface molecules defined by the Workshop antibodies (in groups CD2, CD8, and CD3) and involved in CTL–target cell interaction is altered, e.g., the amount of T11 antigen increases while cells lose T8 antigen and the T3 receptor complex. These phenotypic changes, in particular changes of T8 and T3 antigen density, might be responsible for the reduction of cytotoxic activity.

Acknowledgments. This work was partly supported by the Wellcome Trust. I.A. is a holder of a long-term EMBO Fellowship on leave from the Biological Research Center of the Hungarian Academy of Sciences.

References

1. Reinherz, E.L., S.C. Meuer, and S.F. Schlossman. 1983. The human T-cell receptor: Analysis with cytotoxic T cell clones. *Immunol. Rev.* **74**:83.
2. Dongworth, D.W., F.M. Gotch, N.P. Carter, P.D.K. Hildreth, and A.J.M. McMichael. 1984. Inhibition of virus-specific HLA-restricted, T-cell mediated lysis by monoclonal anti T-cell antibodies. In: Leucocyte typing, A. Bernard, L. Boumsell, J. Dausset, C. Milstein, and S.F. Schlossman, eds. Springer-Verlag, Berlin, Heidelberg, p. 320.

3. Ando, I., G. Hariri, D. Wallace, and P.C.L. Beverley. 1985. Tumor promoter phorbol esters induce unresponsiveness to antigen and expression of inter-leukin-2 receptor on T cells. *Eur. J. Immunol.* **15**:196.
4. Moss, D.J., A.B. Rickinson, L.E. Wallace, and M.A. Epstein. 1981. Sequential appearance of Epstein–Barr virus nuclear and lymphocyte-detected membrane antigens in B cell transformation. *Nature* **291**:664.
5. Delia, D., M.F. Greaves, R.A. Newman, J. Minowada, P. Kung, and G. Goldstein. 1982. Modulation of T leukaemic cell phenotype with phorbol ester. *Int. J. Cancer* **29**:23.
6. Cassel, D.L., J.A. Hoxie, and R.A. Cooper. 1983. Phorbol ester modulation of T-cell antigens in the Jurkat lymphoblastoid leukaemia cell line. *Cancer Res.* **43**:4582.

CHAPTER 14

Analysis of the Monocyte–T Cell Interaction Required for Induction of T Cell Proliferation by Anti-T3 Antibodies

Loran T. Clement

Introduction

The T3 antigen is present on membrane molecules which are expressed by all post-thymic T lymphocytes (1). Studies using monoclonal antibodies reactive with the T3 antigen have provided evidence that this antigen is closely associated with the T cell antigen receptor (2,3). One interesting and perhaps related property of anti-T3 antibodies is their ability to induce T cells to proliferate (4). This response to cross-linkage of T3 antigens is strictly dependent on the presence of accessory cells (5,6). Accordingly, the available evidence suggests that T cell activation produced in this fashion is accomplished by a two-signal mechanism, the first signal being provided by cross-linkage of the T3 antigens on the T cell membrane, while the second signal is derived from antibody-mediated T cell–monocyte interactions.

In the studies described herein, the mitogenic properties of the antibodies in the CD3 Workshop panel have been analyzed. In addition, pan-T cell antibodies from the CD3 and CD5 (anti-p67) Workshop panels have been used in co-culture experiments to analyze the nature of the monocyte receptors and cellular interactions involved in the induction of T cell proliferation by anti-T3 antibodies.

Materials and Methods

Cell Preparations

Peripheral blood mononuclear cells from healthy adults were isolated by Ficoll–Hypaque density gradient centrifugation. Monocytes were isolated by adherence to plastic, then harvested by scraping. T cells were isolated by rosette formation with sheep erythrocytes (E) and density gradient centrifugation (7).

Immunofluorescence Analysis

Methods for indirect immunofluorescent analysis of antigen expression and for determining the heavy-chain isotype of T cell-reactive antibodies have been described (8). Fluorescein (FITC)-conjugated, affinity-purified goat antibodies specific for murine μ, $\gamma 1$, $\gamma 2a$, $\gamma 2b$, and $\gamma 3$ heavy chains were used as the secondary antibodies. Directly conjugated FITC–Leu-4 antibodies were obtained from Becton-Dickson (Mountain View, CA). Reactivity was assessed with a fluorescence-activated cell sorter (FACS IV, Becton-Dickinson) equipped with a logarithmic amplifier.

Assessment of Antibody Reactivity with the Leu-4 Antigen

The reactivity of Workshop antibodies with the Leu-4 antigen was assessed by two methods. First, in direct blocking experiments, E[+] cells[1] (1×10^6) were incubated with a 1 : 100 dilution of the Workshop antibody (predetermined for each antibody to be in excess of that needed for saturating all binding sites). Control cells were incubated in medium alone or in medium containing an excess of the Leu-4 or Leu-1 antibodies. After 30 min on ice, directly conjugated FITC–Leu-4 antibody was added, and cells were incubated an additional 15 min on ice. Cells were then washed, and the relative fluorescent staining intensity of the FITC–Leu-4 antibody determined by flow cytometry. In addition, the ability of the Workshop antibodies to modulate the Leu-4 antigen was assessed. E[+]cells were incubated at 37°C for 24 hr in RPMI 1640 medium containing 10% fetal calf serum and a 1 : 2000 dilution of the test antibody. Control samples included cells in medium only or in suitable dilutions of the Leu-4 and Leu-1 antibodies. After incubation, each cell sample was washed and stained with either FITC–goat anti–mouse Ig antibodies or FITC–Leu-4 antibodies. Modulation of the antigen reactive with the workshop antibody and of the Leu-4 antigen was then determined by flow cytometry.

Assessment of T Cell Proliferation

E[+] cells $(1 \times 10^5/\text{well})$ supplemented with 15% adherent cells were cultured for 72 hr at 37°C in triplicate flat-bottom microtiter wells in RPMI 1640 medium containing 15% fetal calf serum, glutamine, and gentamicin. Antibodies from the CD3 Workshop panel (nos. 117–127) and the CD5 panel (nos. 4, 5, and 7) were dialyzed to remove NaN$_3$, sterilized, and

---

[1] E[+]: expressing receptors for sheep erythrocytes.

added at various dilutions alone or in combination. Cultures were pulsed with [³H]thymidine (³H-TdR, 1 μCi/well) during the final 16–18 hr of culture, and ³H-TdR uptake was determined by scintillation counting.

Results

Selected Characteristics of CD3 Workshop Panel Antibodies

Preliminary analyses of the eleven antibodies comprising the CD3 Workshop panel (antibodies 117–127) were performed to assess their cellular reactivity pattern, heavy chain isotype, and reactivity with the T3/Leu-4 antigen. All eleven antibodies reacted specifically with comparable percentages of E⁺ lymphocytes, although the staining intensity of antibodies 123 and 127 was somewhat lower than that of the other antibodies. When the heavy-chain isotype of the antibodies reactive with E⁺ cells was analyzed with a panel of FITC-conjugated goat antibodies specific for murine heavy chains, nine of the samples contained reactive antibodies of a single isotype, while two samples had two or more classes of T-reactive antibodies (Table 14.1). Antigen modulation experiments and binding inhibition studies using the CD3 antibodies and FITC–Leu-4 antibodies demonstrated that nine of the eleven samples contained antibodies which modulated the T3/Leu-4 antigen from the T cell surface and which blocked (to a variable extent) the binding of FITC–Leu-4 antibodies.

Table 14.1. Selected characteristics of antibodies in the CD3 panel.

CD3 Antibody	Isotype of T cell-reactive antibodies	Modulation of Leu-4 antigen[a]	Blocking of anti–Leu-4 reactivity[b]	Mitogenic properties[c]
117	IgG1	+	+++	+
118	IgG1	+	+++	+
119	IgG1,IgG2a	+	+++	+
120	IgG2a	+	++	+
121	IgG1,2a,2b,3	+	+	+
122	IgM	+	+	0
123	IgG1	0	0	0
124	IgG2b	+	+	0
125	IgG1	+	+	+
126	IgG2a	+	+	+
127	IgG1	0	0	0

[a] E⁺ cells were incubated with a 1 : 200 dilution of the CD3 panel antibody at 37°C for 24 hr, then washed, stained with Leu-4–FITC antibodies, and analyzed with the FACS. The (+) denotes modulation of the Leu-4 antigen; the (0) denotes lack of Leu-4 antigenic modulation.
[b] E⁺ cells were pretreated with an excess of the CD3 panel antibody at 4°C for 30 min, then stained with Leu-4–FITC antibodies and analyzed with the FACS. The relative blocking of Leu-4 reactivity was graded from 0 (= no blocking) to +++ (= complete blocking).
[c] Based on the ability to induce a T cell proliferative response >6,000 cpm in cells from any of nine donors.

The mitogenic properties of these antibodies, which are discussed in detail below, are also summarized in Table 14.1. Seven of the CD3 antibodies were mitogenic for T cells from some, if not all, of the nine donors tested, while four of the antibodies did not induce T cell proliferation in any individual. On the basis of their demonstrated reactivity with the T3/Leu-4 antigen or their isotypic characteristics, eight CD3 antibodies (nos. 117–120, 122, 124–126) were selected for use in the subsequent experiments.

Mitogenic Properties of Anti-T3 Antibodies

The mitogenic properties of the anti-T3 antibodies were assessed by culturing E^+ cells and monocytes with serial tenfold dilutions (ranging from 10^{-3} to 10^{-7}) of dialyzed ascites samples. In Table 14.2, results from four representative donors (and the mean proliferative responses for nine donors) are shown for experiments using antibodies 120, 122, 124, and 126. Antibody 122, an IgM antibody, and antibody 124, and IgG2b reagent, induced virtually no T cell proliferation at any dilution in any individual. In contrast, the two IgG2a antibodies (nos. 120 and 126) had potent mitogenic effects on cells from all subjects.

When the four IgG1 antibodies reactive with the T3/Leu-4 antigen were similarly tested, contrasting results were obtained. Representative results using various dilutions of two of these antibodies (nos. 117 and 118) and cells from eight different donors are shown in Figure 14.1. Two distinct response patterns were observed. At the lowest dilution tested, all donors had a significant proliferative response to these IgG1 anti-T3 antibodies,

Table 14.2. Mitogenic properties of IgM, IgG2b, and IgG2a anti-T3 antibodies.

Anti-T3 antibody	T cell proliferative response (^{3}H-TdR cpm)[a]				
	Donor 1	Donor 2	Donor 3	Donor 4	Mean[b]
None	448	617	550	450	487 ± 156
Antibody 122[c]	412	723	1,226	828	936 ± 432
(IgM)					
Antibody 124[c]	3,317	1,405	3,078	885	2,316 ± 1,040
(IgG2b)					
Antibody 120[d]	109,893	76,576	100,240	85,313	89,346 ± 15,320
(IgG2a)					
Antibody 126[d]	98,243	76,398	110,661	81,594	87,633 ± 17,070
(IgG2a)					

[a] E^+ cells (1×10^5) supplemented with 15% autologous adherent cells were cultured in triplicate wells for 72 hr with the indicated anti-T3 antibodies. Cells were pulsed with [^{3}H]thymidine (^{3}H-TdR) during the final 16 hr of culture, and ^{3}H-TdR uptake determined.
[b] Mean ^{3}H-TdR cpm ± 1SD for cells from 9 donors.
[c] Antibodies 122 and 124 were used at a 1 : 10,000 final dilution. Similar results were obtained using dilutions of 1 : 1000 to 1 : 1,000,000.
[d] Antibodies 120 and 126 were used at dilutions predetermined to induce maximal ^{3}H-TdR incorporation (1 : 200,000 and 1 : 100,000, respectively).

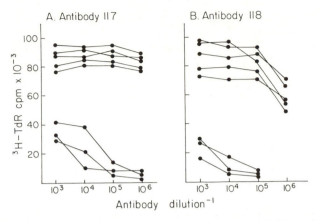

Fig. 14.1. Heterogeneity of T cell proliferative responses to IgG1 anti-T3 antibodies. Dose–response studies using cells from eight donors and varying dilutions of two different IgG1 anti-T3 antibodies reveal two distinct response patterns.

although the magnitude of the responses was variable. As the concentration of IgG1 anti-T3 antibodies declined, the T cell proliferative response of some donors rapidly declined to baseline levels. In other donors, however, maximal ^{3}H-TdR uptake was still observed at antibody concentrations 20,000-fold lower than those required for responses by cells from "low responders." Comparable results were observed with antibodies 119 and 125. These data demonstrate that the mitogenic properties of anti-T3 antibodies are influenced by the heavy-chain isotype of the antibody. Whereas IgG2a antibodies are mitogenic for cells from all subjects, donor heterogeneity is seen for responses to a given concentration of IgG1 anti-T3 antibodies. Antibodies of the IgM and IgG2b classes do not induce T cell proliferation.

Cellular Basis for the Heterogeneity of Proliferative Responses Induced by IgG1 Anti-T3 Antibodies

Previous studies using IgG1 anti-T3 antibodies have demonstrated responder heterogeneity which is determined by the monocyte phenotype (5,6,9,10). To determine whether this observation was also applicable to the IgG1 anti-T3 antibodies in the Workshop panel, cell mixing experiments were performed. E$^+$ cells and monocytes purified from high-responder (HR) and low-responder (LR) donors were co-cultured in various combinations with each IgG1 anti-T3 antibody, and ^{3}H-TdR uptake was determined. One representative experiment is shown in Table 14.3. For each IgG1 anti-T3 antibody, HR monocytes supported a vigorous T cell proliferative response, irrespective of the responder status of the T cell donor. In contrast, monocytes from LR donors were inefficient in this

Table 14.3. The proliferative response of IgG1 anti-T3 antibodies is determined by the phenotype of the monocyte.

Cells in culture[a]		Proliferative response (^{3}H-TdR cpm) induced by:[b]			
T cells	Monocytes	Antibody 117	Antibody 118	Antibody 119	Antibody 125
HR	HR	70,915	71,516	61,848	66,412
HR	LR	20,677	6,880	2,261	1,410
LR	HR	73,255	75,080	76,250	58,222
LR	LR	15,825	4,438	8,242	1,402

[a] T cells and monocytes were isolated from donors who were either high-responders (HR) or low-responders (LR) to IgG1 anti-T3 antibodies, and cell mixing experiments were performed with the four IgG1 anti-T3 antibodies.
[b] All antibodies were present at a 1 : 10,000 final dilution.

regard for all T cells. Experiments using monocytes from two other LR donors gave similar results. Hence, the inability of monocytes from certain individuals to support T cell proliferative responses at lower IgG1 anti-T3 antibody concentrations appears to be generally applicable to all antibodies of this subclass.

Analysis of Monocyte Receptors and T Cell–Monocyte Interactions

To analyze the nature of the interactions of antibody, T cells, and monocytes which result in T cell proliferation, a series of experiments were performed using different anti-T3 antibodies and selected antibodies from the CD5 panel, which was comprised of monoclonal antibodies reactive with the p67 pan-T cell antigen. Three CD5 antibodies were employed: antibody 4 (an IgG1 antibody) and antibodies 5 and 7 (which were IgG2a antibodies). Preliminary analyses indicated that each of these ascites samples contained a single class of T cell-reactive antibodies which did not modulate the Leu-4 antigen or induce T cell proliferation in any donors.

In Table 14.4, composite data from a representative experiment of this nature are presented. Varying concentrations of either antibody 7 (an

Table 14.4. Effects of CD5 (anti-p67) antibodies on the response to anti-T3 antibodies.[a]

CD5 antibody	Dilution^{-1}	Proliferative response (^{3}H-TdR cpm) induced by:[b]			
		Ab.122 (IgM)	Ab.124 (IgG2b)	Ab.126 (IgG2a)	Ab.118 (IgG1)
None	—	816	2,122	118,333	91,688
Antibody 7	10^3	636	3,821	59,124	85,433
(IgG2a)	10^4	916	3,017	78,120	86,573
Antibody 4	10^3	884	2,836	116,076	39,816
(IgG1)	10^4	662	4,032	119,431	58,188

[a] E$^+$ cells and adherent cells were cultured with the indicated anti-T3 antibodies and dilutions of two CD5 (anti-p67) antibodies. ^{3}H-TdR uptake was determined as before.
[b] Antibodies 122 and 124 were used at 1 : 1000 dilutions; antibodies 126 and 118 were used at 1 : 100,000 dilutions.

IgG2a antibody from the CD5 panel) or antibody 4 (an IgG1 CD5 antibody) were added to cultures containing different anti-T3 (CD3) antibodies. The addition of antibody 7 inhibited the mitogenic effect of the IgG2a anti-T3 antibody (no. 126) but did not affect the response induced by antibody 118, an IgG1 anti-T3 reagent. Conversely, antibody 4, an IgG1 monoclonal, inhibited only the proliferation induced by the IgG1 anti-T3 antibody. When these CD5 antibodies were co-cultured with IgM or IgG2b anti-T3 antibodies (nos. 122 or 124), no T cell proliferation was observed. Comparable data were obtained in three other experiments using antibody 5 (IgG2a) from the CD5 panel, cells from different donors, or other mitogenic anti-T3 antibodies. As discussed below, these data suggest that monocytes have two dissimilar Fc receptors for murine IgG2a and IgG1 antibodies. In addition, it appears that the signals required for anti-T3-induced T cell proliferation require an intimate association of the T3 antigen with the monocyte membrane.

Discussion

Monoclonal antibodies from the CD3 and CD5 Workshop panels have been used in a series of experiments investigating several aspects of the interactions between anti-T3 antibodies, T cells, and monocytes which result in T cell proliferation. One factor which determines the mitogenic properties of a murine anti-T3 antibody is its heavy-chain isotype. The two IgG2a anti-T3 antibodies in the CD3 Workshop panel were mitogenic for all individuals tested, a finding consistent with results obtained using other IgG2a anti-T3 antibodies such as OKT3 (4–6). Comparable analyses with four IgG1 antibodies reactive with the T3/Leu-4 antigen revealed two distinct response patterns. Whereas high concentrations of each of these IgG1 antibodies induced T cell proliferative responses >15,000 cpm in all donors, monocytes from high-responder individuals could support vigorous proliferation at concentrations 20,000-fold lower than those required for responses by T cells cultured with low-responder monocytes. Heterogeneity of mitogenic responses to other IgG1 antibodies (i.e., UCHTI and Leu-4) has been previously reported and shown to be determined by the phenotype of the monocyte (5,6,9,10). The results for IgG1 antibodies presented herein are therefore in general agreement with these previous reports. They differ in one regard, however, in that the monocyte defect of low-responder monocytes could induce significant T cell proliferation. Finally, IgM and IgG2b antibodies reactive with the T3/Leu-4 antigen did not induce proliferation of T cells from any donor.

One possible explanation for the isotype-related differences in the mitogenic properties of anti-T3 antibodies is that murine antibodies differ in their ability to bind to Fc receptors on human monocytes. According to this model hypothesis, monocytes from all humans express functional Fc receptors for murine IgG2a antibodies. In contrast, the expression of functional receptors for IgG1 antibodies is heterogeneous, with low-responder individuals having either inadequate numbers of Fc receptors for IgG1 antibodies or receptors with very low affinity for these molecules. In the present studies, CD5 (anti-p67) IgG2a antibodies bound to the T cell surface could inhibit the mitogenic response induced by IgG2a anti-T3 antibodies but did not affect IgG1 anti-T3–induced mitogenesis. Similarly, IgG1 antibodies from the CD5 panel selectively inhibited the effects of IgG1 anti-T3 antibodies. These data therefore suggest that the Fc receptors for murine IgG2a and IgG1 antibodies are distinct from one another. Finally, the data herein suggest that human monocytes do not have functional receptors for murine IgM or IgG2b antibodies.

Previous studies of the mechanism involved in T cell activation by anti-T3 antibodies have indicated that two signals are required (11). One signal is provided by perturbation of T3 membrane antigens by antibody while a second signal is derived from accessory cells (or, in some instances, by treatment with phorbol diesters). Because IgM and IgG2b antibodies reactive with T3 antigens were deficient in their ability to induce T cell proliferation, experiments were performed to determine whether this defect could be circumvented with other antibody-mediated stimuli. When T cells were treated with IgM or IgG2b anti-T3 antibodies (to cross-link T3 antigens) and also IgG2a or IgG1 antibodies from the CD5 panel (to provide T cell-bound antibody molecules capable of binding to monocyte Fc receptors), no T cell proliferation was observed. Hence, the two signals required for T cell activation are not independent of one another, i.e., cross-linkage of T3 antigens with one antibody and Fc receptor-mediated T cell–monocyte interactions by another antibody are not sufficient. Rather, it appears that the cross-linked T3 molecules (or closely associated structures) must be intimately associated with monocyte Fc receptors (or other membrane components) for coordinated expression of the two signals required for T cell proliferation.

Summary

Monoclonal antibodies from the CD5 and CD3 Workshop panels have been used to analyze the T cell–monocyte interactions required for the induction of T cell proliferation by anti-T3 antibodies. Dose–response analyses with eight anti-T3 antibodies indicated that their mitogenic properties were a function of their heavy-chain isotype. IgM and IgG2b anti-T3 antibodies were nonmitogenic for cells from all individuals, while IgG2a antibodies induced proliferation in all donors. Cell mixing experiments and dose–response studies with four IgG1 anti-T3 antibodies revealed donor heterogeneity at the monocyte level. Whereas all individuals responded to very high concentrations of each IgG1 antibody, monocytes from high-responder donors could mediate maximal proliferative responses at concentrations 20,000-fold lower than those required for low responders. Co-culture experiments using the anti-T3 panel and pan-T (anti-p67) antibodies from the CD5 panel demonstrated that 1) CD5 antibodies of the IgG2a class selectively inhibited the mitogenic effects of IgG2a anti-T3 antibodies but could not provide the required signal to monocytes to allow responses to IgG2b or IgM anti-T3 antibodies and 2) CD5 antibodies of the IgG1 isotype selectively inhibited responses induced by IgG1 anti-T3 antibodies. These data suggest that monocytes have two different Fc receptors which mediate anti-T3-induced proliferation: one receptor binds IgG2a antibodies and is functionally homogeneous among humans, while a second receptor site binds IgG1 and shows considerable functional heterogeneity. Furthermore, a direct antibody-mediated interaction of the T3 molecule with the monocyte membrane appears to be necessary for mitogenesis.

Acknowledgment. These studies were supported in part by grants CA 16673, CA 13148, and 5MO1-RR2—DRR/NIH, awarded by the National Institutes of Health.

References

1. Kung, P.C., G. Goldstein, E.L. Reinherz, and S.F. Schlossman. 1979. Monoclonal antibodies defining distinctive human T cell surface antigens. *Science* **206**:347.
2. Meuer, S.C., K.A. Fitzgerald, R.E. Hussey, J.C. Hodgdon, S.F. Schlossman, and E.L. Reinherz. 1983. Clonotype structures involved in antigen-specific human T cell function. Relationship to the T3 molecular complex. *J. Exp. Med.* **157**:705.
3. Meuer, S.C., O. Acuto, R.E. Hussey, J.C. Hodgdon, K.A. Fitzgerald, S.F. Schlossman, and E.L. Reinherz. 1983. Evidence for the T3-associated 90 Kd heterodimer as the T-cell antigen receptor. *Nature* **303**:808.
4. Van Wauwe, J.P., J.R. De Mey, and J.G. Goossens. 1980. OKT3: a monoclonal anti-human T lymphocyte antibody with potent mitogenic properties. *J. Immunol.* **124**:2708.
5. Van Wauwe, J.P., and J.G. Goossens. 1981. Mitogenic actions of orthoclone OKT3 on human peripheral blood lymphocytes: effects of monocytes and serum components. *Int. J. Immunopharmac.* **3**:203.
6. Kanoka, H., G. Perez-Rojas, T. Sasasuki, C.J. Benike, and E.G. Engleman. 1983. Human T lymphocyte proliferation induced by a pan-T monoclonal antibody (anti-Leu 4): heterogeneity of response is a function of monocytes. *J. Immunol.* **131**:158.
7. Pellegrino, M.A., S. Ferrone, M.P. Dierich, and R.A. Reisfield. 1975. Enhancement of sheep red blood cell–human lymphocyte rosette formation by the sulfhydryl compound 2-aminoethylisothiouronium bromide. *Clin. Immunol. Immunopathol.* **23**:324.
8. Tedder, T.F., L.T. Clement, and M.D. Cooper. 1984. Expression of C3d

receptors during human B cell differentiation: Immunofluorescent analysis with the HB-5 monoclonal antibody. *J. Immunol.* **133:**678.

9. Tax, W.J.M., H.W. Willems, P.P.M. Reekers, P.J.A. Capel, and R.A.P. Koene. 1983. Polymorphism in mitogenic effect of IgG monoclonal antibodies against T3 antigen on human T cells. *Nature* **304:**445.

10. Van Wauwe, J.P., and J. Goossens. 1983. The mitogenic activity of OKT3 and anti-Leu 4 monoclonal antibodies: a comparative study. *Cell. Immunol.* **77:**23.

11. Weiss, A., R.L. Wiskocil, and J. Stobo. 1984. The role of T3 surface molecules in the activation of human T-cells. A two-stimulus requirement for IL-2 production reflects events occurring at a pre-translational level. *J. Immunol.* **133:**123.

CHAPTER 15

Evaluation of the T Cell Workshop Monoclonal Antibodies in *In Vitro* Lymphocyte Proliferation Assays

Nicolas L. von Jeney, Katja Olas, and Walter Knapp

Monoclonal antibodies (mAbs) specifically recognizing surface structures of human lymphocytes are potentially useful for the modulation of the immune response. Thus, antibodies directed against CD3, a molecule present on all mature T cells where it is associated with the T cell antigen receptor (1–3), are mitogenic for these cells (4–9). These antibodies, on the other hand, can block the induction and further functioning of T cells (6,9–13), apparently by removing the CD3 molecule and the associated T cell receptor from the surface of the cells (1,14,15). Likewise, antibodies to another pan T cell antigen, CD2, the erythrocyte (E) receptor, can block lymphocyte functions (16–18), and, as has been shown recently, also activates T cells (19). A further set of antigens, CD4 and CD8, are present on separate subpopulations of mature T cells (20,21) and probably serve as associative elements for major histocompatibility complex (MHC) gene products (22–24). Antibodies directed against these antigens can block the effector functions of T cells (12,13,22,25,26). Antibodies to activation markers restricted to lymphocytes, for example the receptor for interleukin-2 (IL-2), can block the binding of this lymphokine (27) and consequently several functions of induced cells (28), without influencing resting cells.

Anti-clonotypic (anti-idiotypic) antibodies against the T cell antigen receptor, the structure of which was unravelled only recently (2,3,23,29), could possibly be used to manipulate the immune response of antigen T cell clones specifically.

The purpose of this study was to evaluate the potential of the panel of anti–human-T-cell mAbs to influence *in vitro* proliferative assays. In order to be able to compare the antibodies with each other, aliquoted stocks of cryopreserved human peripheral blood mononuclear cells (PBMC) from the same donors were employed throughout this study.

Materials and Methods

Cells

Human peripheral blood mononuclear cell (PBMC) concentrates were obtained by leukophoresis from volunteers in the blood bank of the University Hospital, Vienna (Prim. Dr. P. Höcker). The PBMCs were purified by centrifugation over a Ficoll–Hypaque gradient (Pharmacia Fine Chemicals, Uppsala, Sweden). The cells were washed twice, suspended at $3-5 \times 10^7$/ml in freezing medium consisting of RPMI 1640 (Gibco Europe Ltd., Paisley, Scotland) with 20% human heat-inactivated human AB serum (PAA, Linz, Austria) and 12.5% dimethyl sulfoxide (DMSO), aliquoted (1-ml portions), and frozen to $-70°C$ in a Revco freezer. Twelve hours later the vials were transferred to a liquid nitrogen storage tank. Thawing of the cells was done as quickly as possible by dropping the bud of frozen cells into 15 ml of prewarmed medium. The cells were washed twice and the viability was determined by trypan blue exclusion or phase contrast microscopy. Viability usually was between 90–95%.

The cells of three donors, all healthy young males, were used in this study. Volunteer no. 254 had blood group O, Rh positive and HLA antigens A2, B38, C-, DR5, w6. No. 255 had blood group O, Rh positive and HLA antigens A1, 32, B35, Cw4, DR1,4. The cells of donor no. 292, blood group B, Rh positive and HLA antigens A2, B12, Cw5, DR4, w8 were only used as stimulator cells in the one-way mixed lymphocyte reaction (MLR). The serological determinations were done by Prof. Dr. W.R. Mayr of the Institute for Bloodgroup Serology, Vienna, Austria.

The cultivation medium for all the test systems was RPMI 1640, supplemented with 10% heat-inactivated human AB serum, 2 mM glutamine, 100 U/ml penicillin, and 100 μg/ml streptomycin. The medium contained 2 g/liter NaHCO$_3$ and was incubated at 37°C in a mixture of 5% CO$_2$ and 95% air and with maximal humidification.

Immunoglobulins

The antibodies investigated in this study are the T cell panel of the Second International Workshop on Human Leukocyte Differentiation Antigens. They were supplied in 100 μl amounts, mostly in the form of ascites. The various groupings of the antibodies and the number tested in each group are given in Table 15.1 and their names and Ig subclasses (for groups discussed in greater detail) are specified in Tables 15.2–15.8.

A number of control antibodies of known specificity and activity were added to the various groups. Coulter Clone T11 (CC-T11) was obtained from Coulter Electronics Ltd., Hialea, FL, USA. VIP 1, VIP 2b, VIT 3,

VIT 3b, VIT 4, and VIT 13 were developed by W. Knapp, Institute of Immunology, University of Vienna, Vienna, Austria (30,31).

The antibodies were diluted 1 : 20 in phosphate buffered saline (PBS) with 10% heat-inactivated human AB serum. They were portioned in volumes of 0.1 ml and kept frozen at −70°C.

The antibodies were added to the test system at the beginning of the culture period in four final dilutions, either 1 : 200, 1 : 1000, 1 : 5000, and 1 : 25,000 (mitogen-driven assays), or 1 : 400, 1 : 2000, 1 : 10,000, and 1 : 50,000 (MLR, tetanus toxoid assay, and IL-2 assay). In this study report only the results of the 1 : 1000 and 1 : 2000 dilutions are presented. These concentrations of the antibodies yielded the most consistent results and were regarded as the most representative.

Mitogenicity Testing and Mitogen-Driven Proliferation Assay

All mAbs were tested for their mitogenic activity on cells of two donors. In further series of tests the effect of the mAbs was investigated on cells that were mitogen-stimulated with either phytohemagglutinin (PHA) (Pharmacia Fine Chemicals, Uppsala, Sweden; product no. 17-0449-01) at a final dilution of 1 : 100, or pokeweed mitogen (PWM) (Gibco Europe Ltd., Paisley, Scotland; product no. 061-5360) at a final dilution of 1 : 10,000. Both these concentrations induce about one-half of the maximal proliferative responses of the cryopreserved human PBMCs.

The cells, 5×10^4 in a final volume of 0.1 ml per well, were incubated for 72 hr with and without the mAbs in round-bottomed microtiter plates (Greiner, Nürtingen, FRG). One μCi of [^{3}H]thymidine (^{3}H-Tdr) (Amersham International Inc., Amersham, England; TRK 300, specific activity 25 Ci/mmol) was added in 10 μl of medium and incubation commenced for a further 18 hr. The cells were then harvested on a Titertek Cell Harvester (Flow Laboratories, Meckenheim, FRG) and the samples were measured by liquid scintillation in a Packard Tri-Carb 460M (Packard Instrument Co., Inc., Downers Grove, IL, USA). The mean of the triplicate samples, standard deviations, and the stimulation indices (SI) were calculated on a Digital PDP-8 computer.

Mixed Lymphocyte Reaction (MLR)

For the one-way MLR the stimulator cells (donor no. 292) were irradiated with 2000 rad; 2.5×10^4 cells of each of the responder and the stimulator, in a final total volume of 0.1 ml per well, were incubated in round-bottomed microtiter plates (Greiner) for 6 days with and without the mAbs to be tested. One μCi of ^{3}H-Tdr was added for a further 18 hr. The cells were harvested, counted, and evaluated as described above.

Tetanus Toxoid Recall Assay

The cells were incubated at 5×10^4 per well, final volume 0.1 ml, with and without mAbs in the presence of tetanus toxoid (Tet. Tox), supplied as a ready-made solution by the Serotherapeutic Institute, Vienna (Product no. Ch 209/1, 1275 Lf/ml, 1545 Lf/mgN) in a final dilution of 1 : 10,000 for a period of 6 days. ^{3}H-Tdr labeling, harvesting, and evaluation were done as described above.

IL-2 Assay

The donor cells were incubated at a density of 1×10^6 per ml for 5 days in the presence of PHA, final dilution 1 : 100, in 50-ml tissue culture flasks (Nuclon 1 63371, Nunc, Roskilde, Denmark), 10 ml per flask. The supernatant was then removed, the cells were washed once, and then incubated in fresh medium without mitogen for another 1–2 days. They were then distributed at 5×10^4 per well of a round-bottomed microtiter plate (Greiner) and incubated with and without mAbs for 48 hr in the presence of human recombinant IL-2 (Sandoz Forschungsinstitut, Vienna) at a final concentration of 2 ng per ml. After 48 hr, ^{3}H-Tdr labeling, harvesting, and evaluation were done as described above.

Results

Overall Results

All antibodies of the T cell panel were tested in six assay systems. The results are summarized in Table 15.1. Clear differences between certain groups of antibodies are apparent. The mAbs in the groups CD1, CD5–8, and leukemia-specific did not influence the cells' proliferative performance to any appreciable extent and they will not be discussed. Since in group T subset other only a few mAbs caused a small change, with the exception of mAb 101 which suppressed the MLR strongly, this group is also not discussed in greater detail.

Certain mAbs in the groups CD3 and pan T other and unknown were highly mitogenic (SI $\geq$ 3.1), whereas in the activated cell systems the strongest reactions were the suppressions (SI $\leq$ 0.3). Most of the antibodies in group CD2 were inhibitory, 13–15 out of 16 mAbs depending on the test system, while in the group pan T other and unknown only 2–5 out of a total of 19 mAbs and in the T-activation group 4–8 out of 19 mAbs were clearly inhibitory. In each of these groups some of the antibodies were somewhat stimulatory, indicating the heterogeneity of the material under investigation. Of special interest are the results on the IL-2 assay. Eight mAbs of the CD3 group stimulated, while no inhibition occurred; in the T-activation group, on the other hand, 4 mAbs inhibited the reaction while no stimulation was found.

Group CD2

The majority of the SIs in the various assays reported in Table 15.2 are well below 1, demonstrating the general tendency of these mAbs to block proliferation responses of human PBMCs. Only mAbs 15 and 28 were not inhibitory, but rather slightly stimulatory. Antibody 13 enhanced the PHA assay somewhat. The IL-2 assay was not influenced by the CD2 mAbs.

Group CD3

The results in Table 15.3 clearly show that donor no. 254 is an IgG1 nonresponder—the cells reacted only to the mAbs of Ig subclass IgG2a (120, 126) and to the IgG3 (121), whereas donor no. 255 was a good responder to IgG1 (117, 118, 125), IgG2a (120, 126), and to the unknown mAb 119 which thus may be an IgG1. The response to the IgG2b (124) and to the IgG3 (121) was rather weak. The IgM (122) was inhibitory. Two mAbs (123, 127) did not cause any mitogenic stimulation. The control mAb VIT 3, an IgM, did not stimulate, while VIT 3b, an IgG1, very effectively stimulated the cells of donor no. 255 (SI 65.0), while those of donor no. 254 were stimulated to a low degree (5.5). This latter result was unexpected and it was found on repetition that VIT 3b was mitogenic for donor no. 254 only occasionally and then only to a low degree.

Table 15.4 shows the highly variable influence of anti-CD3 mAbs on induced cells. There was no clear correlation between the mitogenic property of a mAb and its inhibitory or stimulatory capacity in these assays. mAbs 117, 118, 119, 122, and 123 were strongly suppressive (SI ≤ 0,3). The two IgG2a mAbs were distinguishable from the others, because they stimulated the IL-2-driven cell proliferation.

Group CD4

The results in Table 15.5 show that 10 mAbs (69–72, 74–79) were inhibatory in the MLR and the tetanus toxoid assay. mAb 76 had the most pronounced effect.

Group Pan T Other and Unknown

Table 15.6 shows that mAb 61 was very mitogenic for both cell donors (SI 40.6 and 20.6) and it probably belongs in the group CD3. Moderate mitogenic reactions were obtained with mAbs 49, 51, 57, 60, 62, 63, and 64. mAb 61 also could be detected by its strong inhibition of the MLR and tetanus toxoid assays and its stimulation of the IL-2 assay (Table 15.7).

Table 15.1. *In vitro* modulation of human lymphocyte functions by the panel of anti–T cell monoclonal antibodies.

| Monoclonal antibody | | Effect in functional test system | | | | | |
| | | Mitogen | | | Antigen | | Lymphokine |
Group	No. tested	None	PHA	PWM	MLR	Tetanus toxoid	IL-2
CD1	7	—	3↑ 3↓	—	—	1↓	—
CD2	16	—	3↑6➤7↓	1↑8➤6↓	1↑8➤7↓	6➤8↓	—
CD3	11	7➤1↑	7↑5➤	5➤3↓	1↑4➤2↓	1↑4➤3↓	2➤6↑
CD4	14	—	—	—	3➤7↓	4➤6↓	—
CD5	9	—	—	—	—	—	—
CD6	2	—	2↑	—	—	—	—
CD7	17	—	3↑	—	—	—	—
CD8	20	—	2↑	4↓	—	1↓	—
Pan T unknown	19	4➤4↑2↓	3↑1➤1↓	2➤3↓	5↑1➤3↓	2↑1➤3↓	2↑
T subset other	16	—	5↑ 1↓	1↑ 1↓	1↑1➤2↓	4↓	—
T-activation	19	—	2↑3➤5↓	1➤5↓	2↑2➤4↓	7↓	2➤2↓
Leukemia	3	—	—	—	1↓	—	—

[a] Stimulation index: ≤ 0.3, ➤; 0.4–0.6, ↓; 0.7–1.4, —; 1.5–3.0, ↑; ≥ 3.1, ➤

Table 15.2. CD2 group of monoclonal anti–human T cell antibodies: modulation of mitogen-, antigen-, or growth factor-induced PBMC cultures.

| Monoclonal antibody | | | Stimulation index in PBMC cultures of 2 donors (254, 255) | | | | | | | | | |
| | | | PHA | | PWM | | Allo-antigen | | Tetanus toxoid | | PHA/rec IL-2 | |
Panel no.	Name	Ig subclass	254	255	254	255	254	255	254	255	254	255
13	9-1	IgG2b	2.1	1.7	0.4	0.6	0.3	0.4	0.3	0.3	1.0	0.9
14	9-2	IgM	0.3	0.3	0.5	0.4	0.8	0.4	0.4	0.5	0.9	0.9
15	G19-3.1	IgG1	1.7	1.8	1.2	1.2	1.3	1.6	0.7	0.8	0.9	0.9
16	S2/Leu 5b	IgG2a	0.3	0.2	0.4	0.3	0.4	0.4	0.2	0.5	1.0	0.9
17	MT 26	IgG1	0.6	0.7	0.3	0.3	0.4	0.2	0.3	0.3	1.2	0.9
18	MT 910	IgG1	0.5	0.6	0.2	0.3	0.3	0.4	0.3	0.3	1.1	0.8
19	MT 1110	IgG1	0.6	0.4	0.4	0.5	0.8	0.4	0.4	0.5	1.1	0.8
20	T11/3Pt2H9	IgG1	0.6	0.5	0.3	0.5	0.5	0.4	0.6	0.7	0.9	0.9
21	T11/ROLD2-1H8	IgG1	0.5	0.6	0.4	0.9	0.8	0.4	0.8	0.6	0.8	0.9
22	T11/3T4-8B5	IgG2a	0.3	0.3	0.4	0.3	0.5	0.2	0.5	0.5	0.7	0.9
23	T11/7T4-7A9	IgM	0.3	0.2	0.5	0.5	0.7	0.0	0.7	0.6	0.7	0.9
24	T11/7T4-7E10	IgG2b	0.3	0.3	0.4	0.5	0.3	0.3	0.5	0.5	0.8	0.9
25	9.6	IgG2a	0.2	0.3	0.3	0.3	0.3	0.2	0.3	0.6	0.8	1.0
26	35.1	IgG2a	0.4	0.6	0.3	0.6	0.2	0.2	0.2	0.4	0.9	1.0
27	T4IIB5	IgG1/G2	0.4	1.0	0.3	0.5	0.4	0.4	0.6	0.6	0.9	1.0
28	KOLT-2	IgG1	2.6	1.6	0.9	1.6	0.4	0.8	0.8	1.1	0.8	1.1
Control	CC-T11	IgG1	0.7	1.1	0.4	0.3	1.0	ND	0.9	0.5	1.0	0.9

Table 15.3. CD3 group of monoclonal anti–human T cell antibodies: mitogenic effect on human PBMCs.

Monoclonal antibody			Stimulation index (final mAb dilution 1:1000)	
Panel no.	Name	Ig subclass	Donor 254	Donor 255
117	G19-4.1	IgG1	0.8	40.2
118	SK7/Leu 4	IgG1	1.0	18.8
119	89b1	NK	0.9	33.7
120	BW264/56	IgG2a	12.0	13.2
121	BW242/55	IgG3	6.3	2.4
122	T3/2Ad2A2	IgM	0.3	0.4
123	T3/2T8-2F4	IgG1	0.3	0.9
124	T3/RW2-4B6	IgG2b	0.6	1.8
125	T3/RW2-8C8	IgG1	1.7	29.4
126	X35-3	IgG2a	26.0	10.2
127	NU-T1	IgG1	1.2	0.7
Control	VIT 3	IgM	1.0	1.0
	VIT 3b	IgG1	5.5	65.0

Table 15.4. CD3 group of monoclonal anti–human T cell antibodies: modulation of mitogen-, antigen-, or growth factor-induced PBMC cultures.

Monoclonal antibody			Stimulation index in PBMC cultures of 2 donors (254, 255)									
			PHA		PWM		Allo-antigen		Tetanus toxoid		PHA/rec IL-2	
Panel no.	Name	Ig subclass	254	255	254	255	254	255	254	255	254	255
117	G19-4.1	IgG1	0.2	1.9	0.1	0.5	0.0	0.4	0.0	0.2	1.4	1.6
118	SK7/Leu 4	IgG1	0.1	1.7	0.2	0.5	0.4	0.3	0.3	0.2	0.8	1.8
119	89b1	NK	0.1	1.7	0.2	0.6	0.3	0.6	0.3	0.4	1.2	1.6
120	BW264/56	IgG2a	0.4	0.8	0.7	0.6	0.5	0.8	0.9	0.8	4.7	3.1
121	BW242/55	IgG3	1.0	0.5	0.7	0.8	1.1	2.1	0.6	0.7	1.7	1.5
122	T3/2Ad2A2	IgM	0.8	0.3	0.2	0.6	1.0	0.9	0.8	0.9	0.9	0.9
123	T3/2T8-2F4	IgG1	0.2	0.1	0.2	0.2	0.2	0.4	0.3	0.6	1.0	1.1
124	T3/RW2-4B6	IgG2b	2.2	0.4	0.4	0.5	0.7	1.3	0.8	2.1	1.7	2.0
125	T3/RW2-8C8	IgG1	0.8	1.6	0.4	0.5	0.8	0.8	1.1	0.5	1.4	1.8
126	X35-3	IgG2a	1.6	0.6	1.0	0.8	0.5	0.9	0.6	1.0	3.2	2.3
127	NU-T1	IgG1	1.5	0.5	0.9	0.8	0.8	0.9	0.7	0.9	1.0	1.3
Control	VIT 3	IgM	0.1	0.0	0.1	0.2	0.0	0.1	0.1	0.1	1.5	0.9
	VIT 3b	IgG1	0.3	0.8	0.2	0.7	0.1	0.2	0.4*	0.2	2.2	2.2

Table 15.5. CD4 group of monoclonal anti–human T cell antibodies: modulation of mitogen-, antigen-, or growth factor-induced PBMC cultures.

Panel no.	Name	Ig subclass	PHA 254	PHA 255	PWM 254	PWM 255	Allo-antigen 254	Allo-antigen 255	Tetanus toxoid 254	Tetanus toxoid 255	PHA/rec IL-2 254	PHA/rec IL-2 255
67	T10C5	IgM	1.2	1.4	1.0	1.0	1.2	1.1	0.9	0.7	0.9	1.0
68	G19-2	IgG1	0.8	1.2	0.8	1.1	0.7	0.9	0.7	0.7	1.2	1.0
69	91d6	IgG2a	0.8	1.1	0.8	1.0	0.6	0.5	0.6	0.4	0.9	0.9
70	94b1	IgG2a	0.7	0.8	1.1	1.0	0.5	0.5	0.6	0.6	1.1	0.9
71	BW264/123	IgM	0.8	0.9	0.9	0.9	0.8	0.5	0.5	0.5	1.3	0.8
72	MT 151	IgG2a	1.2	1.1	0.8	0.8	0.4	0.3	0.3	0.6	0.9	0.7
73	MT 321	IgG1	1.0	1.2	0.9	1.1	1.0	0.8	0.7	0.8	1.0	0.8
74	T4/12T4D11	IgG1	1.3	1.1	0.9	1.2	0.5	0.5	0.6	0.7	0.9	0.8
75	T4/18T3A9	IgG1	1.2	0.8	0.8	1.1	0.6	0.3	0.3	0.5	0.9	0.9
76	MT 310	IgG1	1.1	1.0	0.8	1.2	0.5	0.1	0.2	0.3	0.9	0.8
77	T4/19Thy5D7	IgG2	1.1	0.9	0.9	1.0	0.6	0.4	0.3	0.4	0.9	0.8
78	T4/7T4-6C1	IgM	1.0	1.0	0.8	1.0	0.8	0.6	0.7	0.6	0.8	1.0
79	66.1	IgM	1.0	1.1	0.9	0.9	0.7	0.5	0.7	0.5	0.8	0.9
80	TII19-4-7	NK	1.1	0.9	0.9	0.9	1.1	0.9	0.8	0.9	0.8	0.9
Control	VIT 4	IgG2a	ND	ND	ND	ND	0.6	0.5	0.5	0.6	0.8	0.8

Stimulation index in PBMC cultures of 2 donors (254, 255)

Table 15.6. Pan T other or unknown group of monoclonal anti–human T cell antibodies: mitogenic effect on human PBMCs.

Panel no.	Name	Ig subclass	Donor 254	Donor 255
48	T10B9	IgM	1.0	1.0
49	T12A10	IgM	2.1	1.3
50	E9	IgG	1.1	0.6
51	G3-5	IgG1	3.9	1.4
52	G10-2.1	IgG1	0.9	1.1
53	G19-1.2	IgG1	1.5	1.1
54	T55	IgG2a	0.8	1.5
55	T56	IgM	0.9	1.5
56	T57	IgG	0.9	1.0
57	BW239/347	IgG	5.5	4.3
58	MT 211	IgG1	0.8	1.5
59	MT 421	IgG1	1.1	0.9
60	CRIS-3	IgG	8.1	3.0
61	CRIS-7	IgG	40.6	20.6
62	CRIS-8	IgG	2.0	1.9
63	K20	NK	1.2	1.9
64	K50	NK	1.9	1.3
65	G144	NK	1.2	1.0
66	D47	NK	1.2	0.5

Stimulation index (final mAb dilution 1 : 1000)

Table 15.7. Pan T other or unknown group of monoclonal anti–human T cell antibodies: modulation of mitogen-, antigen-, or growth factor-induced PBMC cultures.

Panel no.	Name	Ig subclass	PHA 254	PHA 255	PWM 254	PWM 255	Allo-antigen 254	Allo-antigen 255	Tetanus toxoid 254	Tetanus toxoid 255	PHA/rec IL-2 254	PHA/rec IL-2 255
			Stimulation index in PBMC cultures of 2 donors (254, 255)									
48	T10B9	IgM	0.8	0.6	0.3	0.3	0.5	0.5	0.7	1.1	ND	1.2
49	T12A10	IgM	1.3	1.4	1.2	1.1	1.1	1.5	0.9	1.1	ND	0.8
50	E9	IgG	1.3	1.3	1.1	1.0	1.1	1.4	0.7	1.2	ND	0.8
51	G3-5	IgG1	1.1	1.2	0.9	1.1	1.1	1.5	0.7	1.0	ND	0.8
52	G10-2.1	IgG1	1.6	1.2	1.2	1.2	1.0	2.4	0.9	1.5	ND	1.0
53	G19-1.2	IgG1	1.3	1.2	1.1	1.0	1.1	1.6	1.0	1.3	ND	0.8
54	T55	IgG2a	1.3	1.2	0.8	0.8	1.2	1.2	0.7	0.7	ND	0.9
55	T56	IgM	1.1	0.8	0.7	0.6	0.7	0.8	0.6	0.8	ND	1.0
56	T57	IgG	0.3	0.3	0.4	0.2	0.5	0.5	0.6	0.5	ND	0.9
57	BW239/347	IgG	1.2	1.1	0.8	0.6	0.9	1.0	1.0	1.5	ND	2.2
58	MT 211	IgG1	1.5	1.3	1.1	1.1	1.2	1.2	0.9	1.0	ND	1.0
59	MT 421	IgG1	1.6	1.8	0.6	0.9	0.6	1.1	0.4	0.5	ND	0.9
60	CRIS-3	IgG	1.4	1.2	0.8	0.9	0.7	1.2	0.7	0.8	ND	1.2
61	CRIS-7	IgG	1.2	0.8	0.4	0.6	0.3	0.3	0.1	0.2	ND	3.8
62	CRIS-8	IgG	1.5	1.0	1.2	1.0	0.9	1.0	1.0	0.9	ND	1.2
63	K20	NK	1.2	1.0	0.8	1.0	0.8	1.0	0.8	0.8	ND	1.0
64	K50	NK	1.2	0.8	0.9	0.9	1.1	1.3	0.8	0.8	ND	0.9
65	G144	NK	0.7	0.7	0.7	0.8	0.9	1.1	0.7	1.0	ND	0.9
66	D47	NK	0.9	1.0	0.8	1.0	0.8	1.5	0.8	0.7	ND	0.8

This again indicates its probable anti-CD3 nature. mAb 56 is distinct from the others by its strong inhibition of the mitogen-driven assays.

Group T-Activation

In this group the results of the IL-2 assay are of interest since inhibition may indicate an anti–Il-2 receptor mAb. This could apply to the mAbs 140, 145, 146, and 153 (Table 15.8). The fact that mAb 159, which is the authentic anti-Tac, could not be detected in this assay was disturbing. It may be due to too high concentration of IL-2 in the assay. This antibody, however, was found to inhibit the PHA stimulation. In all, 6–8 out of 19 mAbs were inhibitory in one assay or another, the strongest being 144, which was not found in the IL-2 assay.

The control mAb VIP 1 is an anti–transferrin receptor antibody—except for the clear inhibition of the tetanus toxoid response of donor no. 255, it had no activity. Similarly VIP 2b and VIT 13 did not influence any of the assays.

Table 15.8. T-activation group of monoclonal anti–human T cell antibodies: modulation of mitogen-, antigen-, or growth factor-induced PBMC cultures.

Panel no.	Name	Ig subclass	PHA 254	PHA 255	PWM 254	PWM 255	Allo-antigen 254	Allo-antigen 255	Tetanus toxoid 254	Tetanus toxoid 255	PHA/rec IL-2 254	PHA/rec IL-2 255
			Stimulation index in PBMC cultures of 2 donors (254,255)									
135	T1A	IgG2	1.1	0.5	0.8	0.7	0.8	0.9	0.7	0.7	0.8	1.0
136	TS145	IgG1	0.9	0.9	1.0	0.8	1.0	1.2	0.9	1.1	1.1	1.0
137	100-1A5	NK	1.0	1.3	0.9	0.8	1.0	1.7	0.8	0.8	1.2	1.0
138	1 MONO 2A6	IgG3	1.5	1.0	0.5	0.6	0.7	1.3	0.6	0.7	1.1	1.0
139	4EL1C7	IgG1	1.1	1.0	1.0	0.9	0.7	1.6	0.8	0.7	1.0	0.9
140	Tac/1HT4-4H3	NK	0.6	0.4	0.8	0.6	ND	1.1	0.7	0.5	0.4	0.6
141	B149.9	IgG2a	0.9	0.9	0.8	0.7	0.7	0.8	0.8	0.7	1.1	1.2
142	B1.19.2	IgG2a	1.5	1.0	0.8	0.8	1.0	1.0	1.0	0.8	1.0	1.0
143	23A9.3	NK	1.1	1.0	0.8	0.7	1.0	1.0	0.9	0.8	0.9	1.0
144	39C1.5	NK	0.3	0.2	0.4	0.4	0.5	0.3	0.7	0.4	1.0	0.9
145	39C6.5	NK	0.5	0.3	0.9	0.8	0.3	0.6	0.6	0.2	0.2	0.4
146	33B3.1	NK	0.6	0.4	0.7	0.7	ND	0.9	0.5	0.6	0.4	0.5
147	33B7.3	NK	1.1	1.0	0.7	0.8	1.2	1.0	1.0	0.8	0.9	1.0
148	39C8.18	NK	0.7	0.5	0.3	0.5	0.5	0.6	0.7	0.5	1.0	1.0
149	39H7.3	NK	0.6	0.5	0.5	0.5	0.7	0.5	0.7	0.7	0.8	0.9
150	41F2.1	NK	0.8	0.8	0.6	1.0	1.0	0.7	1.0	0.7	0.9	0.9
151	KOLT-1	IgG1	1.0	1.4	1.0	0.9	0.9	0.6	1.1	1.0	0.9	0.9
153	AA3	IgG1	1.0	1.2	0.9	0.8	1.0	1.0	0.9	0.8	0.1	0.2
159	TAC	IgG2a	ND	0.3	0.7	0.6	0.6	0.9	0.7	0.6	0.9	0.9
Control	VIP 1	IgG1	ND	ND	1.0	0.8	1.1	1.1	0.9	0.2	0.9	1.0
	VIP 2b	IgM	ND	ND	1.1	0.9	1.2	1.6	1.0	1.2	1.0	1.0
	VIT 13	IgM	ND	1.1	0.9	1.0	1.2	1.4	1.0	0.8	ND	1.0

Discussion

The screening of the workshop T cell mAbs in *in vitro* lymphocyte proliferation assays enabled us to identify certain of the established clusters of mAbs and to distinguish between them. As summarized in Table 15.1, the mitogenicity of the CD3 group of mAbs for normal PBMCs and the general inhibitory effect of the CD2, CD3, and T-activation mAbs in induced cell assays and the CD4 group specific mAbs in the antigen-driven systems could clearly be demonstrated. Antibodies against the groups CD1, CD5, CD6, CD7, Leukemia specific, and the majority of the CD8 group only showed little or no effects in the proliferation assays. An anti–CD4 mAb was recently found to markedly enhance B cell differentiation (32). This property could not be detected in the proliferation assays.

Our results generally are in agreement with those of previous studies. Thus the anti–CD2 mAbs were found to block proliferative lymphocyte responses (16–18). CD2, the E receptor is of special interest, since it has recently been shown to play a role in an alternative pathway of T cell activation (19).

With regard to the group CD3, the mitogenic property of these antibodies (4–9) and the polymorphism of the responses depending on the IgG subclass specificity of the Fc receptors on the accessory cells of a donor (7,8) was also confirmed by our results. Donor no. 255 responded to the anti–CD3 IgG1 and IgG2a+b mAbs, whereas donor no. 254 only responded well to the IgG2a antibodies. Interestingly, the IgG3 was somewhat stimulatory for both donors. The mAb 119, on the basis of its nonmitogenicity for the cells of donor no. 254 and its strong reaction with donor no. 255 probably is of the subclass IgG1.

It is suggested that the mAb 61 from the group pan T other and unknown, because of its strong mitogenicity, belongs in the group CD3, and possibly also the mAbs 57 and 60.

Our results also confirm the finding of previous studies on the blocking effect of certain anti–CD3 mAbs on T cell proliferative responses to soluble and cell surface antigens (10–15). Since the mitogen-driven proliferation also was suppressed by certain of the antibodies, it is possible that CD3 mediates the stimulatory effect of certain mitogens on T cells, as has been indicated previously (33). The enhancement of the proliferation after the combination of a mitogenic anti–CD3 and the T cell growth factor IL-2 was noted previously (1,2,29). This observation was confirmed for the two IgG2a anti–CD3 mAbs. Recent studies in this direction, employing T cell clones, showed that anti–CD3 mAbs activate T cells via the expression of IL-2 receptors and measureable IL-2 production in the cultures (34). A further study with T leukemia cells indicated a two-stimulus requirement for IL-2 production and proliferation (35). Furthermore, a study with human PBMCs showed that mitogenic anti–CD3 mAbs always lead to the expression of IL-2 receptors on the responding cells, but also that proliferation can proceed in the apparent absence of IL-2 given off into the culture medium (36). Clearly, there are several conditions under which the stimulation and induction of proliferation of T cells can take place. A detailed knowledge of these processes may reveal new approaches for the manipulation of the T cell responsiveness to various stimuli.

The results obtained with the anti–CD4 and –CD8 mAbs were partly consistent with reports in the literature. Recent studies (22–25) show that CD4 and CD8 glycoproteins serve as associative recognition elements for class II and class I MHC antigens respectively. mAbs to both CD4 and CD8 inhibit autologous and allogeneic MLR (24,25). We only found significant inhibition of the MLR and the antigen driven system by anti–CD4 mAbs, but observed no effect of the anti–CD8 mAbs. The reason for this discrepancy is not clear.

In the T activation group of mAbs, several blocked the IL-2–driven cell proliferation as one would expect from anti–IL-2 receptor antibodies. Especially the mAbs 145 and 153 fall in this category.

Some technical aspects should be pointed out, for example, too high amounts of IL-2 probably leads to insensitivity of the IL-2–driven cell proliferation test to influences by antibodies. Immunoglobulin-free culture medium may be helpful in the investigation of mAbs, since adverse effects may occur in the presence of serum (37). Also, the physical condition of the mAb preparation is important—aggregated antibodies have been shown to block lymphocyte reactions nonspecifically (38).

The potential usefulness of anti–T-cell mAbs for immunomodulation should not solely rely on the blocking or stimulatory properties of these antibodies per se. The most important property of these molecules is their exquisite capacity to specifically recognize subsets of cells, cellular activation markers, and structures involved in cellular functions. If the antibodies do not influence the cells in any, or the desired way, they may be "activated" by conjugating them to stimulating or suppressive compounds or even to toxins (39). Finally, it should be pointed out that human antibodies will be needed before the envisaged wide-spread clinical application (40) can become reality.

Summary

The Workshop series of anti–T cell mAbs was tested in proliferative lymphocyte assays, employing single large batches of peripheral blood lymphocytes obtained from healthy donors by leukophoresis and maintained frozen in liquid nitrogen.

Most of the 16 mAbs of the CD2 group inhibited the mitogen- (PHA, PWM) and antigen- (MLR, tetanus toxoid) driven assays, 6–8 mAbs being strongly suppressive. The IL-2-driven proliferation of lymphocytes was not influenced. Eight of the 11 CD3 group of mAbs were mitogenic. The IgG1 responder and nonresponder could clearly be identified. Only the 2 IgG2a mAbs enhanced the IL-2 assay. In the stimulated test systems the majority of the CD3 mAbs were suppressive. The mitogenicity and the inhibitory capacity of the mAbs did not correlate. Ten mAbs of the CD4 group suppressed the MLR and tetanus toxoid reaction—no other system was affected. Several mAbs in the pan T other and unknown group were mitogenic, suggesting that they belong in the CD3 group. Three mAbs out of 19 of the T-activation group were strongly suppressive; 4 inhibit the IL-2-dependent cell proliferation, indicating that they may be anti–IL-2 receptor mAbs. Of the other groups of anti–T cell mAbs, only the occasional one showed some activity in these tests.

The overall conclusion is that these assays permit a useful classification of mAbs with regard to their capacity to modulate some *in vitro* immunological responses.

Acknowledgment. The authors wish to acknowledge the technical assistance provided by Elisabeth Harfeldt, Andrea Koulhanek, and Erika Puntigam.

References

1. Reinherz, E.L., S. Meuer, K.A. Fitzgerald, R.E. Hussey, H. Levine, and S. Schlossmann. 1982. Antigen recognition by T lymphocytes is linked to surface expression of the T3 molecular complex. *Cell* **30**:735.
2. Meuer, S., O. Acuto, R. Hussey, et al. 1983. Evidence for the T3-associated 90K heterodimer as the T-cell antigen receptor. *Nature* **303**:808.
3. Reinherz, E., S. Meuer, K. Fitzgerald, et al. 1983. Comparison of T3-associated 49- and 43-Kd cell surface molecules on individual human T-cell clones: evidence for peptide variability in T-cell receptor structures. *Proc. Natl. Acad. Sci. U.S.A.* **80**:4104.
4. Van Wauwe, J.P., J.R. De Mey, and J.G. Goossens. 1980. OKT3: a monoclonal anti-human T lymphocyte antibody with potent mitogenic properties. *J. Immunol.* **124**:2708.
5. Van Wauwe, J.P., and J.G. Goossens. 1981. Mitogenic actions of Orthoclone OKT3 on human peripheral blood lymphocytes: effects of monocytes and serum components. *Int. J. Immunopharmacol.* **3**:203.
6. Burns, G.F., A.W. Boyd, and P.C. Beverley. 1982. Two monoclonal anti-human T lymphocyte antibodies have similar biologic effects and recognize the same antigen. *J. Immunol.* **129**:1451.
7. Tax, W.J.M., H.W. Willems, P.P.M. Reekers, P.J.A. Capel, and R.A.P. Koene. 1983. Polymorphism in mitogenic effect of IgG1 monoclonal antibodies against T3 antigen on human T cells. *Nature* **304**:445.
8. Kaneoka, H., G. Perez-Rojas, T. Sasasuki, C.J. Benike, and E.G. Engleman. 1983. Human T lymphocyte proliferation induced by a pan-T monoclonal antibody (anti-Leu4): heterogeneity of response is a function of monocytes. *J. Immunol.* **131**:158.
9. Van Wauwe, J.P., and J.G. Goossens. 1983. The mitogenic activity of OKT3 and anti-Leu-4 monoclonal antibodies: a comparative study. *Cell Immunol.* **77**:23.
10. Reinherz, E.L., R.E. Hussey, and S.F. Schlossman. 1980. A monoclonal antibody blocking human T cell function. *Eur. J. Immunol.* **10**:758.
11. Chang, T.W., P.C. Kung, S.P. Gingras, and G. Goldstein. 1981. Does OKT3 monoclonal antibody react with an antigen-recognition structure on human T cells? *Proc. Natl. Acad. Sci. U.S.A.* **78**:1805.
12. Platsoucas, C.D., and R.A. Good. 1981. Inhibition of specific cell-mediated cytotoxicity by monoclonal antibodies to human T cell antigens. *Proc. Natl. Acad. Sci. U.S.A.* **78**:4500.
13. Platsoucas, C.D. 1984. Human T cell antigens involved in cytotoxicity against allogeneic or autologous chemically modified targets. Association of the Leu

2a/T8 antigen with effector–target cell binding and of the T3/Leu 4 antigen with triggering. *Eur. J. Immunol.* **14:**566.

14. Van Wauwe, J.P., J. Goossens, and G. van Nyen. 1984. Inhibition of lymphocyte proliferation by monoclonal antibody directed against the T3 antigen on human T cells. *Cell. Immunol.* **86:**525.

15. Kammer, G.M., R. Kurrasch, and J.J. Scillian. 1984. Capping of the surface OKT3 binding molecule prevents the T-cell proliferative response to antigens: evidence that this molecule conveys the activation signal. *Cell Immunol.* **87:**284.

16. Palacios, R., and O. Martinez-Maza. 1982. Is the E receptor on human T lymphocytes a "negative signal receptor?" *J. Immunol.* **129:**2479.

17. Martin, P., G. Longton, J. Ledbetter, W. Newman, M. Braun, P. Beatty, and J. Hansen. 1983. Identification and functional characterization of two distinct epitopes on the human T cell surface protein Tp50. *J. Immunol.* **131:**180.

18. Wilkinson, M., and A. Morris. 1984. The E receptor regulates interferon-gamma production: four-receptor model for human lymphocyte activation. *Eur. J. Immunol.* **14:**708.

19. Meuer, S., R.E. Hussey, M. Fabbi, et al. 1984. An alternative pathway of T cell activation: a functional role for the 50 kd T11 sheep erythrocyte receptor protein. *Cell* **36:**897.

20. Reinherz, E.L., and S.F. Schlossman. 1980. Regulation of the immune response—inducer and suppressor T-lymphocyte subsets in human beings. *New England J. Med.* **303:**370.

21. Hoffman, R.A., P.C. Kung, W.P. Hansen, and G. Goldstein. 1980. Simple and rapid measurement of human T lymphocytes and their subclasses in peripheral blood. *Proc. Natl. Acad. Sci. U.S.A.* **77:**4914.

22. Meuer, S.C., S.F. Schlossman, and E.L. Reinherz. 1982. Clonal analysis of human cytotoxic T lymphocytes: T4$^+$ and T8$^+$ effector T cells recognize products of different major histocompatibility complex regions. *Proc. Natl. Acad. Sci. U.S.A.* **79:**4395.

23. Reinherz, E.L., S. Meuer, and S. Schlossman. 1983. The delineation of antigen receptors on human T lymphocytes. *Immunology Today.* **4:**5.

24. Romain, P.L., S. Schlossman, and E.L. Reinherz. 1984. Surface molecules involved in self-recognition and T cell activation in the autologous mixed lymphocyte reaction. *J. Immunol.* **133:**1093.

25. Engleman, E.G., C.J. Benike, C. Metzler, P.A. Gatenby, and R.L. Lewis. 1983. Blocking of human T lymphocyte functions by anti-Leu-2 and anti-Leu-3 antibodies: differential inhibition of proliferation and suppression. *J. Immunol.* **130:**2623.

26. Reinherz, E.L., R.E. Hussey, K. Fitzgerald, P. Snow, S. Terhorst, and S. Schlossman. 1981. Antibody directed at a surface structure inhibits cytolytic but not suppressor function of human T lymphocytes. *Nature* **294:**168.

27. Depper, J.M., W.J. Leonard, R.J. Robb, T.A. Waldmann, and W.C. Greene. 1983. Blockade of the interleukin 2 receptor by anti-Tac antibody: inhibition of human lymphocyte activation. *J. Immunol.* **131:**690.

28. Depper, J.M., W.J. Leonard, T.A. Waldmann, and W.C. Greene. 1984. A monoclonal antibody which recognizes the human receptor for T cell growth factor: functional effects and use as a probe to investigate receptor regulation. In: *Lymphokines,* Vol. 9, E. Pick, ed. Academic Press, New York, p. 127.

29. Meuer, S., K. Fitzgerald, R. Hussey, J. Hodgdon, S. Schlossman, and E. Reinherz. 1983. Clonotypic structures involved in antigen-specific human T cell function. *J. Exp. Med.* **157**:705.
30. Stockinger, H., O. Majdic, K. Liska, U. Köller, W. Holter, C. Peschel, P. Bettelheim, H. Gisslinger und W. Knapp. 1985. T-14, a non-modulating 150 kd T-cell surface antigen. Proceedings of the Second International Conference on Human Leucocyte Differentiation Antigens. This volume.
31. Holter, W., O. Majdic, K. Liska, H. Stockinger and W. Knapp. 1985. Kinetics of activation antigen expression by in vitro-stimulated human T-lymphocytes. *Cell. Immunol.* **90**:322.
32. Thomas, Y., E. Glickman, J. DeMartino, J. Wang, G. Goldstein, and L. Chess. 1984. Biologic functions of the OKT 1 T cell surface antigen. I. The T1 molecule is involved in helper functions. *J. Immunol.* **133**:724.
33. Fleischer, B. 1984. Activation of human T lymphocytes. II. Involvement of the T3 antigen in polyclonal T cell activation by mitogenic lectins and oxidation. *Eur. J. Immunol.* **14**:748.
34. Meuer, S., R.E. Hussey, D.A. Cantrell, J.C. Hogdon, S. Schlossman, K.A. Smith, and E.L. Reinherz. 1984. Triggering of the T3-Ti antigen-receptor complex results in clonal T-cell proliferations through an interleukin 2-dependent autocrine pathway. *Proc. Natl. Acad. Sci. USA.* **81**:1509.
35. Van Wauwe, J.P., J.G. Goossens, and P.C. Beverley. 1984. Human T lymphocyte activation by monoclonal antibodies; OKT 3, but not UCHT1, triggers mitogenesis via an interleukin 2-dependent mechanism. *J. Immunol.* **133**:129.
36. Weiss, A., R.L. Wiskocil, and J.D. Stobo. 1984. The role of T3 surface molecules in the activation of human T cells: A two-stimulus requirement for IL-2 production reflects events occurring at a pre-translational level. *J. Immunol.* **133**:123.
37. Looney, R.J., and G.N. Abraham. 1984. The Fc portion of intact IgG blocks stimulation of human PBMC by anti-T3. *J. Immunol.* **133**:154.
38. Burns, G.G., T. Triglia, and G.A. Varigos. 1983. Mouse monoclonal antibodies can nonspecifically inhibit the proliferation of human T-cell growth factor-dependent T cells. *Cell. Immunol.* **82**:4.
39. Kernan, N.A., R.W. Knowles, M.J. Burns, et al. 1984. Specific inhibition of in vitro lymphocyte transformation by an anti-pan T cell (gp67) ricin A chain immunotoxin. *J. Immunol.* **133**:137.
40. Goldstein, G., J. Lifter, and R. Mittler. 1982. mAbs to human lymphocyte surface antigens. In: *Monoclonal Antibodies and T Cell Products.* p. 71. D.H. Katz, ed. CRC Press, Inc. Boca Raton, Florida.

CHAPTER 16

The Influence of the Workshop Monoclonal Antibodies on CML, AgTR, PLT, ADCC, and NK Cell Activity. Functional Studies with Workshop Antibodies

Frits Koning, Marrie Kardol, Jan van der Poel,
Annemarie Termijtelen, Els Goulmy, Tom Ottenhoff,
Els Blokland, Dienne Elferink, Jos Pool,
Simin Naipal-van den Berge, and Hans Bruning

The introduction of the hybridoma technique (1) has made it possible to produce monoclonal antibodies against functionally different (T-) lymphocyte subsets. The antigens recognized by monoclonal antibodies from the CD4, CD8, and LFA-1 class appear to play a role in the recognition–adhesion of the target/stimulator cell by the effector cell (for review see Ref. 2). The T3 antigen, associated with the T cell receptor (3), is not involved in the recognition–adhesion step but might transmit signals for the lethal hit or mitogenesis. Recently, it has been found that sheep red blood cell receptors, defined by CD2 mAbs, can also play a role in the activation of T cells (4) while earlier reports indicated that the cytolytic activity of cytotoxic T lymphocytes could be partially blocked by CD2 mAbs (5,6).

Usually, the influence of monoclonal antibodies on functional assays has been investigated using small panels of antibodies. The Workshop therefore offered a unique opportunity to study and compare the effects of a large set of monoclonal antibodies on a number of functional assays.

We have studied the effects of the mAbs on the cytolytic activity of three HLA-class I specific or restricted T cell lines (CML), the proliferative response of PPD-specific T lymphoblasts (AgTR), HLA-class II specific primed lymphocytes (PLT), and on the activity of killer (ADCC) and natural killer cells (NK cells).[1]

---

[1] Abbreviations used in this paper: ADCC, antibody dependent cellular cytotoxicity; AgTR, antigen-specific T-lymphoblast response; APC, antigen presenting cell; MLC, mixed lymphocyte culture; PLT, primed lymphocyte test; PPD, purified protein derivate; TCGF, T cell growth factor.

Materials and Methods

Monoclonal Antibodies

In all assays the final dilution of the mAbs was 1 : 200 and they were present in the reaction mixture throughout. For inhibition studies in AgTR and PLT, NaN_3 was removed by dialysis against RPMI 1640.

Cell Mediated Lympholysis

CML was performed using a nonradioactive assay which has been described previously (7,8) with three modifications: (a) Target cells were three-day Con A blasts (20 μg/ml, Calbioch.). To avoid lectin-dependent cell cytotoxicity, 50 mM α-methyl-D-mannoside was added to the target cell culture on day two to dissociate cell-bound Con A; (b) The test was carried out in Terasaki type trays (Greiner, Cat.no. 726180) with a well volume of 40 μl; (c) Leitz ink, 1 : 300 in isotonic 5% EDTA was used to quench released cellular carboxyfluorescein label. Each combination was tested with two different effector : target cell ratios (i.e., 20 : 1 and 10 : 1). Effector cells were either HLA-A2.1-specific 6-day MLC cultures (9) which were expanded with 20% TCGF (Biotest) for three days or cell lines which were established from lymphocytes from bone marrow transplant recipients and which had been shown to be specific for MHC-restricted minor transplantation antigens (anti-HA-4 and anti-H-Y) (10,11).

Measurement of ADCC and NK Cell Activity

Both assays were carried out using nonradioactive assays which have been described previously (12,13). Freshly isolated PBLs were used as effector cells.

Proliferative Response to Soluble Antigen

PPD-specific T lymphoblasts were generated as described previously (14) and tested as follows : 10,000 PPD-specific T lymphoblasts and 50,000 40-Gy irradiated autologous PBLs as antigen-presenting cells were co-cultured in flat-bottomed microtiter trays in 0.15 ml/well of tissue culture medium (RPMI 1640 supplemented with 15% pooled human AB serum, penicillin 100 U/ml, and streptomycin 100 μg/ml) containing either 5 μg/ml PPD (Statens Serum Institute, Copenhagen, Denmark), 1% PHA (Bacto Difco), or control medium. The cells were cultured in a humified 5% CO_2 incubator at 37°C for 72 hr. Sixteen hours before harvesting, 2-μCi [^{3}H]thymidine was added to each culture.

Primed Lymphocyte Test

Primed lymphocyte typing has been performed using our standard protocol for the secondary MLC (15). The cell lines used were specific for
HLA-SB4 and LB-Q1 (15).

Results

Cell-mediated Lympholysis

The effect of all mAbs in the T cell specific panel (designated T1–T159
hereafter) and the LFA mAbs from the Monocyte/Myeloid specific panel
(M1–M118) on the cytolytic activity of a CTL-line specific for an HLA-A2
variant (HLA-A2.1) was determined. Effector: target cell ratios of 20 : 1
and 10 : 1 were used. Figure 16.1 shows the percent inhibition induced by
the mAbs for the 20 : 1 effector: target cell ratio. The 10 : 1 ratio gave

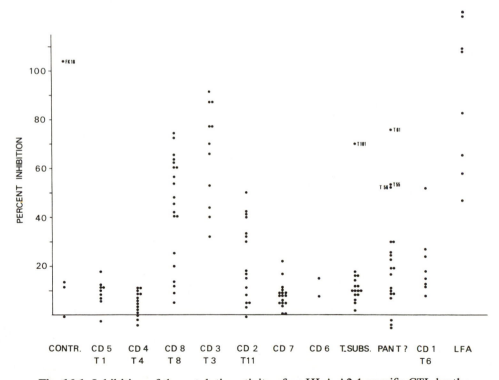

Fig. 16.1. Inhibition of the cytolytic activity of an HLA-A2.1-specific CTL by the
Workshop monoclonal antibodies. Each dot represents the percent inhibition in-
duced by a given mAb from the group indicated at the bottom of the figure.
Effector: target cell ratio 20 : 1. (Percent specific lysis in control was 67.)

similar results (not shown). As control antibodies, T1, T2, and T3 (no inhibition) and the CD8-like mAb FK18 (16) (complete blocking) were used. Little or no inhibition was induced by mAbs in the CD5, CD4, CD7, and CD6 group nor by the majority of mAbs in the CD1 and remaining groups (T48–T66 and T101–T116). Strong inhibition was induced by most mAbs in the CD3 and LFA group as well as by mAbs T61 and T101. Apparent bimodality is found in the inhibition patterns of both the CD2 and CD8 groups which show clusters of non- or weakly inhibiting mAbs and of moderately to strongly inhibiting mAbs. Further analysis of the data showed that the observed bimodality might be due to the IgG sub-class of the mAbs (Fig. 16.2). In the CD2 group mAbs of the IgG1 subclass appear to be ineffective in blocking CML, this in contrast to the CD8 group where most IgG1 mAbs are found in the cluster of blocking antibodies. Such a distribution was not found for the CD3 mAbs. Based on the above results 60 mAbs were selected for a second CML inhibition experiment. For this purpose, two CTL lines directed at MHC-restricted minor transplantation antigens were used (anti-HA-4 and anti-H-Y). The CTL-

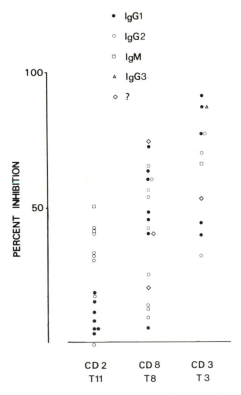

Fig. 16.2. Analysis of the influence of the Ig (sub)class of mAbs from the CD2, CD8, and CD3 groups on inhibition of CTL activity.

line anti-HA-4, like the anti-HLA-A2.1 line, was inhibited by CD3, LFA, and some of the CD8 and CD2 mAbs and not by CD4 or CD1 mAbs [Fig. 16.3(a)]. In contrast, the anti-H-Y CTL was inhibited strongly only by CD3 mAbs, the LFA mAbs blocking to a limited extent [Fig. 16.3 (b)]. These results might be related to a difference in affinity for the target antigen between the anti-H-Y line on one hand and the anti-HLA-A2.1 and anti-HA-4 line on the other hand (see discussion). The mAbs T61 and T101 inhibited all three CTL lines.

Antigen-specific T Lymphoblast Proliferation

The influence of a selected panel of mAbs on the proliferative response of PPD-specific T lymphoblasts (AgTR) was determined. The response of the cell line was inhibited by CD3, CD2, some CD4, and several other less well-characterized mAbs (Fig. 16.4). No inhibition was found with CD7 mAbs, only moderate blocking with most CD8, LFA, and some CD4 mAbs and several antibodies from the "T-activation" group (various). One CD2 mAb (T28) induced a significant increase in [^{3}H]thymidine incorporation.

Primed Lymphocyte Test

Results similar to those in AgTR were obtained in the inhibition study using an L_B-Q1 specific T cell line with most of the mAbs tested (not shown). However, in this case no enhancement of [^{3}H]thymidine incorporation was found with mAb T28.

The influence of the CD3 mAbs on the proliferative response of an HLA-SB4 specific T cell line was studied in more detail. The response of the cell line to several SB4 positive and one SB4 negative stimulator cell was determined in the presence or absence of the CD3 mAbs. Almost complete blocking was found when mAbs T120–T124 were added to the assay (Table 16.1). These mAbs do not induce proliferation of the cell line if tested against an SB4 negative stimulator cell. This is in contrast to mAbs T117–T119, T125, and T126 which block only partially and induce proliferation. However, when the T cell line is stimulated with cells from donor C complete blocking with all mAbs is observed whereas stimulation with cells from donor D results in an enhancement of the reaction if mAbs T117–T119 and T125 are added. Consequently, blocking or enhancement appears to depend not only on the mAb but also on the stimulator cell used.

Antibody-dependent Cellular Cytotoxicity (ADCC) and NK Cell Activity

Both ADCC and NK cell activity were blocked (partially) by very few mAbs only.

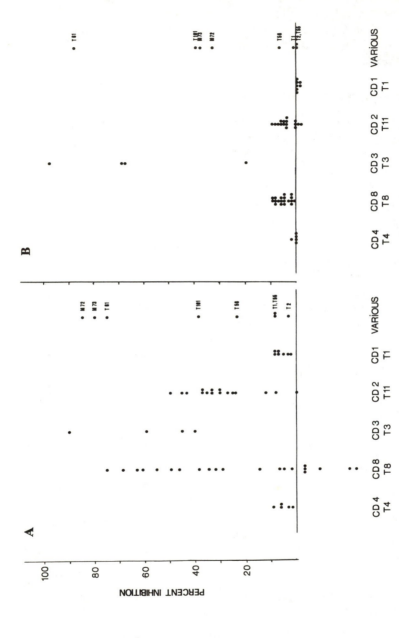

Fig. 16.3. Inhibition of the cytolytic activity of MHC-restricted CTL lines directed against the minor transplantation antigens HA-4 (A) and H-Y (B) by a selected panel of mAbs. Effector : target cell ratio 20 : 1. Percent specific lysis in control was 53 (anti-HE) and 85 (anti-H-Y).

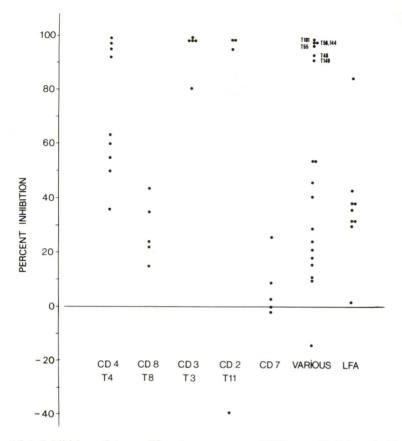

Fig. 16.4. Inhibition of the proliferative response of PPD specific T lymphoblasts to PPD by a panel of workshop mAbs. [³H]thymidine incorporation in control was 85,817 ± 1716 cpm.

Moderate blocking of ADCC was found with some of the LFA mAbs as well as with some others (Fig. 16.5).

NK cell activity was blocked strongly by (some) LFA antibodies (Fig. 16.6). MAbs from the CD2 group, T59, and some mAbs from the CD4 and CD8 groups seemed to be able to block partially. None of the mAbs from the Monocyte/Myeloid panel which were identified as being NK cell specific inhibited the reactivity of these cells.

Several mAbs of the Monocyte/Myeloid panel caused enhanced lysis when added to the NK assay. An explanation for this observation might be that these mAbs bind to the target cell and are therefore able to mediate in ADCC which results in additional lysis.

Table 16.1. The influence of the CD3 mAbs on the proliferative response[a] of an HLA-SB4 (DP4) T cell line when tested against several SB4-positive and one SB4-negative stimulator cells.

Stimulator	mAb added: Control	117 IgG1	118 IgG1	119 NK[b]	120 IgG2a	121 IgG3	122 IgM	123 IgG1	124 IgG2b	125 IgG1	126 IgG2a	127 IgG1
A SB 3/4	29,616	19,510	10,110	34,150	1,155	6,240	195	155	160	16,300	8,350	6,790
B SB 4/4	28,130	8,960	3,345	6,940	240	4,035	170	125	140	10,470	5,040	7,170
C SB 4/4	9,303	705	325	795	150	690	195	120	165	515	500	360
D SB 4/5	13,606	21,550	22,070	29,200	375	1,705	230	180	175	31,370	4,580	2,610
E SB 2/2	250	10,650	6,840	10,300	570	660	180	150	165	10,390	5,880	210

[a] Values in table are [^{3}H]thymidine incorporation. Enhanced reactions are underlined.
[b] NK = not known

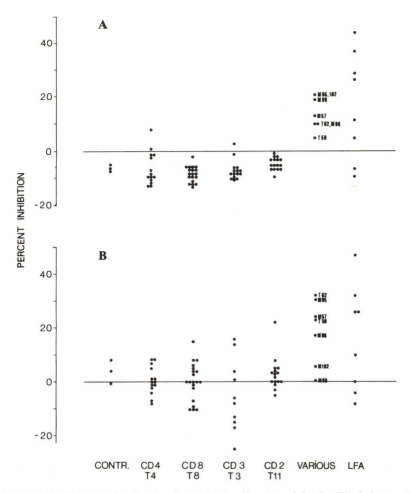

Fig. 16.5. Inhibition of antibody-dependent cell cytotoxicity by Workshop mAbs using two different effector cell suspensions (A and B). Effector : target cell ratio 10 : 1 (74% specific lysis in control).

Discussion

Since all inhibition experiments were performed only once and little is known at present about the precise specificity of or differences in affinity between the antibodies in any given CD group, our results only indicate the inhibitory potential of a certain group of antibodies in the functional assays. Nevertheless, we observed that some mAbs in the CD8, CD3 and LFA groups repeatedly induced a high degree of inhibition in certain assays, indicating that these are either high-affinity antibodies or more concentrated preparations.

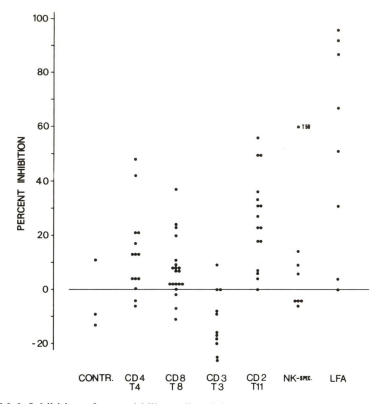

Fig. 16.6. Inhibition of natural killer cell activity by Workshop mAbs. Effector: target cell ratio 20:1 (47% specific lysis in control).

Two out of three cytotoxic T cell lines were inhibited by CD3, LFA, and some of the CD8 and CD2 mAbs. The bimodality in the CD8 group might reflect the difference in blocking capacity between T5- and T8a-like mAbs as described previously (17). Those CTLs which were blocked by CD8 mAbs were inhibited partially also by some CD2 mAbs, which is in good agreement with work of other investigators (5,6). The bimodality observed using the HLA-A2.1-specific CTL clearly correlated with the inability of IgG1 mAbs to induce inhibition. This correlation was less clear with the HA-4 specific CTL. However, all IgG1 mAbs are found in the lower part of the cluster while the remaining mAbs are in the upper part (results not shown). Since other investigators (18) have shown that the mitogenicity of CD3 mAbs of the IgG1 subclass depends on the ability of the monocyte Fc receptor to bind to IgG1, this observation deserves further attention since a similar mechanism might be involved. In contrast to the anti-HLA-A2.1 and anti-HA-4 CTL lines (67 and 55% specific lysis, respectively), the anti-H-Y CTL line (80% specific lysis) was not or only marginally inhibited by CD8 and CD2 mAbs. In addition, the effect of

LFA antibodies was greatly reduced. The highly specific lysis induced by the anti-H-Y CTL makes it likely that this cell line has a higher affinity for its target antigen as compared to the two other cell lines. This result tends to support the hypothesis that the T8 antigen can serve as an adhesion-strengthening molecule which stabilizes the interaction between effector and target cell when the T cell receptor has a low affinity for its target antigen. In case of a high-affinity T cell receptor this would not be necessary (19). The observation that the anti-HLA-A2.1 and HLA-class I restricted anti-HA-4 lines can be blocked by CD8 mAbs is in good agreement with the observation that T8 positive CTLs recognize HLA-class I gene products (20,21).

Proliferation of the HLA-class II specific primed T lymphocytes (PLT) and the PPD specific T lymphoblasts (AgTR) was blocked by CD4, CD2, and CD3 mAbs. The first result agrees with the observation that T4 positive lines recognize or are restricted by HLA-class II gene products (21).

LFA antibodies appeared inefficient in blocking AgTR which may be related to a high affinity of the cell line for its antigen, like in CML. In PLT, blocking or enhancement of the proliferative response by CD3 mAbs was not only dependent on the mAb used (concentration ?, epitope recognized ?) but also on the stimulator cell used. This observation could not be explained on the basis of the IgG subclass as has been described (18) and might therefore indicate an additional heterogeneity within this group of antibodies.

In contrast to the results in PLT, induction of proliferation by CD3 mAbs was not observed in AgTR. Since only one APC has been used, this might, like in PLT, be due to the stimulator cell.

Since CD2 mAbs appear to be able to induce proliferation (4, this report) and to block CML as well as PLT and AgTR the antigen recognized apparently plays a crucial role in T cell function. In contrast to CD3 mAbs, these antibodies did not inhibit the cytolytic activity of the anti-H-Y CTL; therefore, the mechanisms whereby these two groups of mAbs inhibit must be different.

Several other less well characterized antibodies like T55, T56, T61, and T101 were able to (partially) block CML, PLT, and AgTR and are therefore most likely CD3-like mAbs although T101 may be an LFA mAb.

Only very few mAbs blocked ADCC and NK cell activity. In the ADCC assay virtually no effect was exerted by any mAb in the highest effector:target cell ratio used (20:1). Partial blocking was found in the 10:1 ratio. In contrast to CML, neither CD3, CD2, or CD8 mAbs inhibited ADCC, indicating that the antigens recognized by these mAbs do not play a functional role in this assay. Partial inhibition was found with LFA mAbs, confirming the results of other investigators (22). Furthermore, some mAbs from the T cell and Monocyte/Myeloid panel inhibited very weakly. More detailed studies are needed to clarify whether or not these antibodies can inhibit ADCC.

Table 16.2. Summary of workshop monoclonal antibodies inhibiting or enhancing the functional assays indicated.

Antibody group	CML					ADCC	NK-cell activity
	Anti HLA-A2.1	Anti-He	Anti-H-Y	AgTR	PLT		
CD4	—	—	—	68-69,70,72,75, ?67,71,73,74,76	68-80	—	?72,76
CD8	82-84,86-90, 92-97	83,84,86-90,92, 96,97	—	—	—	—	±?
CD3	117-127	117,118,121,123	117,118,121,123	117,118,120-122	117-127	—	—
CD2	14,16,22-24, 26, 27	14-28	—	19,23,27	19,23,27,28	—	±
CD7	—	—	—	—	NT	—	—
CD6	—	NT	NT	NT	NT	—	—
T subs.	101	101	101	101	NT	—	—
Pan T	55,56,61	61	61	48,55,56,?61	55,56,61	62,?50	59
CD1	—	—	—	NT	NT	—	—
T-act.	NT[a]	NT	NT	140,144	NT	—	—
LFA	+	+	±	±	NT	±	+
M1-118	NT	NT	NT	NT	NT	95,96,99,102	—

[a] NT = not tested.

In the NK assay, strong blocking was found with some LFA mAbs and partial blocking by mAbs from the CD4, CD8, and CD2 groups. This latter observation is in agreement with the results from Fast *et al.* (5) which showed that the CD2 mAb 9.6 can partially inhibit NK cell activity.

No inhibition was found with the "NK cell specific" mAbs suggesting that the antigens recognized do not play a role in NK cell activity.

Finally, we conclude that we were able to identify mAbs capable of inhibiting functional assays, to confirm the proposed specificities of most of the CD3, CD8, CD4, and CD2 mAbs, and to provide information on some less well characterized mAbs.

A summary of the results indicating mAbs inhibiting functional assays is given in Table 16.2.

Summary

The results of our studies show that CML could be blocked by CD3, LFA, and part of the CD8 and CD2 mAbs. In the latter group mAbs of the IgG1 subclass appeared ineffective in blocking. One CTL line could only be blocked by CD3 mAbs which might be due to high affinity of this line for its target antigen. AgTR was inhibited by CD4, CD2, and CD3 mAbs; LFA mAbs appeared ineffective. PLT was blocked by CD4 and CD2 mAbs whereas CD3 mAbs occasionally blocked or enhanced the reaction. Additionally several less well characterized mAbs blocked CML as well as PLT and AgTR. Both the ADCC and NK cell activity were blocked by only very few mAbs of which some belonged to the T cell and some to the Monocyte/Myeloid panel.

Acknowledgments. This work was in part supported by the Dutch Foundation for Medical Research (FUNGO) which is subsidized by the Dutch Organization for the Advancement of Pure Research (ZWO) and the J.A. Cohen Institute for Radiopathology and Radiation Protection (IRS).

References

1. Köhler, G., and C. Milstein. 1975. Continuous cultures of fused cells secreting antibody of predefined specificity. *Nature* **256**:495.
2. Martz, E., W. Heagy, and S.H. Gromkowski. 1983. The mechanism of CTL-mediated killing: monoclonal antibody analysis of the roles of killer and target-cell membrane proteins. *Immunol. Rev.* **72**:73.
3. Meuer, S.C., O. Acuto, R.E. Hussey, J.C. Hodgdon, K.A. Fitzgerald, S.F. Schlossman, and E.L. Reinherz. 1983. Evidence for the T3-associated 90K heterodimer as the T-cell antigen receptor. *Nature* **303**:808.
4. Meuer, S.C., R.E. Hussey, M. Fabbi, D. Fox, O. Acuto, K.A. Fitzgerald, J.C. Hodgdon, J.P. Protentis, S.F. Schlossman, and E.L. Reinherz. 1984. An

alternative pathway of T-cell activation: a functional role for the 50 kd T11 sheep red blood cell receptor protein. *Cell* **36:**897.

5. Fast, L.D., J.A. Hansen, and W. Newman. 1981. Human NK, ADCC, and CTL: evidence for shared T cell antigen. *J. Immunol.* **127:**448.

6. Krensky, A.M., F. Sanchez-Madrid, E. Robbins, J.A. Nagy, T.A. Springer, and S.J. Burokoff. 1983. The functional significance, distribution, and structure of LFA-1, LFA-2, and LFA-3: cell surface antigens associated with CTL–target interactions. *J. Immunol.* **131:**611.

7. Bruning, J.W., J.J. van der Poel, and M.J. Kardol. 1982. The fluorochromasia cell mediated lympholysis assay (CML). In: HLA typing: methodology and clinical aspects, Volume II, S. Ferrone and B.G. Solheim, ed. CRC Press, Inc., Boca Raton, Florida 33431.

8. van der Poel, J.J., M.J. Kardol, E. Goulmy, E. Blokland, and J.W. Bruning. 1980. Carboxy fluorescein fluorochromasia cell mediated lympholysis. A comparative study. *Immunol. Lett.* **2:**187.

9. van der Poel, J.J., J. Pool, E. Goulmy, and J.J. van Rood. 1983. Recognition of the serologically defined HLA-A2 antigen by Cytotoxic T-cells. II Definition of three HLA-A2 subtypes by CTLs. *Immunogen.* **17:**599.

10. Goulmy, E., J.D. Hamilton, and B.A. Bradley. 1979. Anti self HLA may be clonally expressed. *J. Exp. Med.* **149:**545.

11. Goulmy, E. 1984. Class I restricted human cytotoxic T lymphocytes directed against minor transplantation antigens and their possible role in organ transplantation. *Prog. Allergy* **36.** In press.

12. Bruning, J.W., M.J. Kardol, R. Arentzen, A. Naipal, and J.J. van der Poel. 1979. Carboxyfluorescein fluorochromasia assays for cell mediated lympholysis (CML) and antibody dependent cellular cytotoxicity (ADCC): a nonradioactive technique. *Trans. Proc.* **11:**1961.

13. Koning, F., M. Dubelaar, A. Bakker, and H. Bruning. MD 2.6. A mouse monoclonal antibody detecting a lymphocyte subset surface antigen which disappears after cell stimulation. Submitted to *Eur. J. Immunol.*

14. Ottenhoff, T.H.M., B.G. Elferink, J. Hermans, and R.R.P. de Vries. HLA class II restriction repertoire of antigen specific T cells. I. The main restriction determinants for antigen presentation are associated with HLA = D/DR and not with DP and DQ. *Hum. Immunol.* in press.

15. Termijtelen, A., S.J. van den Berge, and J.J. van Rood. 1983. LB-Q1 and LB-Q2: two determinants defined in the primed lymphocyte test and independent of HLA-D/DR, MB/LB-E, or SB. *Human Immunol.* **8:**11.

16. Koning, F. 1982. An OKT 8-like mouse monoclonal antibody. In: Abstracts, Fifth European Immunology Meeting.

17. Reinherz, E.L., R.E. Hussey, K. Fitzgerald, P. Snow, C. Terhorst, and S.F. Schlossman. 1981. Antibody directed at a surface structure inhibits cytolytic but not suppressor cell function of human T-lymphocytes. *Nature* **294:**168.

18. Tax, W.J.M., H.W. Willems, P.P.M. Reekers, P.J.A. Capel, and R.A.P. Koene. 1983. Polymorphism in mitogenic effect of IgG1 monoclonal against T3 antigen on human T-cells. *Nature* **304:**445.

19. MacDonald, H.R., A.L. Glasebrook, and J.C. Cerotinni. 1982. Clonal heterogeneity in the functional requirement for lyt-2/3 molecules on cytolytic T-lymphocytes: analysis by antibody blocking and selective trypsinisation. *J. Exp. Med.* **156:**1711.

20. Spits, H., H. IJssel, C. Terhorst, and J.E. de Vries., 1982. Establishment of human T lymphocyte clones highly cytotoxic for an EBV-transformed B cell line in serum free medium: isolation of clones that differ in phenotype and specificity. *J. Immunol.* **128:**95.

21. Meuer, S.C., S.F. Schlossman, and E.L. Reinherz. 1982. Clonal analysis of human cytotoxic T lymphocytes: T4[+] and T8[+] effector T cells recognize products of different major histocompatibility complex regions. *Proc. Natl. Acad. Sci. U.S.A.* **79:**4395.

22. Miedema, F., P.A.T. Tettero, W.G. Hesselink, G. Werner, H. Spits, and C.J.M. Melief. 1984. Both Fc receptors and LFA-1 on human T lymphocytes are required for antibody-dependent cellular cytotoxicity (killer cell activity). *Eur. J. Immunol.* **6:**518.

CHAPTER 17

The Influence of Anti–T Cell Monoclonal Antibodies on Calcium Mobilization: Investigation of Workshop Antibodies

Kieran O'Flynn, Peter C.L. Beverley, and David C. Linch

Anti–T cell monoclonal antibodies may affect a variety of functions (1–4). Antibodies to CD3 and the T cell receptor for antigen (Ti) are mitogenic (5), suggesting that these molecules are important in T cell activation. Several antibodies have been described which block mitogen-induced proliferation and CTL killing (3,4), but these findings are difficult to interpret as T cell activation is a multistep process and the binding of a monoclonal antibody to a surface ligand may interfere at one of a number of stages in this process or activate a suppressor mechanism.

To overcome these problems we have investigated the effects of monoclonal antibodies on intracellular calcium levels, $[Ca^{2+}]i$, as there is a large body of evidence to suggest that early calcium mobilization is a primary event in T cell activation (for review see Ref. 6). Both PHA and Con A induce a rise in $[Ca^{2+}]i$ which is complete within three to four minutes. A similar effect is seen with the anti-CD3 antibodies UCHT1, anti-Leu-4, and WT32 (7,8). The anti-CD2 antibodies OKT11 and anti-LFA-2 had no direct effect on $[Ca^{2+}]i$, but did block subsequent calcium mobilization induced by PHA but not by Con A or the anti-CD3 antibody UCHT1. This suggests that CD2 is an alternative activation pathway to the antigen receptor (Ti) and that it is through this pathway that the effect of PHA is mediated (9).

To confirm and extend these findings we have investigated the ability of a selection of the Workshop anti–pan T monoclonal antibodies to induce a rise in $[Ca^{2+}]i$ and to block PHA-induced calcium mobilization.

Materials and Methods

Cell Preparation

Peripheral blood mononuclear cells (PBMC) were prepared by buoyant density sedimentation on Ficoll–Hypaque. T cells were prepared from this fraction by a standard rosetting procedure with AET-treated sheep red blood cells.

Measurement of Intracellular Calcium

Cells were incubated with 15 μM Quin 2 tetraacetoxymethyl ester (Amersham) for one hour as previously described (7) using a modification of the method of Tsien *et al.* (10). After washing, fluorescence was measured at 37°C in a modified Locarte fluorimeter with excitation at 339 nm and emission measured at 492 nm. $1-2 \times 10^6$ E^+ cells were used per experiment and cell suspensions were continuously stirred. The system was calibrated using the Triton X.100/DTPA/MnCl$_2$ procedure as previously reported (7).

Monoclonal Antibodies

Workshop antibodies tested were the anti-CD3 antibodies with the exception of 125, the anti-CD2 antibodies with the exception of 24, the anti-CD6 antibodies 46 and 47, and the pan T other/unknown antibodies 48–66 with the exception of 60 and 65. Affinity-purified rabbit anti–mouse Ig was obtained from Zymed Laboratories, San Francisco, California and fluoresceinated rabbit anti–mouse Ig was from Nordic Laboratories, UK.

Indirect Immunofluorescence

The fluorescence intensity and profile of PBMC was determined after staining with different dilutions of antibody using an indirect immuno-fluorescence technique (11). Analysis was performed on a FACS IV (Becton-Dickinson, Sunnyvale, California), and the percentage of cells above background and the peak channel number of the positive population recorded.

Blocking of Sheep Erythrocyte Rosette Formation

PBMC were incubated with a 1 : 200 dilution of anti-CD2 ascitic fluid at 4°C for 30 min. Cells were washed three times and incubated in a pellet with AET-treated SRBC for 1 hr at 4°C. Rosettes were scored after gentle resuspension.

Results

Anti-CD3 Antibodies

Test ascites were added to Quin 2-loaded E^+ cells at a dilution of 1 : 200, and the magnitude and kinetics of any rise in [Ca^{2+}]i was determined and compared to that produced by 2.0 μg/ml of UCHT1. A rise comparable to

UCHT1 was designated as ++ (Fig. 17.1). Any rise that was less than that produced by UCHT1, or in which the rise in calcium was significantly slower or unsustained was designated as (+). Six of the ten antibodies tested induced (++) calcium mobilization and one a (+) rise (Table 17.1). Three antibodies had no effect on [Ca^{2+}]i at a dilution of 1 : 200 and 1 : 100. In a previous study the titer of UCHT1 giving rise to calcium mobilization was shown to be similar to that required for optimal fluorescent staining of T cells (7). We therefore compared the titer and intensity of staining of the (−) and (+) antibodies with two of the antibodies giving (++) calcium responses. Antibodies 118 and 120, which gave a (++) calcium response, stained 77% and 73% of PBMC with peak channel values of 108 and 110, respectively.

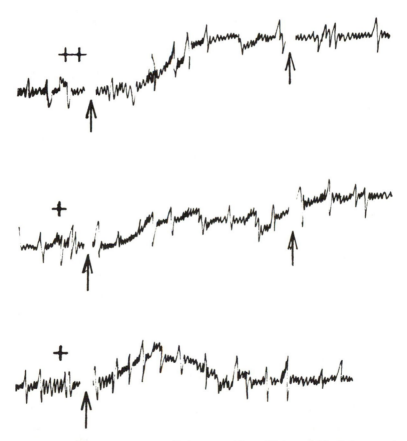

Fig. 17.1. Traces show the rise in (Ca^{2+})i induced by addition of Workshop antibodies to E$^+$ cells. Top, a response equivalent to that to UCHT1 and scored as ++. Addition of UCHT1 (right-hand arrow) had no additional effect. Middle and bottom, responses scored as +. Addition of UCHT1 (right-hand arrow) induced a further rise in (Ca^{2+})i in the middle example.

Table 17.1. Effect of anti-CD3 workshop antibodies on calcium mobilization.

Workshop number	Degree of calcium mobilization[a]	Staining by immunofluorescence	
		Peak channel number	Percentage positive
117	++		
118	++	108	77
119	++		
120	++		
122	++	110	73
123	++		
124	+	98	71
121	−	Atypical profile	
126	−	89	55
127	−	56	7

[a] Degree of calcium mobilization relative to UCHT1: ++ indicates a response approximately equal to that to UCHT1, + indicates a distinct but lesser response.

Antibody 124, which gave a (+) calcium response, stained 71% of PBMC with a peak channel value of 98. Similar values were obtained at dilutions of 1:50 and 1:100. Antibody 127, which gave a (−) calcium response, stained very few T cells at dilutions of 1:50–1:200. Antibody 121, which also gave no calcium response, produced a fluorescence profile not typical of anti-CD3 antibodies. Thirty-one percent of cells were positive, some bright (peak channel 136) and some dim (peak channel 70). The one remaining antibody giving no calcium response (No. 126) stained 55% of PBMC with a peak channel number of 89 at dilutions of 1:50–1:200. The binding of this antibody did not prevent subsequent calcium mobilization by UCHT1.

Anti-CD2 Antibodies

None of these antibodies tested stimulated calcium mobilization at a dilution of 1:200 when added alone or when subsequently cross-linked with rabbit anti–mouse immunoglobulin. Eight of fifteen antibodies tested gave (++) blocking of PHA-induced calcium mobilization and two a (+) blocking effect. Subsequent addition of the anti-CD3 antibody UCHT1 gave a normal rise in $[Ca^{2+}]i$. Five antibodies did not significantly suppress a PHA calcium response. All but two of the ten blocking antibodies inhibited sheep red cell rosette formation by greater than 90% at a dilution of 1:200. Of the five antibodies failing to block a PHA response, the supression of E-rosette formation ranged between 0–73% (Fig. 17.2). The fluorescent staining of these nonblocking antibodies was analyzed at dilutions of 1:50, 1:100, and 1:200, and compared with two (++) antibodies and one (+) antibody. The peak channel numbers were constant at all three dilutions and are circled in Fig. 17.2. In general, there is concordance of

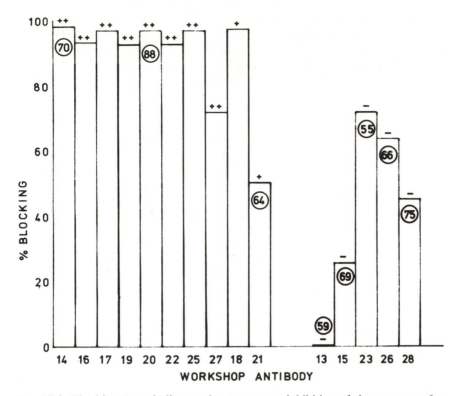

Fig. 17.2. The histogram indicates the percentage inhibition of sheep rosette formation by anti-CD2 monoclonal antibodies at 1 : 200 dilution. Numbers in circles indicate peak channel number (fluorescence intensity) of stained P.B.M.; + + and − indicate degree of blocking of PHA-induced calcium mobilization.

the intensity of antibody staining, the ability to block E-rosettes, and the ability to block PHA-induced calcium mobilization. It is of interest that antibody 28 stained a subset of PBMC (presumably T cells) with a fluorescence intensity and profile similar to that seen by the PHA-calcium response blocking antibodies, and yet showed only moderate blocking of E-rosette formation and no blocking of the PHA calcium response.

Anti-CD6 Antibodies

Neither of the anti-CD6 antibodies, Workshop numbers 46 and 47, caused calcium mobilization or blocked a PHA calcium response.

Pan T Other or Unknown

Two antibodies (Workshop numbers 48 and 61) caused calcium mobilization directly at a dilution of 1 : 200, although the rise in $[Ca^{2+}]i$ was not

210 K. O'Flynn, P.C.L. Beverley, D.C. Linch

Table 17.2. Effect of pan T other/unknown antibodies on calcium mobilization.

Workshop number	Degree of direct calcium mobilization		Blocking of PHA-induced calcium mobilization
	Alone	Cross-linked	
48	+		
61	+		
53	−	+	
59	−	+*	
56	−	−	+
57	−	−	+
49	−	−	−
50	−	−	−
51	−	−	−
52	−	−	−
54	−	−	−
55	−	−	−
58	−	−	−
62	−	−	ND
63	−	−	−
64	−	−	−
66	−	−	−

* This experiment was performed only once.

well sustained and is therefore designated as a (+) response (Table 17.2). These findings would be compatible with anti-CD3 antibodies. Two other antibodies (Workshop numbers 53 and 59) gave no response alone but produced a small rise in $[Ca^{2+}]i$ upon cross-linking with rabbit anti–mouse immunoglobulin. One antibody (number 56) blocked a PHA calcium response (+), and a similar effect was probably produced by antibody number 57 (+/−). Neither antibody affected UCHT1-induced calcium mobilization, suggesting that these antibodies may bind to CD2.

Discussion

The results with the anti-CD3 panel confirm our previous findings that these antibodies induce calcium mobilization (7,8). Of the three antibodies not causing a rise in $[Ca^{2+}]i$, one (Workshop number 121) was clearly shown not to be an anti-CD3 antibody by fluorescence analysis of PBMC. The other two antibodies, if anti-CD3s, gave very low-intensity staining. This was not due to a concentration effect, and either represents low-affinity antibody or degradation of reagent prior to use.

Ten of the anti-CD3 antibodies inhibited PHA-induced calcium mobilization but not the calcium response to the anti-CD3 antibody UCHT1. This is in agreement with our previous findings with OKT11 and anti-LFA-2 (9). These findings clearly implicate CD2 as a T cell activation molecule that is involved in the stimulation of T cells by PHA. This is in accord with the findings of Meuer *et al.* that the combination of antibodies to specific epitopes of CD2 can be mitogenic (12). Anti-T11$_2$ binds to an epitope of CD2 distinct from the sheep red cell receptor (T11$_1$), and this causes exposure of the neo-epitope T11$_3$. Reactivity with an anti-T11$_3$ antibody then induces proliferation. We have suggested that PHA binds to CD2, creates a conformational change which exposes T11$_3$, and then reacts with this epitope (9). The relationship between the T11 activation pathway and the Ti-T$_3$ pathway is still unclear.

There was general concordance between the ability to block E-rosette formation and the ability to block the PHA calcium response and the intensity of T cell binding. Those antibodies showing some degree of discordance are worthy of further study. The differences may be due to differences in avidity, but may reveal informative CD2 epitopes. For instance, antibody number 23 appeared to block sheep red cell rosette formation moderately well but did not bind avidly to T cells or block PHA-stimulated calcium mobilization. In contrast, antibody 28 bound avidly to T cells, but inhibited E-rosette formation less well and did not block a PHA calcium response.

The anti-CD6 antibodies did not influence calcium mobilization in these studies. Similar results have been previously obtained with the anti-CD5 antibodies UCHT2 and Leu-1, and the anti-CD5 antibodies were not therefore screened in this study.

Of the pan T other/unknown antibodies, two (Workshop numbers 48 and 61) have effects similar to anti-CD3 antibodies. The finding that anti-bodies 53 and 59 cause calcium mobilization when cross-linked, but not alone, is not at present interpretable. We have previously noticed this phenomenon with the anti-Ti antibody WT-31 on T cell lines, but not on peripheral blood T cells (8). Antibody 56 and, to a lesser extent, 57 block PHA calcium mobilization, suggesting that they react with CD2. The other antibodies tested in this study did not influence calcium mobilization.

Summary

The investigation of rapid changes in [Ca^{2+}]i using Quin 2 is a useful tool for the investigation of T cell surface antigens involved in cell activation, and is suitable for screening large numbers of antibodies.

References

1. Reinherz, E.L., S.C. Meuer, and S.F. Schlossman. 1983. The human T cell receptor: analysis with cytotoxic T cell clones. *Immunol. Rev.* **74,** 83.
2. Smith, K.A. 1984. Interleukin 2. *Annu. Rev. Immunol.* **2,** 319.

3. Palacios, R. and O. Martinez-Maza. 1982. Is the E receptor on human T lymphocytes a "negative signal receptor"? *J. Immunol.* **129,** 2479.
4. Krensky, A.M., R. Sanchez-Madrid, E. Robbins, J.A. Nagy, T. Springer, and S. Burakoff. 1983. The functional significance, distribution and structure of LFA-1, LFA-2 and LFA-3: cell surface antigens associated with CTL target interactions. *J. Immunol.* **131,** 611.
5. Burns, G.F., A.W. Boyd, and P.C.L. Beverley. 1982. Two monoclonal anti-human T lymphocyte antibodies have similar biologic effects and recognise the same surface antigen. *J. Immunol.* **129,** 1451.
6. Lichtman, A.H., G.B. Segel, and M.A. Lichtman. 1983. The role of calcium in lymphocyte proliferation—(an interpretive review). *Blood* **61,** 413.
7. O'Flynn, K., D.C. Linch, and P.E.R. Tatham. 1984. The effect of mitogenic lectins and monoclonal antibodies on intracellular free calcium concentration in human T-lymphocytes. *Biochem. J.* **219,** 661.
8. O'Flynn, K., E.D. Zanders, J.R. Lamb, P.C.L. Beverley, D.L. Wallace, P.E.R. Tatham, W.J.M. Tax, and D.C. Linch. 1985. Investigation of early T-cell activation: analysis of the effect of specific antigen, IL-2 and mono-clonal antibodies on intracellular free calcium concentration. *Eur. J. Immunol.* **15,** 7.
9. O'Flynn, K., A.M. Krensky, P.C.L. Beverley, S.J. Burakoff, and D.C. Linch. 1984. T-cell calcium mobilisation induced by PHA is mediated through the T11 antigen, the sheep red blood cell receptor. *Nature* **313,** 686.
10. Tsien, R.Y., T. Pozzan, and T.J. Rink. 1982. T-cell mitogens cause early changes in cytoplasmic free Ca^{2+} and membrane potential in lymphocytes. *Nature* **295,** 68.
11. Beverley, P.C.L. and R.E. Callard. 1981. Distinctive functional characteristics of human "T" lymphocytes defined by E rosetting or a monoclonal anti-T cell antibody. *Eur. J. Immunol.* **11,** 329.
12. Meuer, S.C., R.E. Hussey, M. Fabbi, D. Fox, O. Acuto, K.A. Fitzgerald, J.C. Hodgdon, J.P. Protentis, S.F. Schlossman, and E.L. Reinherz. 1984. An alternative pathway of T-cell activation; A functional role for the 50 kd T11 sheep erythrocyte receptor protein. *Cell* **36,** 897.

CHAPTER 18

T Cell-Dependent Immunoglobulin Synthesis in the Human System. Studies with T Cell-Specific Monoclonal Antibodies

Frank Miedema, Fokke G. Terpstra, and
Cornelis J.M. Melief

Introduction

The immunoregulatory activity of T cell subsets on human B cell differentiation has been amply studied in the pokeweed mitogen (PWM)-driven culture system (1,2). PWM-driven immunoglobulin (Ig) synthesis is strictly T cell-dependent and helper activity is only provided by $T4^+8^-$ cells, whereas $T4^-8^+$ cells have suppressor activity (1,2). We demonstrated that interleukin-2 (IL-2) plays an important role in T cell-dependent Ig synthesis (3). It was found that PWM-induced IL-2 synthesis is an early and necessary event in PWM-driven Ig synthesis. This was confirmed by the finding that anti-Tac, an anti-IL-2 receptor antibody (4), fully abrogated PWM-driven Ig synthesis, and moreover, by the innate Ig-inducing capacity of IL-2 itself, dependent on $T4^+8^-$ cells (3).

It has been shown that anti-T3 monoclonal antibody (mAb) inhibits T cell activation and blocks T helper activity in the PWM system (5,6). Some anti-T4 mAbs inhibit T helper activity in autologous mixed lymphocyte reactions (AMLR) but not PWM-induced Ig synthesis (2).

We studied the inhibiting effects on T cell-dependent Ig synthesis of the CD3, CD4, and T-activation clusters in both the PWM- and the IL-2-driven system. It was furthermore tested which subsets of normal T cells are recognized by mAbs in CD4 and how depletion of T cells for these T cell subsets affects the helper activity in PWM-driven Ig synthesis.

Materials and Methods

Lymphocyte Preparation and Cell Separations

Healthy donor peripheral blood leukocytes (PBL) were obtained by leukapheresis. Mononuclear cells were isolated by Ficoll–Isopaque density gradient centrifugation. T and non-T cells were separated by the E-rosette sedimentation technique, using neuraminidase-treated sheep erythrocytes (7). For the separation of T cell subpopulations based on their reactivity with mAbs, a panning technique was used (8). Briefly, plastic dishes (Falcon 3002 F) were coated overnight with 300 μg affinity purified sheep anti–mouse Ig in PBS. Pelleted T cells (10 × 10^6) were incubated for 30 min on ice with 50 μl of a 1 : 300 dilution of mAbs that was previously freed of sodium azide by dialysis against PBS. As a control OKT4 and OKT8 mAbs at a 1 : 1000 dilution were used (9). The cells were washed twice and 15 × 10^6 cells were applied to a single sheep anti–mouse IgG-coated plate. After 60-min incubation on ice, the nonadherent fraction was harvested.

Flow Cytofluorography

Phenotypic analysis of cell populations was performed by indirect immunofluorescence using as second antibody fluorescein-conjugated goat anti–mouse Ig, produced in our laboratory. Fluorescence was evaluated by means of cytofluorometry with an Ortho FC200 cytofluorograph. Workshop mAbs were used in a 1 : 600 dilution.

Assay of T Cell-Dependent Immunoglobulin Production *In Vitro*

PWM- and IL-2-induced polyclonal IgM synthesis by 20,000 non-T cells was performed in a microculture system and measured with an ELISA as described before (10). In all experiments 20,000 non-T cells were cultured for 7 days in wells of round-bottomed microtiter plates (Greiner) in a final volume of 170-μl Iscove's modified Dulbecco's medium supplemented with 20% fetal calf serum (Gibco cat. no. 629 H 1) and antibiotics. PWM (Gibco lot no. C 477102) was used at a final concentration of 50 μg/ml and IL-2, kindly provided by Dr. L.A. Aarden, at a final concentration of 30 U/ml, one Unit (U) being defined as the amount of IL-2 that induces half-maximal [^{3}H]thymidine incorporation in an IL-2-dependent murine T cell line. Helper activity was tested by co-culturing graded numbers of T cells with 20,000 normal non-T cells in this culture system.

Blocking Studies with Monoclonal Antibodies

The inhibiting effect of mAbs on T cell-dependent Ig production was evaluated by adding serial dilutions of ascites to cultures containing

20,000 non-T cells and 20,000 T cells in the presence of PWM or IL-2. The ascites had been dialyzed overnight against PBS to dialyze out the sodium azide. The final dilutions applied were 1:200, 1:2,000, and 1:20,000, respectively.

Ig production was measured after 7 days of culture. IgM production in control cultures without ascites ranged from 200–2000 ng/well.

Results

Inhibiting Effect of CD4 mAbs

Results of blocking studies with CD4 mAbs are shown in Table 18.1. Most mAbs had a weak inhibiting effect on both PWM- and IL-2-induced Ig synthesis. mAbs 72 and 75 had a strong inhibitory effect on PWM- and IL-2-driven Ig synthesis. mAbs 67 and 71 clearly inhibited the PWM system whereas Mab 73 and 76 only inhibited the IL-2 system.

Inhibiting Effect of CD3 mAbs

In the CD3 cluster 4 groups of mAbs could be distinguished on the basis of the inhibition studies (Table 18.2).

 I. mAbs that inhibited both systems: mAbs 118, 120, 126, and 127.
 II. mAbs that inhibited only the PWM system: mAbs 122, 123, and
 125.

Table 18.1. Inhibiting effect of CD4 mAbs on T cell-dependent Ig synthesis.

| mAb code number | Inhibiting effect (%)[a] | | | | | |
| | PWM-driven | | | IL-2-driven | | |
	1:20,000[b]	1:2000[b]	1:200[b]	1:20,000[b]	1:2000[b]	1:200[b]
67	40	26	71	−15	−32	22
68	40	42	39	17	−2	26
69	42	15	−4	29	41	−6
70	26	24	15	51	49	30
71	42	50	61	64	36	31
72	37	57	71	66	64	71
73	49	22	15	36	51	53
74	53	−3	36	51	44	34
75	37	61	82	54	58	68
76	21	51	33	49	34	51
77	28	0	62	48	52	42
78	37	32	31	34	24	30
79	57	−8	26	47	43	42
80	29	9	26	36	44	41

[a] Data shown are mean of 2 experiments.
[b] Final ascites dilution.

Table 18.2. Inhibiting effect of CD3 mAbs on T cell-dependent Ig synthesis.

| | Inhibition (%)[a] | | | | | | |
| | PWM-driven | | | IL-2-driven | | | |
mAb	1:20,000[b]	1:2000[b]	1:200[b]	1:20.000[b]	1:2000[b]	1:200[b]	Group no.
118 (SK7/Leu 4)	66	88	94	74	76	78	
120 (BW264/56)	51	67	93	59	80	90	I
126 (X35-3)	50	90	95	52	54	61	
127 (NU-T1)	69	67	77	33	30	67	
122 (T3/2Ad2A2)	3	35	74	−85	−17	23	
123 (T3/2T8-2F4)	68	80	95	10	−31	33	II
125 (T3/RW2-8C8)	33	64	93	60	15	−2	
117 (G19-4.1)	−22	−21	62	23	13	39	III
119 (89b1)	11	8	39	75	65	78	
121 (BW242/55)	2	2	40	8	3	22	IV
124 (T3/RW2-4B6)	−80	2	22	−34	−5	20	

[a] Results are the mean of 2 experiments.
[b] Final ascites dilution.

III. mAbs that inhibited only the IL-2 system: mAbs 117, and 119.
IV. mAbs that did not inhibit at all: mAbs 121 and 124.

Inhibiting Effect of T-activation mAbs

A subgroup (I) of the T-activation cluster, mAbs 141, 144, 145, and 150, showed a very pronounced inhibition of both PWM- and- IL-2-driven Ig synthesis. Even at very low concentrations of mAb a significant blocking was observed. A second subgroup (II), mAbs 135, 137, 138, and 143, inhibited exclusively the PWM system, whereas mAbs 136 and 139 (subgroup III) inhibited preferentially the IL-2 system. The remainder did not inhibit or only weakly inhibited Ig synthesis (Table 18.3).

Immunofluorescence Studies with CD4 and CD8 mAbs

Studies were undertaken to determine which portion of normal T cells reacted with the mAbs in CD4 and CD8 and, in comparison, with OKT4 and OKT8 mAbs. In the CD4 cluster all mAbs except mAbs 67, 74, and 80 reacted with approximately 44% of normal T cells [range 33–54%, mean (SD) 44% (±6)] (Table 18.4). The percentage of T4[+] cells as measured by the OKT4 mAbs was 43%. mAbs 67 and 80 did not stain above background whereas mAb 74 reacted with 60% of the T cells, although very weakly. In the CD8 cluster all mAbs, except mAbs 85, 86, 98, and 100, reacted with approximately 26% of the T cells [range 22–30, mean (SD) 26 (±2)] (Table 18.5).

Table 18.3. Inhibiting effect of T-activation mAbs on T cell-dependent Ig synthesis.

mAb	Inhibition (%)[a]						Group no.
	PWM-driven			IL-2-driven			
	1:20,000[a]	1:2000[a]	1:200[a]	1:20,000[a]	1:2000[a]	1:200[a]	
141 B149.9	80	79	94	57	92	95	
144 39C1.5	81	89	95	69	92	97	I
145 39C6.5	26	58	83	31	60	79	
150 41F2.1	31	27	79	11	38	63	
135 T1A	15	60	63	−7	−20	17	
137 100-1A5	10	24	70	−14	−2	49	II
138 1 MONO 2A6	12	41	85	−5	3	53	
143 23A9.3	2	61	79	−6	20	23	
136 TS145	−40	−6	45	16	32	69	III
139 4EL1C7	−2	0	52	16	56	67	
140 Tac/1HT4	−61	27	81	−13	5	26	
142 B1.19.2	−2	15	78	7	16	43	
146 33B3.1	37	0	83	−19	−3	75	
147 33B7.3	−7	10	83	−38	9	85	IV
148 39C8.18	17	14	83	0	−66	55	
149 39H7.3	−68	−37	72	−51	−28	27	
151 KOLT-1	−42	29	68	15	−11	46	

[a] Final ascites dilution.

Table 18.4. Immunofluorescence studies with CD4 mAbs on normal T cells.

mAb		%	mAb		%
Code	Name	Positive	Code	Name	Positive
—	OKT4	43	73	MT 321	43
—	OKT8	26	74	T4/12T	60[a]
67	T10C5	1	75	T4/18T	48
68	G19-2	44	76	MT 310	37
69	91d6	54	77	T4/19THY	48
70	94b1	45	78	T4/7T4	33
71	BW264/123	38	79	66.1	48
72	MT 151	46	80	TII19	2

[a] Very weak staining.

Table 18.5. Immunofluorescence studies with CD8 mAbs on normal T cells.

mAb		%	mAb		%
Code	Name	Positive	Code	Name	Positive
81	14	24	91	T8/7Pt	26
82	M236	28	92	T8/2T8	26
83	G10-1.1	30	93	T8-2T8	27
84	C12/D3	29	94	T8/2T8	24
85	BW264/162	2	95	T8/2ST8	22
86	BW135/80	1	96	66.2	25
87	MT 415	29	97	51.2	27
88	MT 1014	24	98	T411E1	4
89	MT 122	27	99	T41D8	24
90	T8/21THY	26	100	BL-TS1	2

Effect of Depletion of T Cells Binding CD4 mAbs on Helper Activity

Panning experiments were performed with CD4 mAbs. T cells, depleted in cells binding a specific CD4 mAb, were reexamined with the CD4 mAb used for depletion and OKT4 and OKT8 mAbs by cytofluorography (Table 18.6).

In most cases a small rest population of cells binding the mAbs used for depletion was demonstrable. In most cases a fairly good correlation between the depletion for OKT4$^+$ cells and a depletion for cells binding the specific CD4 mAb was obtained. Depletion with mAbs 67 and 80 did not result in a depletion of T4$^+$ cells. T cells depleted in cells positive for mAbs 74 and 78 still contained a considerable proportion of OKT4$^+$ cells—19 and 15%, respectively.

These T cell populations were tested for helper activity on PWM-driven Ig synthesis. Graded numbers of T cells were added to 20,000 non-T cells and cultured for 7 days in the presence of PWM. T cells depleted in OKT4$^+$ or OKT8$^+$ cells were included as controls (Table 18.7). The results clearly show that in most cases the helper activity of the depleted T cells was strongly decreased and even completely abrogated in the T-69, T-70, T-72, T-74, T-75, T-76, T-77 populations. No effect was observed when T cells were depleted with mAbs 67 and 80. In some cases helper activity was detectable at high cell numbers, most likely due to a small subset of T helper cells in the population (T-78, f.i.).

Table 18.6. Depletion of T cells with CD4 mAbs by a panning technique. Surface marker analysis.

T cell population	Percentage of positive cells			
	Control	OKT4	OKT8	CD4 mAb used for depletion
T-OKT4	6	9	58	—
T-OKT8	4	88	16	—
T-67	2	44	19	2
T-68	2	10	41	12
T-69	5	9	52	14
T-70	1	6	49	9
T-71	2	10	26	6
T-72	3	3	47	3
T-73	3	8	55	6
T-74	1	14	32	5
T-75	3	6	61	7
T-76	2	5	55	5
T-77	4	4	53	5
T-78	2	15	36	9
T-79	6	10	53	14
T-80	2	59	26	1

Table 18.7. Helper activity of T cell populations depleted in CD4-mAb-positive cells in PWM-driven Ig synthesis.

T cell population added	Number of T cells added (X10^{-3})			
	10	20	40	80
T-OKT4	93	80	100	121
T-OKT8	637	1816	3284	2304
T-67	328	739	1326	1359
T-68	62	101	242	335
T-69	34	70	78	181
T-70	71	52	124	159
T-71	71	188	214	420
T-72	20	35	56	101
T-73	53	108	203	176
T-74	35	116	166	127
T-75	37	61	80	83
T-76	29	66	97	133
T-77	37	60	92	76
T-78	115	174	277	455
T-79	52	162	182	278
T-80	567	1125	1486	1767

[a] Values in table are helper activity (ng Ig/well). 20,000 non-T cells alone, in the presence of PWM, produced less than 8.5 ng IgM/well.

Table 18.8. Depletion of T cells with the CD8 mAbs by a panning technique. Surface marker analysis.

T cell population	Percentage of positive cells		
	OKT4	OKT8	CD8 mAb used for depletion
T-OKT4	8	55	—
T-OKT8	69	8	—
T-81	75	8	5
T-82	70	9	6
T-83	86	3	5
T-84	83	6	5
T-85	60	27	2
T-86	61	21	2
T-87	81	6	5
T-88	79	8	8
T-89	84	7	6
T-90	86	6	6
T-91	80	5	5
T-92	72	15	12
T-93	76	7	7
T-94	80	9	10
T-95	66	17	14
T-96	74	6	7
T-97	68	8	12
T-98	61	21	3
T-99	63	11	8
T-100	49	30	2

Depletion of T Cells Binding CD8 mAbs

T cells were depleted in cells binding CD8 mAbs by a panning technique. The depleted T cells were treated with OKT4, OKT8, and the mAb used for the panning procedure, and the percentage positive cells was evaluated by cytofluorometry. With the majority of mAbs a severe depletion of OKT8$^+$ cells was achieved, comparable to a panning step with OKT8 mAbs (Table 18.8). mAbs 85, 86, 98, and 100 were shown not to bind to T cells (Table 18.5) and no depletions of T8$^+$ cells were observed with these mAbs.

Panning with mAbs 92 and 95 only resulted in a partial depletion of OKT8$^+$ T cells. An increase of helper activity of the depleted T cells compared to unseparated T cells, corresponding to the depletion in T8$^+$ cells and enrichment in OKT4$^+$ cells, was observed (data not shown). T cells depleted in mAb 85, 86, 98, and 100 positive cells did not show a significantly increased helper activity. T cells panned with mAbs 92 and 95 only showed a marginally increased helper activity.

Discussion

mAbs allow a more precise investigation of membrane structures involved in functional activities mediated by leukocytes. Anti-T4, anti-T8, and anti-T3 antibodies have been shown to inhibit cytotoxic T lymphocyte activity (CTL) (5). Some anti-T4 mAbs were shown to inhibit helper activity in Ig synthesis in autologous mixed lymphocyte reaction (AMLR), but not PWM-induced T cell-dependent Ig synthesis (2). Anti-T3 mAbs inhibit T cell proliferation and T cell-dependent Ig synthesis (5,6). Anti-Tac, a mAb directed against the human IL-2 receptor, has been shown to inhibit T cell activation by a functional blockade of the receptor (4). We have shown that anti-Tac inhibits T cell-dependent Ig synthesis induced by both PWM and IL-2 (3).

In the present study we showed that three CD4 mAbs strongly inhibited PWM-induced Ig synthesis and four CD4 mAbs inhibited IL-2-driven Ig synthesis. mAbs 72 and 75 abrogated Ig synthesis in both systems. It is unclear what the role of the T4 molecule is in the delivery of helper activity for B cell differentiation. Our results show that some mAbs against the T4 molecule significantly abrogate the delivery of the helper signal, even in the presence of exogenous IL-2. Whether this reflects a role in T–B interaction for T4, or has a more trivial explanation, remains to be elucidated.

It is well established that T3 is associated with the T cell receptor for antigen (5). The major functional effects of anti-T3 antibodies have been explained as a direct effect on the antigen recognition complex on T cells.

The majority of the CD3 mAbs inhibited PWM-induced Ig synthesis as described for OKT3 (6). Perhaps mAbs of group I, that inhibited both PWM- and IL-2-driven Ig synthesis, have an inhibiting effect on the delivery of the actual helper activity induced by IL-2 and inhibit one of the later steps of T-dependent Ig synthesis, whereas mAbs that inhibit only PWM- and not IL-2-induced Ig synthesis may do so by inhibiting PWM-induced IL-2 synthesis, the first necessary step in this system (3). We have demonstrated that anti-LFA-1 mAbs inhibit PWM-induced IL-2 synthesis and thus Ig synthesis, but not IL-2-driven Ig synthesis (see Vol. III, Chapter 5, Miedema, Terpstra, and Melief). This may also hold for the mAbs in the T-activation group. In addition, mAbs in subgroup I, which strongly abrogated Ig synthesis in both systems, possibly inhibit by a total blockade of the IL-2 receptor. Anti-Tac mAb (4) fully abrogates PWM- and IL-2-driven Ig synthesis (3). Inhibition of the PWM system by mAbs in the T-activation cluster may point to activation molecules on T cells involved in T cell–macrophage interactions, probably also resulting in IL-2-production inhibition (early activation antigens). mAbs in this cluster that only inhibited IL-2-driven Ig synthesis probably interfere with a late stage of T cell activation in the delivery of helper activity, only resulting in a weak effect on the PWM system.

Some mAbs in the CD4 cluster may define a previously not recognized subset of T cells that harbors helper activity. This was investigated by depletion studies in which T cells were depleted for cells binding the specific CD4 mAb. Immunofluorescence studies showed that of the CD4 mAbs only mAbs 67, and 80 did not react with 33–54% of normal T-cells. With all other mAbs, depletion resulted in complete abolition of helper activity or severely decreased helper activity corresponding to a depletion of OKT4$^+$ cells. T cells depleted for 74$^+$ and 78$^+$ cells lacked helper activity but still contained up to 15% OKT4$^+$ cells. This indicates that mAbs 74 and 78 bind to a subset of OKT4$^+$ cells that harbors all helper activity. Depletion with 67 and 80 did not affect the helper activity, in accord with the finding that these mAbs did not bind to T cells. Depletion studies with the CD8 mAbs demonstrated that indeed the majority of mAbs reacted with the T8$^+$ subset. In the CD8 series 4 mAbs (85, 86, 90, and 100) did not bind T cells and did not result in a decrease of T8$^+$ cells when used in depletion experiments.

Summary

The inhibiting effect of CD4, CD3, and T-activation monoclonal antibodies (mAbs) on T cell-dependent Ig synthesis was studied in a pokeweed mitogen (PWM)- and an interleukin-2 (IL-2)-driven system. In the CD4 cluster, 2 mAbs (72 & 75) inhibited both systems; mAb 67 only inhibited the PWM-driven Ig synthesis. The remainder of mAbs only weakly blocked Ig synthesis. Four groups of mAbs could be distinguished in the CD3 and T-activation clusters:

I. mAbs that inhibited both systems.
II. mAbs that inhibited PWM-induced Ig synthesis.
III. mAbs that inhibited IL-2-driven Ig synthesis.
IV. mAbs that did not inhibit Ig synthesis.

The majority of CD4 mAbs bound to a subpopulation of T cells identified by OKT4[+]. T cells depleted in 74[+] cells and 78[+] cells contained up to 15% OKT4[+] cells, but were devoid of helper activity. Depletion of T cells in cells reactive with CD8 mAbs resulted in a depletion of OKT8[+] cells.

Acknowledgment. This work was supported in part by grant CLB-80-2, Koningin Wilhelmina Fonds/Netherlands Cancer Organization.

References

1. Waldmann, T.A., and S. Broder. 1982. Polyclonal B-cell activation in the study of immunoglobulin synthesis in the human system. *Adv. Immunol.* **32:**1.
2. Thomas, Y., L. Rogozinski, and L. Chess. 1983. Relationship between human T cell functional heterogeneity and human T cell surface molecules. *Immunol. Rev.* **74:**113.
3. Miedema, F., J.W. van Oostveen, R.W. Sauerwein, F.G. Terpstra, L.A. Aarden, and C.J.M. Melief. 1984. Induction of immunoglobulin synthesis by Interleukin-2 is T4+8−cell dependent. A role for Interleukin-2 in the pokeweed-mitogen-driven system. *Eur. J. Immunol.* **15:**107.
4. Depper, J.M., W.J. Leonard, R.J. Robb, T.A. Waldmann, and W.C. Greene. 1983. Blockade of the Interleukin-2 receptor by anti-Tac antibody; inhibition of human lymphocyte activation. *J. Immunol.* **131:**690.
5. Reinherz, E.L., S.C. Meuer, and S.F. Schlossman. 1983. The human T cell receptor; analysis with cytotoxic T cell clones. *Immunol. Rev.* **74:**83.
6. Reinherz, E.L., R.E. Hussey, and S.F. Schlossman. 1980. A monoclonal antibody blocking human T-cell function. *Eur. J. Immunol.* **10:**758.
7. Van Oers, M.H.J., W.P. Zeijlemaker, and P.Th.A. Schellekens. 1979. Separation and properties of EA-rosette-forming lymphocytes in humans. *Eur. J. Immunol.* **7:**143.
8. Reinherz, E.L., A.C. Penta, R.E. Hussey, and S.F. Schlossman. 1981. A rapid method for separating functionally intact human T lymphocytes with monoclonal antibodies. *Clin. Immunol. Immunopathol.* **21:**257.
9. Reinherz, E.L., and S.F. Schlossman. 1980. The differentiation and function of human T lymphocytes. *Cell* **19:**821.
10. Rümke, H.C., F.G. Terpstra, B. Huis, T.A. Out, and W.P. Zeijlemaker. 1982. Immunoglobulin production in human mixed lymphocyte cultures. *J. Immunol.* **128:**696.

CHAPTER 19

Monoclonal Antibodies Recognizing the T3/Leu 4 T Cell Differentiation Antigen Induce Suppressor Cells

Jolanta E. Kunicka and Chris D. Platsoucas

The OKT3 and anti-Leu 4 monoclonal antibodies define a T cell surface differentiation antigen selectively expressed on functionally mature T cells (1,2). This antigen exhibits a complex biochemical structure consisting of at least three polypeptides with molecular weight in the range of 19–26 Kd (3–5). Monoclonal antibodies recognizing the T3/Leu 4 antigen exhibit profound effects on various T cell functions, including: (a) inhibition of proliferative responses of human peripheral blood lymphocytes to mitogens and allogeneic cells in mixed lymphocyte culture (6,7); (b) inhibition of T cell helper function to B cell responses (6); (c) inhibition of specific T cell-mediated cytotoxicity at the effector phase (7,8) and at a post-adhesion stage of the cytolytic process (9–12). It has been suggested that the T3 antigen may be associated with triggering of T cell functions and signal transfer or transduction (12).

We report here that *in vitro* treatment of human peripheral blood mononuclear leukocytes with the OKT3 or anti-Leu 4 monoclonal antibodies resulted in induction of suppressor cells to proliferative responses to mitogens and allogeneic cells in mixed lymphocyte culture and to *de novo* immunoglobulin synthesis and secretion in the PWM-induced differentiation system.

Materials and Methods

Preparation of Mononuclear Leukocytes

Human peripheral blood mononuclear leukocytes from normal donors were prepared by centrifugation on a Ficoll–Hypaque density cushion at room temperature. The cells were washed three times with Hank's balanced salt solution (HBSS).

Induction of Suppressor Cells

Peripheral blood mononuclear leukocytes were resuspended at a concentration of 3×10^6 cells/ml in RPMI 1640 containing 10% heat-inactivated fetal calf serum (HIFCS), 25 mM Hepes buffer, 2 mM L-glutamine, 100 U/ml penicillin, and 100 μg/ml streptomycin and incubated with various concentrations of (azide-free) OKT3 or anti-Leu 4 monoclonal antibodies for 24, 48 or 72 hr at 37°C, in a humidified incubator with 5% CO_2. The cells were washed three times with RPMI 1640 supplemented with 10% HIFCS and incubated with 50 μg/ml of mitomycin C for 45 min at 37° C. Subsequently, the cells were washed three times with RPMI-1640 supplemented with 10% HIFCS.

Determination of Suppressor Cell Activity to Proliferative Responses to Mitogens and Allogeneic Cells in MLC

Mononuclear leukocytes treated with the OKT3 or anti-Leu 4 monoclonal antibodies and mitomycin C (as previously described) were resuspended at a concentration of 1×10^6 cells/ml in RPMI 1640 containing 10% HIFCS, 25 mM Hepes buffer, 2 mM L-glutamine, 100 U/ml penicillin, and 100 μg/ml streptomycin. These cells were added to autologous or allogeneic peripheral blood mononuclear leukocytes (responder cells) resuspended in the same medium, at suppressor/responder cell ratio (S/R) of 2:1 or 1:1 in round-bottomed microtiter plates. PHA (5 μg/ml) or irradiated (2500 R) allogeneic mononuclear leukocytes (stimulating cells) were added and the cultures were incubated, respectively, for 3 or 6 days at 37°C in a humidified incubator with 5% CO_2. The cells were pulsed with [³H]thymidine (specific activity 6.7 Ci/mmol, New England Nuclear, Boston, MA) during the last 18 hr of culture and harvested using an automatic harvester. Percent suppression was calculated by the formula:

$$\% \text{ Suppression} = \left(1 - \frac{(S_p - S)}{(C_p - C)}\right) \times 100$$

where: S_p = cpm of responder cells, cultured with mitomycin C-treated OKT3- or anti-Leu 4-induced suppressor cells and PHA or allogeneic mononuclear cells; S = cpm of responder cells, cultured with mitomycin C-treated OKT3- or anti-Leu 4-induced suppressor cells; C_p = cpm of responder cells, cultured with mitomycin C-treated control cells and PHA or allogeneic mononuclear cells; C = cpm of responder cells, cultured with mitomycin C-treated control mononuclear cells.

Determination of Suppressor Cell Activity to de novo Immunoglobulin Synthesis and Secretion

Mononuclear leukocytes treated with the OKT3 or anti-Leu 4 monoclonal antibodies for 48 hr and with mitomycin C (as previously described) were resuspended at a concentration of 2×10^6 cells/ml in RPMI 1640 supplemented with 10% HIFCS, 25 mM Hepes buffer, 2 mM L-glutamine, 100 U/ml penicillin, and 100 μg/ml streptomycin. One hundred microliters of these cells were added to 1×10^5 freshly prepared, autologous mononuclear leukocytes in the previously described medium (suppressor/responder ratio 2 : 1) in round-bottomed microtiter plates. Control cultures of freshly prepared mononuclear leukocytes received mitomycin C-treated autologous mononuclear cells, which were not exposed to the OKT3 or anti-Leu 4 monoclonals. PWM (5 μg/ml) was added and the mixtures were cultured for 7 days at 37°C. Supernatants were collected and *de novo* synthesized IgM, IgA, and IgG were determined by a heavy chain-specific ELISA, as previously described (13). Results are expressed as μg/ml of either IgM, IgA, or IgG produced by mononuclear leukocytes cultured with PWM and in the presence of one of the following: (a) autologous mononuclear cells treated for 48 hr with the OKT3 or anti-Leu 4 monoclonal antibodies and with mitomycin C; (b) control autologous mononuclear leukocytes incubated in medium for 48 hrs and treated with mitomycin C.

Results

Inhibition of Proliferative Responses to PHA and Allogeneic Cells in MLC by OKT 3/anti-Leu 4-Induced Suppressor Cells

Treatment of peripheral blood mononuclear leukocytes for 24 or 48 hr resulted in the induction of suppressor cells inhibiting proliferative response of autologous or allogeneic mononuclear cells to PHA. Representative results are shown in Table 19.1. Induction for 24 hr was sufficient for the generation of suppressor activity. Both OKT3 and anti-Leu 4 monoclonal antibodies were able to induce suppressor cells in the majority of the donors examined. However, the OKT3 monoclonal antibody was superior in inducing suppressor cells in certain donors (Table 19.1, donors 2, 4, and 5), whereas the anti-Leu 4 monoclonal was more effective in others (donor 8 and Table 19.3).

Monoclonal antibodies recognizing other T cell differentiation antigens (anti-Leu 2a, anti-Leu 3a, and anti-Leu 5) did not induce the generation of suppressor cells to the proliferative responses to PHA by autologous or allogeneic mononuclear cells, even at very high antibody concentrations (10 μg/ml) (Table 19.2).

OKT3/anti-Leu 4-induced suppressor cells also inhibited the proliferative responses of autologous mononuclear leukocytes to allogeneic cells in mixed lymphocyte culture. Representative experiments are shown in Table 19.3. The ability of these monoclonal antibodies to induce suppressor cells was donor-dependent.

Table 19.1. Inhibition of proliferative responses of autologous or allogeneic mononuclear leukocytes to PHA by OKT3/Anti-Leu 4-induced suppressor cells.

| | % Suppression[a] | | | |
| | Induction for 24 hr | | Induction for 48 hr | |
Donors	OKT3[b]	Anti-Leu 4[b]	OKT3[b]	Anti-Leu-4[b]
1.	17	23	50	59
2.	31	2	34	7
3.	48	36	30	32
4.	+3[c] (32)[d]	1 (26)[d]	35	6
5.	36 (26)[d]	+29[c] (17)[d]	11	+38[c]
6.	39	44	34	ND
7.	55 (20)[d]	29 (12)[d]	27	ND
8.	ND[e]	ND	13 (36)[d]	+43[c] (9)[d]
9.	ND	ND	53 (27)[d]	67 (14)[d]
10.	ND	ND	59	61
11.	ND	ND	60 (57)[d]	13 (20)[d]
12.	ND	ND	60 (54)[d]	31 (8)[d]

[a] Percent suppression was calculated as described in Materials and Methods.
[b] OKT3 or anti-Leu 4 monoclonal antibodies were used at a concentration of 0.06 μg/ml.
[c] Increase of proliferative responses, instead of suppression, was observed in these experiments.
[d] Numbers in parentheses represent percent suppression of proliferative responses to PHA of allogeneic mononuclear leukocytes. Remaining numbers represent percent suppression of proliferative responses to PHA of autologous mononuclear leukocytes.
[e] ND = Not done.

Table 19.2. Monoclonal antibodies recognizing T cell differentiation antigens other than the T3/Leu 4 did not induce suppressor cells.

Monoclonal antibodies[b]	% Suppression[a]			
	Donor 1[c]	Donor 2[c]	Donor 3[d]	Donor 4[d]
OKT3	37	57	19	36
Anti-Leu 4	ND[e]	36	39	9
Anti-Leu 2a	7	3	+8[f]	+9
Anti-Leu 3a	13	25	+21	+4
Anti-Leu 5	13	16	ND	+28

[a] Percent suppression was calculated by the formula previously described.
[b] Monoclonal antibodies were used at a concentration of 10 μg/ml.
[c] Percent suppression of the proliferative responses of autologous mononuclear leukocytes to PHA is shown. Suppressor/responder ratio was 2:1.
[d] Percent suppression of the proliferative responses of allogeneic mononuclear leukocytes to PHA is shown. Suppressor/responder ratio was 2:1.
[e] ND = Not done.
[f] Increase of proliferative responses instead of suppression was observed in these experiments.

Table 19.3. Inhibition of proliferative responses of autologous mononuclear leukocytes to allogeneic cells in MLC by OKT3/Anti-Leu 4-induced suppressor cells.

Donors	S/R ratio[b]	% Suppression[a]			
		Induction for 24 hr		Induction for 48 hr	
		OKT3[c]	Anti-Leu 4[c]	OKT3	Anti-Leu 4
1.	2:1	+18[d]	44	+38	31
2.	2:1	+5	5	+14	44
3.	2:1	+8	65	66	73
4.	2:1	53	42	ND	ND
5.	2:1	55	51	ND	ND
6.	1:1	ND[e]	22	ND	98
	2:1	ND	14	ND	96
7.	2:1	ND	43	ND	84

[a] Percent suppression was determined and calculated as previously described.
[b] S/R ratio = Suppressor to responder cell ratio.
[c] OKT3 and anti-Leu 4 monoclonal antibodies were used at a concentration of 0.06 μg/ml.
[d] Increase of the proliferative response, instead of suppression was observed in these experiments.
[e] ND = Not done.

Experiments using ^{51}Cr-labeled responding cells strongly suggested that suppression was not due to lysis of these cells by the suppressor cells. Even at very high effector/target ratios (such as 500 : 1 and 250 : 1) OKT3/anti-Leu 4-induced suppressor cells did not lyse ^{51}Cr-labeled mononuclear responding cells (% cytotoxicity: 0%; data not shown). Furthermore, inhibition of proliferative responses by the OKT3/anti-Leu 4-induced suppressor cells by a mechanism involving depletion of interleukin-2 is unlikely, because PHA blasts, expressing interleukin-2 receptors, did not exhibit any suppressor activity (data not shown).

Inhibition of *de novo* Immunoglobulin Production by OKT3/Anti-Leu 4-Induced Suppressor Cells

OKT3/anti-Leu 4-induced suppressor cells inhibited *de novo* immunoglobulin synthesis and secretion by mononuclear leukocytes in the PWM-induced differentiation system. Representative results are shown in Table 19.4. Secreted IgA, IgM, and IgG were determined by heavy chain-specific ELISA. The ability of these monoclonal antibodies to induce suppressor cells appears to be donor-dependent.

Induction of Suppressor Cells Precedes Proliferation in Response to OKT3 or anti-Leu-4 Monoclonal Antibodies

In other experiments we investigated if proliferation, as determined by [^{3}H]thymidine incorporation, is required for generation of suppressor

Table 19.4. OKT3/Anti-Leu 4-induced suppressor cells inhibit *de novo* immunoglobulin synthesis and secretion by mononuclear leukocytes in the PWM-induced differentiation system.

Donors	Monoclonal antibodies	Immunoglobulin (μg/ml)[a]		
		IgM	IgA	IgG
1.	None	130.4 ± 12	129.4 ± 4.2	151.5 ± 12
	Anti-Leu 4[b]	43.0 ± 2.4	49.7 ± 12.1	82.0 ± 5.4
2.	None	62.5 ± 4.0	ND[c]	25.0 ± 2.0
	Anti-Leu 4	15.0 ± 2.3	ND	3.0 ± 0.7
3.	None	187.8 ± 13.7	66.5 ± 3.6	ND
	Anti-Leu 4	124.9 ± 39.9	36.3 ± 6.3	ND
4.	None	76.2 ± 16	72.0 ± 11	ND
	Anti-Leu 4	59.3 ± 2.9	27.8 ± 7.8	ND
	OKT3[b]	56.2 ± 4.1	35.5 ± 5.4	ND

[a] Cultures were set up as described in Materials and Methods. IgM, IgA, and IgG were determined in tissue culture supernatants by heavy-chain-specific ELISA as described in Materials and Methods.
[b] Monoclonal antibodies were used at a concentration of 0.06 μg/ml.
[c] ND = Not done.

cells (Table 19.5). We observed that induction of suppressor cells was achieved within 24 hr of treatment with these monoclonal antibodies, whereas proliferation was observed after longer treatment (48 hr).

Discussion

We report here that human peripheral blood lymphocytes from normal donors can be induced *in vitro* by monoclonal antibodies recognizing the T3/Leu 4 T cell differentiation antigen to manifest suppressor functions. These monoclonal antibodies exhibit mitogenic properties (14) and induce the production of lymphokines (15). Human peripheral blood lymphocytes treated *in vitro* with Con A exhibit suppressor functions to proliferative responses of T cells and to immunoglobulin production (16,17). Staphylococcal enterotoxin A (SEA) also induces the generation of suppressor cells (18), whereas PHA and other mitogens do not. It has been suggested that the generation of suppressor cells by Con A may represent a functional property of T cells and that loss of this activity may be related to autoimmune responses observed in systemic lupus erythematosus (19). Con A-induced suppressor cells are T lymphocytes and reside primarily within the cytotoxic/suppressor subset of T cells, previously identified by the anti-TH$_2$ sera (20). The OKT3/anti-Leu 4-induced suppressor cells described here are E-rosette forming cells (unpublished results). It is of interest that although the binding site(s) of Con A on the surface of the T cells has not been identified, it has been suggested that Con A competes with the OKT3 monoclonal antibody for the same binding site on the cell surface (21).

Table 19.5. Kinetics of proliferative responses and induction of suppressor cells by monoclonal antibodies recognizing the T3/Leu 4 T cell differentiation antigen.

Donors	Induction time	OKT3			Anti-Leu 4		
		Proliferative responses[a] (cpm ± SD)		Suppression[c] (%)	Proliferative responses[a] (cpm ± SD)		Suppression[c] (%)
		Medium	OKT3[b]		Medium	Anti-Leu-4[b]	
1.	24 hr	414 ± 89	719 ± 76	36	414 ± 89	856 ± 342	+29
	48 hr	573 ± 104	30,225 ± 5670	59	573 ± 104	26,533 ± 4694	61
	72 hr	2103 ± 1262	35,988 ± 8732	61	2103 ± 1262	18,386 ± 3267	54
2.	24 hr	409 ± 94	702 ± 157	+3	409 ± 94	708 ± 133	1
	48 hr	1495 ± 243	21,371 ± 4263	35	1495 ± 243	19,566 ± 4001	6
	72 hr	1049 ± 100	27,317 ± 4287	43	1049 ± 100	26,263 ± 4753	31
3.	24 hr	334 ± 31	535 ± 105	55	334 ± 31	515 ± 178	29
	48 hr	1233 ± 659	45,285 ± 12345	27	1233 ± 659	37,019 ± 6264	ND
	72 hr	1115 ± 161	32,999 ± 3280	40	1115 ± 161	38,610 ± 1266	38

[a] Human peripheral blood mononuclear leukocytes were incubated at 37°C with monoclonal antibodies for 24 hr, 48 hr, or 72 hr and pulsed with [^{3}H]thymidine 12 hr before harvesting.
[b] OKT3 and anti-Leu 4 monoclonal antibodies were used at a concentration of 0.06 μg/ml.
[c] Percent suppression was determined and calculated as previously described. Suppressor to responder cell ratio was 1:1.

Proliferation was not required for the induction of suppressor cells by the OKT3 or anti-Leu 4 monoclonal antibodies. Induction of suppressor cells preceded proliferation and was observed within 24 hr of treatment with these monoclonals. Similar findings have been reported with Con A-induced suppressor cells (22).

OKT3/anti-Leu 4-induced suppressor cells may be responsible in part for inhibition by the OKT3/anti-Leu 4 monoclonals of: (a) proliferative responses to mitogens and alloantigens in mixed lymphocyte culture (6,7); (b) T cell helper function to immunoglobulin production in the PWM-induced differentiation system (6); (c) generation of specific T cell-mediated cytotoxicity in MLC (proliferative phase) (6,8). Furthermore, these monoclonal antibodies exhibit mitogenic properties (14), induce the production of lymphokines (15), and block specific T cell-mediated cytotoxicity at the effector phase (7,8) and at a post-binding stage of the cytolytic process (9–12). In consideration of these properties of monoclonal antibodies recognizing the T3/Leu 4 antigen we proposed that this antigen may be involved in triggering of T cell functions and signal transfer or transduction (12). This hypothesis is compatible with recent reports that the T3 antigen is noncovalently associated on the cell surface with the T cell antigen receptor. The two antigens co-modulate (23) and anti-T3 monoclonal antibodies, under appropriately selected conditions, co-immunoprecipitate the T cell receptor molecules from certain T cell clones (24).

Studies are in progress to investigate the mechanism of action of these suppressor cells. They may act by suppressing directly both the T4 and T8 populations of the responding cells, or they may activate responder T8 cells to exercise suppression.

Summary

In vitro treatment of human peripheral blood mononuclear leukocytes with monoclonal antibodies recognizing the T3/Leu 4 T cell differentiation antigen resulted in induction of suppressor cells. OKT3/anti-Leu 4-treated cells were able to suppress proliferative responses of human peripheral blood mononuclear leukocytes to mitogens and allogeneic cells in mixed lymphocyte culture and *de novo* immunoglobulin synthesis and secretion by human mononuclear leukocytes in the PWM-induced differentiation system. Induction of suppressor cells preceded proliferation and was observed within 24 hours of treatment with these monoclonal antibodies.

Acknowledgments. This work was supported by grants CA 32070 from the National Cancer Institute and CH-151 from the American Cancer Society.

References

1. Kung, P.C., G. Goldstein, E.L. Reinherz, and S.F. Schlossman. 1979. Monoclonal antibodies defining distinctive human T cell surface antigens. *Science* **206**:347.
2. Evans, R.L., D.W. Wall, C.D. Platsoucas, F.P. Siegal, S.M. Fikrig, C.M. Testa, and R.A. Good. 1981. Thymus-dependent membrane antigens in man: Inhibitions of cell-mediated lympholysis by monoclonal antibodies to the TH_2 antigen. *Proc. Natl. Acad. Sci. U.S.A.* **78**:544.
3. van Agthoven, A., C. Terhorst, E.L. Reinherz, and S.F. Schlossman. 1981. Characterization of T cell surface glycoproteins T1 and T3 present on all human peripheral T lymphocytes and functionally mature thymocytes. *Eur. J. Immunol.* **11**:18.
4. Borst, J., M.A. Prendiville, and C. Terhorst. 1982. Complexity of the human T lymphocyte-specific cell surface antigen T3. *J. Immunol.* **128**:1560.
5. Borst, J., S. Alexander, J. Elder, and C. Terhorst. 1983. The T3 complex on human T lymphocytes involves four structurally distinct glycoproteins. *J. Biol. Chem.* **258**:5153.
6. Reinherz, E.L., R.E. Hussey, and S.F. Schlossman. 1980. A monoclonal antibody blocking human T cell function. *Eur. J. Immunol.* **10**:758.
7. Platsoucas, C.D., and R.A. Good. 1981. Inhibition of specific cell-mediated cytotoxicity by monoclonal antibodies to human T cell antigens. *Proc. Natl. Acad. Sci. U.S.A.* **78**:4500.
8. Chang, T.W., P.C. Kung, S.T. Gingras, and G. Goldstein. 1981. Does OKT3 monoclonal antibody react with an antigen-recognition structure on human T cells? *Proc. Natl. Acad. Sci. U.S.A.* **78**:1805.
9. Landegren, U., U. Ramstedt, I. Axberg, M. Ullberg, M. Jondal, and H. Wigzell. 1982. Selective inhibition of human T cell cytotoxicity at levels of target recognition or initiation of lysis by monoclonal OKT3 and Leu 2a antibodies. *J. Exp. Med.* **155**:1579.
10. Tsoucas, C.D., D.A. Carson, S. Fong, and J.H. Vaughan. 1982. Molecular interactions in human T cell-mediated cytotoxicity to EBV. II. Monoclonal antibody OKT3 inhibits a post-killer-target recognition/adhesion step. *J. Immunol.* **129**:1421.
11. Platsoucas, C.D. 1982. Inhibition of specific T-cell mediated cytotoxicity by the OKT3/anti-Leu 4 and anti-Leu 2a/OKT8 monoclonal antibodies occurs at different stages of the cytolytic process. *Immunobiology* **163**:329.
12. Platsoucas, C.D. 1984. Human T cell antigens involved in cytotoxicity against allogeneic or autologous chemically modified targets. Association of the Leu 2a/T8 antigen with effector–target cell binding and of the T3/Leu 4 antigen with triggering. *Eur. J. Immunol.* **14**:566.
13. Wasserman, J., L.-V. von Stedingk, G. Biberfeld, B. Petrini, H. Blomgren, and E. Baral. 1979. The effect of irradiation on T-cell suppression of ELISA-determined Ig production by human blood B-cells *in vitro*. *Clin. Exp. Immunol.* **38**:366.
14. Van Wauwe, J.P., J.R. De May, and J.G. Goossens. 1980. A monoclonal anti-human T lymphocyte antibody with potent mitogenic properties. *J. Immunol.* **124**:2708.

15. von Wussow, P., C.D. Platsoucas, M. Wiranowska-Stewart, and W.E. Stewart. 1981. Human γ-interferon production by leukocytes induced with monoclonal antibodies recognizing T cells. *J. Immunol.* **127**:1197.
16. Shou, L., S.A. Schwartz, and R.A. Good. 1976. Suppressor cell activity after Concanavalin A treatment of lymphocytes from normal donors. *J. Exp. Med.* **143**:1100.
17. Schwartz, S.A., L. Shou, R.A. Good, and Y.S. Choi. 1979. Suppression of immunoglobulin synthesis and secretion by peripheral blood lymphocytes from normal donors. *Proc. Natl. Acad. Sci. U.S.A.* **74**:2099.
18. Platsoucas, C.D., E.L. Oleszak, and R.A. Good. Immunomodulation of human leukocytes by staphylococcal enterotoxin A. Augmentation of natural killer cells and induction of suppressor cells. *Cell. Immunol.* in press.
19. Fauci, A.S., A.D. Steinberg, B.F. Haynes, and G. Whalen. 1978. Immunoregulatory aberrations in systemic lupus erythematosus. *J. Immunol.* **121**:1473.
20. Reinherz, E.L., and S.F. Schlossman. 1979. Con-A-inducible suppression of MLC: Evidence for mediation by the TH_2^+ T cell subset in man. *J. Immunol.* **122**:1335.
21. Palacios, R. 1982. Concanavalin A triggers T lymphocytes by directly interacting with their receptors for activation. *J. Immunol.* **128**:337.
22. Gupta, S., S.A. Schwartz, and R.A. Good. 1979. Subpopulations of human T lymphocytes. VII. Cellular basis of Concanavalin A-induced T cell-mediated suppression of immunoglobulin production by B lymphocytes from normal donors. *Cell. Immunol.* **44**:242.
23. Meuer, S.C., K.A. Fitzgerald, R.E. Hussey, J.C. Hodgdon, S.F. Schlossman, and E.L. Reinherz. 1983. Clonotypic structures involved in antigen-specific human T cell function. *J. Exp. Med.* **157**:705.
24. Reinherz, E.L., S.C. Meuer, K.A. Fitzgerald, R.E. Hussey, J.C. Hodgdon, O. Acuto, and S.F. Schlossman. 1983. Comparison of T3-associated 49- and 43-kilodalton cell surface molecules on individual human T-cell clones: Evidence for peptide variability in T-cell receptor structures. *Proc. Natl. Acad. Sci. U.S.A.* **80**:4104.

CHAPTER 20

Modulation of T Cell Functions by Monoclonal "Pan T Cell" Antibodies Not Directed Against the T Cell Receptor Complex

Peter Rieber, Gerti Rank, Sybille Wirth, Martin Wilhelm, Eugen Kopp, and Gert Riethmüller

Introduction

Several membrane glycoproteins have been identified by monoclonal antibodies (mAbs) which serve as specific markers for the various human lymphocyte differentiation pathways (1). Some of the T lineage associated antigens are expressed on all mature and immature T lymphocytes, such as the CD2, Tp50 sheep erythrocyte receptor (E-receptor) (1) or the Tp40 antigen recognized by the WT1 mAb (2). Other pan-T markers appear with increasing density during thymic maturation and are fully expressed only when T cells have acquired immunocompetence. Examples are the CD3, Tp20 molecule or the closely associated 90-Kd heterodimer representing the specific antigen receptor on T cells (3). Other pan-T markers are the CD5, Tp67 and the CD6, Tp120 glycoproteins. In normal tissue their expression seems to be restricted to mature T lymphocytes. However, they are not T lineage specific markers, since they can also be found on malignant B lymphocytes and on a small subpopulation of normal B lymphocytes (1).

In spite of the selective expression of these different membrane molecules on a major functional lymphocyte subset the physiologic role of most of them is hardly understood. A clue as to their biologic function is derived from experiments in which the effect of various mAbs on distinct T cell functions is studied. Several investigators reported that mAbs against the Tp50 E-receptor are able to inhibit the mitogen- or antigen-induced T cell proliferation (4–7) as well as the T cell-mediated and the natural killer cell cytotoxicity (4,5). The Tp50 molecule was therefore regarded as an "inhibitory signal receptor" for T cell activation (6). Recently, however, Meuer et al. (8) reported that mAbs against the same Tp50 molecule can be potent inducers of T cell proliferation. Less data are available on the Tp67 and the Tp120 pan-T marker glycoproteins.

Here we report on the modulation of T cell functions by a series of mAbs raised against the Tp50, Tp67, and Tp120 pan T cell antigens. Three mAbs obtained against the E-rosette receptor proved to be inhibitors of antigen- and mitogen-induced T cell proliferation, whereas mAbs to the Tp67 and Tp120 molecules were found to be mitogenic for T lymphocytes.

Materials and Methods

Isolation of Cells

Mononuclear cells (PBL) were isolated from defibrinated peripheral blood by centrifugation on Ficoll–Paque (Pharmacia, Uppsala, Sweden).

Monoclonal Antibodies

Monoclonal antibodies against the Tp50, Tp67, and Tp120 T cell glyco-proteins were obtained from fusions of P3x63-Ag8.653 myeloma cells with spleen cells from BALB/c mice immunized with the T cells from patients with chronic lymphocytic leukemia of T type. Purified mAbs were pre-pared from malignant ascites by pevicon-block electrophoresis followed by gel filtration through Sephacryl-S200 (Pharmacia). The CD3 mAb BW-264/56 used in some experiments was a kind gift of Drs. R. Kurrle and F. Seiler, Behringwerke, Marburg, FRG. Immobilized mAbs were prepared by coupling purified mAbs to CNBr-activated Sepharose (Pharmacia) at a concentration of 20 mg protein/ml Sepharose.

Lymphocyte Proliferation Assays

For mitogen- and antigen-induced responses 2×10^5 PBLs were incubated in 200-μl RPMI 1640 medium with 10% fetal calf serum in U-shaped microculture wells (microtiter plates, Nunc, Roskilde, Denmark) together with 1% phytohemagglutinin (PHA) (PHA-M, Difco, Detroit, MI, USA) or tetanus toxoid, 1 μg/ml (Behringwerke) or purified mAb at various concentrations. Cell proliferation was assayed after the predetermined optimal incubation time by a terminal 18-hr [^{3}H]thymidine (NEN, Boston, MA, USA) pulse, 1 μCi/well.

IL-2-Sensitive Cells

IL-2-sensitive cells were obtained from mixed lymphocyte reaction (MLR) activated cells which were kept in culture with 10% IL-2 containing supernatant until response to PHA was lost.

Cell-Mediated Cytotoxicity

Alloantigen sensitization and lysis of ^{51}Cr-labeled PHA blast target cells were performed as described previously (9).

Results

Characterization of Monoclonal Antibodies

Table 20.1 shows the assignment of mAbs used in this study to clusters of differentiation as defined by the First International Workshop on Human Leucocyte Differentiation Antigens (1), their isotype, and their capacity to block E-rosette formation. The three anti-Tp50 antibodies showed 100% inhibition of E-rosette formation at a concentration of 10 ng/ml.

Cross-blocking experiments (data not shown) suggested that the MT 910 and MT 1110 antibodies bind to the same or a closely related epitope that is located at some distance from the determinant recognized by the MT 26 antibody. The anti-Tp120 mAbs MT 411 and MT 211 seem to recognize either identical or adjacent epitopes whereas the MT 421 reacts with a more remote determinant on the TP120 molecule.

Inhibition of T Cell Proliferation by Anti-Tp50 mAbs

In view of the reported inhibitory effects of anti-Tp50 mAbs on T cell activation the three anti–E-rosette receptor mAbs were first tested for their ability to block the mitogen- and antigen-induced proliferation of T lymphocytes. As indicated in Table 20.2 each of the three mAbs significantly diminished the activation of T cells by PHA when present at a concentration of 50 μg/ml. However, when non-cross-reactive antibodies were combined, an almost complete reduction of the proliferative response was obtained. On the other hand, when the anti-Tp120 mAb MT

Table 20.1. Monoclonal antibodies used in the study.

Cluster of differentiation	Mol. weight (Kd)	Antibody name	Isotype	Inhibition of E-rosette formation
CD2	50	MT 910	IgG1, k	+
		MT 1110	IgG1, k	+
		MT 26	IgG1, k	+
CD6	120	MT 411	IgG1, k	−
		MT 211	IgG1, k	−
		MT 421	IgG1, k	−
CD5	67	MT 61	IgG2b, k	−

Table 20.2. Inhibition of the PHA-induced proliferation of T lymphocytes by monoclonal anti-Tp50 antibodies.

Stimulus	Monoclonal antibody	µg/ml	^{3}H-TdR uptake (cpm)	% Inhibition
Medium	—	—	428[a]	—
PHA[b]	—	—	146.082	—
PHA	MT 910	50	86.072	41
PHA	MT 1110	50	54.315	63
PHA	MT 26	50	86.033	41
PHA	MT 910 + MT 26	25 25	3.503	98
PHA	MT 1110 + MT 26	25 25	2.172	99
PHA	MT 421	50	137.835	6

[a] Results represent means of triplicate cultures. Standard deviations were ≤10%
[b] PHA-M (Difco), 1%

211 was used as T cell activator, each of the anti-Tp50 mAbs was capable alone to suppress the T cell proliferation at lower concentrations, as can be seen from Table 20.3. The specific proliferative response to tetanus toxoid was also inhibited by the anti-Tp50 mAbs in a dose-dependent manner as indicated in Fig. 20.1. The suppressive capacity of the three mAbs was comparable. Other pan T mAbs, such as the anti-TP120 antibody MT 211, applied at equal concentrations had no effect on the antigen-specific T cell response.

In order to find out at which step the anti-Tp50 mAbs interfere with the T cell activation, T lymphocytes already rendered sensitive to IL-2 were incubated with a supportive concentration of IL-2 in the presence of mAbs. As can be seen from Table 20.4, the inhibition of the IL-2-induced proliferation by the anti-Tp50 mAbs was only marginal, even when the antibodies were present at high concentrations (50 µg/ml), whereas a

Table 20.3. Inhibition of the anti-Tp120-induced T cell proliferation by monoclonal anti-Tp50 antibodies.

Stimulus	Monoclonal antibody (1 µg/ml)	^{3}H-TdR uptake (cpm)	% Inhibition
Media	—	487[a]	—
MT 211[b]	—	30.317	—
MT 211	MT 910	3.395	89
MT 211	MT 1110	1.934	94
MT 211	MT 26	1.598	95
Media	MT 910	843	—

[a] Results represent means of triplicate cultures. Standard deviations were ≤10%
[b] PBL were stimulated with 1 µg/ml of purified anti-Tp120 antibody MT 211

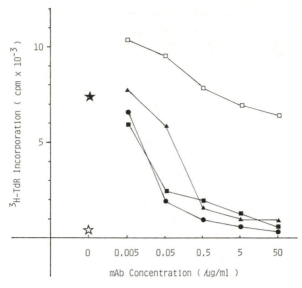

Fig. 20.1. Inhibition of the tetanus toxoid-induced T cell proliferation by monoclonal anti-Tp50 antibodies. PBLs were stimulated with 1 µg/ml-tetanus toxoid in the presence of various amounts of purified mAbs. After 5 days the cultures were pulsed for 18 hr with 1 µCi/well ^{3}H-TdR. Medium control (☆), cells with tetanus antigen in the absence of mAb (★), MT 910 (●), MT 1110 (■), MT 26 (▲), MT 211 (□). Results represent means of triplicate cultures. Standard deviations were ≤10%.

Table 20.4. Effects of monoclonal anti-Tp50 antibodies on the IL-2-supported proliferation of IL-2-sensitive T lymphocytes.

Stimulus	Monoclonal antibody	µg/ml	^{3}H-TdR uptake[a] (cpm)	% Inhibition
Media	—	—	783 ± 102	—
IL-2 (10%)	—	—	31.414 ± 2.559	—
IL-2	MT 910	50	22.883 ± 3.446	27
IL-2	MT 1110	50	25.383 ± 2.953	19
IL-2	MT 26	50	30.914 ± 1.450	2
IL-2	MT 910 + MT 26	25 / 25	17.779 ± 4.185	43
IL-2	MT 1110 + MT 26	25 / 25	13.615 ± 2.931	57
IL-2	MT 411	50	30.089 ± 2.224	4

[a] Results represent means of triplicate cultures ± standard deviation.

Table 20.5. Effects of monoclonal anti-Tp50 antibodies on the cytotoxicity of alloantigen-sensitized T lymphocytes.

Monoclonal antibody used for incubation	μg/ml	%Specific lysis[a]
Media	—	27[b]
MT 910	20	24
MT 1110	20	24
MT 26	20	23
MT 910	10	
+		22
MT 26	10	
MT 1110	10	
+		23
MT 26	10	
MT 811 (anti-Tp32)	10	14

[a] Specific cytotoxicity against ^{51}Cr-labeled stimulator PHA blasts at a 25:1 effector-to-target cell ratio.
[b] Results represent means of four determinations. The standard deviations were ≤8%.

combination of two non-cross-reactive antibodies reduced the T cell proliferation by about 50%. Similar data were obtained in several other experiments. These findings suggest that T cells are less sensitive to the inhibitory effect of anti-Tp50 mAbs when IL-2 receptors are already expressed.

The effect of anti–E-receptor mAbs on a pure effector function of T cells was investigated in MLR-induced cytotoxicity. In the experiments shown in Table 20.5, cytotoxic T cells sensitized against class I alloantigens were not inhibited by single anti-Tp50 mAbs, nor by combinations of non-cross-reactive mAbs, even when added at high concentrations. On the other hand, cytolysis was significantly diminished by the anti-Tp32/33 antibody MT 811, as has been shown before (10). In some other MLR combinations, however, a slight to moderate reduction of cytotoxicity by anti-Tp50 mAbs was observed (data not shown).

Induction of T Cell Proliferation by Anti-Tp120 and Tp67 mAbs

Incubation of PBLs with the different anti-Tp120 mAbs caused a strong proliferative response of T lymphocytes as indicated in Fig. 20.2. Also the anti-Tp67 mAb MT 61 induced a moderate, but distinct T cell activation. The proliferation triggered by the CD6 antibodies was comparable to that obtained with the CD3 mAb BW264/56. An unspecific stimulation by the mAbs was unlikely, since other mAbs of the same isotype but with different specificity, such as the CD4 antibody MT 310, did not induce proliferation. A strong stimulation was also observed when the CD6 mAbs were immobilized on Sepharose, as shown in Fig. 20.3. Optimal proliferation

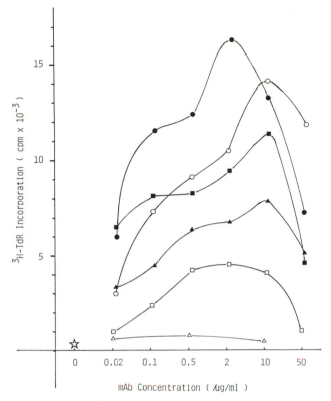

Fig. 20.2. Stimulation of T lymphocytes by monoclonal anti-Tp120 and anti-Tp67 antibodies. PBLs were cultured in the presence of various amounts of purified mAbs. After 5 days the cultures were pulsed for 18 hr with 1 μCi/well ^{3}H-TdR. Medium control (☆), MT 211 (●), MT 411 (■), MT 421 (▲), MT 61 (□), MT 310 (CD 4) (△), BW-264/56 (CD3) (○). Results represent means of triplicate cultures. Standard deviations were ≤15%.

was obtained with about 500 Sepharose beads per microtiter well. Other immobilized anti–T cell mAbs of the same isotype, such as CD2 or CD4 antibodies, presented at comparable concentrations, were inactive. These data also suggest that the CD6, Tp120 and CD5, Tp67 surface molecules can serve as receptors for activation signals.

Discussion

In the present study the effect of various mAbs against different pan-T marker proteins on T cell functions was investigated. The ability of all three anti-Tp50 mAbs to inhibit mitogen- and antigen-driven T cell proliferation is in agreement with other reports (4–7), although the blocking of

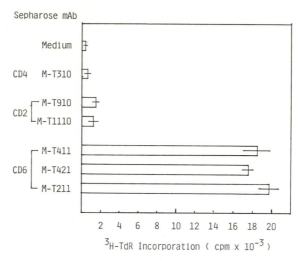

Fig. 20.3. Stimulation of T lymphocytes by immobilized monoclonal anti-Tp120 antibodies. PBLs were cultured with Sepharose-bound mAbs, about 500 beads/ well. After 4 days the cultures were pulsed with ^{3}H-TdR, 1 μCi/well for 18 hr. Results are given as means of triplicates ± standard deviation.

the PHA response was weaker than that reported for other anti–E-receptor antibodies, OKT11A (6), LFA-2 (5), or 9.6 (7). The blocking capacity, however, could definitely be increased by combination of two non-cross-reactive anti-Tp50 mAbs. Furthermore, the IL-2-supported proliferation of already activated T cells could be reduced by anti-Tp50 mAbs, but only when two antibodies were combined. This finding together with the blocking of cytotoxic effector T cells reported by others argues against the view held by Wilkinson and Morris (7) that the main effect of anti-Tp50 antibody is the inhibition of IL-2 receptor expression. A new light on the biologic role of the E-receptor molecule was shed by the findings of Meuer *et al.* (8) that simultaneous triggering of two different epitopes on the Tp50 glycoprotein induces T lymphocytes to proliferate. This observation suggests that this molecule functions as a receptor for activation signals. The ''negative signals'' provided by other anti-Tp50 mAbs might be explained by their blocking the binding of an as yet unknown natural ligand to the Tp50 molecules. The reactivity with all mature and immature T lymphocytes and the strong inhibitory capacity of certain anti-Tp50 mAbs recommend these antibodies as possibly strong immunosuppressive agents *in vivo*.

A new finding reported here is the stimulating capacity of anti-Tp120 and anti-Tp67 mAbs. The antigens recognized by these antibodies appear on T lymphocytes at a relatively late stage of differentiation. Their expression is not restricted to cells of the T lineage, since they can also be found on a small subset of normal B lymphocytes and on malignant B cells

(1,11). The stimulation of T lymphocytes by the MT 61 antibody indicates that the Tp67 molecule can be involved in the modulation of T cell functions. This view is supported by the recent finding of Thomas et al. (12) that the T4$^+$ T cell-assisted differentiation of B cells is enhanced by addition of the mAb OKT1.

Little is known about the biologic function of the Tp120 membrane molecules. Reinherz et al. (13) used the anti-Tp120 mAb T12 for successful in vivo suppression of graft-versus-host disease. This mAb which cross-blocked the MT 411 antibody (data not shown) was not mitogenic for T lymphocytes and did not modulate the Tp120 molecule. In contrast, the three anti-Tp 120 mAbs reported on here activated T lymphocytes and modulated the Tp120 molecule, but did not co-modulate other T lineage associated surface molecules such as the Tp20 (T3) or Tp50 (T11) glycoproteins (unpublished observation). The exact mechanism by which the anti-TP120 mAbs exert their stimulatory effect awaits further elucidation. Taken together, the data demonstrate that the decision whether a positive or a negative signal is transmitted to the cell interior after interaction with an individual mAb depends on the receptor molecule or the particular epitope that is recognized. When dealing with antibodies as functional probes of natural signals to the lymphocyte surface, the role of the Fc isotype in the stimulation or inhibition process has to be separately analyzed, since the interaction with Fc receptors may further complicate the picture. The use of a panel of diverse mAbs against functional surface molecules opens a new field in the analysis of membrane-controlled cell functions.

Acknowledgment. This work was supported by the Deutsche Forschungs-gemeinschaft, Bonn, SFB 37.

References

1. Bernard, A., L. Boumsell, J. Dausset, C. Milstein, and S.F. Schlossman, eds. 1984. *Leucocyte typing*. Springer-Verlag, Berlin, Heidelberg.
2. Tax, W.J.M., N. Tidman, G. Janossy, L. Trejdosiewicz, R. Willems, J. Leeuwenberg, T.J.M. DeWitte, P.J.A. Capel, and R.A.P. Koene. 1984. Monoclonal antibody (WT1) directed against a T cell surface glycoprotein: characteristics and immunosuppressive activity. *Clin. Exp. Immunol.* **55**:427.
3. Meuer, S.C., O. Acuto, R.E. Hussey, J.C. Hodgdon, K.A. Fitzgerald, S.F. Schlossman, and E.L. Reinherz. 1983. Evidence for the T3-associated 90 kd heterodimer as the T cell antigen receptor. *Nature* **303**:808.
4. Martin, P.J., G. Longton, J.A. Ledbetter, W. Newman, M.P. Braun, P.G. Beatty, and J.A. Hansen. 1983. Identification and functional characterization of two distinct epitopes on the human T cell surface protein Tp50. *J. Immunol.* **131**:180.
5. Krensky, A.M., F. Sanchez-Madrid, E. Robbins, J.A. Nagy, T.A. Springer, and S.J. Burakoff. 1983. The functional significance, distribution, and struc-

ture of LFA-1, LFA-2, and LFA-3: Cell surface antigens associated with CTL-target interactions. *J. Immunol.* **131**:611.

6. Palacios, R., and O. Martinez-Maza. 1982. Is the E receptor on human T lymphocytes a "negative signal receptor"? *J. Immunol.* **129**:2479.

7. Wilkinson, M., and A. Morris. 1984. The E receptor regulates interferon-gamma production: four-receptor model for human lymphocyte activation. *Eur. J. Immunol.* **14**:708.

8. Meuer, S.C., R.E. Hussey, M. Fabbi, D. Fox, O. Acuto, K.A. Fitzgerald, J.C. Hodgdon, J.P. Protentis, S.F. Schlossman, and E.L. Reinherz. 1984. An alternative pathway of T-cell activation: A functional role for the 50 kD T11 sheep erythrocyte receptor protein. *Cell* **36**:897.

9. Schendel, D.J., R. Wank, and G.D. Bonnard. 1980. Genetic specificity of primary and secondary proliferative and cytotoxic responses of human lymphocytes grown in continued culture. *Scand. J. Immunol.* **11**:99.

10. Rieber, P., J. Lohmeyer, D.J. Schendel, H. Göttlinger, S. Brodmann, G. Rank, S. Heydecke, E. Kopp, and G. Riethmüller. 1984. Characterization of functional human T cell subsets by monoclonal antibodies. In: *Leucocyte typing,* A. Bernard, L. Boumsell, J. Dausset, C. Milstein, and S.F. Schlossman, eds. Springer-Verlag, Berlin, Heidelberg, p. 303.

11. Kamoun, M., M.E. Kadin, P.J. Martin, J. Nettleton, and J.A. Hansen. 1981. A novel human T cell antigen preferentially expressed on mature T cells and shared by both well and poorly differentiated B cell leukemias and lymphomas. *J. Immunol.* **127**:987.

12. Thomas, Y., E. Glickman, J. DeMartino, J. Wang, G. Goldstein, and L. Chess. 1984. Biologic functions of the OKT1 T cell surface antigen. I. The T1 molecule is involved in helper function. *J. Immunol.* **133**:724.

13. Reinherz, E.L., R. Geha, J.M. Rappeport, M. Wilson, A.C. Penta, R.E. Hussey, K.A. Fitzgerald, J.F. Daley, H. Levine, F.S. Rosen, and S.F. Schlossman. 1982. Reconstitution after transplantation with T-lymphocyte-depleted HLA haplotype-mismatched bone marrow for severe combined immunodeficiency. *Proc. Natl. Acad. Sci. U.S.A.* **79**:6047.

CHAPTER 21

Determinant Heterogeneity of CD5, CD8, and CD4 Antigen Molecules as Defined by Monoclonal Antibodies

Takashi Takei, Yoshifumi Ishii, Shinichiro Kon, Junichiro Fujimoto, and Kokichi Kikuchi

Introduction

A variety of human T cell surface antigens have been discovered through the use of monoclonal antibodies (mAbs) (1). Some of them have been postulated to play important roles in immunoregulation. T8 (Leu-2) and T4 (Leu-3) antigens, for example, which were originally thought to be suppressor/cytotoxic and helper/inducer T cell markers, respectively, have been analyzed in detail and the results indicate that T8 and T4 antigens serve as receptors for class I and class II major histocompatibility complex (MHC) antigens, respectively (2–4).

In our laboratories several mAbs which define unique T and B cell antigens have been developed (5,6). In this study, we report the production of twelve mAbs that define three T cell antigens, L1, L2, and L3. Tissue distribution studies and immunochemical studies indicate that they belong to CD5, CD8, and CD4 groups, respectively (1). Determinant heterogeneities defined by these mAbs and functional roles of these antigens are also discussed.

Materials and Methods

Cell Preparations

Normal human thymocytes and tonsil lymphocytes were prepared according to the method previously described (5). Peripheral blood lymphocytes (PBLs) from healthy donors were also used. Cells were suspended in RPMI 1640 medium after collecting viable cells by Ficoll–Conray gradient (specific gravity = 1.080) centrifugation. Cultured human lympho-hematopoietic cell lines used in this study were all maintained in RPMI 1640 medium supplemented with 10% fetal calf serum and penicillin–streptomycin. T cell- and B cell-enriched fractions were obtained from tonsil cells by means of nylon fiber column and E-rosette depletion methods (5). Purity of T cell- and B cell-enriched fractions was 90–95% and more than 95%, respectively.

Production of Monoclonal Antibodies

mAbs were obtained from hybridomas made between NS-1 myeloma cells and splenocytes from BALB/c mouse immunized three times i.p. and once i.v. with either human thymocytes or tonsil T cells.

Immunofluorescence Assays

Binding of mAbs to cell surfaces was examined by indirect immuno-fluorescence and FACS analysis (Becton-Dickinson Co., Mountain View, CA).

Determination of Molecular Weight of Antigens Defined by mAbs

Molecular weights (M.W.) of the antigens defined by mAbs were determined by SDS polyacrylamide gel electrophoresis following thymocyte cell surface radioiodination, cell solubilization, and immunoprecipitation according to methods described previously (5).

Cell Binding Inhibition Assays

Determinant heterogeneities of antigens defined by mAbs were examined by cross-blocking study using unlabeled and FITC- or ^{3}H-labeled mAbs. Briefly, PBLs were incubated with unlabeled mAbs and, after washing out free mAbs, FITC- or internally ^{3}H-labeled mAbs were reacted. Binding of FITC and ^{3}H to cell surfaces was detected by FACS analysis and by liquid scintillation counter, respectively.

Autologous Mixed Leukocyte Culture (AMLC) and Cytotoxicity Tests

PBLs and autologous EB virus-transformed B cells (mytomycin-C treated) were co-cultured in a 4 : 1 ratio for six days. Proliferation responses were determined by [^{3}H]thymidine uptake. Cytotoxic activity mediated by killer cells generated in AMLC was measured by ^{51}Cr-release assay using autologous B cells as targets at effector: target ratio of 20 : 1. In experiments where the effects of mAbs on the generation of killer cells were examined, viable cell counts were adjusted after AMLC were cultured in the presence of mAbs. mAbs used in cultures were purified from hybridoma containing ascites.

Results and Discussion

Development of mAbs and Their Reactivities on Lympho-hematopoietic Cells

Out of four fusions, 12 clones were selected by their staining patterns on PBLs and thymocytes. Reactivities of these 12 clones with normal lymphocytes and with various cultured human cell lines determined by FACS are shown in Table 21.1 and Fig. 21.1. Patterns of reactivities could be divided into three groups, L1, L2, and L3, according to their staining profiles on PBLs and thymocytes. L1 mAbs, 5B3 and 7C6, reacted with

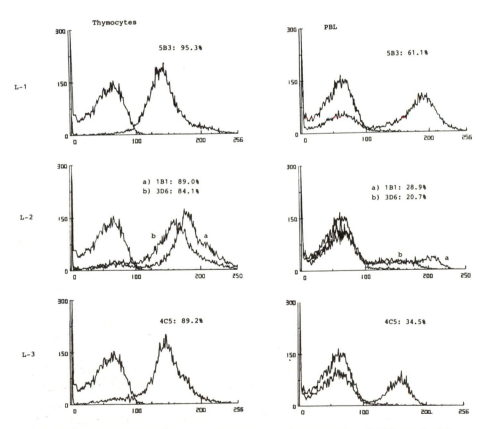

Fig. 21.1. Cytofluorographic analysis of human thymocytes and PBLs stained by L1(5B3), L2(1B1 and 3D6), and L3(4C5) mAbs.

Table 21.1. Reactivity of mAbs with various human normal lymphocytes and with cell lines as defined by immunofluorescence.

		mAbs		
		L2		
		1B1(G1) 3A2(G2b) 4A2(G2a) 4C6(G1) 7D2(G1) 9C6(G1)	3D6(G1)	L3 1A3(G1) 4C5(G1) 3A4(G1)
	L1 5B3(G2a) 7C6(G2b)			
Normal lymphoid cells				
Thymus	>95%	80–90%	75–80%	80–90%
Peripheral blood	60–75%	25–35%	20–25%	35–45%
Tonsil T enriched	>95%	30–40%	20–30%	60–70%
Tonsil B enriched	<5%	0%	0%	0%
Cultured lympho-hemopoietic cell lines				
T cell lines				
CCRF-CEM	+	−	−	+
MOLT-4F	+	+	−	±
TALL-1	+	+	−	−
HPB-ALL	+	+	−	+
MT-1	+	−	−	−
Peer	+	−	−	−
SKW-3	+	±	−	+
B cell lines				
Normal				
RPMI-6410	−	−	−	−
RPMI-8075	−	−	−	−
Burkitt				
Raji	−	−	−	−
Daudi	−	−	−	−
Pre-B				
NALM-1	−	−	ND	−
Non-T non-B				
KM-3	−	−	−	−
Reh	−	−	ND	−
Myeloid				
KG-1	−	−	−	−
ML-2	−	−	−	−
Monocytic				
U-937	−	−	−	±
Erythroid				
K-562	−	−	−	−

almost all the thymocytes and T cells but not with the majority of B cells. On cultured cell lines these mAbs reacted with all T cell lines but not with cell lines of other types, suggesting their pan-T specificities. When the reactivities of these mAbs on fresh leukemia cells were examined, B-CLL cells as well as T-ALL, T-CLL, and adult T cell leukemia cells were found to be positive for this antigen (data not shown).

L2 mAbs, which include 1B1, 3A2, 3D6, 4A2, 4C6, 7D2, and 9C6 also showed T cell specificities. They stained the majority (80–90%) of thymocytes but stained only a subpopulation (20–35%) of PBL cells. Among this group, 3D6 always stained a fewer number of PBL cells and with less intensity than other L2 mAbs. On cultured T cell lines, 3D6 failed to stain some T cells which were reactive with other L2 mAbs. Judging from the low-intensity staining on PBL cells, 3D6 staining may not reach the threshold level on cultured T cells lines which express a low amount of L2 antigens compared with normal PBL cells. Alternatively, on cultured T cells, 3D6-defined determinant may be somewhat hidden or missing due to a different biosynthesis process.

L3 mAbs, 1A3, 3A4, and 4C5, reacted with 80–90% of thymocytes and with 60–70% of PBL-T cells. The relationship between L2 and L3 was examined by their reactivities on PBL-T cells and they were found to stain nonoverlapping subpopulations (data not shown). The same observation was reported for CD8 and CD4 antigens (7). On cell lines, L3 mAbs were found to react with some T cells and with a monocytic cell line, U937, which is T4 (Leu-3) positive (8).

Immunochemical Characterizations of Antigens Defined by L1 and L2 mAbs

Immunochemical analyses of CD5, CD8, and CD4 antigens have been investigated in detail and were found to be glycoproteins having M.W. of 67,000, 34,000 plus 46,000, and 55,000 on thymocytes, respectively. Thus, the molecular natures of L1, L2, and L3 antigens were analyzed. Both L1 mAbs precipitated 67,000 and 65,000 M.W. antigens from thymocytes under both reducing and non-reducing conditions (Fig. 2.2), which was identical to the Leu-1 antigen defined by clone 17F12 (Fig. 21.2) (9). Occasionally, the low M.W. component did not appear, suggesting that this component might be a precursor form of the L1 antigen (10).

L2 mAbs, on the other hand, recognized 32,000 and 30,000 M.W. antigens on thymocytes under reducing conditions (Fig. 21.2). Furthermore, all mAbs in the L2 group detected the same M.W. antigens (Fig. 21.3). Clone 3D6 precipitated a lesser amount of L2 antigen, as judged by radioactivity, compared with other L2 mAbs. This result seems to be inconsistent with that observed in fluorescence studies. Under non-reducing conditions, the L2 antigen was replaced by a 70,000 and a much higher M.W. complex (Fig. 21.2), indicating that L2 has subunit structures bound by disulfide bonds. In a parallel experiment, the T8 antigen defined by OKT8 bound to the same MW antigen (Fig. 21.3). The T8 antigen was reported to be an antigen having subunit structures of 34,000 and 46,000 M.W. on thymocytes (11). Very occasionally, in our experiments, a 45,000 M.W. component could be identified but it was not conclusive that the 45,000 M.W. antigen was a subunit of the L2 molecule.

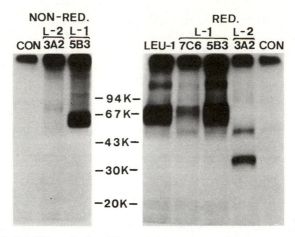

Fig. 21.2. SDS–PAGE analysis of L1 and L2 antigens on human thymocytes. L1 and L2 antigens were precipitated from ^{125}I-labeled thymocyte lysates and were analyzed under reducing (right panel) or non-reducing conditions (left panel). Monoclonal antibody which did not react with human thymocytes was used as control.

With regard to the L3 antigen, in spite of our several trials, this antigen could not be identified by the method used.

Identification of Determinant Heterogeneities Defined by mAbs

Tissue distributions and molecular characterizations of L1, L2, and L3 antigens emphasized that these antigens belong to CD5, CD8, and CD4,

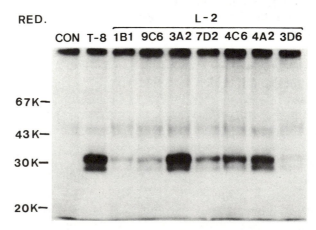

Fig. 21.3. SDS–PAGE analysis of L2 antigen analyzed on human thymocytes under reducing conditions.

respectively. Various determinant heterogeneities were found on these antigens (12) and some epitopes, especially in the CD4 group, were shown to be closely related to T cell functions (13). Thus, cross-blocking studies using unlabeled and FITC- or ^{3}H-internally labeled mAbs were undertaken to examine whether determinant heterogeneities could be separated by our mAbs. As is shown in Table 21.2, 5B3 in the L1 group did not block subsequent binding of 7C6 to PBL and vice versa, suggesting that they recognized different epitopes on the same molecule. In addition, 7C6 seemed to define the same epitope as was defined by 17F12 (anti-Leu-1). Using L2 mAbs, a variety of inhibitions were seen. 1B1 and 9C6 detected the same epitope as defined by OKT8. Other L2 mAbs recognized differ-

Table 21.2. Determinant heterogeneities of L1, L2, and L3 antigen molecules defined by binding inhibition assay.

L1

	Second mAb			
	Leu-1	7C6	5B3	Group
Leu-1	++	++	−	
7C6	++	++	±	A
5B3	−	−	++	B

L2

	Second mAb								
	OKT8	1B1	9C6	3A2	7D2	4C6	4A2	3D6	Group
OKT8	++	++	++	−	−	−	−	−	
1B1	++	++	++	±	−	−	±	−	A
9C6	++	++	++	±	−	−	±	−	A
3A2	−	±	±	++	++	++	−	−	B
7D2	−	−	−	++	++	++	−	−	B
4C6	−	−	−	++	++	++	−	−	B
4A2	−	±	±	−	−	−	++	−	C
3D6	−	−	−	−	−	−	−	++	D

L3

	Second mAb				
	OKT4	OKT4A	1A3	3A4	4C5	Group
OKT4	++	−	−	−	−	
OKT4A	−	++	++	++	++	
1A3	−	++	++	++	++	A
3A4	−	++	+	++	++	A
4C5	−	++	+	++	++	A

ent determinants from that defined by OKT8. From various cross-blocking studies at least four antigenic epitopes could be separated by L2
mAbs; one defined by clone 1B1 and 9C6, one by 3A2, 7D2, and 4C6, one
by 4A2, and one by 3D6. Lastly, determinant heterogeneity in L3 was
studied and all three mAbs seemed to detect the same epitope as defined
by OKT4A. Cross-blocking study must be done to examine whether our
L1 and L2 mAbs define newly discovered epitope(s) on CD5 and CD8
antigens.

Effects of mAbs on Various T Cell Functions

Many observations have been accumulated which indicate the functional
importance of T cell antigens defined by mAbs (14). The T1 antigen (CD5)
was recently reported to be involved in helper function (15). T8 (Leu-2)
and T4 (Leu-3) antigens have been postulated to serve as receptors for
class I and class II MHC antigens, respectively (2,3). Although mAbs
reacting with different determinants on CD8 have similar inhibitory effects on T cell functions (16,17), mAbs defining different epitopes on CD4
were shown to have quite different effects on T cell functions (13). Thus
our mAbs were examined for their effects on AMLC and killer cells to
determine whether they have different effects on T cell functions. Consistent with previous observations, L1 mAbs had no inhibitory effects on T
cell functions as evidenced by the following observations: 1. L1 mAbs did
not significantly suppress the proliferative response in AMLC (Fig. 21.4);
2. L1 mAbs did not influence the generation of cytotoxic cells in AMLC

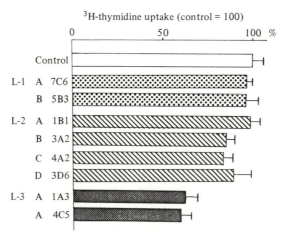

Fig. 21.4. Cell proliferation response in autologous MLC in the presence of mAbs.
Cell proliferation was significantly suppressed by L3 reagents (p 0.05).

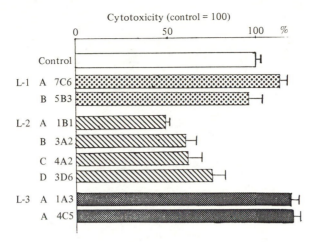

Fig. 21.5. Cytotoxic activity induced in autologous MLC with mAbs. Cytotoxic cell induction was moderately inhibited by each L2 mAb (1B1: p 0.001; 3A2: p 0.01; 4A2 and 3D6: p 0.05).

(Fig. 21.5); 3. L1 mAbs did not abrogate the killing of target cells mediated by cytotoxic cells (Fig. 21.6).

L2 mAbs, on the other hand, had inhibitory effects on T cell functions in AMLC. L2 mAbs significantly blocked the cytotoxic cell killing generated in AMLC (Fig. 21.6). In order to demonstrate these blocking effects more clearly, AMLC primed effector cells were fractionated by complement-dependent cell lysis. OKT4 and 3A2 were used to deplete their reactive populations and the effects of L2 mAbs on each effector population were examined. L2 mAbs clearly blocked the OKT4-depleted (L2-enriched) effector cell killing but had little effects on 3A2-depleted (L3-enriched) effector cell killing (Fig. 21.6). Since these results indicated the presence of L2-positive killer T cells, a cold target inhibition study was done to determine the specificity of such effector cells. These L2-sensitive killer cells were found to have class I MHC restriction (data not shown). Effects of L2 mAbs on the generation of killer cells were also studied and all L2 mAbs equally inhibited the generation of killer cells in AMLC (Fig. 21.5). This observation seems to be significant. The functional importance of the L2 molecule in target cell recognition by cytotoxic T cells has been demonstrated but the active role of this molecule in the induction of cytotoxic T cells has not been reported. Our result, thus, may point to a definite role of the L2 molecule in the generation of L2-positive cytotoxic T cells.

Finally, the effects of L3 mAbs on the T cell functions were examined. L3 mAbs also blocked the killing of target cells by cytotoxic cells (Fig.

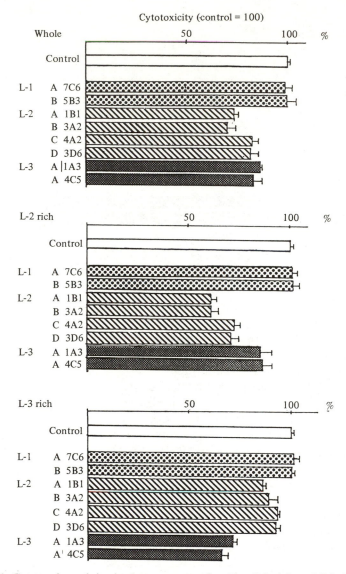

Fig. 21.6. Cytotoxic activity in the presence of mAbs. L2-rich and L3-rich fractions were obtained by complement-dependent cell lysis using OKT4 and 3A2 mAbs, respectively. Cytotoxicity of whole effector cells was significantly inhibited by each of L2 and L3 mAbs (1B1 and 3A2: p 0.01; A42 and 3D6: p 0.05; 1A3 and 4C5: p 0.05). This inhibition was enhanced by fractionation of effector cell populations.

21.6). This inhibitory effect was more clearly demonstrated by the fractionation of effector cells. L3 mAbs clearly blocked the 3A2-depleted (L3-enriched) effector cell killing and had little effect on OKT4-depleted (L2-enriched) effector cell killing (Fig. 21.6), indicating that our AMLC generated L3-positive killer cells. But, since T4 (Leu-3) was shown to be present on macrophages/monocytes, the possibility cannot be formally excluded that the L3-sensitive killer cells may represent activated macrophages which may kill a wide spectrum of cells. In agreement with previous observations on OKT4 and anti-Leu-3, L3 mAbs inhibited the proliferative response in AMLC (Fig. 21.4). In spite of the inhibitory effect of L3 mAbs on AMLC-induced proliferation, they did not inhibit the generation of cytotoxic cells in AMLC (Fig. 21.5). The precise mechanism involved in this phenomenon is not known but it is noteworthy in this regard that OX-19 mAb recognizing the rat homologue of mouse Lyt-1 enhances alloantigen-induced proliferation of rat T cells but reduces the generation of cytotoxic T cells in culture (18).

Summary

Twelve monoclonal antibodies (mAbs) have been developed which define three distinct antigens, L1, L2, and L3, on human T cells. Tissue distributions and immunochemical studies suggest that they belong to CD5, CD8, and CD4 antigens, respectively. Determinant heterogeneities defined by these mAbs were investigated. Two determinants were identified in the L1 antigen and one of them was identical to that defined by anti-Leu-1. At least four different determinants were separated in the L2 antigen and all L3 mAbs were found to react with the same epitope as defined by OKT4A. The effects of these mAbs on T cell functions were also examined. While L1 mAbs did not show significant effect, L2 and L3 mAbs had inhibitory effects. L2 mAbs blocked cytotoxic cell killing generated in autologous mixed leukocyte cultures (AMLC). Furthermore, all of L2 mAbs equally inhibited the generation of killer cells, suggesting that the L2 molecule is involved in the induction phase in AMLC. L3 mAbs also blocked cytotoxic cell killing. Although L3 mAbs inhibited proliferation in AMLC, they did not affect the generation of cytotoxic cells.

References

1. Bernard, A., L. Boumsell, and C. Hill. 1984. Joint report of the First International Workshop on Human Leucocyte Differentiation Antigens by the investigators of the participating laboratories. In: A. Bernard, L. Boumsell, J. Dausset, C. Milstein, and S.F. Schlossman, eds. *Leukocyte typing,* Springer-Verlag, Berlin, Heidelberg, p. 9.

2. Krensky, A.M., C. Clayberger, C.S. Reiss, J.L. Strominger, and S.J. Burakoff. 1982. Specificity of OKT4⁺ cytotoxic T lymphocyte clones. *J. Immunol.* **129**:2001.
3. Meuer, S.C., S.F. Schlossman, and E.L. Reinherz. 1982. Clonal analysis of human cytotoxic T lymphocytes: T4⁺ and T8⁺ effector cells recognize products of different major histocompatibility complex regions. *Proc. Natl. Acad. Sci. U.S.A.* **79**:4395.
4. Engleman, E.G., C.J. Benike, F.C. Grumet, R.L. Evans. 1981. Activation of human T lyphocytes subsets: helper and suppressor/cytotoxic T cells recognize and respond to distinct histocompatibility antigens. *J. Immunol.* **127**:2124.
5. Ishii, Y., S. Kon, T. Takei, J. Fujimoto, and K. Kikuchi. 1983. Four distinct antigen systems on human thymus and T cells defined by monoclonal antibodies: Immunohistological and immunochemical studies. *Clin. Exp. Immunol.* **53**:31.
6. Ishii, Y., T. Takami, H. Yuasa, T. Takei, and K. Kikuchi. 1984. Two distinct antigen systems in human B lymphocytes: identification of cell surface and intracellular antigens using monoclonal antibodies. *Clin. Exp. Immunol.* **58**: in press.
7. Reinherz, E.L., P.C. Kung, G. Goldstein, and R.H. Levey, and S.F. Schlossman. 1980. Discrete stages of human intrathymic differentiation. Analysis of normal thymocytes and leukemic lymphoblasts of T cell lineage. *Proc. Natl. Acad. Sci. U.S.A.* **77**:1588.
8. Mosciki, R.A., E.P. Amento, S.M. Krane, J.T. Kurnick, R.B. Colvin. 1983. Modulation of surface antigens of a human monocyte cell line, U937, during incubating with lymphocyte-conditioned medium: detection of T4 antigen and its presence on normal blood monocytes. *J. Immunol.* **131**:743.
9. Engleman, E.G., R.I. Warnke, R.I. Fox, J. Dilley, C.J. Benike, and R. Levy. 1981. Studies of a human T lymphocyte antigen recognized by a monoclonal antibody. *Proc. Natl. Acad. Sci. U.S.A.* **78**:1971.
10. Bergman, Y., and R. Levy. 1982. Biosynthesis and processing of a human T lymphocyte antigen. *J. Immunol.* **128**:1334.
11. Snow, P., and C. Terhorst. 1983. The T8 antigen is a multimeric complex of two distinct subunits on human thymocytes but consists of homomultimeric forms on peripheral blood T lymphocytes. *J. Biol. Chem.* **258**:14675.
12. Hansen, J.A., P.J. Martin, P.G. Beatty, E.A. Clark, and J.A. Ledbetter. 1984. Human T lymphocyte cell surface molecules defined by the workshop monoclonal antibodies ("T cell protocol"). In: *Leukocyte typing,* A. Bernard, L. Boumsell, J. Dausset, C. Milstein, and S.F. Schlossman, eds. Springer-Verlag, Berlin, Heidelberg, p. 195.
13. Biddison, W., P.E. Rao, M.A. Talle, G. Goldstein, and S. Shaw. 1982. Possible involvement of the T4 molecule in T cell recognition of class II HLA antigens. Evidence from studies of cytotoxic T lymphocytes specific for SB antigens. *J. Exp. Med.* **156**:1065.
14. Reinherz, E.L., S.C. Meuer, and Schlossman, S.F. 1983. The human T cell receptor: analysis with cytotoxic T cell clones. *Immunol. Rev.* **74**:83.
15. Thomas, Y., E. Glickman, J. Demartino, J. Wang, G. Goldstein, and L. Chess. 1984. Biological functions of the OKT1 T cell surface antigen. I. The T1 molecule is involved in helper function. *J. Immunol.* **133**:724.

16. Snow, P., H. Spits, J.D. Vries, and C. Terhorst. 1983. Comparison of target antigens of monoclonal reagents OKT5, OKT8 and anti-Leu-2A, which inhibit effector function of human cytotoxic T lymphocytes. *Hybridoma* **2**:187.

17. Martin, P.J., J.A. Ledbetter, E.A. Clark, P.G. Beatty, and J.A. Hansen. 1984. Epitope mapping of the human surface suppressor/cytotoxic T cell molecule Tp32. *J. Immunol.* **132**:752.

18. Dallman, M.J., M.L. Thomas, J.R. Green. 1984. MRC OX-19: a monoclonal antibody that labels rat T lymphocytes and augments *in vitro* proliferative responses. *Eur. J. Immunol.* **14**:260.

Part III. Biochemical Studies

CHAPTER 22

Immunochemical Analysis of the T Cell-Specific Antigens

Robert W. Knowles

During the First International Workshop on Human Leucocyte Differentiation Antigens, eight T cell-specific clusters of differentiation were defined serologically using 70 monoclonal antibodies tested on a large panel
of target cells by each of the participating laboratories as described in the
joint report of the Workshop (1). Immunochemical analysis of the cell
surface antigens recognized by these monoclonal antibodies, performed
by two laboratories, showed a strong correlation with the clusters established by the serological analysis (2,3). There are certain limitations in the
interpretation of immunochemical results due to the weak affinity of some
antibodies to detergent-solubilized antigens under the conditions used for
immunoprecipitation. However, the demonstration that two monoclonal
antibodies bind to the same cell surface molecule provides the strongest
evidence that they belong in the same cluster of differentiation. For this
reason, each of the monoclonal antibodies included in the T cell section of
the second Workshop was analyzed for its ability to immunoprecipitate
specific radiolabeled cell surface T cell antigens. This study provides a
molecular basis for interpreting the serological and functional studies performed during the Workshop.

Materials and Methods

Cells

The T cell line, MOLT-4, derived from a patient with acute lymphocytic
leukemia (4), was obtained from Dr. W.F. Bodmer, who obtained it from
Dr. J. Minowada. Activated human T cells isolated from the peripheral
blood of a healthy individual were provided by Dr. N. Flomenberg.
Mononuclear cells were isolated by discontinuous density gradient centrifugation using Lymphoprep (Nyegaard, Oslo, Norway), activated with

PHA-M (Difco, Detroit, MI), and placed in continuous culture in the presence of conditioned medium as a source of IL-2. Production of the conditioned medium is described in Chapter 9 of this volume. Two allo-reactive, HLA-class II-specific, IL-2-dependent, cytotoxic T cell clones, KID and KIG, isolated by Dr. Flomenberg, were used in this study. Details of their isolation and characterization are described in Chapter 9 of this volume. Both clones are phenotypically CD4 positive and CD8 negative.

Cell Surface Protein Labeling and Production of Cell Lysates

Cells were washed 3 times with PBS to remove serum proteins. Twenty million cells were surface labeled in a volume of 0.5 ml with 5 mCi of Na^{125}I (New England Nuclear, Boston, MA) using 100 μg of lactoperox-idase (Sigma, St. Louis, MO) and 0.5 units of glucose oxidase (Sigma) in PBS containing 5 mM glucose for 15 min with frequent agitation. Labeled cells were washed 3 times with PBS and lysed with 0.5 ml of lysis buffer containing 0.5% (w/v) NP-40 in NET buffer (Ref. 6; 0.15 M NaCl, 5 mM EDTA, 50 mM Tris, pH 7.4, and 1 mM phenylmethyl sulfonyl fluoride) for 30 min at 4°C. Nuclei and insoluble material were removed by centrifuga-tion at 13,000 × g for 5 min at 4°C.

Preclearing Cell Lysates

Lysates were cleared by incubation with *S. aureus* (IgGSORB, Enzyme Center, Boston, MA) precoated with rabbit antibodies to mouse IgG (RaMIg) and washed prior to use. Lysates were incubated with 0.5 ml of a 20% (w/v) suspension of RaMIg-coated *S. aureus* in lysis buffer for 16 hr at 4°C. The *S. aureus* were removed by centrifugation and the lysates were then cleared for 1 hr at 4°C using an additional 0.5 ml of the 20% suspension of RaMIg-coated *S. aureus*. Cleared lysates were stored at −70°C.

Immunoprecipitation

Frozen cleared lysates were thawed, diluted with lysis buffer, and filtered through Millex-GV filters with a 0.22-μ pore size (Millipore, Bedford, MA). Immunoprecipitation was performed using a modification of the procedure described by Kessler (6), using 1 μl of the antibody-contain-ing samples provided for the Workshop. Generally, 1 μl of ascites fluid, 100 μl of culture supernatant, or 10 μg of purified antibody were used. The monoclonal antibodies were added to 0.5-ml aliquots of cleared, di-luted, and filtered lysates. After 30 min at 4°C, 50 μl of a 10% suspension of RaMIg-coated *S. aureus* were added. After an additional 30 min at 4°C, the *S. aureus* were pelleted by centrifugation at 13,000 × g for 2 min and washed three times with lysis buffer. Washed pellets were eluted with an SDS electrophoresis sample buffer containing 0.05 M Tris, pH 6.8, 2% (w/w) SDS, 20% (w/w) sucrose, and 5% (w/w) 2-mercaptoethanol for 30 min at room temperature. The *S. aureus* were removed by centrifugation, and the eluted material was heated at 100°C for 5 min.

One-dimensional SDS Slab Gel Electrophoresis

Proteins were separated on SDS polacrylamide slab gels using the buffer system of Laemmli (7). Radiolabeled antigens were detected by the exposure of dried gels to AR 5 X-ray film (Kodak, Rochester, NY) at −70°C using Cronex fluorescent intensifying screens (DuPont, Wilmington, DE). Radioactive ^{14}C-methylated proteins (Amersham, Arlington Heights, IL) were included on each slab gel as molecular weight markers.

Two-dimensional Isoelectric Focusing and SDS Slab Gel Electrophoresis

Two-dimensional gel electrophoresis of the CD1 antigens was performed according to the procedures described by O'Farrell (8). Following immunoprecipitation, the washed pellets were resuspended in an IEF sample buffer instead of the SDS electrophoresis sample buffer described above. This IEF sample buffer contained 1.75 g urea, 400 μl of a 10% (w/v) NP-40 stock, 100 μl of the ampholyte mixture used for the IEF gels, 100 μl of 2-mercaptoethanol, 700 μl of NET buffer (6), and 0.2 g of sucrose. Pellets were eluted with 50 μl of this solution at 50°C for 30 min. The *S. aureus* were removed by centrifugation, and the eluted material was loaded on the basic end of 12 × 0.3 cm tube gels prepared as described by O'Farrell (8), containing a mixture of ampholytes, (Servalytes, Accurate Chemical, Westbury, NY) with pH ranges 2–11, 3–5, 5–7 and 7–9 (in a ratio of 1:3:3:1). After isoelectric focusing, the tube gels were equilibrated with SDS electrophoresis sample buffer and loaded onto 12.5% polyacrylamide slab gels (8). The radioactive ^{14}C-methylated proteins were included on each slab gel as molecular weight markers.

Results

Molecular Weight Determinations

The antigens detected by each of the 157 monoclonal antibodies submitted to the T cell section of the Workshop were examined on one-dimensional SDS gels following immunoprecipitation from lysates of cell surface labeled T cells. Surface ^{125}I-labeled antigens were detected with 106 of these antibodies, while 47 failed to immunoprecipitate any detectable antigen.

Table 22.1. Molecular weight determination for the antigens detected by the T cell workshop antibodies.

Original CD5 group		Original CD6 group		Original CD8 group		Original CD1 group	
Ab#	M.W.	Ab#	M.W.	Ab#	M.W.	Ab#	M.W.
T4	67	T46	85, 130	T81	32	T128	43, 16, 12
T5	67	T47	85, 130	T82	32	T129	49, 12
T6	ND			T83	32	T130	49, 12
T7	67	**Original pan T other**		T84	32	T131	46, 12w
T8	67	**or unknown group**		T85	ND	T132	49, 12
T9	ND	Ab#	M.W.	T86	32w	T133	46, 12w
T10	ND	T48	ND	T87	32	T134	49, 12w
T11	ND	T49	ND	T88	32w		
T12	ND	T50	ND	T89	32	**Original T-activation**	
		T51	ND	T90	32	**group**	
Original CD2 group		T52	90	T91	32	Ab#	M.W.
Ab#	M.W.	T53	90	T92	32	T135	55, 46
T13	46, 43, 55, 32, 25	T54	40	T93	32	T136	120, 200
T14	46w	T55	46w	T94	45, 32, 25	T137	ND
T15	46w, 55w	T56	46, 55, 25	T95	32w	T138	46, 25
T16	46, 55, 25	T57	ND	T96	32	T139	120, 200
T17	46, 55, 25	T58	ND	T97	32	T140	55, 46, 25
T18	46, 55, 25	T59	ND	T98	ND	T141	55, 46
T19	46, 55, 25	T60	90, 160	T99	32	T142	250
T20	46, 55, 25	T61	19–28	T100	ND	T143	55, 46
T21	46w	T62	ND			T144	46, 55, 25
T22	46, 55, 25	T63	120, 130, 200	**Original T cell subset**		T145	55, 46
T23	46w	T64	ND	**other group**		T146	55, 46, 25
T24	46, 55, 25	T65	ND	Ab#	M.W.	T147	ND
T25	46, 55, 25	T66	ND	T101	19–28	T148	46, 55, 25
T26	46, 55, 25			T102	ND	T149	46, 55, 25
T27	46w	**Original CD4 group**		T103	ND	T150	46, 55, 25
T28	ND	Ab#	M.W.	T104	ND	T151	55w
		T67	ND	T105	ND	T153	ND
Original CD7 group		T68	55	T106	ND	T159	55, 46, 25
Ab#	M.W.	T69	55	T107	55		
T29	48	T70	55	T108	46, 55, 25	**Original leukemia**	
T30	40	T71	55	T109	ND	**associated group**	
T31	40w	T72	55	T110	ND	Ab#	M.W.
T32	ND	T73	55	T111	ND	T152	90, 160, 40w
T33	ND	T74	55	T112	46, 55, 25	T154	40
T34	ND	T75	55	T113	55	T155	42
T35	ND	T76	55	T114	ND		
T36	ND	T77	55	T115	ND	**Original positive**	
T37	32	T78	46w	T116	ND	**control**	
T38	40	T79	ND			Ab#	M.W.
T39	40	T80	120, 200	**Original CD3 group**		156	85
T40	40			Ab#	M.W.		
T41	40			T117	19–28		
T42	ND			T118	19–28		
T43	40			T119	55, 19w		
T44	40			T120	19–28		
T45	40			T121	ND		
				T122	ND		
				T123	ND		
				T124	19w		
				T125	ND		
				T126	ND		
				T127	46, 55, 25		

Antibodies T4–28, T48–80, T101–127, T135–151, T153, and T159 were examined with lysates from the two CD4$^+$ alloreactive T cell clones described in the Materials and Methods section. Antibodies T29–47, T81–100, and T152 were examined using a lysate from a culture of IL-2-expanded PHA-activated peripheral blood T cells. Antibodies T66, T128–134, T154, and T155 were examined using a lysate from the T cell line MOLT-4 derived from an acute lymphocytic leukemia patient. A summary of these results is presented in Table 22.1 in the order in which the antibodies were originally grouped at the time of distribution.

CD1 [Thy,p45,12] TL-like Antigens

The seven antibodies grouped in the CD1 cluster, T128–134, were examined immunochemically using lysates of the CD1-positive T cell line, MOLT-4. Three different cell surface molecules were immunoprecipitated with these antibodies, providing evidence for three biochemically defined subclusters of CD1 antigens, as shown in Fig. 22.1. The first subcluster is defined by three mAbs, NA1/34 (T129), SK9/Leu 6 (T130), and 10D12 (T132), which recognize the same CD1 molecule characterized

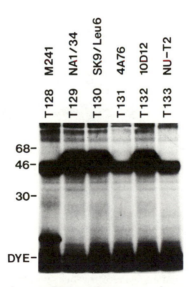

Fig. 22.1. The CD1 antigens. CD1 antigens were immunoprecipitated from a MOLT-4 lysate and separated by SDS gel electrophoresis under reducing conditions as described in Materials and Methods. Three distinct patterns of heavy chains were found with this group of antibodies as shown on the autoradiogram of the SDS slab gel shown here. Standard proteins were run on the same gel with the immunoprecipitates, and the relative mobilities and molecular weights ($\times 10^{-3}$) of these standards are indicated. β_2-microglobulin co-migrated with the nonspecifically precipitated material found at the dye front on this gel.

previously (9). This CD1 molecule migrated with the slowest relative mobility on these one-dimensional SDS gels. The second CD1 molecule was recognized by one mAb, M241 (T128), shown previously to be distinct in sequential immunoprecipitation studies (10) and by two-dimensional gel electrophoresis (11). It was the fastest migrating molecule as shown in Fig. 22.1. This 43-Kd CD1 heavy chain is also associated with a 16-Kd subunit not found with any of the other CD1 molecules. This molecule can be resolved into two spots on two-dimensional gels, with isoelectric points that are somewhat more basic than human β_2-microglobulin (data not shown). The identity and function of this subunit are unknown. A third CD1 molecule with an intermediate mobility was recognized by 4A76 (T131) and NU-T2 (T133). The heavy chains of all three antigens formed heterogeneous and somewhat overlapping patterns on one-dimensional gels but could be distinguished by their patterns on two-dimensional gels. A comparison of the heavy-chain patterns of the molecules immunoprecipitated by NA1/34, M241, and NU-T2 is shown in Fig. 22.2. Since the molecules recognized by M241 and NU-T2 are highly glycosyla-

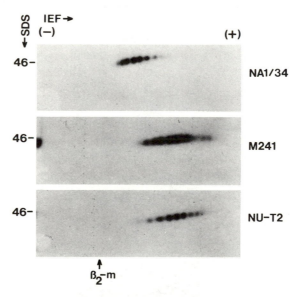

Fig. 22.2. Two-dimensional analysis of the heavy chains of three CD1 antigens. CD1 antigens were immunoprecipitated with NA/134, M241, or NU-T2 and separated by isoelectric focusing (IEF), followed by SDS gel electrophoresis. Only the heavy chain portion of the patterns are shown for the comparison in this figure after alignment of the horizontal pH gradients. Alignment was based on the position of the human β_2-microglobulin subunits which were found at a pI of 5.5, as indicated by the arrow, in the lower portions of each gel which are not shown in this figure. The horizontal pH gradient is from approximately pH 7 (left) to pH 4 (right).

ted and showed very similar but distinct patterns, the possibility that they might represent different glycosylated forms of the same gene product was examined. A comparison of their polypeptide backbones and partially glycosylated intermediates was made by treating the immunoprecipitates with the endoglycosidase, endo F, which cleaves carbohydrate oligosaccharide side chains from glycoproteins at their attachment sites near the polypeptide backbone (12). When endo F-treated samples were compared in parallel with untreated samples on one-dimensional gels, the pattern of partially glycosylated intermediates was found to be distinct for each of these three CD1 molecules (Fig. 22.3). In addition, the fastest migrating molecule in each of the endo F-treated samples, which was shown to correspond to the unglycosylated polypeptide backbone in a previous study (13), was also distinct, suggesting that each polypeptide represents a distinct gene product. Since proteolytic degradation or other post-translational modifications might also explain these observed patterns, sequential immunoprecipitation studies and structural comparisons of the polypeptides similar to those reported for the NA1/34 molecule and

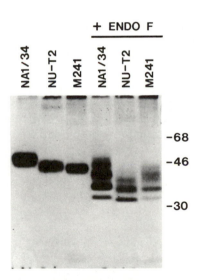

Fig. 22.3. Endo F treatment of CD1 antigens. Following immunoprecipitation, the CD1 antigens were eluted and treated with endo F. [Samples were eluted by boiling with 0.2% SDS and 2% β-mercaptoethanol, adjusted to a volume of 25 μl containing 0.1% SDS, 1% β-mercaptoethanol, and 1% NP-40 in phosphate buffer pH 6.1, and treated with 1 unit of endo F (New England Nuclear, Boston, MA) at 37°C for 16 hr.] Untreated samples are shown on the left and treated samples are shown on the right. Treated samples appear as a mixture of molecules with varying numbers of oligosaccharides removed. The fastest migrating molecules correspond to polypeptide backbones of approximately 32–34 Kd, as discussed in the text.

the M241 molecule (10,11) are needed to demonstrate that the molecule recognized by 4A76 and NU-T2 is distinct from the previously defined CD1 molecules. In a recent report describing the specificity of 4A76, sequential immunoprecipitation studies were used to demonstrate that the CD1 molecule recognized by 4A76 is distinct from the CD1 molecule recognized by NA1/34 (14), but a similar comparison with the molecule recognized by M241 was not performed.

Another antibody in this group, I19 (T134), reacted weakly but appears to bind to a molecule with a heavy chain indistinguishable on two-dimensional gels from the molecule recognized by NA1/34, SK9/Leu 6, and 10D12 (data not shown). Two additional mAbs, D47 and T4111E1, clustered serologically with the CD1 antibodies, but D47 (T66), tested in parallel, failed to immunoprecipitate any surface labeled molecules from MOLT-4 lysates, as observed in the first Workshop (2), and T411E1 (T98) was not examined with the MOLT-4 lysate in this study. A summary of these results is shown in Table 22.2, with the biochemically defined subclusters designated CD1 A,B, and C, based on the chronological order in which they were described (9,10,14).

CD2 [T,p50] Sheep RBC Receptor, Pan T Cell Antigen

A large number of the antibodies included in this workshop showed a pan T cell pattern of reactivity characteristic of the previously defined CD2 cluster (15). Eighteen were found to immunoprecipitate the p50 sheep RBC receptor molecule identified in the 1982 Workshop as the CD2 antigen (Table 22.3). This antigen showed a heterogeneous molecular weight of approximately 46 Kd when immunoprecipitated from two IL-2-dependent T cell clones (Fig. 22.4). Most of the immunoprecipitates also contained labeled molecules of 25 Kd and 55Kd. These may represent additional weakly labeled subunits of the CD2 molecule or co-precipitation of weakly associated molecules which form complexes on the cell surface.

Table 22.2. Biochemically defined CD1 subclusters.

mAb name	Workshop no.	Molecular weight	Lysate	Biochemical cluster	Serological cluster
NA1/34	T129	49, 12	MOLT-4	CD1 A	CD1
SK9/Leu 6	T130	49, 12	MOLT-4	CD1 A	CD1
10D12.2	T132	49, 12	MOLT-4	CD1 A	CD1
I19	T134	49, 12	MOLT-4	CD1 A	CD1
M241	T128	43, 16, 12	MOLT-4	CD1 B	CD1
4A76	T131	46, 12	MOLT-4	CD1 C	CD1
NU-T2	T133	46, 12	MOLT-4	CD1 C	CD1
D47	T66	ND	MOLT-4		CD1
T411E1	T98	ND	T clones		CD1

Table 22.3. CD2 antigens.

mAb name	Workshop no.	Molecular weight	Biochemical cluster	Serological cluster
9-1	T13	46, 43, 55, 32, 25	CD2	CD2
9-2	T14	46w	CD2w	CD2
S2/Leu 5b	T16	46, 55, 25	CD2	CD2
MT 26	T17	46, 55, 25	CD2	CD2
MT 910	T18	46, 55, 25	CD2	CD2
MT 1110	T19	46, 55, 25	CD2	CD2
T11/3Pt2H9	T20	46, 55, 25	CD2	CD2
T11/ROLD2-1H8	T21	46w	CD2w	CD2
T11/3T4-8B5	T22	46, 55, 25	CD2	CD2
T11/7T4-7A9	T23	46w	CD2w	CD2
T11/7T4-7E10	T24	46, 55, 25	CD2	CD2
9.6	T25	46, 55, 25	CD2	CD2
35.1	T26	46, 55, 25	CD2	CD2
T4IIB5	T27	46w	CD2w	CD2
T57	T56	46, 55, 25	CD2	CD2
6F10.3	T112	46, 55, 25	CD2	CD2
NU-T1	T127	46, 55, 25	CD2	CD2
39C1.5	T144	46, 55, 25	CD2	CD2
T56	T55	46w	CD2w	VII
1 MONO 2A6	T138	46, 25	CD2	VII
39C8.18	T148	46, 55, 25	CD2	VII
G144(D66)	T65	ND		VII
39H7.3	T149	46, 55, 25	CD2	CD3 A
41F2.1	T150	46, 55, 25	CD2	CD3 A
TQ1/28T17G6	T108	46, 55, 25	CD2	XVII
T4/7T4-6C1	T78	46w	CD2w	CD4
G19-3.1	T15	46w, 55w	CD2w+CD4w	CD5
89b1	T119	55, 19w	CD4+CD3	CD2

The 25-Kd molecule was first observed during the First Workshop in precipitates from resting PBL T cells (2), but it has not been identified as any previously known cell surface antigen. The 55-Kd molecule has not been previously reported and could simply represent part of the heterogeneous pattern normally observed for the 50-Kd molecule on SDS gels. It does, however, co-migrate on these gels with the p55 molecule immunoprecipitated with mAbs, such as TAC (T159), recognizing the IL-2 receptor. The possibility of weak interactions between these two cell surface molecules will be discussed in more detail below.

Several additional antibodies were found to immunoprecipitate the same 46-Kd molecules from lysates of these T cell clones. Three of these antibodies, T56 (T55), 1 MONO 2A6 (T138), and 39C8.18 (T148), were grouped with G144 (T65) in the serological analysis. They formed a cluster, designated VII, distinct from CD2, because they reacted weakly with

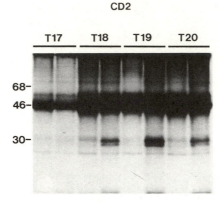

Fig. 22.4. The CD2 antigen. The CD2 antigen was immunoprecipitated from ly-sates of two IL-2-dependent alloreactive T cell clones by 25 of the Workshop antibodies. The CD2 antigens immunoprecipitated from both of these clones with each antibody were analyzed on adjacent wells of SDS slab gels. The autoradio-gram of one gel is shown here for the immunoprecipitates using the T17–20 Workshop antibodies. These patterns are typical of the patterns obtained with the other CD2 specific antibodies listed in Table 22.3. The amount of labeled 46-Kd antigen found on the gels varied with the antibody, as can be seen for T17, which immunoprecipitated less antigen than other antibodies but similar amounts from each T cell clone. In addition to the strongly labeled 46-Kd molecule, weakly labeled molecules of 55 Kd and 25 Kd and variable amounts of 30-Kd material were also found on the autoradiograms. The patterns of CD2 antigens immuno-precipitated by antibodies originally grouped with the "T-activated" antibodies can be found in Figs. 22.12 and 22.13.

resting PBL T cells, which are CD2-positive, but reacted strongly with activated T cells (15). By immunoprecipitation these antibodies could not be distinguished from those which showed the expected CD2 serological pattern. Like the previously reported D66 antigenic determinant (16), the epitopes recognized by these antibodies are only expressed on activated T cells, but structural differences in the CD2 molecules on resting and acti-vated cells have not been reported. An apparent decrease in the size of these molecules (46 Kd) on activated T cell clones used in this immuno-chemical analysis suggests that differences in glycosylation might explain the increased expression of these epitopes. Further structural compari-sons using the same gel system will be required but were not performed in this study. Immunoprecipitation of the CD2 molecule from these lysates was not observed with G144 (T65), although this antibody clustered sero-logically with the cluster VII antibodies. This antibody is, in fact, an IgM subclone of the D66 antibody, recognizing the same epitope (17), but may have a weak affinity for detergent-solubilized molecules. It did, however, show the expected functional reactivity against the same T cell clones used for the immunochemical studies (5).

Three antibodies which did not cluster with the CD2 or VII serological clusters did immunoprecipitate the CD2 molecules. Two of these antibodies, 39H7.3 (T149) and 41F2.1 (T150), were clustered with the CD3 pan T cell cluster. They showed reactivity with a large percentage of thymocytes and subclustered with the CD3 A antibodies (15). The third antibody, TQ1/28T17G6 (T108), which has been reported to define functional subpopulations of peripheral T cells (18), was also found to immunoprecipitate the CD2 molecule. In functional studies it was also found to block the formation of sheep RBC rosettes (17) and blocked the cytotoxic activity of the T cell clones used for the immunochemical analysis (5). One of the CD4 antibodies, T4/7T4-6C1 (T78), appeared to react weakly with the CD2 molecule but showed the expected CD4 serological pattern (15).

The only antibody which was clustered with the CD2 antibodies serologically but immunoprecipitated different molecules in this study was 89b1 (T119). It appeared to recognize the CD4 antigen and a small amount of the CD3 antigen (Fig. 22.5). It was originally grouped with the anti-CD3 antibodies because of its reactivity in the First Workshop (T36 in the First Workshop). Although 89b1 was capable of blocking the binding of three other mAbs recognizing the CD3 antigen in the First Workshop (3), the CD3 antigen was not detected by immunoprecipitation (2). The weak precipitation of CD3 antigens in the present study (Fig. 22.5), is consistent with the previous results indicating that this antibody has a very weak affinity for solubilized antigen. The appearance of the 55-Kd molecule in

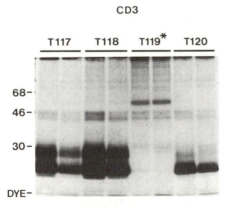

Fig. 22.5. The CD3 antigen. The CD3 antigen was immunoprecipitated from lysates of two T cell clones with six Workshop antibodies and analyzed on SDS gels. The molecules immunoprecipitated from both of the T cell clones were separated in adjacent wells for the antibodies T117–120 as shown here. The CD3 patterns were complex and somewhat variable, but appear to correspond to the typical patterns of 19- and 28-Kd subunits. *(T119 immunoprecipitated a 55-Kd molecule which may correspond to the CD4 antigen and a very weakly labeled 19-Kd molecule which may correspond to the CD3 19-Kd subunit. Possible explanations for this pattern are discussed in the text.)

these precipitates suggests reactivity with the CD4 antigen (Fig. 22.5), which may be due to a second antibody in this preparation. During this workshop, the T119 preparation was found to contain both IgG1 and IgG2a antibodies by subclass analysis (19). The serological clustering of T119 with the CD2 antibodies may reflect the combined serological pattern of the two antibodies.

Hence, it would appear that the immunochemical cluster for antibodies recognizing the CD2 antigen based on immunoprecipitation alone (Table 22.3) correlates extremely well with the serological cluster for CD2 (15). The few notable exceptions provide an important link between the cluster "VII" epitopes expressed only on activated T cells and other epitopes on the CD2 molecule.

CD3 [T,p19,29] Pan T Cell Antigens

A group of 16 mAbs in the Workshop clustered serologically in one of three CD3 subclusters, based on the percentage of thymocytes which reacted with each antibody (15). Only five of these antibodies were found to immunoprecipitate detectable amounts of the CD3 molecule from lysates of two T cell clones (Table 22.4). Most of the other 11 antibodies in this serological cluster did not precipitate other cell surface molecules and may simply have a low affinity for the detergent-solubilized molecule. Two of the antibodies in the CD3 A subcluster, 39H7.3 (T149) and 41F2.1

Table 22.4. CD3 Antigens.

mAb name	Workshop no.	Molecular weight	Biochemical cluster	Serological cluster
G19-4.1	T117	19–28	CD3	CD3 B
SK7/Leu 4	T118	19–28	CD3	CD3 A
BW264/56	T120	19–28	CD3	CD3 B
BW242/55	T121	ND		CD3 A
T3/2Ad2A2	T122	ND		CD3 A
T3/2T8-2F4	T123	ND		CD3 C
T3/RW2-4B6	T124	19w	CD3w	CD3 B
T3/RW2-8C8	T125	ND		CD3 B
X35-3	T126	ND		CD3 B
KOLT-2	T28	ND		CD3 B
T10B9	T48	ND		CD3 B
BW239/347	T57	ND		CD3 B
CRIS-7	T61	19–28	CD3	CD3 B
T10C5	T67	ND		CD3 C
BRC-T1	T101	19–28	CD3	ND
89b1	T119	55, 19w	CD4+CD3w	CD2
39H7.3	T149	46, 55, 25	CD2	CD3 A
41F2.1	T150	46, 55, 25	CD2	CD3 A

(T150), did however clearly immunoprecipitate the CD2 molecule and behaved like CD2 mAbs in competitive binding and E-rosette inhibition studies (17). One other antibody, 89b1 (T119), clustered serologically with the CD2 antibodies but appeared to be a mixture of antibodies recognizing CD4 and CD3, based on the immunochemical analysis, as discussed previously.

CD4 [T,p55] T Cell Subset Antigens

A group of 12 mAbs were found to recognize the 55-Kd CD4 molecule in the immunochemical analysis (Table 22.5), and all 12 were found to cluster serologically with the CD4 pattern of reactivity (15). Two additional antibodies, T4/7T4-6C1 (T78) and 66.1 (T79), which also clustered serologically as CD4, did not immunoprecipitate detectable amounts of antigen. It should be noted, however, that immunochemical detection of the CD4 molecule was difficult throughout this study due to weak labeling or weak expression of the antigen on both of these CD4-positive T cell clones (Fig. 22.6). Additional labeled material was found with these antibodies at the 46- and 43-Kd positions on the gels, when long exposure times were used to detect the weak CD4 antigens. The significance of this material to the CD4 antigen is unclear, but it was especially noticeable with one of the antibodies (T78) where detectable CD4 antigen was not found (Fig. 22.6). Only one other antibody, 89b1 (T119), was found to immunoprecipitate a CD4-like molecule, but it also appeared to have anti-CD3 activity, as discussed previously.

Table 22.5. CD4 Antigens.

mAb name	Workshop no.	Molecular weight	Biochemical cluster	Serological cluster
G19-2	T68	55	CD4	CD4
91d6	T69	55	CD4	CD4
94b1	T70	55	CD4	CD4
BW264/123	T71	55	CD4	CD4
MT 151	T72	55	CD4	CD4
MT 321	T73	55	CD4	CD4
T4/12T4D11	T74	55	CD4	CD4
T4/18T3A9	T75	55	CD4	CD4
MT 310	T76	55	CD4	CD4
T4/19Thy 5D7	T77	55	CD4	CD4
T4/7T4-6C1	T78	ND		CD4
66.1	T79	ND		CD4
EDU-2	T107	55	CD4	CD4
13B8.2	T113	55	CD4	CD4
89b1	T119	55, 19w	CD4+CD3w	CD2

CD4

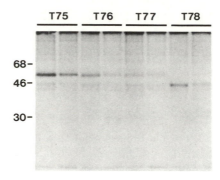

Fig. 22.6. The CD4 antigen. The CD4 antigen was immunoprecipitated by 12 of the Workshop antibodies from both of the CD4$^+$ T cell clones examined. The weakly labeled antigens precipitated with T75–77 are shown, but the pattern immunoprecipitated by T78 does not appear to include detectable amounts of the CD4 antigen. A small amount of 46-Kd material was found to be immunoprecipitated with this antibody, although variable amounts of background material were also found in this position.

CD5 (T,p67] Pan T Cell Antigens

Only 4 of the 9 antibodies originally grouped as CD5 were found to immunoprecipitate the 67-Kd CD5 molecule (Table 22.6). The same four antibodies were also found to cluster serologically with the expected CD5 reactivity (15). There was significantly more of the CD5 antigen immunoprecipitated from one of the two T cell clones examined using each of the four antibodies (Fig. 22.7). This could result from better labeling or higher expression on one of the clones. This effect was not observed for any of the other major T cell antigens studied. One other workshop antibody, (T15), clustered serologically with these CD5 antibodies (15) but did not immunoprecipitate the CD5 antigen. It appeared to react weakly with CD2- and CD4-like molecules.

Table 22.6. CD5 Antigens.

mAb name	Workshop no.	Molecular weight	Biochemical cluster	Serological cluster
H65	T4	67	CD5	CD5
6-2	T5	67	CD5	CD5
L17F12/Leu 1	T7	67	CD5	CD5
MT 61	T8	67	CD5	CD5
G19-3.1	T15	46, 55	CD2w+CD4w	CD5

CD5

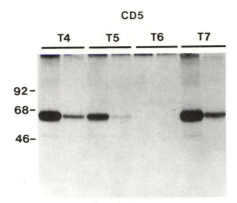

Fig. 22.7. The CD5 antigen. The CD5 antigen was immunoprecipitated by four of the workshop antibodies. The amount of this 67-Kd molecule immunoprecipitated with each of the CD5 antibodies from the lysate of one of the T cell clones was consistently higher than the amount obtained from the other clone. The immunoprecipitates from these two clones were run in adjacent wells on the slab gel shown here.

CD6 [T,p120] Pan T Cell Antigens

As in the First Workshop, the CD6 antigens were, again, difficult to immunoprecipitate. For this reason, the two antibodies, T12/3Pt12B8 (T46) and 12.1.5 (T47), were examined using lysates of resting PBL in the same experiment with four of the CD6 antibodies from the First Workshop (T411,12.1, WT31, and B614). These antibodies immunoprecipitated weakly labeled molecules of approximately 100 Kd from these PBL lysates. When the two CD6 antibodies from the Second Workshop (T46 and T47) were examined using a culture of IL-2-expanded PHA-activated T cells, they immunoprecipitated two labeled molecules of approximately 85 and 130 Kd (Fig. 22.8). Serologically, five additional antibodies of the Second Workshop clustered with the two known CD6 antibodies (Table 22.7) (15). When examined using lysates from two T cell clones, these five

Table 22.7. CD6 Antigens.

mAb name	Workshop no.	Molecular weight	Biochemical cluster	Serological cluster
T12/3Pt12B8	T46	85, 130	CD6	CD6
12.1.5	T47	85, 130	CD6	CD6
SJ10-2H10	T6	ND		CD6
T12A10	T49	ND		CD6
G3-5	T51	ND		CD6
MT 211	T58	ND		CD6
MT 421	T59	ND		CD6

CD6

T46 T47 T52

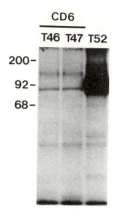

Fig. 22.8. The CD6 antigens. The CD6 ? igens were immunoprecipitated from a lysate of IL-2-expanded, PHA-activated peripheral blood T cells, with two Workshop antibodies, T46 and T47. Molecules with subunit molecular weights of approximately 85 and 130 Kd were found as shown here. In contrast the antibodies T52 (shown here) and T53 immunoprecipitated a strongly labeled 90-Kd molecule which is not T cell specific, as described in the text.

antibodies did not immunoprecipitate any detectable labeled molecules. They were not, however, examined in comparative immunochemical studies with T46 and T47, so the amount of labeled CD6 antigen in these lysates was not controlled for in this experiment. Further immunochemical analysis of these antibodies will be necessary to demonstrate their specificity for the p120 CD6 molecule.

CD7 [T,p41] Pan T Cell Antigens

Ten antibodies were found to immunoprecipitate the CD7 p41 molecule from an IL-2-expanded PHA-activated T cell culture (Table 22.8) and were all found in the CD7 serological cluster (15). One Workshop antibody, MT 215 (T9), also clustered with these antibodies serologically but did not immunoprecipitate the CD7 antigen.

The CD7 antigen has a heterogeneous subunit size of approximately 40 Kd with an additional molecule of approximately 30 Kd found in the immunoprecipitates. This was first observed and reported in the First Workshop for the CD7 antigen (2). This additional 30-Kd molecule has been found in lysates of the ^{125}I surface-labeled T cell lines, MOLT-4 and HSB-2 (2), as well as resting PBL (2) and IL-2-expanded, PHA-activated T cell cultures (Fig. 22.9). This 30-Kd molecule may represent a partially glycosylated form of the 40-Kd glycoprotein. This is further suggested by the recent report that the molecular weight of the precursor form is approximately 29 Kd (20). Because surface-labeled cells were used for the

Table 22.8. CD7 Antigens.

mAb name	Workshop no.	Molecular weight	Biochemical cluster	Serological cluster
G3-7	T30	40	CD7	CD7
4H9/Leu 9	T31	40w	CD7	CD7
8H8.1	T38	40	CD7	CD7
3A1A	T39	40	CD7	CD7
3A1A(irrad.)	T40	40	CD7	CD7
3A1B-4G6	T41	40	CD7	CD7
4A	T43	40	CD7	CD7
1-3	T44	40	CD7	CD7
I21	T45	40	CD7	CD7
T55	T54	40	CD7	CD7
MT 215	T9	ND		CD7

Workshop analysis, the 30-Kd molecule appears to be expressed on the cell surface. This is somewhat unexpected and it is possible that some internal proteins were labeled due to a small percentage of dead cells in these cultures. It is also possible that the 30-Kd molecule represents a distinct surface molecule which does not express the CD7 antigenic determinant but is physically associated with the CD7 molecule. More detailed comparisons of these two molecules will be required to demonstrate structural homology.

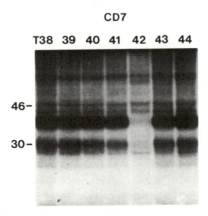

Fig. 22.9. The CD7 antigen. The CD7 antigen was immunoprecipitated from a lysate of IL-2-expanded, PHA-activated peripheral blood T cells with 10 Workshop antibodies. When analyzed by SDS gel electrophoresis a major subunit of approximately 40 Kd and a minor labeled molecule of 30 Kd were found. The patterns found with T38–44 are shown, where T42 was not reactive with this antigen. Serologically T42 did not show a CD7 pattern of reactivity during the Workshop analysis (this volume, Chapter 1).

CD8 [T,p32–33] T Cell Subset Antigens

There were 18 mAbs which immunoprecipitated the CD8 T cell subset antigen (Table 22.9) and were included in the cluster of 21 mAbs which showed the expected CD8 serological reactivity (15). The CD8 antigen was immunoprecipitated from lysates of ^{125}I-labeled T cells from IL-2-expanded, PHA-activated cultures and showed a somewhat heterogeneous subunit molecular weight of 32 Kd under reduced conditions used for the SDS gel analysis (Fig. 22.10). One antibody, BW264/162 (T85), did not immunoprecipitate any detectable molecules when tested with the other antibodies. Two other antibodies 10B4.6 (T110) and 8E-1.7 (T111) were only tested with lysates from CD4$^+$ T cell clones which do not express the CD8 antigen. The antigen immunoprecipitated by one of the CD8 antibodies, T8/2T8-2A1 (T94), appeared to contain labeled material with subunit molecular weights of approximately 46, 43, and 25 Kd, in addition to the 32-Kd CD8 molecule. Variable amounts of this weakly labeled material were also found to be associated with the CD8 molecule when other antibodies were used. Similar results were reported previously with CD8 antibodies, when thymocytes or peripheral blood lymphocytes were used (21).

Table 22.9. CD8 Antigens.

mAb name	Workshop no.	Molecular weight	Biochemical cluster	Serological cluster
4D12.1	T37	32	CD8	CD8
14	T81	32	CD8	CD8
M236	T82	32	CD8	CD8
G10-1.1	T83	32	CD8	CD8
C12/D3	T84	32	CD8	CD8
BW264/162	T85	ND		CD8
BW135/80	T86	32w	CD8	CD8
MT 415	T87	32	CD8	CD8
MT 1014	T88	32w	CD8	CD8
MT 122	T89	32	CD8	CD8
T8/21Thy2D3	T90	32	CD8	CD8
T8/7Pt3F9	T91	32	CD8	CD8
T8/2T8-1B5	T92	32	CD8	CD8
T8/2T8-1C1	T93	32	CD8	CD8
T8/2T8-2A1	T94	32	CD8	CD8
T8/2ST8-5H7	T95	32w	CD8	CD8
66.2	T96	32	CD8	CD8
51.1	T97	32	CD8	CD8
T41D8	T99	32	CD8	CD8
10B4.6	T110	NT[a]		CD8
8E-1.7	T111	NT		CD8

[a] NT: not tested on lysates from CD8$^+$ cells. No labeled antigens were immunoprecipitated by T110 or T111 from lysates of CD4$^+$ T cell clones.

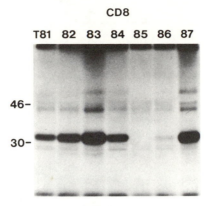

Fig. 22.10. The CD8 antigens. The CD8 antigens were immunoprecipitated from a lysate of IL-2-expanded, PHA-activated peripheral blood T cells with 18 of the Workshop antibodies. Patterns for T81–87 are shown with a major labeled subunit at 32 Kd and weakly labeled material at 45, 43, and 55 Kd. These antibodies showed considerable variation in the amount of labeled antigen which they immunoprecipitated. T85 did not precipitate detectable amounts of antigen but was found to react with a CD8 serological pattern of reactivity during the workshop (this volume, Chapter 1).

CD25 [p55] IL-2 Receptor Antigens

A group of seven mAbs (Table 22.10) formed a new cluster of differentiation, which could be defined biochemically, by reactivity with a 55-Kd cell surface molecule strongly expressed on the T cell clones which were examined in this immunochemical analysis (Fig. 22.11). These antibodies were also found to form a new serological cluster (XI), which was designated CD25 by the Second Workshop (15). One additional antibody, AA3 (T153), which was clustered with the other CD25 antibodies serologically (15), did not immunoprecipitate any detectable labeled antigens from these lysates.

Table 22.10. CD25 Antigens.

mAb name	Workshop no.	Molecular weight	Biochemical cluster	Serological cluster
T1A	T135	55, 46	TAC	XI
Tac/1HT4-4H3	T140	55, 46, 25	TAC	XI
B149.9	T141	55, 46	TAC	XI
23A9.3	T143	55, 46	TAC	XI
39C6.5	T145	55, 46	TAC	XI
33B3.1	T146	55, 46, 25	TAC	XI
TAC	T159	55, 46, 25	TAC	XI
AA3	T153	ND		XI

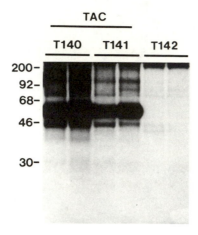

Fig. 22.11. The CD25 antigen. A new cluster designated CD25 in the Workshop (this volume, Chapter 1) corresponds to the p55 IL-2 receptor recognized by seven Workshop antibodies including the TAC antibody (T159). Each of the antibodies in the original "T-activated" group of Workshop antibodies was examined by immunoprecipitation with lysates of two IL-2-dependent T cell clones which express the IL-2 receptor. Two of the three antibodies analyzed on the gel shown here were found to immunoprecipitate the strongly labeled p55 molecule with a minor band at 46 Kd. Other antibodies in this cluster are shown in Fig. 22.12 (T143) and Fig. 22.13 (T135). The T142 antibody was found in the CDw26 serological cluster (this volume, Chapter 1) but, unlike the other CDw26 antibodies, T142 immunoprecipitated a 250-Kd molecule which ran near the origin on this gel. On gels of lower acrylamide concentration, this molecule appeared as a single band migrating slower than the 200-Kd marker protein (data not shown).

The p55 antigen has been shown to be closely associated with the IL-2 receptor in studies using the TAC antibody (included in the workshop as T159) (22) and has been characterized biochemically as a cell surface glycoprotein of approximately 50 Kd with a precursor polypeptide of 33 Kd (23). Variations in the pattern of glycosylation have also been reported (24,25). The Workshop antibodies which were found to recognize this 55-Kd antigen were also found to immunoprecipitate weakly labeled material with a molecular weight of 46 Kd which co-migrates on these SDS gels with the major subunit of the CD2 antigens. The antibodies recognizing the CD2 antigen were similarly found to immunoprecipitate weakly labeled material with a subunit molecular weight of 55 Kd which co-migrates with the TAC antigen. The reciprocal nature of the intensity of bands in these patterns is clearly shown in Fig. 22.12, which compares the patterns found with 23A9.3 (T143) and 39C1.5 (T144), which recognize the TAC and CD2 antigens, respectively. Although the weakly labeled molecules which co-precipitate with either CD2 or TAC antigens have not been identified, the similarities in these SDS gel patterns lead to specula-

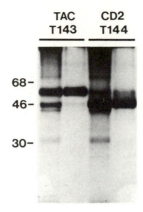

Fig. 22.12. A comparison of the CD25 and CD2 antigens. Two Workshop antibodies, T143 and T144, from the "T-activated" group were examined in parallel by immunoprecipitation using lysates of two T cell clones. Both immunoprecipitates of the antigens which these antibodies recognize were run in adjacent wells on the same slab gel. The major and minor bands of the CD25 and CD2 immunoprecipitates can be compared in this way.

tion that a physical association between these molecules on the surface of IL-2-dependent allocytotoxic T cell clones may have functional significance.

CDw26 [p120,200] Activation Antigens

Another new cluster of differentiation was defined biochemically by antibodies which recognized a molecule, with subunit molecular weights of 120 Kd and 200 Kd, which was strongly expressed on the T cell clones examined in this study (Fig. 22.13). Three antibodies, TII19-4-7 (T80), TS145 (T136), and 4EL1C7 (T139), were found to recognize this antigen (Table 22.11) and formed a new serological cluster, (X), given the workshop designation CDw26 (15).

A fourth antibody, B1.19.2 (T142), was clustered with the others serologically (15) but immunoprecipitated a molecule with a single subunit of

Table 22.11. CDw26 Antigens.

mAb name	Workshop no.	Molecular weight	Biochemical cluster	Serological cluster
TII19-4-7	T80	120, 200	p120, 200	X
TS145	T136	120, 200	p120, 200	X
4EL1C7	T139	120, 200	p120, 200	X
B1.19.2	T142	250		X
K20	T63	120, 130, 200		XXI

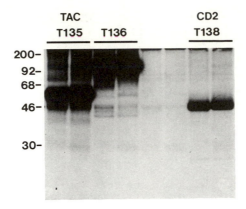

Fig. 22.13. The p120, 200 antigens expressed on activated T cells. The p120, 200 antigens are shown with two other antigens from distinct serological clusters which are also preferentially expressed on activated T cells. The p120, 200 antigens were recognized by T136 (shown here) and two other antibodies (Table 22.11) which formed a new serological cluster designated CDw26 (this volume, Chapter 1). T135 recognized the CD25 p55 antigen and T138 recognized an epitope on the CD2 molecule which is weakly expressed on resting T cells (this volume, Chapter 1). Similar antigens for each of these antibodies were immunoprecipitated from both IL-2-dependent T cell clones examined and analyzed on adjacent wells of the gel shown here.

approximately 250 Kd (Fig. 22.11). A fifth antibody, K20 (T63), recognized a molecule with subunit molecular weights of 120, 130, and 200 Kd which appeared very similar to the p120,200 antigen recognized by the three CDw26 antibodies but reacted serologically with a unique pattern of binding, designated XXI (15). Similar T cell activation antigens have been described (26,27), but the antibodies used in those studies were not included in the Workshop.

[p48] Pan T Cell Antigen

One antibody, 9-3 (T29) (Table 22.12) was found to immunoprecipitate a molecule of approximately 48 Kd, which migrated slower than the CD2 antigens on these SDS gels (data not shown). During the Workshop 9-3 was found to have a serological pattern distinct from other Workshop antibodies (cluster XXIV) (15).

Table 22.12. [p48] Antigen.

mAb name	Workshop no.	Molecular weight	Biochemical cluster	Serological cluster
9-3	T29	48		XXIV

Table 22.13. Leukemia associated antigens.

mAb name	Workshop no.	Molecular weight	Biochemical cluster	Serological cluster
3-40	T154	40		NEG
3-3	T155	42		NEG
6-4	T152	160, 90, 40w		XV

Leukemia-Associated Antigens

Three antibodies were included in the Workshop as potential leukemia-associated antigens. Two of these, 3-40 (T154) and 3-3 (T155), have been reported previously (28) to react with T cell acute lymphocytic leukemia cells but not with normal hematopoietic cells and to immunoprecipitate cell surface molecules of approximately 35–40 Kd from the MOLT-4 cell line. Immunochemical analysis using a MOLT-4 lysate showed that these antibodies recognized weakly labeled molecules as reported previously (Table 22.13). Their serological clustering with the negative controls in this Workshop (15) may reflect weak reactivity by indirect fluorescence analysis with the small number of T ALL leukemias examined.

[p90,160] LFA-1 Antigen

One antibody included in the Workshop, CRIS-3 (T60) (Table 22.14), immunoprecipitated an antigen with characteristic subunit molecular weights of the p90,160 LFA-1 antigen described previously (29). Like the LFA-1 antigens, the antigen recognized by T60 is not T cell specific and was identified on SDS gels following immunoprecipitation from a variety of cells including cultures of IL-2-expanded PBL T cells, allocytotoxic T cell clones, the T cell line HSB-2, EBV-transformed B cells lines, and peripheral blood granulocytes (data not shown). On granulocytes, the antigen had the same structure as the antigen recognized by the LFA-1 specific antibody MHM 24 (M56 in the myeloid workshop) which could be distinguished from the pattern of molecules recognized by MHM 23 (M55) and several other antibodies which immunoprecipitate the whole family of LFA-1-related molecules expressed on these cells (30). This antibody, CRIS-3, was also found to block some cytotoxic T cell clones as found with other antibodies specific for this antigen (5,30). This group of antigens was designated CDw18 in the myeloid section of the Workshop (31).

Table 22.14. LFA-1 Antigen.

mAb name	Workshop no.	Molecular weight	Biochemical cluster	Serological cluster
CRIS-3	T60	90, 160		XV

Table 22.15. [p90] Hematopoietic-common antigens.

mAb name	Workshop no.	Molecular weight	Biochemical cluster	Serological cluster
G10-2.1	T52	90	p90	XIV
G19-1.2	T53	90	p90	XIV

[p90] Hematopoietic-Common Antigens

Two antibodies, G10-2.1 (T52) and G19-1.2 (T53), immunoprecipitated a 90-Kd subunit molecule (Table 22.15). This antigen appears to have the structure and tissue distribution expected for the transferrin receptor, recognized by the antibody OKT9 (32). The 90-Kd molecule was immuno-precipitated from cultures of IL-2-expanded PBL T cells (shown in Fig. 22.8 for G10-2.1) and a variety of activated cells and cultured cell lines of various hematopoietic lineages including allocytotoxic T cell clones, the T cell line HSB-2, EBV-transformed B cell lines, and the erythroblastoid cell line K562 (data not shown). In the serological analysis, these two antibodies were identical, forming a unique cluster (XIV) (15).

Discussion

A total of 153 monoclonal antibodies submitted to the T cell section of the Workshop were examined immunochemically. Cell surface ^{125}I-labeled antigens were detected with 106 of these antibodies, while 47 failed to immunoprecipitate any detectable antigen. The Workshop antibodies could be clustered from the results of this analysis based on the molecular weight of the separated subunits of the antigens which they immunopre-cipitated. When analyzed on one-dimensional SDS gels under reducing conditions, distinctive patterns were obtained for each of the eight clusters of differentiation, CD1–8, defined by the First Workshop in 1982 (1–3).

There is a good correlation between the results of the immunochemical analysis presented here and the results of the Workshop serological analysis (15) for most of the antibodies in these clusters. Agreement was found for 7 of 9 CD1 antibodies, although these antigens could be further sub-clustered biochemically using a two-dimensional gel analysis and enzymatic removal of the carbohydrate chains from the polypeptides. Agreement was found for 18 of the 25 CD2 antibodies while three antibodies clustering separately from CD2 (cluster VII) were found to immunopreci-pitate the CD2 molecule. They appear to define a distinct CD2 determinant only expressed on activated T cells. Agreement was found for only 5 out of 16 CD3 antibodies since most of the antibodies in this cluster failed to immunoprecipitate any detectable antigen. Agreement was also found for 12 out of 14 CD4 antibodies, 4 out of 5 CD5 antibodies, 2 out of 7 CD6 antibodies, 10 out of 11 CD7 antibodies, and 18 out of 21 CD8 antibodies. Some of the possible reasons for the discrepancies between these two types of analysis are discussed below.

In addition to these previously defined T cell clusters, two new clusters were identified from the immunochemical analysis. Seven antibodies recognized the p55 IL-2 receptor, and three antibodies recognized the distinct p120,200 antigen. During the Workshop serological analysis these two groups of antibodies were also found to identify two distinct clusters of differentiation given the designations CD25 and CDw26 based on their patterns of reactivity with a large panel of hematopoietic cells (15).

Several additional antigens were identified immunochemically, but only a single Workshop antibody was found to react with each antigen. Therefore, these antibodies are not yet considered to define new clusters of differentiation. These antigens include the p48 defined by 9-3 (T29), p120,130,200 defined by K20 (T63), and p250 defined by B1.19.2 (T142). Comparative studies using additional antibodies recognizing these antigens will be necessary in future workshops to define them as clusters of differentiation. Although the 9-3 and K20 antibodies were found to have unique serological patterns during this workshop, the B1.19.2 antibody reacted with the same pattern as the CDw26 antibodies which immunoprecipitate the distinct p120,200 molecule. Two leukemia-associated antigens, defined by 3-40 (T154) and 3-3 (T155), were immunoprecipitated from MOLT-4 lysates, as described previously (28), although the Workshop serological study found them to be negative with all cells tested (15).

Two additional antigens which are also expressed on non-T cells were identified in this immunochemical analysis. The LFA-1 antigen was recognized by CRIS-3 (T60), and the p90 antigen was recognized by G10-2.1 (T52) and G19-1.2 (T53).

One of the serious limitations of this immunochemical analysis was the inability to immunoprecipitate any detectable antigen with 47 of the 153 Workshop antibodies examined. One reason for this problem may be that these antibodies bind antigen with relatively weak affinity during immunoprecipitation even though they bind to the cell surface with sufficient affinity to be useful in serological assays. The effect of affinity may be more important during immunoprecipitation, which requires strong independent binding with one of the antigen binding sites of the antibody, because the antigen has been solubilized in detergent. Binding in solution may not take advantage of the cooperative effects which can result from the use of both of the antigen binding sites of IgG antibodies, as is the case when the antigens are held on the cell surface in the two-dimensional matrix formed by the lipid bilayer. This differential effect of affinity may be even more pronounced for IgM antibodies with ten antigen binding sites which can be used together on the cell surface. Thus, two antibodies binding to the same antigen with different affinities in solution may show identical serological patterns, but they would not be clustered together biochemically if the labeled antigen could not be detected by the weak-affinity antibody. With some antibodies which were found to immunoprecipitate the same antigen, quantitative differences were also seen in the amount of labeled antigen found on the gels. This could result from differences in the concentration of the antibodies in these preparations or differences in affinity as discussed above.

In addition to the problems of weak affinity to known antigens, other antibodies which fail to immunoprecipitate detectable antigens may recognize new antigens, which are not labeled under these conditions or are not solubilized by the detergent (NP-40) used to make the cell lysates. Failure in immunoprecipitation will also result when the antigens are not expressed on the cells used for the immunochemical analysis. Many of the unknown pan T and unknown T subset antibodies were only examined with lysates of two $CD4^+$ alloreactive T cell clones which may not express certain antigens found on other T cell subpopulations. The CD6, CD7, and CD8 groups of antibodies were tested on uncloned cultures of IL-2-expanded, PHA-activated peripheral blood lymphocytes, but even these cultures may not equally represent all subpopulations of lymphocytes recognized by some of the individual antibodies. For these reasons, the lack of reactivity for a given antibody in the immunochemical analysis is difficult to interpret, and additional biochemical studies will be needed in the characterization of the antigens which they recognize.

Despite these limitations, the definitive placement of a given antibody in one of the established clusters of differentiation is best justified by biochemical evidence that it immunoprecipitates the correct molecule. In some cases antibodies recognizing clusters which can be distinguished serologically from each other may still recognize the same molecule through different epitopes. Understanding the molecular relationship between these clusters will be central to the understanding of their functional relationship.

The finding that distinct cell surface antigens can form molecular complexes on the cell surface suggests that they may function as a complex transferring signals from one molecule to the other. This has been found for the CD3 antigen which complexes with the T cell receptor (33). The observation reported here that CD2 antibodies immunoprecipitate additional molecules of 55 Kd and 25 Kd suggests that these molecules may form a complex involved in the function of the CD2 antigens. These additional molecules have not been characterized, but the 55 Kd molecule co-migrates on these SDS gels with the CD25 IL-2 receptor. Further studies are necessary to establish the exact structural and functional relationship between these molecules.

Summary

T cell-specific antigens recognized by the Workshop antibodies were analyzed immunochemically with lysates of surface-labeled activated T lymphocytes or T cell lines. Analysis of the antibodies grouped in the eight T cell clusters of differentiation, CD1–8, defined in the First Workshop demonstrated that each of these groups included several antibodies which immunoprecipitated the expected antigen. Heterogeneity in the CD1 cluster was examined in more detail, and subclustering of the antibodies was possible based on the biochemical structure of these molecules. Analysis of the unclustered antibodies grouped as "pan T unknown," "T subset unknown," or "T-activated" indicated that these groups included several antibodies recognizing previously defined antigens. Two new clusters of differentiation did emerge, however, in the group of antibodies designated "T-activated." One cluster contained several antibodies which, like the TAC antibody, recognize the 55-Kd IL-2 receptor found on activated T cells. The other cluster contained antibodies which recognize a molecule with apparent subunit molecular weights of 120 and 200 Kd also found on activated T cells. Another antibody recognized a molecule with an apparent molecular weight of 250 Kd. Several of the other antibodies included in the "T-activated" group were found to recognize the CD2 [T,p50] "sheep red blood cell receptor." These appear to recognize a new epitope expressed on activated cells which is not found on this molecule when it is present on resting T lymphocytes. In addition to these clusters, one antibody was found which immunoprecipitated a molecule with the 90- and 160-Kd subunit structure characteristic of the LFA-1 antigen but is not T cell-specific. Other antibodies were found in each group which failed to immunoprecipitate any detectable antigens. This may be due to a variation in the concentration or affinity of individual antibodies. While generally confirming the conclusions of the First Workshop, this immunochemical analysis of the Second Workshop antibodies has also revealed two clusters of differentiation which were not defined in the First Workshop. The results provide a molecular basis for interpreting the serological and functional studies performed during the Workshop.

Acknowledgments. This study was supported by grants from the US Public Health Service, CA 22507 and CA 23766, and a grant from the Xoma Corporation. Dr. Bo Dupont has also provided support and encouragement throughout this project. The T cell clones used in this study were provided by Dr. Neal Flomenberg and details of the Workshop functional studies which have been cited were kindly provided by Drs. Alain Bernard, Laurence Boumsell, Frits Koning, and Neal Flomenberg. Dr. Barton Haynes provided details of the Workshop serological analysis performed by the participating laboratories. They have been included in this report along with the immunochemical results of this study for comparative purposes. The expert technical assistance of Mr. Michael Moon and Ms. Bernadette Kienzle is gratefully acknowledged.

References

1. Bernard, A., L. Boumsell, and C. Hill. 1984. Joint report of the First International Workshop on Human Leucocyte Differentiation Antigens by the investigators of the participating laboratories. In: *Leucocyte typing,* A. Bernard, L. Boumsell, J. Dausset, C. Milstein, and S.F. Schlossman, eds. Springer-Verlag, Berlin, Heidelberg, pp. 9–143.
2. Horibe, K., R.W. Knowles, K. Naito, Y. Morishima, and B. Dupont. 1984. Analysis of T lymphocyte antibody specificities: comparison of serology with immunoprecipitation patterns. In: *Leucocyte typing,* A. Bernard, L. Boumsell, J. Dausset, C. Milstein, and S.F. Schlossman, eds. Springer-Verlag. Berlin, Heidelberg, pp. 212–223.
3. Hansen, J.A., P.J. Martin, P.G. Beatty, E.A. Clark, and J.A. Ledbetter. 1984. Human T lymphocyte cell surface molecules defined by the workshop monoclonal antibodies. In: *Leucocyte typing,* A. Bernard, L. Boumsell, J. Dausset, C. Milstein, and S.F. Schlossman, eds. Springer-Verlag. Berlin, Heidelberg, pp. 195–212.
4. Minowada, J., T. Ohnuma, G.E. Moore. 1972. Rosette-forming human lymphoid cell lines. I. Establishment and evidence for origin of thymus-derived lymphocytes. *J. Natl. Cancer Inst.* **49:**891.
5. This volume, Chapter 9.
6. Kessler, S.W. 1975. Rapid isolation of antigens from cells with a staphylococcal protein A-antibody adsorbent: parameters of the interaction of antibody–antigen complexes with protein A. *J. Immunol.* **115:** 1617.
7. Laemmli, U.K. 1970. Cleavage of structural proteins during the assembly of the head of baceriophage T4. *Nature* **227:**680.
8. O'Farrell, P.H. 1975. High resolution two-dimensional electrophoresis of proteins. *J. Biol. Chem.* **250:**4007.
9. McMichael, A.J., J.R. Pilch, G. Galfre, D.Y. Mason, J.W. Fabre, and C. Milstein. 1979. A human thymocyte antigen defined by a hybrid myeloma monoclonal antibody. *Eur. J. Immunol.* **9:**205.
10. Knowles, R.W., and W.F. Bodmer. 1982. A monoclonal antibody recognizing a human thymus leukemia-like antigen associated with β_2-microglobulin. *Eur. J. Immunol.* **12:**676.
11. Knowles, R.W. 1984. Biochemical analysis of human thymus leukemia-like antigens. In: *Leucocyte typing,* A. Bernard, L. Boumsell, J. Dausset, C. Milstein, and S.F. Schlossman, eds. Springer-Verlag, Berlin, Heidelberg, pp. 248–256.
12. Elder, J.H., and S. Alexander. 1982. Endo-β-N-acetylglucosaminidase F: endoglycosidase from *Flavobacterium meningosepticum* that cleaves both high-mannose and complex type glycoproteins. *Proc. Natl. Acad. Sci. U.S.A.* **79:**4540.
13. Van de Rijn, M., P.G. Lerch, R.W. Knowles, and C. Terhorst. 1983. The thymic differentiation markers T6 and M241 are two unusual MHC class I antigens. *J. Immunol.* **131:**851.
14. Olive, D., P. Dubreuil, and C. Mawas. 1984. Two distinct TL-like molecular

subsets defined by monoclonal antibodies on the surface of human thymocytes with different expression on leukemia lines. *Immunogen.* **20**:253.

15. This volume, Chapter 2.

16. Bernard, A., C. Gelin, B. Raynal, D. Pham, C. Gosse, and L. Boumsell. 1982. Phenomenon of human T cells rosetting with sheep erythrocytes analyzed with monoclonal antibodies. *J. Exp. Med.* **155**:1317.

17. This volume, Chapter 4.

18. Reinherz, E.L., C. Morimoto, K.A. Fitzgerald, R.E. Hussey, J.F. Daley, and S.F. Schlossman. 1982. Heterogeneity of human T4$^+$ inducer T cells defined by a monoclonal antibody that delineates two functional subpopulations. *J. Immunol.* **128**:463.

19. Clement, L.T. (personal communication).

20. Sutherland, D.R., C. Rudd, M.F. Greaves. 1984. Isolation and characterization of human T lymphocyte-associated glycoprotein (gp40). *J. Immunol.* **133**:327.

21. Martin, P.J., J.A. Ledbetter, E.A. Clark, P.G. Beatty, J.A. Hansen. 1984. Epitope mapping of the human surface suppressor/cytotoxic T cell molecule Tp32. *J. Immunol.* **132**:759.

22. Leonard, W.J., J.M. Depper, T. Uchiyama, K.A. Smith, T.A. Waldmann, and W.C. Greene. 1982. A monoclonal antibody that appears to recognize the receptor for human T-cell growth factor: partial characterization of the receptor. *Nature* **300**:267.

23. Leonard, W.J., J.M. Depper, R.J. Robb, T.A. Waldmann, and W.C. Greene. 1983. Characterization of the human receptor for T-cell growth factor. *Proc. Natl. Acad. Sci. U.S.A.* **80**:6957.

24. Wano, Y., T. Uchiyama, K. Fukui, M. Maeda, H. Uchino, and J. Yodoi. 1984. Characterization of human interleukin 2 receptor (Tac antigen) in normal and leukemic T cells: coexpression of normal and aberrant receptors on HUT-102 cells. *J. Immunol.* **132**:3005.

25. Hemler, M.E., B. Malissen, N. Rebai, A. Liabeuf, C. Mawas, F.M. Kourilsky, and J.L. Strominger. 1983. A 55,000 M_r surface antigen on activated human T lymphocytes defined by a monoclonal antibody *Hum. Immunol.* **8**:153.

26. Hemler, M.E., F. Sanchez-Madrid, T.J. Flotte, A.M. Krensky, S.J. Burakoff, A.K. Bahn, T.A. Springer, and J.L. Strominger. 1984. Glycoproteins of 210,000 and 130,000 M.W. on activated T cells: cell distribution and antigenic relation to components on resting cells and T cell lines. *J. Immunol.* **132**:3011.

27. Fox, D.A., R.E. Hussey, K.A. Fitzgerald, O. Acuto, C. Poole, L. Palley, J.F. Daley, S.F. Schlossman, and E.L. Reinherz. 1984. Ta$_1$, a novel 105 KD human T cell activation antigen defined by a monoclonal antibody. *J. Immunol.* **133**:1250.

28. Naito, K., R.W. Knowles, F.X. Real, Y. Morishima, K. Kawashima, and B. Dupont. 1983. Analysis of two new leukemia-associated antigens detected on human T-cell acute lymphoblastic leukemia using monoclonal antibodies. *Blood* **62**:852.

29. Sanchez-Madrid, F., A.M. Krensky, C.F. Ware, E. Robbins, J.L. Strominger, S.J. Burakoff, and T.A. Springer. 1982. Three distinct antigens associated with human T lymphocyte-mediated cytolysis: LFA-1, LFA-2, and LFA-3. *Proc. Natl. Acad. Sci. U.S.A.* **79**:7485.

30. Flomenberg N, N.A. Kernan, B. Dupont, R.W. Knowles (Volume 3. Chapter 7.).
31. Bernstein, I.D. (Volume 3. Chapter 7.) Summary of the myeloid workshop.
32. Sutherland, R., D. Delia, C. Schneider, R. Newman, J. Kemshead, and M. Greaves. 1981. Ubiquitous cell-surface glycoprotein on tumor cells is proliferation-associated receptor for transferrin. *Proc. Natl. Acad. Sci. U.S.A.* **78:**4515.
33. Meuer, S.C., O. Acuto, R.E. Hussey, J.C. Hodgdon, K.A. Fitzgerald, S.F. Schlossman, E.L. Reinherz. 1983. Evidence for the T3-associated 90KD heterodimer as the T cell antigen receptor. *Nature* **303:**808.

CHAPTER 23

Epitopic Groups of CD1 Molecules

Laurence Boumsell, Martine Amiot, Brigitte Raynal,
Véronique Gay-Bellile, Bernard Caillou, and Alain Bernard

The first cluster of differentiation, CD1 [Thy, gp45,12], defined by the
First International Workshop on Human Leucocyte Differentiation Antigens (1) included antibodies NA1/34, T6, D47, and M241. The antibodies
reacted with thymocytes, but not peripheral T cells, with some T-ALL
cells from both children and adults, and with some T-lymphoid cell lines.
Antibodies D47 (2) and M241 (3) particularly were dissociated from NA1/
34 (4) and T6 (5) in, respectively, T-ALL cells from adults and T-ALL
cells from children. Biochemically all of the CD1 antibodies recognize a
structure which is similar to that of human HLA-class I molecules with
approximately 45,000-M_r heavy chains attached to β2-microglobulin.

Further biochemical studies have demonstrated that the heavy chains
can be variously associated with human or bovine β2-microglobulin (6,7)
and that the association with β2-microglobulin is labile (8,9). Studies on
skin tissue section also revealed differences: one of the molecules could
be detected on epidermal Langerhans cells (10) while only one of the
antibodies stained all eccrine sweat glands (11).

However precise definition of epitopes of CD1 molecules and their
variants remained to be established with the obtention of additional monoclonal antibodies to the CD1 molecules.

Therefore, the antibodies of the T cell panel of the Second Workshop
on Human Leukocyte Differentiation Antigens as well as new locally
produced antibodies provided us with the opportunity to study CD1 molecules and their variants. We show the existence of at least four different
molecular species and of at least eight different epitopes on CD1 molecules.

Materials and Methods

Monoclonal Antibodies Used in This Study

The T cell battery of the Second International Workshop on Human Leu-kocyte Differentiation Antigens was used for this study. Additionally, five locally produced monoclonal antibodies L76, L119, L161, L232, L298 obtained after hyperimmunization with human thymus cells (12), and re-acting with cortical thymus cells only, were systematically studied (13). Monoclonal antibodies NA1/34, M241, and M28 (14) were also kindly provided by Drs. C. Milstein, R. Knowles, and J. Colombani while fluoresceinated OKT6 was a kind gift of Dr. G. Golstein (Ortho).

Cell Preparations and Tissue Sections

Procedure for cell separations, cryopreservations, serological analysis, and tissue sections have been described elsewhere (12,15,16).

Cross-blocking and Co-capping

Procedures for biotinylation, cross-blocking, and co-capping have been described in detail elsewhere (2,15,16).

Labeling and Immunoprecipitation of Cell Surface Molecules

Human thymus cells were surface-labeled with ^{125}I using lactoperoxidase and lysed with 0.5 or 1% NP40 as described (2). The lysates were pre-cleared with irrelevant mouse ascitis, a goat anti–mouse Ig, and SACI

Table 23.1. Reactivity of "CD1" antibodies on a discriminative panel of cells.

	Cell tested						
Antibodies	Thymus (3)[b]	E+ (3)	E− (3)	T-ALL (1)	B-CLL (1)	T-LL (1)	PHA (2)
NC[a]	2–13[c]	7–29	0–20	50–89	0–20	0–9	8–13
PC	76–97	62–91	54–81	88–92	48–51	80	57–65
CD1	73–98[d]	7–27	0–19	5–10[f]	0–23	0–9	2–20
Other CD(s)	50–98	>30[e]	0–39	0–99	0–59	0–99	30–59

[a] Abbreviations used: Negative controls, NC; positive controls, PC; cluster of differentiation, CD; T-acute lymphoblastic leukemia, T-ALL; B-chronic lymphocytic leukemia, B-CLL; T-lymphoblastic lymphoma, T-LL; 3 days PHA-activated PBL, PHA.
[b] Number in parentheses represents the number of individuals tested.
[c] Numbers represent the lowest and the highest values of the antibodies in the group in terms of percent positive cells.
[d] The shape of the curve was also typical for some "CD1" antibodies (see text).
[e] The shape of the curve obtained with "CD8" antibodies which gave the lowest percent positive cells of well-defined CD(s) was typical.
[f] This T-ALL was stained by T128.

before use for immunoprecipitation. Immunoprecipitations were performed using 5λ of the monoclonal antibody (neat or as provided in the Workshop battery), 5λ of a goat anti–mouse Ig, and 60–100 λ of a 10% solution of SACI. In preliminary experiments, we established for sequential immunoprecipitations the adequate conditions for total removal of the relevant molecule by the various antibodies. After dissociation, the immunoprecipitates and molecular weight standards (Pharmacia) were analyzed on 30 cm long, 13–15% acrylamide gel containing 0.1% SDS (17). The stained and dried gels were exposed at $-70°C$ with Kodak XO Mat AR5 films and intensifying screens for various length of time (18).

Results

Selection of Antibodies

Selection of Antibodies from the Workshop Panel

The selection of antibodies from the T cell Workshop panel was first made according to their % reactivity by indirect immunofluorescence with cell suspensions. The antibodies T34 (BW 264/215), T66 (D47), T98 (T411E1), T128 (M241), T129 (NA1/34), T130 (SK9/Leu 6), T131 (4A7.6), T132 (10D12.2), T133 (NU-T2) and T134 (I19) were thus selected on the basis of their reactivity with human thymus cells, and their lack of reactivity with human E^+ cells, E^- cells, and 3-day PHA blast cells (Table 23.1). Careful examination of the shape of the curve of the fluorescence intensity in microflow-fluorometry given by the various antibodies also revealed that antibodies T34 and T128 had different profiles than the other antibodies. All these antibodies were easily distinguished from antibodies in well-characterized CD groups as shown in Table 23.1, as well as from most antibodies classified as "Pan T, other or unknown" or as "T-cell activation." A second criterion in the selection of the antibodies to be studied was based on their ability to immunoprecipitate ^{125}I-labeled human thymus cells. As shown in Figs. 23.1 and 23.2, antibodies T128 to T134 all precipitated $\simeq$45,000 M_r heavy chains. Of note, the precipitate obtained with T128 showed a slightly lower $\simeq$43,000 M_r protein band and a 46,000 M_r band. No precipitate was observed with antibodies T34, T66, and T98, while T131 and T133 precipitates were more easily obtained in 0.5% NP40 (Fig. 23.2) than in 1% NP40 (Fig. 23.1) thymocyte lysates. The protein band obtained with T131 was also diffuse and extended lower than the band obtained with T129.

Selection of Local Monoclonal Antibodies

Local monoclonal antibodies were selected on the basis of (a) their reactivity with cortical thymus cells on tissue section and (b) their reactivity

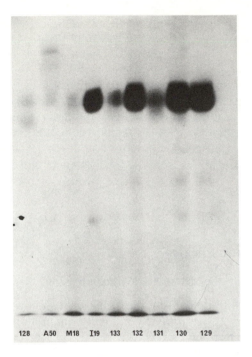

Fig. 23.1. Immunoprecipitations of ^{125}I thymus cells. From left to right, immuno-precipitates obtained from equivalent amount of the same 1% NP40 lysate of ^{125}I thymus cells with T128 (M241), A50, M18, T134 (I19), T133 (NU-T2), T132 (10D12.2), T131 (4A76), T130 (SK9/Leu 6), T129 (NA1/34). Exposure time was 5 days.

with human thymus cells, and their lack of reactivity with human E^+ cells, E^- cells, and 3-day PHA blast cells. Additionally, these antibodies were found to stain human T cell lines known to express CD1 molecules, and not other T or B cell lines lacking CD1 molecules. Antibodies L76, L119, L232, L298, and L161 were thus selected. Of interest to note, while antibodies L76, L119, L232, and L298 gave fluorescence curves with a shape similar to T129–T134, L161 gave a curve with a shape identical to T128 (results not shown).

Epitopes and Epitopic Groups Defined by Cross-blocking

Cross-blocking of the fixation of biotinylated NA1/34 (T129), M241 (T128), D47 (T66), I19 (T134), L161, L76, L119, L232, or of fluoresceina-ted OKT6 was systematically performed with the Workshop antibodies T128–T134, the aforementioned antibodies, L298, and one antibody to $\beta 2$-microglobulin M28. Results are summarized in Table 23.2. We could thus delineate, on the basis of complete or almost complete cross-block-

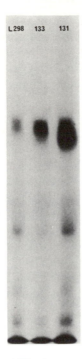

Fig. 23.2. Immunoprecipitations of ^{125}I thymus cells. From left to right, immuno-precipitates obtained from equivalent amount of the same 0.5% NP40 lysate of ^{125}I thymus cells with L298, T133 (NU-T2), T131 (4A76). Exposure time was 5 days.

Table 23.2. Cross-blocking of labeled "CD1" antibodies.[a]

Unlabeled antibody	Labeled antibodies								
	D47	NA1/34	L76	L119	I19	OKT6	L232	M241	L161
D47	±	±	±	±	−	−	−	−	−
T129 (NA1/34)	+ +	+ +	−	+	−	−	−	±	−
L76	+ +	+ +	+ +	+ +	−	−	±	−	±
L119	+ +	+ +	+ +	+ +	−	−	−	±	±
L298	+ +	+ +	+ +	+ +	−	−	±	±	±
T134 (I19)	±	−	−	±	+	+	+ +	−	−
OKT6	−	−	−	−	+ +	+ +	+ +	−	−
L232	−	−	−	−	+ +	+ +	+ +	±	±
T132	−	−	−	−	+ +	+ +	+ +	−	−
T128 (M241)	±	−	−	−	−	−	−	+ +	+ +
L161	−	−	−	−	−	±	−	+ +	+ +
T130	−	−	−	−	−	−	−	−	−
T131	−	−	−	−	−	−	−	−	−
T133	±	±	−	−	−	−	−	±	−
M28	−	−	−	−	−	−	−	−	−

[a] + + Complete cross-blocking; + almost complete cross-blocking; ± slight cross-blocking; − no cross-blocking.

ing, a first epitopic group with T128 and L161, a second group with T129, L119, L76, L298, and D47, and a third group with T132, T134, L232, and OKT6. Antibodies T130, T131, and T133 did not inhibit the fixation of the directly labeled antibodies. Similarly the anti-β2-microglobulin did not block the fixation of these directly labeled antibodies.

Molecules or Molecular Complexes Defined by Co-capping

Capping of the cells bearing the molecules recognized by L161, T128, T131, T133, T130, T129, T132, L119, and M28 was achieved and results of relabeling with all antibodies are summarized in Table 23.3. The three molecular complexes which were thus delineated are L161 and T128, T131 and T133, and T129, L119, L298, L76, D47, T134, T132, L232. In addition, after capping of all the β2-microglobulin with M28 we observed that the molecular complex recognized by L161 and T128 was totally associated with β2-microglobulin as was the molecular complex recognized by L76, L298, and D47 while the molecular complex recognized by T129, L119, T134, T132, L232 and the molecular complex recognized by T131 and T133 were not.

Molecules and Molecular Variants Defined by Sequential Immunoprecipitation

First we immunoprecipitated the molecules recognized by L119, L76, L161, and L232 (Fig. 23.3), whereas the molecules recognized by L298 were weakly immunoprecipitated from ^{125}I human thymus cells. L232 and L119 precipitated molecules of similar size as T129. As L119 immunoprecipitated protein bands similar to T129, sequential and reciprocal immunoprecipitations were performed and showed the identity of the molecules precipitated by both antibodies (not shown). T130 also immunoprecipitated protein bands similar to T129 and removal of T129 totally removed T130 (Fig. 23.4). In contrast the T131 protein bands were still visible after removal of the T129 protein bands (Fig. 23.4).

L161 immunoprecipitated similar protein bands to those obtained with T128 as expected from the co-capping, cross-blocking, and staining pattern of both antibodies. Reciprocal sequential immunoprecipitation performed with T128 and L161 showed the identity of the molecules precipitated by both antibodies (not shown).

L76 immunoprecipitated also two protein bands of similar size to those precipitated by T128 and L161 (Fig. 23.3). This is in contrast with the results of cross-blocking and co-capping which had shown that L76 belonged to the same epitopic group as T129 and recognized the same molecular complex as T129. Therefore, we performed series of sequential immunoprecipitations. First, after removal of T129 precipitable material from a thymus cell lysate we observed only the 43,000 Mr. band in L76

Table 23.3. Molecular complexes defined by capping of "CD1" antibodies.

Capped antibody	Labeling by second antibody outside the cap													
	T128	L161	T129	L119	L298	L76	T134	T132	L232	T130	D47	T131	T133	M28
T128	−[a]	−	+	+	+	+	+	+	+	+	+	+	+	+
L161	−	−	+	+	+	+	+	+	+	+	+	+	+	+
T129	−	+	−	±	−	−	−	−	−	−	−	+	+	±
L119	−	+	−	−	−	−	−	−	−	±	−	+	+	+
T132	±	+	−	−	−	−	−	−	−	±	−	+	+	±
T130	+	+	−	−	−	−	−	±	−	−	−	+	+	±
T131	+	+	+	+	+	+	+	+	+	+	+	−	−	+
T133	+	+	+	+	+	+	+	+	+	+	+	−	−	+
M28	−	−	±	+	−	−	+	+	+	+	−	+	+	−

[a] + Diffuse labeling of most capped cells was observed; ± diffuse labeling of an intermediate proportion of capped cells; − no diffuse labeling of capped cells.

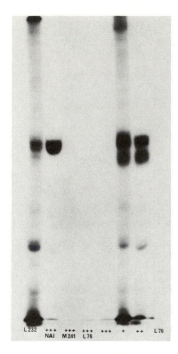

Fig. 23.3. Sequential immunoprecipitation of ^{125}I thymus cells. From the right to the left lane:

- Immunoprecipitation of 1% NP40 lysate with L76 (2nd time) (++).
- Immunoprecipitation with L76 (1st time) (+).
- Immunoprecipitation with L76 (3rd time) (+++).
- Immunoprecipitation with L76 (3rd time) (+++) followed by immunoprecipitation with L76.
- Immunoprecipitation with L76 (3rd time) (+++) followed by immunoprecipitation with M241 (T128).
- Immunoprecipitation with L76 (3rd time) (+++) followed by immunoprecipitation with NA1/34 (T129)
- Last lane: immunoprecipitation with L232.

immunoprecipitates (Fig. 23.4). Conversely after removal of L76 protein bands we still observed a diffuse 49,000 Mr. protein band in T129 immunoprecipitates (Fig. 24.3). Similarly after removal of T128 or L161 a diffuse 49,000 Mr. protein band was observed in T129 immunoprecipitates (not shown). Thus, in order to clarify the relationships between the molecule(s) recognized by L76 and T128 or L161 we removed from thymus cell lysates the material precipitable by L76 and then we could no longer precipitate any protein band with L161 or T128 (Fig. 23.3).

In conclusion, we could immunoprecipitate a diffuse and broad protein band (46–49,000 M_r with T129, T130, T132, T134, L119, and L232. T131

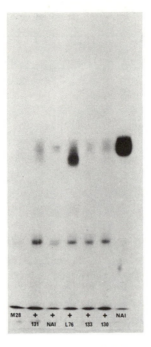

Fig. 23.4. Sequential immunoprecipitation of ^{125}I thymus cells. From the right to the left:

- Immunoprecipitation of 1% NP40 lysate with NA1/34 (T129).
- Immunoprecipitation of 1% NP40 lysate with NA1/34 (T129) followed by T130 (SK9/Leu 6).
- Immunoprecipitation of 1% NP40 lysate with NA1/34 (T129) followed by T133 (NU-T2).
- Immunoprecipitation of 1% NP40 lysate with NA1/34 (T129) followed by L76.
- Immunoprecipitation of 1% NP40 lysate with NA1/34 (T129) followed by NA1/ 34 (T129).
- Immunoprecipitation of 1% NP40 lysate with NA1/34 (T129) followed by T131 (4A76).
- Immunoprecipitation with M28.

was shown to immunoprecipitate another protein band of $\approx$45,000–48,000 M_r of lower intensity than that immunoprecipitated by T129 which could be precipitated after removal of the T129 protein band. T128 and L161 were shown to immunoprecipitate the same protein bands of $\approx$43,000–45,000 M_r (strong) and 46,000–48,000 M_r (weak). L76 was shown to precipitate two strong protein bands of 43,000–45,000 M_r and 46,000–49,000 M_r. The fact that L76 recognizes part of the 46,000–49,000 M_r molecules and all of the 43,000–45,000 M_r molecules was shown by the aforementioned sequential immunoprecipitations.

Table 23.4. Staining of skin tissue section by "CD1" antibodies.[a]

mAb	Eccrine sweat glands		Langerhans cells	
	Paraffin	Frozen	Paraffin	Frozen
T128	±	±	−	−
L161	−	−	−	−
OKT6	−	−	−	+
T129	−	−	−	+
L119	−	−	−	+
L298	−	−	−	+
L76	−	−	−	+
T134	−	−	−	+
T132	−	−	−	+
L232	−	−	−	+
T130	−	−	−	−
D47	+	+	−	−
T131	−	−	−	−
T133	−	−	−	−

[a] + Positive; − negative; ± only some cells were stained.

Further Dissection of Epitopes and Molecular Variants by Studies of Skin Tissue Section

CD1 antibodies from the Workshop as well as local antibodies were studied both on paraffin-fixed skin sections by immunoperoxydase and on frozen skin sections by immunofluorescence. After paraffin fixation all eccrine sweat glands were stained by D47 while only some eccrine sweat glands were stained by T128. On frozen skin sections similar staining of the sweat glands was observed with D47 and T128 while the epidermal Langerhans cells of the skin were stained by T129, L119, L76, L298, T134, T132, L232, and OKT6. In contrast, T130, T131 and T133 stained no cells in the skin. The results are summarized in Table 23.4.

Discussion

Results from systematic blind studies of 14 monoclonal antibodies belonging to CD1 and of one monoclonal antibody recognizing human β2-microglobulin shows the existence of eight epitopes which can be variously associated on four molecular variants on normal human thymus cells.

The utilization of several technical approaches permitted the precise definition of at least eight epitopes on these molecules. First systematic cross-blocking permitted the definition of three epitopic groups.

The first group was made up of antibodies L161 and T128 (M241) which showed reciprocal cross-blocking. However, studies of skin section revealed that only antibody T128 recognizes some eccrine sweat glands and must therefore define an epitope different from but close to L161. Reciprocal co-capping then revealed that T128 and L161 must recognize the same or associated molecules which are associated with β2-microglobulin. Finally sequential and reciprocal immunoprecipitation confirmed that T128 and L161 recognize identical molecules.

The second epitopic group consisted of antibodies T129 (NA1/34), L119, L76, L298, and D47. While the first three antibodies showed reciprocal cross-blocking and L298 totally blocked their fixation, D47, whose fixation was totally abolished by these other four antibodies in the group did not block completely the fixation of T129, L119, and L76 nor its own. This could reflect an intrinsic property of antibody D47 itself (low affinity) or that the epitope recognized by D47 induces a positive modulation of CD1 molecules.

Studies of skin section revealed that only D47 recognizes eccrine sweat glands, as already described (11), while the four other antibodies recognized Langerhans cells. D47 must therefore recognize a different epitope. Co-capping showed that the five antibodies must recognize the same or associated molecules and also that only the molecules recognized by L76, L298, and D47 were totally associated with β2-microglobulin. This indicated that three epitopes are infact defined in this second epitopic group: T129–L119, L76–L298, and D47. While L298 and D47 did not immunoprecipitate ^{125}I thymus cells, we could show that the L76 epitope is expressed on part of the molecules defined by T129–L119 and also on all the molecules defined by L161–T128. L76 could thus detect an epitope created by the association of these CD1 heavy chains with β2-microglobulin, as has been reported for the association of HLA with β2-microglobulin. Cross-blocking results would also indicate that all L76, L298, and D47 epitopes are close to the T129–L119 epitope, also they are not expressed on the same molecule on the cell surface (19).

Co-capping had previously shown that after capping L161–T128 molecules, T129–L119, L76–L298, and D47 still stained molecules dispersed on whole cell surface. Surprisingly only L161 stained dispersed molecules on the surface of cells capped for T129 or L119 while we could not detect such staining with T128, D47, L298, and L76 as would be expected. This can be explained as an artifact in that T129–L119 give a very large cap which can occupy almost 2/3 of the cell diameter and may prevent good examination of the remaining staining due to antibodies recognizing lower-density surface molecules. Alternatively this observation can be explained by the fact that during the formation of large caps, in particular, certain molecules may be unspecifically trapped. Finally it can also reflect the existence of biologically significant molecular complexes (20,21), or biologically significant modifications of uncapped molecules detected at the level of their epitopes.

The third epitopic group consisted of T132, T134, L232, and OKT6. Co-capping indicated that these antibodies may recognize the same molecule or molecular complex as T129–L119 while all these antibodies stained skin Langerhans cells. These results are in agreement with previous reports showing that NA1/34 (T129) and OKT6 recognize the same molecule (22) and that the molecule recognized by OKT6 can be immunoprecipitated from human Langerhans cells (10).

Finally, three antibodies—T130, T131, T133—did not cross-block any of the labeled antibody and did not stain cells in the skin. That T130 recognizes the same molecule as T129 was shown by co-capping and sequential immunoprecipitation. In summary, ten antibodies define five epitopes on this 46,000–49,000 M_r CD1 molecule. Two variants of this molecule can be detected on thymus cells, one variant with no detectable β2-microglobulin and lacking L76–L298 and D47 epitopes and another variant molecule with the five epitopes. On the skin a variant lacking T130 and D47 epitopes can also be detected.

T131 and T133 were shown to co-cap and T131 was shown to recognize a molecule distinct from T129. Further studies will be required to demonstrate that T131 and T133 recognize the same molecule and to analyze directly the relationships of the epitope(s) they define on this molecule.

CD1 molecules were originally thought to recognize class I molecules analogous to the mouse TL antigens. Numerous class I genes have been identified in the human genome whereas only six gene products (HLA A, B, C) have been isolated. Search for expression of CD1 molecules after transfection of class I genes into mouse L cells and mouse L cells containing human β2-microglobulin, including ours with the Workshop battery, have been so far unsuccessful (23). This leaves open the question of whether CD1 molecules are encoded by class I genes or whether β2-microglobulin is associated with non-class I gene products.

CD1 [Thy, gp45,12] now appears to be constituted of numerous antibodies defining a complex family of glycoproteins with variants which share some epitopes while others are private. This illustrates the interest of blind exchanges of numerous well-characterized monoclonal antibodies.

Summary

The results from systematic studies of tissue distribution, staining of skin sections, cross-blocking, co-capping, and immunoprecipitations performed with 14 different monoclonal antibodies (local products and workshop antibodies) recognizing the first cluster of differentiation are presented. CD1 [Thy, gp45,12] can presently be defined as composed of eight different epitopes which can be variously associated into four molecular variants on the surface of normal human thymus cells. We were also able to show that some of these epitopes are shared while others are unique to given molecular variant molecules.

References

1. Bernard, A., L. Boumsell, J. Dausset, C. Milstein, and S.F. Schlossman, eds. 1984. *Leucocyte typing.* Springer-Verlag, Berlin, Heidelberg.
2. Boumsell, L., C. Gelin, H. Coppin, P. Caudan, J. Kalil, D. Pham B. Raynal, and A. Bernard. 1984. Diversity of class I molecules heavy and light chains on human thymus cells. In: *Leucocyte typing,* A. Bernard, L. Boumsell, J. Dausset, C. Milstein, and S.F. Schlossman, eds. Springer-Verlag, Berlin, Heidelberg.
3. Knowles, R.K., and W.F. Bodmer. 1982. A monoclonal antibody recognizing a human TL-like antigen. *Eur. J. Immunol.* **12:**676.
4. McMichael, A.J., J.R. Pilch, G. Galfre, D.Y. Mason, J.W. Fabre, and C. Milstein. 1979. A human thymocyte antigen defined by a hybrid myeloma monoclonal antibody. *Eur. J. Immunol.* **9:**205.
5. Reinherz, E.L., P.C. Kung, G. Goldstein, R.L. Levey, and S.F. Schlossman. 1980. Discrete stages of intrathymic differentiation analysis of normal thymocytes and leukemic lymphoblasts of T lineage. *Proc. Natl. Acad. Sci. U.S.A.* **77:**1588.
6. Bernaben, C., M. Van de Rijn, P.G. Lerch, and C.P. Terhorst. 1984. β2-Microglobulin from serum associates with MHC class I antigens on the surface of cultured cells. *Nature* **308:**642.
7. Kefford, R.F., F. Calabi, I.M. Fearnely, O.R. Burrone, and C. Milstein. 1984. Serum β2-microglobulin binds to a T-cell differentiation antigen and increases its expression. *Nature* **308:**641.
8. Ziegler, A., and C. Milstein. 1979. A small polypeptide different from β2-microglobulin associated with a human cell surface antigen. *Nature* **279:**243.
9. Knowles, R.W. 1984. Biochemical analysis of human thymus leukemia-like antigens. In: *Leucocyte typing,* A. Bernard, L. Boumsell, J. Dausset, C. Milstein, and S.F. Schlossman, eds. Springer-Verlag, Berlin, Heidelberg.
10. Takezaki, S., S.L. Morrison, C.L. Berger, G. Goldstein, A.C. Chu, and R.L. Edelson. 1982. Biochemical characterization of a differentiation antigen shared by human epidermal langerhans cells and cortical thymocytes. *J. Clin. Immunol.* **2:**1288.
11. Kanitakis, J., D. Schmitt, A. Bernard, L. Boumsell, and J. Thivolet. 1983. Anti-D47: a monoclonal antibody reacting with the secretory cells of human eccrine sweat glands. *Brit. J. Dermatol.* **109:**509.
12. Boumsell, L., and A. Bernard. 1980. High efficiency of Biozzi's high responder mouse strain in the generation of antibody secreting hybridomas. *J. Immunol. Methods* **138:**225.
13. Boumsell, L., M. Amiot, B. Raynal, V. Gay-Bellile, and A. Bernard. Manuscript in preparation.
14. Teillaud, J.L., D. Crevat, P. Chardon, J. Kalil, C. Goujet-Zali, G. Mahony, M. Vaiman, M. Fellous, and D. Pious. 1982. Monoclonal antibodies as a tool for phylogenetic studies of major histocompatibility antigens and B$_2$ microglobulin. *Immunogen.* **15:**377.
15. Bernard, A., C. Gelin, B. Raynal, D. Pham, C. Goose, and L. Boumsell. 1982. Phenomenon of human T-cells rosetting with sheep erythrocytes analyzed with monoclonal antibodies. "Modulation" of a partially hidden epitope determining the conditions of interactions between T-cells and erythrocytes. *J. Exp. Med.* **155:**1317.

16. Bernard, A., V. Gay-Bellile, M. Amiot, B. Caillou, P. Charbord, and L. Boumsell. 1984. A novel human leukocyte differentiation antigen: monoclonal antibody anti-D44 defines a 28 Kd molecule present on immature hematologic cells and a subpopulation of mature T-cells. *J. Immunol.* **132:**2338.

17. Laemmli, U.K. 1970. Cleavage of structural proteins during the assembly of the head of bacteriophage T4. *Nature* **227:**680.

18. Bonner, W.M., and R.A. Laskey. 1974. A film detection method for tritium-labeled proteins and nucleic acids in polyaorylamide gels. *Eur. J. Biochem.* **46:**83.

19. Flaherty, L., and D. Zimmerman. 1979. Surface mapping of mouse thymocytes. *Proc. Natl. Acad. Sci. U.S.A.* **76:**1990.

20. Bourguignon, L.Y.W., R. Hyman, I. Trowbridge, and S.J. Singer. 1978. Participation of histocompatibility antigens in copping of molecularly independant cell surface components by their specific antibodies. Proc. Natl. Acad. Sci. U.S.A. **75:**2406.

21. Meuer, S.C., O. Acuto, R.E. Hussey, J.C. Hodgton, K.A. Fitzgerald, S.F. Schlossman, and E.L. Reinherz. 1983. Evidence for the T3 associated 90 Kd heterodimer as the T-cell antigen receptor. *Nature* **303:**808.

22. Cotner, T., H. Mashimo, P.C. Kung, G. Goldstein, and J.L. Strominger. 1981. Human T-cell surface antigens bearing a structural relationship to HLA antigens. *Proc. Natl. Acad. Sci. U.S.A.* **78:**3858.

23. Lemonnier, F.A., P. Le Bouteiller, B. Malissen, P. Golstein, M. Malissen, Z. Mishal, D.H. Caillol, B.R. Jordan, and F.M. Kourilsky. 1983. Transformation of murine LMTK⁻ cells with purified HLA class I genes. *J. Immunol.* **130:**1432.

CHAPTER 24

Comparison of the CD7 (3A1) Group of T Cell Workshop Antibodies

Thomas J. Palker, Richard M. Scearce,
Lucinda L. Hensley, Winifred Ho, and Barton F. Haynes

Introduction

The CD7 group of Workshop antibodies react with a 40-Kd glycoprotein (gp40) on the surface of 85% of peripheral blood T cells, essentially all thymocytes, and leukemias of T cell precursors (1–5). Prototypical monoclonal antibodies for the CD7 group described by Haynes et al. (antibodies $3A1_A$ and $3A1_B$) (1–3) and Morishima et al. (antibody 4A) (4) all identified a 40-Kd T lymphocyte antigen present on both $T4^+$ and $T8^+$ T cell subsets. Subsets of $gp40^+$ T cells enhanced immunoglobulin (Ig) synthesis by B cells (1–4), suppressed B cell Ig synthesis when stimulated with Con A (1–3), responded optimally to PHA and Con A stimulation (1,2), and gave rise to alloreactive, cytotoxic T cells in allogeneic mixed leukocyte culture (4). Antibodies to gp40 did not induce [^{3}H]thymidine incorporation in $gp40^+$ T cells (1–4). Importantly, monoclonal antibodies to the gp40 T lymphocyte glycoprotein have been shown to be the most reliable diagnostic markers for the identification of T cell acute lymphoblastic leukemia (5,6).

For the T cell Workshop, 16 coded monoclonal antibodies which had been provisionally assigned to the CD7 group were evaluated for reactivity to the gp40 T cell antigen identified by monoclonal antibody 3A1 in competition radioimmunoassay (RIA), radioimmunoprecipitation (RIP) assays, and indirect immunofluorescence assays. In this study, we report the identification of nine antibodies in the Workshop panel which definitely belong to the CD7 group [T30 (G3-7), T31 (4H9/Leu 9), T38 (8H8.1), T39 ($3A1_A$), T40 ($3A1_A$ irradiated), T41 ($3A1_B$-4G6), T43 (4A), T44 (I-3), T45 (I21)], six antibodies which do not [T29 (9–3), T32 (BW264/50), T33 (BW264/217), T34 (BW264/215), T36 (A1), T37 (4D12.1)], and one antibody which may be a member of this group [T42 ($3A1_C$-5A12)].

Materials and Methods

Monoclonal Antibodies

Sixteen monoclonal antibodies provisionally assigned to the CD7 (3A1) Workshop group from the coded T cell Workshop panel were used in this study (see Table 24.1).

Radioimmunoassays (RIA)

Monoclonal antibodies assigned to the CD7 group were tested for the ability to inhibit binding of ^{125}I-labeled $3A1_A$ (1,2) antibody to HSB-2 T cells in a competition RIA. Monoclonal antibody $3A1_A$ was purified by preparative isoelectric focusing (2), and 250 μg were iodinated using 0.5 mCi ^{125}I and Iodobeads (Pierce Chemical Co., Rockford, IL). For the assay, HSB-2 T cells (5×10^5/sample) were incubated for 30 min at 4°C with serial dilutions of CD7 group antibodies in RPMI media with 20% heat-inactivated fetal calf serum (HIFCS), washed 3 times with media, and then further incubated with 2×10^5 cpm of radiolabeled $3A1_A$ antibody. After washing, cell pellets were evaluated for [125]I-3AI$_A$ binding in a gamma counter.

CD7 group antibodies were also tested for the ability to bind to HSB-2 T cells in an RIA. HSB-2 T cells (5×10^5/sample) were incubated for 30 min at 4°C with 1:100 dilutions of CD7 antibodies in RPMI–20% HIFCS. After washing, cells were then incubated with rabbit anti–mouse IgG +M (Cappel Laboratories, Cochranville, PA), followed by washing and further incubation with ^{125}I-labeled protein A (10^5 cpm/sample).

Radioimmunoprecipitation (RIP) Assay

HSB-2 T cells or peripheral blood leukocytes (PBL) obtained from Ficoll–Hypaque gradients were cell-surface-labeled with ^{125}I using the lactoperoxidase procedure (7) and extracted with 1.0% Nonidet P-40/0.5% deoxycholate/0.05% SDS in 10 mM Tris, pH 8.0/5 mM phenylmethyl sulfonyl fluoride$_{(PMSF)}$/5 mM iodoacetamide for 30 min at 4°C as previously described (8). Extracts were centrifuged at $20,000 \times g$ for 15 min, and supernatants were used in the RIP assay performed as follows. Samples containing 10^7 cpm of radiolabeled cell extracts in 500 μl of extraction buffer were precleared by incubation with 5-μl P3X63 ascites fluid (20 min at 23°C) and then with 100 μl of 10% fixed *S. aureus* Cowan I (SAC) strain (Pansorbin, Calbiochem, La Jolla, CA), preloaded with rabbit anti–mouse IgG +M (H & L chain, Cappel Laboratories). After preclearing, samples were incubated overnight at 4°C with 10 μl of CD7 workshop antibodies, and immune complexes were precipitated with SAC preloaded with rabbit anti–mouse IgG +M as described. SAC pellets were washed three times in extraction buffer, and immune precipitates were extracted by boiling the SAC pellets for 2 min in 0.1 M Tris, pH 6.8 with 10% glycerol, 2% SDS, and 5% β-mercaptoethanol. Supernatants containing the immune precipitates were subjected to SDS–PAGE (9) on 10% polyacrylamide gels followed by autoradiography.

Indirect Immunofluorescence Assays

Acetone-fixed 4-micron cryostat sections of normal human thymus were incubated with dilutions of CD7 antibodies in phosphate-buffered saline (PBS) (pH 7.4) containing 2% BSA for 30 min at 23°C. Samples were then washed three times in PBS and further incubated for 30 min with fluores-ceinated goat anti–mouse IgG +M (H & L chain, Kirkegaard and Perry Laboratories, Inc., Gaithersburg, MD). After additional washing, tissue sections were overlaid with 30% glycerol in PBS and viewed on a Nikon Optiphot fluorescent microscope.

[³H]Thymidine Uptake Studies

The ability of CD7 antibodies to induce [³H]thymidine incorporation into either unstimulated, PHA-, or Con A-activated peripheral blood leuko-cytes (PBL) was evaluated as described previously (1). Briefly, Ficoll–Hypaque purified PBLs were incubated with either CD7 antibodies alone or in the presence of PHA (1 and 5 μg/ml) or concanavalin A (50 and 100 μg/ml) plus [³H]thymidine. After 3 days, peak [³H]thymidine incorpora-tion was determined.

Results

Competitive Inhibition of ¹²⁵I-Labeled 3A1 Binding to HSB-2 T Cells by CD7 Monoclonal Antibodies

In competition RIA experiments, nine CD7 monoclonal antibodies inhib-ited the binding of ¹²⁵I-labeled 3A1 antibody to the cell surface of HSB-2 T cells. For example, Fig. 24.1 shows that Workshop antibodies T31 (4H9/Leu 9), T39 (3A1$_A$), and T41 (3A1$_B$-4G6) all inhibited the binding of ¹²⁵I-labeled 3A1 antibody to HSB-2 T cells, while negative control antibody T1 (P3X63 ascites fluid) did not. With this assay, it was possible to subdi-vide the CD7 antibodies into two groups: those antibodies which inhibited ¹²⁵I-labeled 3A1 binding to HSB-2 T cells (T30, 31, 38, 40, 41, 43, 44 and 45) and those which did not (T29, 32, 33, 34, 36, 37, and 42).

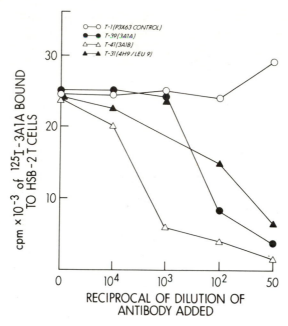

Fig. 24.1. Ability of T41 (3A1$_B$) and T31 (4H9/Leu 9) antibodies to block ^{125}I-labeled T39 (3A1$_A$) binding to HSB-2 T cells. The results of a competition radioimmunoassay (RIA) using HSB-2 T cells, ^{125}I-labeled T39 (3A1$_A$) antibody, and unlabeled CD7 Workshop antibodies are shown. When preincubated with HSB-2 T cells, unlabeled antibodies T41, T31, and T39 all inhibited the binding of ^{125}I-labeled T39 antibodies to HSB-2 T cells while T1 (P3X63) antibodies did not. With this assay, it was possible to subdivide the CD7 group antibodies into two groups: those antibodies which inhibited ^{125}I-labeled T39 binding (T30, 31, 38, 39, 40, 41, 43, 44, 45) and those which did not (T29, 32, 33, 34, 36, 37, 42).

Radioimmunoprecipitation (RIP) of gp40 by CD7 Workshop Antibodies

To further characterize the reactivities of CD7 antibodies, RIP experiments were performed with extracts of ^{125}I-labeled HSB-2 T cells and Ficoll–Hypaque purified peripheral blood leukocytes (PBL). As shown in Fig. 24.2, the same CD7 antibodies that competed with ^{125}I-labeled 3A1 binding to HSB-2 T cells (T30,31,38,39,40,41,43,44, and 45) also precipitated a 40-Kd protein from extracts of HSB cells. In contrast, those CD7 antibodies which did not compete with 3A1 binding (T29, 32, 33, 34, 36, 37, and 42) also did not precipitate gp40. Instead, antibodies in this latter group showed no or weak reactivity to HSB-2 T cell surface proteins in RIP assays (not shown).

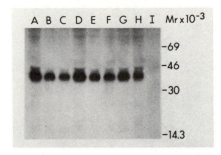

Fig. 24.2. Immunoprecipitation of gp40 with CD7 antibodies that blocked T39 binding to HSB-2 T cells. Lysates of ^{125}I-labeled HSB-2 T cells were incubated with CD7 group antibodies, and precipitated immune complexes were subjected to SDS–PAGE. All CD7 antibodies which inhibited T39 binding to HSB-2 T cells in a competition RIA (see Fig. 24.1) also precipitated gp40. Shown here are proteins precipitated by CD7 antibodies T38 (A), T39 (B), T41 (C), T43 (D), T44 (E), T45 (F), T30 (G), and T31 (H). Lane I: precipitation with T1 (P3X63 negative control). CD7 antibodies that did not block T39 binding in competition RIA also did not precipitate gp40 (not shown).

CD7 antibodies precipitated two proteins of 36 and 40 Kd from extracts of ^{125}I-labeled PBL or thoracic duct drainage cells taken from two of six subjects [two of five shown in Fig. 24.3(A), (B)]. As shown in Fig. 24.3(A), CD7 antibody T39 (3A1$_A$ precipitated both p36 and gp40 from extracts of PBL taken from one normal subject (lane A), while precipitating only gp40 from extracts of PBL obtained from three other normal subjects (lanes B–D). The corresponding negative control RIP experiments performed with P3X63 ascites fluid and extracts of PBLs are shown in lanes E–H. In Fig. 24.3(B), antibodies T39 (lane A) and T41 (lane B) also precipitated both p36 and gp40 from extracts of normal thoracic duct drainage cells.

Reactivity of CD7 Workshop Antibodies with Thymus

To further define the reactivities of CD7 Workshop antibodies, they were reacted with 4-micron, acetone-fixed cryostat sections of human thymus in an indirect immunofluorescence assay. As shown in Fig. 24.4, antibody 3A1$_A$ (T39, T40) reacted with essentially all thymocytes and with foci of brightly staining thymocytes in the subcapsular cortex and cortex. All CD7 antibodies that inhibited [125]I-3A1 binding to HSB-2 T cells and precipitated gp40 in RIP assays gave similar fluorescent-staining patterns on thymus. Antibody T42 (3A1$_C$-5A12) also reacted with thymus in a 3A1-like pattern, although it did not block [125]I-3A1 binding to HSB-2 T-cells nor did it immunoprecipitate gp40. Antibody T37 (4D12.1) reacted in a T8-like pattern on thymus with all cortical and approximately 30% of medul-

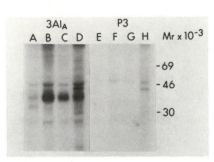
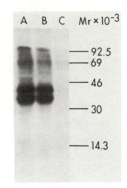

Fig. 24.3. Immunoprecipitation of p36 and gp40 from ^{125}I-labeled PBLs or thoracic duct drainage cells with CD7 antibodies. (A) CD7 antibody T39 (3A1$_A$) precipitated either p36 and gp40 (lane A) or only gp40 (lanes B–D) from extracts of PBLs taken from four normal subjects (lanes A–D). Negative control immunoprecipitations with P3X63 ascites fluid and the extracts of four PBL samples are shown in lanes E–H. (B) CD7 antibodies T39 (3A1$_A$) (lane A) and T41 (3A1$_B$) (lane B) precipitated both p36 and gp40 from extracts of normal thoracic duct drainage cells while P3X63 ascites fluid (lane C) did not.

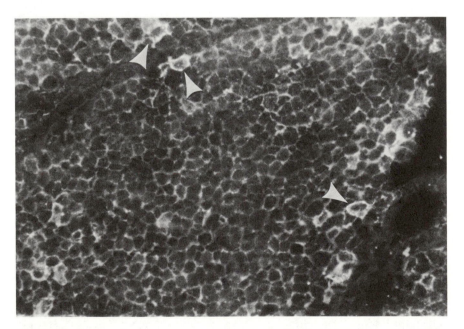

Fig. 24.4. Immune fluorescence of CD7 group antibody T39 (3A1$_A$) on 4-micron cryostat section of thymus. All subcapsular, cortical, and medullary thymocytes were positive. Also present were foci of brightly staining thymocytes in the subcapsular cortex and cortex (arrow heads). All CD7 group antibodies that precipitated gp40 (see Fig. 24.2), as well as antibody T42, gave similar staining patterns on thymus.

lary thymocytes positive, while antibody T29 reacted in an OKT1-like pattern with all medullary thymocytes positive and approximately 5% of cortical thymocytes positive. Other antibodies provisionally assigned to the CD7 group either reacted with thymus in an HLA-like pattern [antibody T33 (BW264/217); cortical and medullary thymic epithelium positive, medullary thymocytes positive] or did not react at all with thymus [T32 (BW264/50), T34 (BW264/215), T36 (A1)].

Effect of CD7 Antibodies on [³H]Thymidine Incorporation into Either Unstimulated, PHA-, or Con A-Stimulated PBLs

To determine if the CD7 antibodies had any mitogenic effects when bound to the cell surface of peripheral blood T cells, Ficoll–Hypaque purified PBLs were incubated either with CD7 antibodies alone, with CD7 antibodies and PHA, or with CD7 antibodies and Con A. After 4 days in culture, peak [³H]thymidine incorporation was monitored. As shown in Fig. 24.5, none of the CD7 antibodies which had previously been shown to inhibit ¹²⁵I-3A1 binding to HSB cells (solid bars) enhanced [³H]thymidine incorporation into Con A-activated peripheral blood T cells. Similar

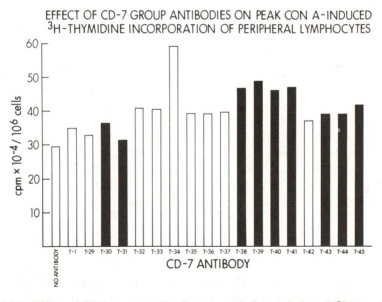

Fig. 24.5. Effect of CD7 group antibodies on peak Con A-induced [³H]thymidine incorporation of peripheral blood leukocytes (PBL). Ficoll–Hypaque purified PBLs were incubated with CD7 group antibodies and Con A, and peak [³H]thymidine was monitored. None of the antibodies except T34 (BW264/215) appeared to stimulate [³H]thymidine incorporation in Con A-stimulated PBLs. Solid bars: CD7 antibodies that inhibited T39 (3A1$_A$) binding to HSB-2 T cells. Open bars: CD7 antibodies that did not inhibit T39 (3A1$_A$) binding to HSB-2 T cells.

results were obtained with unstimulated and PHA-stimulated PBLs (not shown). Of those CD7 antibodies that did not competitively inhibit [125]I-3A1 binding (open bars), only one antibody (T34) appeared to enhance [3H]thymidine uptake into Con A-stimulated PBL. However, since antibody T34 did not react with acetone-fixed frozen sections of thymus (Table 24.1) or with viable PBLs in indirect immunofluorescence assays (not shown), it is likely that the mitogenic effects were mediated by non-immunoglobulin factors in this antibody preparation.

Summary of Reactivities of Monoclonal Antibodies Provisionally Assigned to the CD7 Group

Based on data from competition RIA, RIP assays, and indirect immuno-fluorescence assays, nine monoclonal antibodies provisionally assigned to the CD7 group were shown to be definite CD7 antibodies (Table 24.1). These antibodies (T30, 31, 38, 39, 40, 41, 43, 44, and 45) all competed with ^{125}I-labeled 3A1 antibody for binding to HSB-2 T cells, as well as precipitated gp40 from extracts of radiolabeled PBLs and HSB cells, and also had identical patterns of reactivity to acetone-fixed sections of thymus in indirect immunofluorescence assays. Antibody T42 was classified as a probable CD7 antibody based on its reactivity to thymocytes in fluorescence assays, although this antibody did not competitively inhibit ^{125}I-labeled 3A1 binding to HSB-2 T cells or precipitate gp40. Six antibodies (T29, 32, 33, 34, 36, 37) could be excluded from the CD7 group since none of these antibodies competed with [125]I-3A1 binding, nor did they precipitate gp40 or react with thymus sections in a 3A1-like fluorescence pattern. One of these antibodies, T37, reacted in a T8-like pattern on thymic sections (all cortical and approximately 30% medullary thymocytes positive) and was later found to cluster with the CD8 group of Workshop antibodies after computer analysis of Workshop results (see this volume, Chapter 1). The reactivities of other non-CD7 antibodies are listed in Table 24.1. Thus, 9 of 16 antibodies provisionally assigned to the CD7 group could be classified as definite CD7 antibodies.

Discussion

By using monoclonal antibodies assigned to the CD7 group in RIA, RIP assays, and indirect immunofluorescence assays, we have identified nine antibodies which precipitated gp40 from peripheral blood T cells and HSB-2 T cells, competitively inhibited binding of a known CD7 antibody, 3A1, to HSB-2 T cells, and reacted in a 3A1-like pattern to thymocytes in an indirect immunofluorescence assay. In addition, none of these nine CD7 antibodies induced [3H]thymidine incorporation into resting or lec-tin-activated PBL, in accord with previous data (1) indicating that CD7

Table 24.1. Summary of characterization of CD7 group of anti–T cell monoclonal antibodies.

Workshop number	Antibody	Investigator	Antigen ($M_r \times 10^{-3}$)	Blocks binding of ^{125}I-3A1$_A$	Thymus reactivity by IF[a]	HSB reactivity in radioimmunoassay	Assessment
Definite CD7 antibodies							
T39, T40	3A1$_A$	Haynes	40	Yes	3A1 pattern[c]	Yes	CD7 antibody
T38	8H8.1	Mawas	40	Yes	3A1 pattern	Yes	CD7 antibody
T41	3A1$_B$-4G6	Haynes	40	Yes	3A1 pattern	Yes	CD7 antibody
T43	4A	Naito, Dupont	40	Yes	3A1 pattern	Yes	CD7 antibody
T44	I-3	Naito, Dupont	40	Yes	3A1 pattern	Yes	CD7 antibody
T45	I21	Bernard, Boumsell	40	Yes	3A1 pattern	Yes	CD7 antibody
T30	G3-7	Ledbetter	40	Yes	3A1 pattern	Yes	CD7 antibody
T31	4H9/Leu 9	Warner	40	Yes	3A1 pattern	Yes	CD7 antibody
Probable CD7 antibodies							
T42	3A1$_C$-5A12	Haynes	—[b]	No	3A1 pattern	Yes	Probably CD7 antibody
Not CD7 antibodies							
T37	4D12.1	Mawas	—	No	T8 pattern[d]	No	Probably CD8 antibody
T29	9-3	Naito	—	No	T1 pattern[e]	No	Not CD7 antibody
T32	BW264/50	Kurrle	—	No	None	Yes	Not CD7 antibody
T33	BW264/217	Kurrle	—	No	[f]HLA pattern	Weak yes	Not CD7 antibody
T34	BW264/215	Kurrle	—	No	None	Yes	Not CD7 antibody
T36	A1	Girardet	—	No	None	Weak yes	Not CD7 antibody

[a] IF = Indirect immunofluorescence on thymus frozen sections.
[b] No bands seen in radioimmunoprecipitation assays using SDS–PAGE.
[c] 3A1 pattern = all cortical and medullary thymocytes + with foci of bright cells.
[d] T8 pattern = All cortical and medullary thymocytes +.
[e] T1 pattern = All medullary thymocytes and ~30% of cortical thymocytes +.
[f] HLA pattern = Cortical and medullary epithelium +, medullary thymocytes +.

antibody 3A1 is nonmitogenic. Taken together, these nine CD7 antibodies exhibited reactivity patterns which matched those of prototypical CD7 antibodies $3A1_A$ and $3A1_B$ (1–3) and 4A (4). Indeed, inclusion of 3A1 and 4A in the CD7 antibody panel provided essential internal positive controls for the methods used to identify additional CD7 group antibodies.

In RIP assays with peripheral blood leukocytes and thoracic duct drainage cells, CD7 group antibodies T39 (3A1) and T41 ($3A1_B$-4G6) immunoprecipitated proteins of 36 and 40 Kd from T cells obtained from two of six subjects. In another study, protein bands of 36 and 40 Kd were also immunoprecipitated with a CD7 antibody from 40–50% of PBL samples obtained (S.M. Fu and T. Hara, personal communication). Although it is not clear why in some cases a 36-Kd protein was precipitated by CD7 antibodies in addition to gp40, several explanations may be proposed. The molecular weight of p36 corresponds to that of gp35 precipitated from human T lymphocytes by anti-gp40 antibody WT1 (10). In this study, Sutherland et al. provided evidence that gp35 was a partially glycosylated high-mannose precursor of the mature gp40 complex-type glycoprotein. Moreover, since antibodies WT1 and 3A1 were shown to react with the same gp40 T lymphocyte glycoprotein, it is probable that antibody 3A1 also reacts with the partially glycosylated intermediate of gp40 identified by antibody WT1. Thus, immunoprecipitation of p36 and gp40 from extracts of some PBL samples may reflect variations in the ability to process the high-mannose type N-linked glycan into the mature complex-type gp40 glycoprotein. Alternately the p36 molecule may possess a truncated polypeptide chain due to partial proteolytic degradation of gp40 during the processing of extracts for the RIP assay. Since the proteinase inhibitors PMSF and iodoacetamide included in the extraction buffer would not inhibit metallo- or carboxyl proteinases (11), proteolytic degradation of gp40 remains a possibility. The biochemistry of the p36 molecule is currently under investigation.

Future research related to gp40 and the CD7 group of Workshop antibodies may need to address the biochemical nature of p36 as well as the functional role of the gp40 molecule on T cells.

Acknowledgments. Ms. Joyce Lowery is acknowledged for expert secretarial assistance. This work was supported by Grants CA 28936 and KO400695 from the National Cancer Institute, National Institutes of Health, Bethesda, MD 20205.

References

1. Haynes, B.F., G.S. Eisenbarth, and A.S. Fauci. 1979. Human lymphocyte antigens: Production of a monoclonal antibody that defines functional thymus-derived lymphocyte subsets. *Proc. Natl. Acad. Sci.* **76:**5829.
2. Haynes, B.F., D.L. Mann, M.E. Hemler, J.A. Schroer, J.H. Shelhamer, G.S. Eisenbarth, J.L. Strominger, C.A. Thomas, H.S. Mostowski, and A.S. Fauci.

1980. Characterization of a monoclonal antibody that defines an immunoregulatory T-cell subset for immunoglobulin synthesis in humans. *Proc. Natl. Acad. Sci.* **77**:2914.

3. Haynes, B.F. 1981. Human T-lymphocyte antigens as defined by monoclonal antibodies. *Immunol. Rev.* **57**:127.

4. Morishima, Y., M. Kobayashi, S.Y. Yang, N.H. Collins, M.K. Hoffmann, and B. Dupont. 1982. Functionally different T lymphocyte subpopulations determined by their sensitivity to complement-dependent cell lysis with the monoclonal antibody 4A. *J. Immunol.* **129**:1091.

5. Vodinelich, L., W. Tax, Y. Bai, S. Pegram, P. Capel, and M.F. Greaves. 1983. A monoclonal antibody (WT1) for detecting leukemias of T-cell precursors (T-ALL). *Blood* **62**:1108.

6. Haynes, B.F., R.S. Metzgar, J.D. Minna, and P.A. Bunn. 1981. Phenotypic characterization of cutaneous T-cell lymphoma. *New England J. Med.* **304**:1319.

7. Jones, P.P. 1980. Analysis of radiolabeled lymphocyte proteins by one- and two-dimensional polyacrylamide gel electrophoresis. In: *Selected Methods in Cellular Immunology.* B.B. Mishell and S.M. Shiigi, eds. W.H. Freeman and Co., San Francisco, pp. 398–439.

8. Haynes, B.F., E.G. Reisner, M.E. Hemler, J.L. Strominger, and G.S. Eisenbarth. 1982. Description of a monoclonal antibody defining an HLA allotypic determinant that includes specificities within the B5 cross-reacting group. *Human Immunol.* **4**:273.

9. Laemmli, U.K. 1970. Cleavage of structural proteins during the assembly of the head of bacteriophage T4. *Nature* **227**:680.

10. Sutherland, D.R., C.E. Rudd, and M.F. Greaves. 1984. Isolation and characterization of a human T lymphocyte-associated glycoprotein (gp40). *J. Immunol.* **133**:327.

11. Barrett, A.J. 1980. The many forms and functions of cellular proteinases. *Fed. Proc.* **39**:9.

Part IV. Phenotypic Characterization of T Cell Leukemias and Lymphomas

CHAPTER 25

Study on Human T Leukemia–Lymphoma Cell Lines by the Second International Workshop Monoclonal Antibodies of the T Cell Protocol

Jun Minowada, Mira Menon, Hans Guenter Drexler, Suzanne Gignac, Bishnupriya Misra, and Lisa Skowron

Introduction

The First International Workshop and Conference on Human Leukocyte Differentiation Antigens was held in November, 1982 in Paris, France; this conference provided means and emphasized the need for a worldwide collaboration in the study of human leukocyte antigens (1). Among numerous impacts of the Workshop, uses of murine monoclonal hybridoma antibodies (mAbs) and of leukemia–lymphoma cell lines as consistent cells were amply recognized (1,2). Limitations and difficulties associated with the use of both mAbs and leukemia–lymphoma cell lines have already been documented (3). Large numbers of growth factor-independent human leukemia–lymphoma cell lines of diverse cell lineages have continued to play significant roles in the research of leukocyte differentiation antigens (4). During the First Workshop 165 coded mAbs were tested on 30 leukemia–lymphoma cell lines (10 T, 10 B, and 10 myelomonocytic or non-T/non-B cell lines) (5).

As increasing numbers of new mAbs and leukemia–lymphoma cell lines are developed, we report here the analysis of 159 new mAbs in the T cell protocol provided by the Second Workshop using 22 selected hemopoietic cell lines.

Materials and Methods

Monoclonal Antibodies (mAbs)

A total of 159 mAbs, with code numbers 1 through 159, in the T cell protocol were provided by the organizing committee of the Second International Workshop and Conference on Human Leukocyte Differentiation Antigens. According to the instructions provided, the antibody dilutions (1/100) were prepared in a single preparation and were used throughout the blind Workshop testing. A single known monoclonal antibody reagent which was known to be reactive with each target cell line was added in the testing (mAb no. 160). The mAbs were identified after the completion of the blind testing.

Fluorescein Isothiocyanate (FITC)-Conjugated Goat Anti–mouse Immunoglobulin Reagent

A single pool of the FITC-conjugated anti–mouse immunoglobulin reagent (FITC-conjugated anti–polyvalent mouse Ig; FITC-GAM, Coulter Immunology, Hialeah, FL) was first titrated and standardized to optimal dilution for both IgG- and IgM-primary mouse antibodies using a few known positive primary mAbs.

Test Cells

A total of 22 growth factor-independent leukemia–lymphoma cell lines, which included 16 T cell lines and 6 non-T cell lines, were used. Origin, establishment, characteristics, and marker profiles with a panel of known mAbs were previously described in detail (6,7). According to the marker profiles, these 16 T cell lines and 6 non-T cell lines are further characterized for their lineages and differentiation stages (6–9). As illustrated in Fig. 25.1, four cell lines each in the T-Blast II, T-Blast III, and T-Blast IV and three cell lines in the T-Blast V categories were chosen for the T cells. For the non-T, three cell lines in the Erythroid, two cell lines in the Myelomonocyte, and one cell line in the Pre-B cell categories were chosen. While none of the 16 T cell lines used have Fc receptors, five of the six non-T cell lines except 1 Pre-B cell line (NALM-1) show strong Fc receptors binding, as detected by EA-rosette assay.

All cell lines were grown in suspension in RPMI 1640 nutrient medium supplemented with 5–10% heat-inactivated fetal calf serum at 37°C in 5% CO_2/95% air. Care was taken to use the cells in an exponential growth phase, since the optimal expression of all membrane antigens is known to be in the log growth phase (10). The cell lines had viability ranging from 80 to 99% at the time of testing. A few cell lines, such as MT-1 and C5/MJ lines, were at 60–70% viability level. Viability was determined by trypan

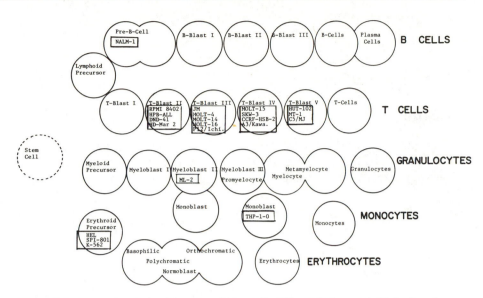

Fig. 25.1. Scheme of the hematopoietic cell differentiation and 22 leukemia–lymphoma cell lines used in the study. According to the marker profiles, 16 T cell lines and 6 non-T cell lines are assigned to respective lineage and differentiation stages (Refs. 4–6,8 and 9).

blue dye exclusion. In addition to the Workshop mAbs, a single known antibody (designated as no. 160) and E- or EA-rosette assay were included for each cell line tested.

The cultured cells were harvested and washed twice with phosphate-buffered saline (PBS). The washed cells were adjusted for a cell concentration ranging from 1.0×10^6 to 5×10^6/ml in PBS.

Indirect Membrane Immunofluorescence

The procedure used has been described in detail earlier (9). Fifty μl of cell suspension in a glass test tube ($7 \times$ mm) were incubated with 50 μl of each primary mAb at room temperature (22°C) for 30 min. A single wash with 0.7 ml of PBS was followed by a 30-min staining with 50 μl of FITC-conjugated anti–mouse Ig reagent at 22°C. After the second wash, the stained cell pellet was suspended in a drop of glycerol–PBS (50% vol) and mounted on a microscope slide with a cover slip. Visual enumeration for positive cells was carried out under $\times 1000$ magnification in an epifluorescent microscope. In this study, results were expressed as 0%, 10%, 50%, and 100% fluorescent cells. A total of at least 100 cells were scanned.

According to the Workshop instructions ("a single test for all mAbs at the same time on the same test cell population"), blind test in this study was performed by a team of five individuals in the laboratory.

Results and Discussion

Overall Results

Table 25.1 shows the overall results. Several points of general consideration can be made in order to evaluate the results. It has been shown in an earlier study (9) that the marker expression remains stable for each cell

Table 25.1. Second International Workshop Data

							T							
							T-Blast II				T-Blast III			
mAb (Code #)	Ig subclass	Fixes C	Binds SPA	Antibody name	Lab number	RPMI 8402	HPB-ALL	DND-41	HD-MAR-2	JM	MOLT-4	MOLT-14	MOLT-16	P12/Ichi.
Controls														
1	−IgG1	N	No	P3X63	105	10	50	0	0	0	10	100	0	0
2	−NA	NA	NA	PBS-BSA*	105	10	0	0	0	0	0	10	0	0
3	+IgG1	Y	No	A3D8	105	100	100	100	100	100	100	100	100	50
CD5														
4	IgG1	N	No	H65	26	100	100	50	100	100	100	100	100	100
5	IgG2a	Y	Yes	6-2	28	100	100	50	100	100	100	100	100	100
6	IgG1	NK	NK	SJ10-2H10	31	10	50	0	50	0	10	100	50	50
7	IgG2a	Y	NK	L17F12/Leu 1	47	100	100	50	100	100	100	100	100	100
8	IgG2b	NK	Yes	MT 61	61	100	100	50	100	100	100	100	100	100
9	IgG1	NK	No	MT 215	61	100	50	100	100	100	100	100	100	100
10	IgG1	N	NK	2H4	75	10	100	100	0	100	100	100	100	10
11	IgG2a	Y	Yes	X1X102-3	96	0	10	0	10	0	0	50	50	10
12	IgG2b	N	NK	BL-T2	116	0	10	50	50	100	50	50	50	50
CD2														
13	IgG2b	Y	NK	9-1	28	50	100	10	100	100	100	100	100	50
14	IgM	Y	NK	9-2	28	50	100	50	100	100	100	100	100	50
15	IgG1	N	No	G19-3.1	36	100	100	50	100	100	100	100	100	100
16	IgG2a	NK	NK	S2/Leu 5b	47	100	100	50	50	100	100	10	100	50
17	IgG1	NK	No	MT 26	61	50	100	10	100	100	100	50	100	50
18	IgG1	NK	No	MT 910	61	100	100	10	100	100	100	50	100	100
19	IgG1	NK	No	MT 1110	61	50	100	50	100	100	100	50	100	50
20	IgG1	N	No	T11/3Pt2H9	72	100	100	50	100	100	100	10	100	50
21	IgG1	N	Yes	T11/ROLD2-IH8	72	50	100	50	100	100	100	10	100	50
22	IgG2a	Y	Yes	T11/3T4-8B5	72	50	100	10	100	100	100	10	100	50
23	IgM	Y	No	T11/7T4-7A9	72	10	100	10	50	100	100	10	100	50
24	IgG2b	Y	Yes	T11/7T4-7E10	72	50	100	10	100	100	100	10	100	50
25	IgG2a	Y	Yes	96	79	100	100	50	100	100	100	10	100	100
26	IgG2a	Y	Yes	35.1	79	50	100	50	100	100	100	10	100	100
27	IgG1/2	Y	NK	T4IIB5	88	50	100	10	100	100	100	100	100	50
28	IgG1	N	NK	KOLT-2	71	100	100	50	100	100	100	10	100	50

line in long-term culture. Nevertheless, it is not always easy to achieve the consistent culture conditions where all markers are expressed optimally. Subtle deviations from the optimal culture conditions at any given time might have existed. Indeed, in another paper being presented in the Workshop study, we found that an overall discrepancy of 12% existed with 11 mAbs (11), when other variables such as individual observer, inherent properties of each cell line, suboptimal concentration, or biological properties of individual mAbs are excluded. It is not possible to rule out the chance that a single or several variables may well have existed in our study. It will be interesting to reevaluate our data when the final results of the entire Workshop study become available.

It should be noted, however, that only a few of the 159 mAbs are restricted to the T cell lineage. Keeping in mind the possible Fc binding of

| T | | | | | | | Non-T | | | | | |
| T-Blast IV | | | | T-Blast V | | | EL | | Ery. | PreB | AML | AMoL |
MOLT-15	SKW-3	CCRF-HSB-2	A3/Kawa.	HUT-102	MT-1	C5/MJ	HEL	SP1-801	K-562	NALM-1	ML-2	THP-1-0
10	10	100	50	0	10	50	0	0	0	0	0	100
0	0	10	10	0	0	10	0	0	0	0	0	0
50	100	100	100	100	10	100	100	0	100	50	100	100
50	100	100	100	100	100	100	0	0	0	0	0	0
50	100	50	100	100	100	100	100	50	0	10	0	100
50	100	50	100	10	50	50	100	10	10	100	0	100
50	100	10	10	100	100	100	0	10	0	0	0	100
50	100	50	100	100	100	100	0	50	0	0	0	100
100	100	100	100	50	50	50	100	100	10	100	0	100
50	50	50	100	10	50	50	100	50	0	100	100	100
0	10	10	100	10	100	100	0	0	0	0	0	0
0	100	10	100	10	50	50	100	10	0	0	0	50
10	100	50	100	50	100	100	100	50	10	50	0	100
10	100	10	100	50	50	100	100	50	0	0	0	100
50	100	50	100	100	100	100	0	50	0	0	0	100
0	100	10	100	10	50	100	0	50	0	0	0	100
10	100	50	100	50	100	100	100	50	50	0	0	100
10	100	50	100	10	100	100	100	50	0	0	0	100
50	100	50	100	50	100	100	100	100	100	0	0	100
50	100	50	100	10	100	50	100	50	0	0	0	100
50	100	50	100	10	50	100	0	10	0	0	0	100
50	100	50	100	10	50	100	100	50	0	0	0	100
50	100	50	100	10	10	100	0	10	0	0	0	100
50	100	50	50	0	50	100	100	50	50	50	0	100
0	100	50	100	0	50	100	100	50	0	0	100	100
0	100	50	100	50	50	100	100	50	0	0	100	100
10	100	10	100	10	50	100	100	50	10	0	0	100
0	100	50	100	50	100	10	0	50	0	100	100	100

Table 25.1. *Continued*

						T-Blast II				T-Blast III				T
mAb (Code #)	Ig subclass	Fixes C	Binds SPA	Antibody name	Lab number	RPMI 8402	HPB-ALL	DND-41	HD-MAR-2	JM	MOLT-4	MOLT-14	MOLT-16	P12/Ichi.
CD7														
29	IgG2b	Y	NK	9-3	28	50	100	10	100	100	50	100	100	50
30	IgG1	N	No	G3-7	36	100	100	100	100	100	100	100	100	100
31	IgG2a	NK	Yes	4H9/Leu 9	47	100	50	100	100	100	100	100	100	100
32	IgM	Y	No	BW264/50	53	0	50	10	50	50	0	10	50	50
33	IgM	Y	No	BW264/217	53	100	100	50	100	100	100	100	100	100
34	IgM	Y	No	BW264/215	53	0	50	50	100	100	100	0	100	100
35	NA	N	No	PBS-BSA*	105	0	0	0	0	0	0	0	0	0
36	IgG2	NK	Yes	A1	88	0	0	0	0	0	0	0	10	0
37	IgG1	NK	NK	4D12.1	100	0	100	0	50	100	50	0	0	0
38	IgG2a	NK	Yes	8H8.1	100	50	100	100	100	100	100	100	100	100
39	IgG1	Y	Yes	3A1A	105	100	50	100	100	100	100	100	100	100
40	IgG1	Y	Yes	3A1A(irrad.)	105	100	50	100	100	100	100	100	100	100
41	IgG2	Y	Yes	3A1B-4G6	105	50	50	100	100	100	100	100	100	100
42	IgM	Y	No	3A1C-5A12	105	50	0	100	100	100	100	100	100	0
43	IgG2	Y	Yes	4A	107,28	100	50	100	100	100	100	100	100	100
44	IgG2a	Y	Yes	1-3	107,28	100	50	100	100	100	100	100	100	100
45	IgG	NK	Yes	I21	103	100	100	100	100	100	100	100	100	100
CD6														
46	IgM	Y	No	T12/3Pt12B8	72	100	50	50	100	100	100	0	100	100
47	IgG2a	Y	Yes	12.1.5	79	50	100	50	100	100	100	50	100	100
Pan T														
48	IgM	Y	NK	T10B9	21	0	100	0	10	100	0	50	100	0
49	IgM	Y	NK	T12A10	21	50	0	0	0	0	0	0	100	0
50	IgG	NK	NK	E9	27	0	0	10	50	100	100	100	50	100
51	IgG1	N	No	G3-5	36	100	100	100	100	100	100	100	100	100
52	IgG1	N	No	G10-2.1	36	100	100	100	100	100	100	100	100	100
53	IgG1	N	No	G19-1.2	36	100	100	100	100	100	100	100	100	100
54	IgG2a	Y	Yes	T55	46	50	100	100	100	100	100	100	100	100
55	IgM	Y	No	T56	46	0	100	10	50	100	100	0	50	10
56	IgG	Y	NK	T57	46	100	100	50	100	100	100	0	100	50
57	IgG	Y	Yes	BW239/347	53	0	100	0	100	100	0	0	100	0
58	IgG1	NK	No	MT 211	61	50	100	0	100	100	100	0	100	100
59	IgG1	NK	No	MT 421	61	100	100	50	100	100	100	100	100	100
60	IgG	Y	Yes	CRIS-3	69	100	100	100	100	100	100	100	100	100
61	IgG	Y	Yes	CRIS-7	69	0	100	50	100	100	10	100	100	50
62	IgG	Y	Yes	CRIS-8	69	10	100	0	10	10	0	10	100	50
63	NK	NK	NK	K20	103	100	100	100	100	100	100	100	100	100
64	NK	NK	NK	K50	103	100	100	100	100	0	0	0	0	0
65	NK	NK	NK	G144	103	0	100	10	100	100	100	0	100	50
66	NK	NK	NK	D47	103	0	100	50	0	100	10	0	10	50
CD4														
67	IgM	Y	NK	T10C5	21	0	100	0	0	0	0	0	100	100
68	IgG1	N	No	G19-2	36	50	100	50	100	100	50	0	10	100
69	IgG2a	NK	Yes	91d6	42	50	100	50	100	100	10	10	10	100
70	IgG2a	NK	Yes	94b1	42	50	100	50	100	100	50	0	10	100
71	IgM	Y	No	BW264/123	53	50	100	50	100	100	50	0	50	100
72	IgG2a	Y	Yes	MT 151	61	50	100	50	100	100	50	10	10	100
73	IgG1	N	No	MT 321	61	50	100	50	100	100	50	10	10	100
74	IgG1	N	Yes	T4/12T4D11	72	50	100	50	100	100	50	0	50	100
75	IgG1	N	Yes	T4/18T3A9	72	100	100	50	100	100	50	0	50	100

								Non-T				
T-Blast IV				T-Blast V			EL		Ery.	PreB	AML	AMoL
MOLT-15	SKW-3	CCRF-HSB-2	A3/Kawa.	HUT-102	MT-1	C5/MJ	HEL	SP1-801	K-562	NALM-1	ML-2	THP-1-0
0	100	50	100	10	50	0	100	50	10	0	10	100
10	100	100	100	50	10	50	0	50	0	100	100	100
50	100	50	10	0	0	50	0	50	0	100	100	100
10	50	10	100	50	100	50	0	10	0	0	0	0
0	100	0	100	100	100	100	0	0	0	10	0	0
0	100	0	100	100	50	100	0	0	0	0	0	0
0	0	0	0	0	0	0	0	0	0	0	0	0
0	0	10	0	0	0	0	100	50	0	0	0	100
0	100	0	0	0	0	0	0	10	0	0	0	100
100	100	50	0	0	0	0	0	100	0	100	0	100
100	100	100	10	0	0	100	100	100	0	100	50	100
100	100	100	0	0	0	50	100	100	0	100	100	100
50	100	100	0	0	0	0	0	50	0	100	0	100
50	0	50	0	50	0	0	0	50	0	50	0	100
50	100	100	0	0	0	50	0	50	0	100	100	100
50	100	100	0	0	0	0	0	50	0	100	100	100
50	100	100	0	10	0	100	100	50	0	100	0	50
100	100	10	0	0	100	100	0	10	0	0	0	100
100	100	100	0	0	100	100	100	10	10	100	0	100
10	0	10	0	0	0	0	0	0	0	0	0	100
50	100	0	0	0	100	0	0	0	0	0	0	100
50	100	50	0	0	10	100	0	10	0	50	0	100
100	100	100	0	50	100	100	100	50	0	100	0	100
100	100	100	100	100	100	100	100	100	100	100	100	100
50	100	100	100	100	100	100	100	100	100	100	100	100
50	100	50	0	0	0	100	0	10	0	100	0	100
0	100	0	0	0	0	100	0	0	0	0	0	10
0	100	0	0	0	0	100	100	0	0	0	0	100
100	0	50	0	50	100	0	0	50	50	0	0	100
100	100	0	0	10	100	50	0	100	0	0	0	100
100	100	50	0	0	0	50	100	10	0	0	0	100
100	100	100	0	100	0	100	100	10	0	100	100	100
0	0	0	100	0	0	0	0	10	0	0	0	100
10	100	50	0	0	0	0	100	0	10	10	0	100
100	100	100	100	100	0	100	100	100	100	100	100	100
0	0	0	0	0	0	0	0	0	0	10	0	100
10	100	0	0	0	0	100	0	0	0	0	0	100
10	0	0	100	0	0	0	0	50	0	0	0	100
0	100	10	0	0	100	50	0	50	0	0	0	100
10	100	10	100	100	0	100	100	100	50	0	0	100
50	100	10	100	100	0	100	100	50	0	0	0	100
50	100	10	100	100	0	100	100	0	0	0	0	50
0	100	10	100	100	10	100	100	50	0	0	0	100
50	100	50	100	100	10	100	100	100	10	0	0	100
50	100	50	100	100	100	100	100	100	0	0	0	100
10	100	50	100	100	0	100	50	50	0	0	0	100
50	100	50	100	100	0	100	100	50	0	0	0	100

Table 25.1. *Continued*

mAb (Code #)	Ig subclass	Fixes C	Binds SPA	Antibody name	Lab number	T-Blast II					T-Blast III			T
						RPMI 8402	HPB-ALL	DND-41	HD-MAR-2	JM	MOLT-4	MOLT-14	MOLT-16	P12/Ichi.
76	IgG1	N	No	MT 310	61	100	100	50	100	100	50	0	10	100
77	IgG2	Y	Yes	T4/19Thy 5D7	72	100	100	50	100	100	50	0	10	100
78	IgM	Y	No	T4/7T4-6C1	72	50	100	50	100	100	50	0	50	100
79	IgM	Y	No	66.1	79	50	100	50	100	100	50	10	50	100
80	NK	NK	NK	TII19-4-7	94	50	50	100	100	0	0	0	50	0
CD8														
81	IgG1	NK	NK	14	25	50	100	0	100	100	100	0	10	0
82	IgG1	NK	No	M236	26	10	100	0	100	100	100	0	10	0
83	IgG2a	Y	Yes	G10-1.1	36	50	100	0	100	100	100	10	10	10
84	IgG1	Y	Yes	C12/D3	43	50	100	10	100	100	100	10	10	0
85	IgG2a	Y	Yes	BW 264/162	53	0	100	0	10	100	10	0	10	0
86	IgG2a	Y	Yes	BW 135/80	53	0	100	0	50	100	50	0	10	0
87	IgG1	N	No	MT 415	61	50	100	0	100	100	100	0	10	10
88	IgM	Y	No	MT 1014	61	0	100	0	100	100	50	10	10	10
89	IgG1	N	No	MT 122	61	10	100	0	100	100	100	10	10	0
90	IgG1	N	No	T8/21Thy2D3	72	0	100	0	100	100	100	10	10	10
91	IgG2	Y	Yes	T8/7Pt3F9	72	0	100	0	100	100	100	0	10	0
92	IgG2b	Y	Yes	T8/2T8-1B5	72	10	100	0	100	100	100	10	10	10
93	IgG1	N	Yes	T8-2T8-1C1	72	10	100	0	50	100	50	10	10	0
94	IgG2b	Y	Yes	T8/2T8-2A1	72	0	100	0	50	100	50	10	10	0
95	NK	NK	NK	T8/2ST8-5H7	72	10	100	0	0	0	0	0	10	0
96	IgG	Y	Yes	66.2	79	10	100	10	100	100	100	50	10	0
97	IgG2a	Y	Yes	51.1	79	10	100	10	100	100	100	10	10	10
98	IgG2	Y	Yes	T411E1	88	0	100	100	100	100	100	10	50	100
99	IgG2	N	Yes	T41D8	88	0	100	0	100	100	100	10	10	10
100	IgG	NK	NK	BL-TS1	116	0	0	0	0	0	0	0	0	0
T subset														
101	IgG1	Y	Yes	BRC-T1	23	10	100	100	100	100	10	100	100	10
102	IgG2b	Y	Yes	D44	103	100	100	100	100	100	100	100	50	50
103	IgG2a	N	Yes	SK11/Leu 8	47	100	0	100	100	10	100	100	100	100
104	IgG1	NK	No	3AC5	66	50	100	50	100	100	100	50	100	100
105	IgG	Y	No	CRIS-4	69	0	100	0	0	0	0	0	10	0
106	IgM	Y	No	CRIS-5	69	10	100	10	0	0	0	0	50	10
107	IgG	Y	Yes	EDU-2	69	100	100	50	100	100	50	0	10	100
108	IgG1	N	Yes	TQ1/28T17G6	72	100	100	100	100	100	100	100	100	100
109	IgG1	NK	NK	GM1	78	100	100	100	10	100	100	100	100	100
110	IgG1	NK	NK	10B4.6	100	0	100	0	100	100	50	10	10	0
111	IgG2b	N	Yes	8E-1.7	100	0	100	0	100	100	100	0	10	0
112	IgG1	NK	NK	6F10.3	100	50	100	50	100	100	100	0	100	100
113	IgG1	NK	NK	13B8.2	100	0	100	50	100	100	10	0	10	100
114	NK	NK	NK	K51	103	100	100	100	100	100	50	100	50	100
115	IgG	NK	NK	BL-TS20	116	0	0	0	0	0	0	0	0	0
116	IgG	NK	NK	BL-TS14	116	0	0	0	0	0	0	0	0	0
CD3														
117	IgG1	N	No	G19-4.1	36	0	100	10	100	100	10	100	100	10
118	IgG1	N	No	SK7/Leu 4	47	0	100	50	100	100	10	100	100	10
119	NK	NK	NK	89b1	42	0	100	100	100	100	50	100	100	100
120	IgG2a	Y	Yes	BW264/56	53	0	100	10	100	100	10	100	100	10
121	IgG3	N	Yes	BW242/55	53	0	100	0	100	100	100	10	100	10
122	IgM	Y	No	T3/2Ad2A2	72	0	100	10	100	100	0	100	100	0
123	IgG1	N	No	T3/2T8-2F4	72	0	100	10	50	100	0	100	100	10

| | T-Blast IV | | | T-Blast V | | | Non-T | | | | | |
| | | | | | | | EL | | Ery. | PreB | AML | AMoL |
MOLT-15	SKW-3	CCRF-HSB-2	A3/Kawa.	HUT-102	MT-1	C5/MJ	HEL	SP1-801	K-562	NALM-1	ML-2	THP-1-0
10	100	50	100	100	10	100	100	50	0	0	0	100
0	100	10	100	100	10	100	100	50	0	0	100	100
0	50	50	50	0	0	100	0	10	0	0	0	100
10	50	50	100	50	0	100	0	50	0	0	100	100
100	0	100	0	0	50	100	0	50	0	100	0	100
0	100	50	0	0	0	50	0	50	0	0	0	100
0	100	50	0	0	0	10	0	50	0	0	0	10
50	100	50	0	0	10	50	0	50	0	0	100	100
50	100	50	0	0	0	100	0	100	0	0	0	100
0	50	0	0	0	0	0	0	0	0	0	0	100
0	100	0	0	0	0	10	0	0	0	0	0	100
50	100	50	100	0	10	100	100	100	10	0	0	100
50	100	50	50	0	0	0	0	50	0	0	0	100
10	100	50	0	10	0	50	0	50	0	0	0	50
10	100	50	0	0	0	50	0	50	0	0	0	10
0	100	50	100	0	0	50	0	50	0	0	0	100
0	100	50	0	0	0	100	0	100	0	0	0	50
0	100	50	0	0	0	50	100	50	10	0	0	100
0	100	50	0	0	0	100	100	100	0	0	0	100
0	10	50	0	0	10	0	0	50	0	0	0	100
10	100	50	0	10	10	100	100	50	0	0	0	100
0	100	50	0	0	0	50	100	50	10	0	0	100
50	100	50	0	0	0	10	100	100	0	0	0	100
0	100	50	100	0	0	100	0	50	0	0	0	100
0	0	10	0	0	0	0	0	0	0	0	0	0
0	0	10	10	0	0	0	0	50	0	0	0	100
100	100	100	0	0	100	0	0	10	0	100	0	50
0	100	10	0	0	100	0	0	10	0	0	0	100
100	100	100	0	0	100	10	100	50	10	100	0	100
0	0	50	10	0	0	0	0	50	10	0	0	10
10	0	50	100	100	0	100	0	50	0	0	0	50
0	100	50	100	100	10	100	100	50	10	0	0	100
10	100	50	0	0	100	100	100	50	10	0	0	50
100	100	100	100	10	0	0	100	50	0	100	100	100
0	100	10	0	0	0	10	0	50	0	0	0	10
0	100	0	50	0	0	10	0	50	0	0	0	100
0	100	0	0	0	0	100	100	50	0	0	0	0
0	100	0	100	100	0	100	100	0	0	0	0	50
0	100	100	0	0	0	0	0	50	0	0	0	100
0	0	0	0	0	0	0	0	0	0	0	0	0
0	0	0	0	0	0	0	0	0	0	0	0	0
0	0	0	0	0	0	0	100	100	0	0	0	100
0	0	0	0	0	0	0	0	0	0	0	0	0
0	100	100	100	100	0	100	100	50	0	0	0	100
0	0	0	0	0	0	0	0	0	0	0	0	50
0	100	0	0	0	0	0	0	0	0	0	0	50
0	0	0	0	0	0	0	0	100	10	0	0	100
0	0	50	0	0	0	0	0	0	0	0	0	100

Table 25.1. *Continued*

mAb (Code #)	Ig subclass	Fixes C	Binds SPA	Antibody name	Lab number	RPMI 8402	HPB-ALL	DND-41	HD-MAR-2	JM	MOLT-4	MOLT-14	MOLT-16	P12/Ichi.
						\<- T-Blast II ->				\<- T-Blast III ->				T
124	IgG2b	Y	Yes	T3/RW2-4B6	72	0	100	10	100	100	0	100	100	10
125	IgG1	N	Yes	T3/RW2-8C8	72	0	100	0	100	100	0	100	100	10
126	IgG2a	Y	Yes	X35-3	96	0	100	0	100	100	0	100	100	10
127	IgG1	N	NK	NU-T1	71	0	100	10	100	100	100	0	100	100
CD1														
128	IgG1	N	No	M241	26	0	100	0	100	100	100	0	10	100
129	IgG2a	Y	Yes	Na1/34	27	0	100	100	100	100	100	10	10	100
130	IgG2b	Y	Yes	SK9/Leu 6	47	0	100	50	100	100	50	0	10	50
131	IgG2a	Y	Yes	4A76	100	0	100	100	100	100	100	10	10	100
132	IgG1	NK	NK	10D12.2	100	0	100	100	100	100	100	0	10	100
133	IgG1	N	NK	NU-T2	71	0	100	100	100	100	100	0	10	100
134	IgG	Y	NK	I 19	103	0	100	100	100	100	50	0	10	10
T-Activation														
135	IgG2	Y	NK	T1A	9	0	0	0	0	0	10	50	0	0
136	IgG1	NK	Yes	TS145	10	0	0	100	100	0	0	0	0	0
137	NK	NK	NK	100-1A5	69	100	100	100	100	100	100	100	0	50
138	IgG3	Y	Yes	1 MONO 2A6	72	0	100	0	100	100	100	0	10	0
139	IgG1	N	Yes	4EL1C7	72	0	0	100	100	0	50	0	0	0
140	NK	NK	NK	Tac/2HT4-4H3	72	0	0	0	0	0	0	50	0	0
141	IgG2a	Y	Yes	B149.9	100	0	0	0	0	0	0	0	0	0
142	IgG2	Y	Yes	B1.19.2	100	0	0	10	0	10	0	0	0	0
143	NK	NK	NK	23A9.3	100	0	0	0	0	0	0	0	0	0
144	NK	NK	NK	39C1.5	100	50	100	10	100	100	100	0	100	100
145	NK	NK	NK	39C6.5	100	0	0	0	0	0	0	0	0	0
146	NK	NK	NK	33B3.1	100	0	0	0	0	0	0	10	0	0
147	NK	NK	NK	33B7.3	100	0	0	0	0	0	0	0	0	0
148	NK	NK	NK	39C8.18	100	50	100	10	100	100	100	0	100	50
149	NK	NK	NK	39H7.3	100	0	100	10	100	100	100	0	100	100
150	NK	NK	NK	41F2.1	100	10	100	10	100	100	100	0	100	100
151	IgG1	N	NK	KOLT-1	71	0	100	100	100	50	10	0	0	100
Leuk. specific														
152	IgG2a	Y	Yes	6-4	28	100	100	100	100	100	100	100	100	100
T-Activation														
153	IgG1	NK	NK	AA3	89	100	0	50	100	100	100	100	100	100
Leuk. specific														
154	IgM	Y	No	3-40	107,28	100	100	0	100	100	100	100	100	100
155	IgG2b	Y	Yes	3-3	107,28	100	100	100	100	100	100	100	100	100
Controls														
156	IgG1	Y	+No	A3D8(irrad.)	105	100	100	100	100	100	100	100	100	100
157	IgG1	N	−No	P3 (irrad.)	105	0	0	0	0	0	0	0	0	0
158	IgG2	Y	−Yes	11G6(HTLV-8)	105	0	0	0	10	0	0	0	0	0
T-Activation														
159	IgG2a	Y	Yes	TAC	106	0	0	0	0	0	0	50	0	0
Lab C+														
160				T-101		100	100	50	100	100		100	100	100
				MCS-2										
				Leu-1							100			
				1/12/13										
				Leu-M1										
				J-5										

| | | | | | | | | | Non-T | | | |
| T-Blast IV | | | | T-Blast V | | | EL | | Ery. | PreB | AML | AMoL |
MOLT-15	SKW-3	CCRF-HSB-2	A3/Kawa.	HUT-102	MT-1	C5/MJ	HEL	SP1-801	K-562	NALM-1	ML-2	THP-1-0
0	0	0	0	0	0	0	0	50	0	0	0	100
50	0	0	0	0	0	0	0	50	0	0	0	50
0	0	0	0	0	0	0	0	0	0	0	0	100
0	100	0	0	0	10	100	0	50	10	0	0	100
0	0	50	0	0	0	0	0	50	0	0	0	100
0	10	0	0	0	0	0	0	100	0	0	10	100
0	0	0	0	0	0	0	0	50	0	0	0	0
10	100	0	0	0	0	0	0	10	0	0	0	100
0	0	0	0	0	0	0	0	10	0	0	0	0
50	100	50	0	0	0	0	0	50	0	0	0	50
50	0	50	0	0	0	0	0	50	0	0	0	0
0	0	50	0	100	100	100	0	50	0	0	100	100
100	0	100	0	0	0	100	0	100	0	100	0	10
50	100	100	0	0	100	0	0	0	0	0	0	0
0	100	0	0	0	0	0	0	10	0	0	0	100
100	0	100	0	0	0	100	0	100	10	100	10	100
0	0	0	0	100	100	100	0	50	0	0	0	100
0	0	0	0	100	100	100	0	10	0	0	0	100
0	0	100	100	100	100	100	0	100	100	0	0	100
0	0	0	0	100	100	100	0	0	0	0	0	0
0	100	0	0	0	0	100	0	0	0	0	0	0
0	0	0	0	100	100	100	0	10	0	0	0	50
0	0	0	0	100	100	100	0	0	0	0	0	10
0	0	0	0	100	100	100	0	0	0	0	0	0
0	100	0	0	0	10	100	0	0	0	0	0	0
0	100	0	0	0	10	100	0	0	0	0	0	0
0	100	0	0	0	10	100	0	0	0	0	0	0
0	50	0	100	0	0	10	0	0	0	0	0	0
100	100	100	0	100	100	100	0	50	0	100	100	100
100	100	100	100	100	100	100	0	100	0	100	0	10
100	100	100	100	100	100	50	100	100	0	100	0	50
100	100	100	0	100	0	0	100	100	0	100	0	100
50	100	100	100	100	0	100	100	100	100	50	100	100
0	0	0	0	0	0	0	0	50	0	0	100	50
0	0	0	0	0	0	0	100	50	0	0	0	100
0	0	0	0	100	100	100	0	100	0	0	100	100
0	100	10		100	100							
							100				100	100
		0	100									
									100			
								100				
										50		

the mAbs in five out of six non-T cell lines, the overall data shown in Table 25.1 can be evaluated as follows.

Nonreactive mAbs (4/159 : 2.5%)

Four mAbs (nos. 35, 100, 115, and 116) did not react at all with any of the 22 cell lines tested. Except for mAb no. 35, which is a PBS-BSA, the reason for this nonreactivity was not clear.

mAbs Reacting Only with T Cell Lines (14/159 : 8.8%)

Table 25.2 summarizes 14 mAbs which react with all or some T cell lines, but not at all with any of the six non-T cell lines. As regards mAb no. 2 (PBS-BSA in the control group) showing reactivity at a 10% level for four T cell lines, this appears to be an erroneous reading. mAb no. 35 (also PBS-BSA in the CD7 group) was found to be nonreactive with all 22 cell lines. Of the remaining 13 mAbs, only mAb no. 4 (H65) reacted with all 16 T cell lines of T-Blasts II–V and therefore this may be regarded as a pan T antibody. This antibody of the CD5 group may also be reactive with a subset of B cells as this has been observed for other mAbs of the CD5 group. mAb no. 7 (L17F12/Leu 1) of the CD5 group is a pan T antibody, reacting with a B-subset and was positive with two Fc receptor-positive non-T cell lines (ML-2 and THP-1-0). mAb no. 118 (SK7/Leu 4) in the CD3 group reacted with all T-Blast II (except RPMI 8402) and T-Blast III cell lines. In this regard, this mAb is similar to the reactivity pattern seen in the CD1 group (cortical thymocytes). Seven mAbs in the CD1 group (nos. 128–134), however, reacted with some of the Fc receptor-positive non-T cell lines. Using a different preparation of FITC-conjugated goat anti–mouse IgG reagent and the standardized dilution of the three mAbs (nos. 129, 130, and 133), these three mAbs did not react with non-T cell lines in previous studies. This shows the importance of standardization of reagents in fluorescence test. Two mAbs (nos. 143 and 147) in the T-activation group reacted only with the three T-Blast V cell lines tested. Further characterization of these two mAbs is necessary to conclude whether these are antibodies recognizing an antigen associated with activation of mature T cells or a mature T cell antigen. mAb no. 100 in the CD8 group reacted only with one of the four T-Blast IV cell lines (CCRF-HSB-2) at a 10% level. Further characterization of this antibody is also required. The remaining eight mAbs (nos. 11, 34, 137, 144, 148–151) were reactive with variable numbers of T cell lines, not necessarily associated with any particular T-Blast stages. A reactivity pattern was identified for mAbs nos. 141, 143, 145, and 147 (mature-activated T cells). mAbs nos. 144, 148, 149, and 150 are very similar in reactivity (random distribution in the T cell lineages). It is, however, possible to associate these patterns with certain types of T cell malignancies, i.e., ALL versus non-Hodgkin's lymphoma T cell characteristics. It is equally conceivable that these anti-

Table 25.2. Monoclonal antibodies reacting only with T-cell lines.

Antibody group	Code number	Antibody name	Ig subclass[a]	Laboratory number	Incidence of positivity[b]	Remarks
Controls	2	PBS-BSA	NA	105	5/16 = 31%	
CD5	4	H65	IgG1	26	16/16 = 100%	Pan T
CD5	11	X1X102-3	IgG2a	96	11/16 = 69%	Random
CD7	34	BW264/215	IgM	53	12/16 = 75%	Random
CD8	100	BL-TS1	IgG	116	1/16 = 6%	Reactive with CCRF-HSB-2 (T-IV) only
CD3	118	SK7/Leu 4	IgG1	47	8/16 = 50%	Limited to T-II and III
T-Activation	137	100-1A5	NK	69	12/16 = 75%	Random
T-Activation	143	23A9.3	NK	100	3/16 = 19%	Random
T-Activation	144	39C1.5	NK	100	10/16 = 63%	Random
T-Activation	147	33B7.3	NK	100	3/16 = 19%	Reactive with T-V only
T-Activation	148	39C8.18	NK	100	11/16 = 69%	Random
T-Activation	149	39H7.3	NK	100	10/16 = 63%	Random
T-Activation	150	41F2.1	NK	100	11/16 = 69%	Random
T-Activation	151	KOLT-1	IgG1	71	9/16 = 56%	Random

[a] NA = not applicable; NK = not known.
[b] Numerator = number of positive T cell lines; denominator = number of total T cell lines tested.

Table 25.3. Reactivity of control antibodies.

Positive or negative control antibody	Code number	Antibody name	Ig subclass[a]	Laboratory number	Incidence of positivity[b]	Remarks
Negative	1	P3X63	IgG1	105	11/22 = 50%	Random
Negative	2	PBS-BSA	NA	105	5/22 = 23%	Reactive only with T cell lines
Negative	157	P3(irrad.)	IgG1	105	3/22 = 14%	Reactive only with non-T lines
Negative	158	11G6(HTLV-8)	IgG2	105	4/22 = 18%	Random
Positive	3	A3D8	IgG1	105	21/22 = 94%	Only SPI-802 negative
Positive	156	A3D8(irrad.)	IgG1	105	21/22 = 95%	Only MT-1 negative

[a] and [b] See explanation in Table 25.2.

gen expressions may not necessarily be associated with any status of differentiation or activation in the T cell lineage.

mAbs Reactive with All 22 Cell Lines (2/159 : 1.3%)

Two mAbs (nos. 52 and 53) reacted with all 22 cell lines tested.

Positive and Negative Control mAbs

Two positive mAbs (nos. 3 and 156) and four negative control mAbs (nos. 1, 2, 157, and 158) were provided; some unexpected results were seen with these reagents. Table 25.3 summarizes the observed results. Two negative results, each with two positive control mAbs, appear to be due to one or more variables discussed earlier. Several positive readings with four negative control mAbs appear to be due to the same variables.

Possibility of Fc Receptor-Binding of mAbs

It has been known that the Fc receptors on the cell membrane bind readily with the Fc portion of immunoglobulin molecules, in particular in the IgG class. Since the cell line NALM-1 in the group of six non-T cell lines was the only Fc-negative cell line, the results of the 159 mAbs on NALM-1 were evaluated in detail. One has to assume that all 159 mAbs used in this analysis were T cell specific. Table 25.4 demonstrates clearly that not only IgG mAbs but also IgM mAbs did react with the Fc-negative non-T cell line NALM-1. Although not completely conclusive, this finding appears to suggest that some mAbs tested may not be T cell specific. It is of

Table 25.4. Reactivity of the "T-specific" 159 monoclonal antibodies according to immunoglobulin subclasses.

Immunoglobulin subclass of monoclonal antibodies	Incidence of positivity
IgG	3/12 = 25%
IgG1	15/54 = 28%
IgG2	2/10 = 20%
IgG2a	7/25 = 28%
IgG2b	4/13 = 31%
IgG3	0/2 = 0%
IgM	3/20 = 15%
NK (not known)	4/21 = 19%
PBS-BSA	0/2 = 0%

Table 25.5. Reactivity of monoclonal antibodies with T cell lines.

Type of reactivity	Stages of T-blast category with which reactive	Antibody group	Positive/total number (%)
Pan-T reactive	T-II–T-V	CD5	5/9 = 56%
		CD2	11/16 = 69%
		CD7	1/17 = 6%
		Pan T	2/19 = 11%
		CD4	2/14 = 14%
		Others	= 0%
Partial-T reactive	T-II–T-IV	CD7	3/17 = 28%
		Pan T	4/19 = 21%
		CD8	2/20 = 10%
		T subset	3/16 = 19%
		CD3	3/11 = 27%
		CD1	6/7 = 86%
		Others	= 0%
	T-II–T-III	CD3	6/11 = 55%
		CD1	1/7 = 14%
	T-II	Pan T	1/19 = 5%
	T-V	T-activated	4/19 = 21%

interest to reevaluate those mAbs when all other data of the entire workshop become available.

Data Regarding Only 16 T-Cell Lines

Although it was not established that the reactivity with non-T cell lines was largely attributable to the Fc-binding of the mAbs, it might be worthwhile to evaluate the data for only T cell reactivity. Table 25.5 summarizes the overall results.

Implications

This study emphasizes again that the serological identification of leukocyte antigens requires careful consideration in a number of aspects. For example, a single antibody reagent is not sufficient as a positive probe. Multiple antigen identifications for both positive and negative antigens are the most practical and sensible approaches at the present time. Also, it is highly desirable to combine other parameters with the serological methods. Despite obvious merits of using mAbs as standard reagents, the individual characteristics (for example, antibody specificity, epitope binding rather than conventional antigen recognition by polyclonal antiserum) have to be kept in mind. State of target cell population, standardization of the procedure, choice of the analytical equipment, and perhaps the most significant aspect, user's experience, are other important parameters. All of these factors are involved in one way or another in the overall results.

Summary

The 159 mAbs of the T cell protocol of the Second International Workshop and Conference on Human Leukocyte Differentiation Antigens were analyzed on 22 growth factor-independent human leukemia–lymphoma cell lines.

Although the final evaluation of the present data requires the completion of the entire Workshop data analysis, several mAbs appear to be unique and useful for the study of leukocyte differentiation antigens. This investigation further confirms that mAbs are exquisite reagents for immunological studies and that leukemia–lymphoma cell lines are irreplaceable tools in any kind of leukemia research.

References

1. Bernard, A., L. Boumsell, J. Dausset, C. Milstein, and S.F. Schlossman, eds. 1984. Leucocyte Typing. Springer-Verlag, Berlin, Heidelberg.
2. McMichael, A.J., and J.W. Fabre. 1982. *Monoclonal antibodies in clinical medicine*. Academic Press, New York.
3. Royston, I., J. Minowada, T.W. LeBien, G. Pavlov, G. Vosika, C.D. Bloomfield, and R.R. Ellison. 1984. Phenotypes of adult lymphoblastic leukemia defined by monoclonal antibodies. In: *Leucocyte typing*, A. Bernard, L. Boumsell, J. Dausset, C. Milstein, and S.F. Schlossman. eds. Springer-Verlag, Berlin, Heidelberg pp. 558–564.
4. Minowada, J. 1983. Immunology of leukemic cells. In: Leukemia, F. Gunz and E.S. Henderson, eds. Grune & Stratton, New York, pp. 119–139.
5. Minowada, J., E. Tatsumi, W. Sagawa, M.S. Lok, T. Sugimoto, K. Minato, L. Zgoda, L. Prestine, L. Kover, and D. Gould. 1984. A scheme of human hematopoietic differentiation based on the marker profiles of the cultured and fresh leukemia–lymphomas: The result of Workshop Study. In: *Leucocyte typing,* A. Bernard, L. Boumsell, J. Dausset, C. Milstein, and S.F. Schlossman, eds. Springer-Verlag, Berlin, Heidelberg, pp. 519–527.
6. Minowada, J. 1983. Membrane and other phenotypes of leukemia cells. In: *13th International Cancer Congress, Part E Cancer management*, E.A. Mirand, W.B. Hutchinson, and E. Mihich, eds. Alan R. Liss, New York, pp. 215–227.
7. Drexler, H.G., G. Gaedicke, and J. Minowada. 1985. Isoenzyme studies on human leukemia–lymphoma cell lines. I. Carboxylic esterase. *Leukemia Res., 9:*209–229.
8. Minowada, J., K. Minato, B.I.S. Srivastava, S. Nakazawa, I. Kubonishi, E. Tatsumi, T. Ohnuma, H. Ozer, A.I. Freeman, E.S. Henderson, and R.C. Gallo. 1982. A model scheme of human hematopoietic cell differentiation as determined by leukemia–lymphoma study. T-cell lineage. In: *International Symposium on Current Concepts in Human Immunology and Cancer Immunomodulation,* B. Serrou and C. Rosenfeld, eds. Elsevier/North Holland Biomedical Press, Amsterdam, pp. 75–84.

9. Minowada, J., K. Sagawa, I.S. Trowbridge, P.D. Kung, and G. Goldstein. 1982. Marker profiles of 55 human leukemia–lymphoma cell lines. *In:* Malignant lymphomas. Etiology, immunology, pathology and treatment, S.A. Rosenberg and H.S. Kaplan, eds. Academic Press, New York, pp. 53–74.
10. Srivastava, B.I.S., and J. Minowada. 1983. Terminal transferase immunofluorescence, enzyme markers and immunological profile of human leukemia–lymphoma cell lines representing different levels of differentiation. *Leukemia Res.* **7**:331.
11. Drexler, H.G., M. Menon, S. Gignac, B. Misra, L. Skowron, and J. Minowada. High concordance between marker profiles of 22 human leukemia–lymphoma cell lines tested with the same monoclonal antibodies before and during the 2nd Workshop. Presented at Second International Workshop and Conference on Human Leukocyte Differentiation Antigens, Boston, Sept. 1984.

CHAPTER 26

Expression of T Cell-Related Antigens on Cells from the Myelo-Monocytic Lineage

Patrice Dubreuil, Patrice Mannoni, Daniel Olive,
Bonnie Winkler-Lowen, and Claude Mawas

Monoclonal antibodies (mAbs) have become basic tools to study cell surface antigens and their relationship with the process of differentiation. Cellular differentiation involves not only morphological and antigenic changes but also acquisition of specific functions. Relationships between cell proliferation, cell maturation, and differentiation are complex and multifactorial, involving extra- and intracellular factors. The modification of cell surface antigens during the differentiation pathway has been known for decades. More recently, availability of monoclonal antibodies specific for lineage-specific antigens has led to the possibility of exploring these mechanisms with such powerful and specific tools. For example it has been clearly established that the expression of some T cell antigens defined by monoclonal antibodies is associated with the process of T cell differentiation which in turn results in acquisition of specific functions. However, it has been observed that some of these markers like the transferrin receptor, LFA antigens, or the T_4gp55 molecule are also expressed on cells from other lineages (1–3). Thus the definition of differentiation antigen specific for one lineage can be questionable, and it appears interesting to determine which antigens are specifically related to a maturation–differentiation process that is restricted to one lineage, and which others could identify structures or functions related to cell proliferation and differentiation.

In this study we investigated the reactivity of all the T cell Workshop monoclonal antibodies on some selected cells belonging to the myelo-monocytic pathway. Since it was difficult to obtain from normal bone marrows a sufficient amount of cells corresponding to precise stages of myelo-monocytic differentiation, we selected human cell lines originating from patients with leukemia or lymphoma, each corresponding to different stages of differentiation. The results led us to the conclusion that several antigens defined as T specific were also expressed on myelo-monocytic cells at some stage of differentiation.

Materials and Methods

The whole panel of mAbs from the T cell Workshop was tested on selected target cells. Cell lines and cells were selected to represent as much
as possible different stages of differentiation in the myelo-monocytic
pathway. Assignment of leukemia–lymphoma cell lines used in this study
according to lineage and stage of differentiation is presented in Fig. 26.1.

U937 cell line and monocytes isolated from normal peripheral blood
were used as representative of the monocytic pathway. The myeloid pathway was studied by testing mAb reactivity on AML (M1 and M2) cells,
KG1 (poorly differentiated myeloblasts), ML1, and HL60, known to express more features of myeloid differentiation, and on mature granulocytes. All cell lines were grown in our laboratory in RPMI–10% FCS.
HL60 cells were induced to differentiate by incubation with recombinant
gamma interferon. Expression of some specific T cell antigens (generous
gift of Dr. E. Falcoff, Institut P. et M. Curie, Paris) was studied before
and after treatment with interferon. In brief HL60 cells were seeded to a
concentration of 1×10^5/ml in RPM1-FCS 10% supplemented with 500 to
1,000 μ of gamma interferon. HL60 cells were tested on day 2, 4, and 6 for
the expression of T cell markers defined by CD1, 2, 3, 4, 5, 6, and 7 mAbs.

To compare the reactivity observed on myeloid or erythroid cell lines
with cells from the T and B lineage, mAb binding was also assessed on the
following cell lines: REH (non-T, non-B), 1301, RPMI 8402, CCRF-CEM,
MOLT4, ICHIGAWA (T ALL cell lines), as well as on NALM6 (pre-B)
and B cells.

K562 and HEL, both erythroleukemia cell lines, and red blood cells
were selected to study expression of Workshop antibodies reactive with

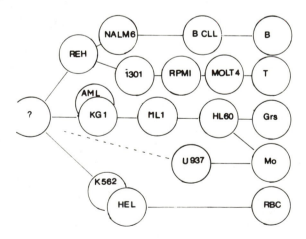

Fig. 26.1. Assignment of the different target cell lines used in this study according
to the classical scheme of human hematopoietic differentiation.

myeloid cells on cells from the erythroid pathway. A schematic representation of the position of these cell lines in the differentiation pathway is presented in Fig. 26.1.

Expression of cell surface antigens was studied by immunofluorescence. FITC-coupled secondary antibody was a mixture of goat (Fab'$_2$ fragment) anti–mouse IgG and goat (Fab'$_2$ fragment) anti–rat IgG (Cappel Laboratory, Chester, PA). Analysis was performed on an EPICS V (Coulter-Coultronics) cell analyzer and sorter. 10,000 cells were counted and positivity was compared to negative controls including irrelevant mAbs, PBS–FCS medium, and mouse immunoglobulins.

Results

An overview of the results obtained in this study show that antibodies defining the clusters of differentiation CD1, CD2, CD3, CD5, CD6, and CD8 and activated T antigens were not found to be reactive with the cells derived from the myelo-monocytic or erythroid pathways. Two exceptions were noticed: T9 (MT 215) and T153 (AA3) stained K562 and KG1 cells. On the other hand, structures defined by CD4 mAbs were found expressed on HL60, U937, and monocytes as well as antigens defined by CD7 mAbs which reacted with K562, K61, and leukemic cells isolated from a patient with acute myeloid leukemia of M1 type (FAB classification).

Expression of CD4 antigens on myeloid cells has already been reported by Minowada *et al.* during the First International Workshop on Leucocyte Differentiation Antigens (3).

Besides the reactivity observed with the above clusters, several monoclonal antibodies defining all T cells or T cell subsets were found positive on some cells from non-T origin. Table 26.1 summarizes their reactivity. All antibodies presented in the table reacted with some myeloid or erythroid cells. They have been subsequently classified according to their reactivity on T or T-derived cells for instance. The first three (T52, 53, 63) reacted with all tested cells from the T lineage but also with cell lines corresponding to B, myeloid, erythroid, or monocytic differentiation. Probably these antibodies define common determinants expressed on the majority of leukocytes like LFA or LFA-structures (2).

Although they recognized more peculiarly T cell lineage or mature T cells, some mAbs stained cells from the myelo-monocytic lineage (T9, 106, 61, 121, 105, 32, 114). Antibody T153, positive on activated T but not on resting T cells, can be distinguished from the other classical anti-Tac antibodies which were found not to be reactive with the myelo-monocytic cells. The last three mAbs, T64, 102, and 109, are only positive on cell lines corresponding to the T cell lineage.

This type of cross-reactivity could define either antigenic identity due

Table 26.1. Workshop mAbs reactive with non-T derived cells.

mAb	Reactive with
T52	All lineages (except U937 cells)
T53	All lineages
T63	T, myeloid, erythroid lineages
T152	Lymphoid, myelo-monocytic lineages
T60	Lymphoid, myelo-monocytic lineages
T10	Lymphoid, monocytic, granulocyte, AML
T62	Lymphoid, monocytic, HEL, NALM6
T104	Lymphoid, monocytic, HEL, ML1, AML
T50	Lymphoid, myelo-monocytic lineage
T9	T lineage, K562, KG1, AML, monocytes
T106	T, REH, B cells, ML1, HL60
T61, T121	T, MOLT4, U937
T105	T, B CLL, K562, monocytes
T32	T, HEL, RPMI, monocytes
T114	T, MOLT4, CEM, AML
T153	activated T, REH, RPMI, CEM, K562, KG1, ML1
T64	REH, T cell lines, U937, REH, NALM6, granulocytes
T102	T cell lines, HEL
T109	RPMI, monocytes, myeloid, HEL, NALM6

to the presence of the same determinant on different carriers (carbohydrates, glycoproteins, or glycolipids) or a true antigenic identity between unrelated cells. In such cases this true antigenic identity should be related to unique differentiation patterns or a common function. To test this hypothesis, we analyzed the results obtained in terms of lineage differentiation by studying the evolution of cross-reactive antigens on KG1, AML cells, ML1, HL60, and granulocytes seen as models for different stages of the myeloid pathway (Fig. 26.2). Analyzing the results in such a way it was possible to observe a certain oriented expression of some antigens during cell differentiation. For instance, antigens defined by CD7 antibodies were expressed on KG1, poorly differentiated AML cells (M1), and K562. These markers are no longer expressed on more differentiated cells as demonstrated by their absence on ML1, HL60, granulocytes, and monocytes. The antigen recognized by the CD4 cluster (T_4gp) was expressed only on HL60, U937, and monocytes and seemed to be linked to monocytic differentiation since it is known that HL60 can easily be induced to differentiate either along the myeloid or monocytic pathway (4). The expression of the CD4 molecule on myelo-monocytic cells is probably weak since not all CD4 mAbs were positive. Clear reactivity was only obtained with T69, 72, 73, 74, 75, 76, and 77. T107 and 119, not included in the CD4 cluster, were also reactive and led us to the conclusion that they probably have the same CD4 specificity. The pattern of reactivity of positive mAbs was quite uniform, all staining the target cells with the same intensity when tested by FACS analysis.

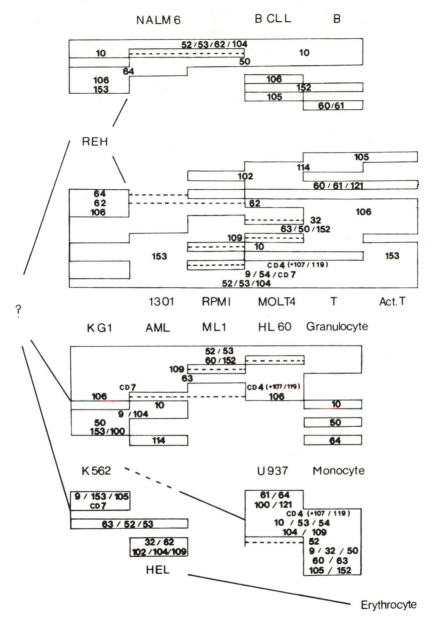

Fig. 26.2. Cross-reactivity of Workshop mAbs as a function of the different lineages and stages of differentiation.

Among other mAbs reactive with non-T-derived cells, T9 appeared to recognize a structure related to undifferentiated cells since it was not expressed on differentiated cells of myeloid origin. On the contrary, T10 stained mostly terminal cells and the corresponding antigen was not expressed on poorly differentiated cell lines like K562 and KG1.

Interestingly, T64 which appeared to be a marker of early differentiation in the T lineage is only expressed on granulocytes. This pattern has been observed with several mAbs detecting late myeolid or granulocytic antigens which were found also reactive with early or immature T cells (5,6). T152 appeared to react mainly with differentiated cells in all lineages.

Some antigenic homology was also clearly detected between monocytes and U937, HEL, and K562. When tested on cells from the T or B cell lineage (upper part of Fig. 26.2), these mAbs displayed a different reactivity pattern showing that the antigenic modulation identified along the myeloid differentiation pathway is not comparable to the one observed along the T or B cell differentiation pathway.

The last results concern the expression of T cell markers on HL60 cells induced to differentiate by gamma interferon. It has been shown that gamma interferon can induce monocytic-like differentiation in HL60 (4). In our hands, after treatment with gamma interferon for 4 days (500 μ/ml in final concentration), HL60 cells strongly express not only HLA-class II molecules, but also several T cell antigens (7). Table 26.2 summarizes the results. After induction we observed a clear expression of antigens defined by CD1, CD2, CD7, as well as the Tac antigen defined by T159 (TAC), T141 (B149.9), and T145 (39C6.5) (7). Expression of CD4 antigens was considerably enhanced by incubation with gamma interferon. Altogether these data support the notion that gamma interferon acts as a differentiation-inducing agent on the HL60 cell line, driving it to a pheno-

Table 26.2. Expression of T cell markers on HL60 cells: effects of treatment with gamma interferon.

	Constitutive HL60	HL60 induced by gamma interferon
CD1	−	+ +
CD2	−	+ +
CD3	−	− or weak
CD4	+	+ +
CD5	−	+
CD6	−	+
CD7	−	+
CD8	−	− or weak
Anti-Tac	−	+

type closer to early or poorly differentiated T cells. More precisely, this antigenic modulation induced by gamma interferon demonstrates that the expression of some T cell markers can be induced on cells from the myeloid lineage. However, HL60 and all myeloid cell lines were derived from patients with leukemia and express many karyotypic abnormalities. Thus it is difficult to relate directly the observed phenotypes to a strict physiological pathway of differentiation. On the other hand, evidence showing that leukemic cell lines can be used as models for studying normal differentiation is accumulating. The fact that no leukemic or tumor-associated antigen has been shown to be exclusively expressed on leukemic or tumor cells and not on normal cells supports this hypothesis. This allows us to study differentiation by using leukemic or tumor cells or cell lines. The fact that myeloid cells and T cells share several common antigenic determinants not only supports the concept of unique pluripotential hematopoietic stem cells, but also suggests some preferential cell cooperation between T cells and cells from the myelo-monocytic lineage. Although the support for the concept that T lymphocytes play a role in regulating *in vitro* hemopoiesis has grown, definitive proofs are still lacking (8).

Another approach could be to show that the expression of T cell markers on myeloid cells will result in the myeloid cells acquiring functions mediated through these receptors or antigens. It is tempting, although still premature, to make the hypothesis that the control of cell proliferation and cell differentiation could be regulated by a relatively small number of membrane receptors presenting some structural homology when expressed on cells committed to different differentiation pathways.

Acknowledgments. This work was supported in part by a grant from the Alberta Heritage Foundation for Medical Research (P. Mannoni, AHFMR Scholar and INSERM contract (C. Mawas). P. Dubreuil received a Fellowship from the Union Internationale Contre le Cancer (UICC).

References

1. Haynes, B.F., M. Hemler, T. Cotner, D. Mann, G.S. Eisenbarth, J.L. Strominger, and A. Fauci. 1981. Characterization of a monoclonal antibody (5E9) that defines a human cell surface antigen of cell activation. *J. Immunol.* **127:**347.
2. Krensky, A.M., F. Sanchez-Madrid, E. Robbins, J.A. Nagy, T.A. Springer, and S.J. Burakoff. 1983. The functional significance, distribution, and structure of LFA-1, LFA-2, and LFA-3: cell surface antigen associated with CTL–target interactions. *J. Immunol.* **131:**611.
3. Minowada, J., E. Tatsumi, K. Sagawa, M.S. Lok, T. Sugimoto, K. Minato, L. Zgoda, L. Prestine, L. Kover, and D. Gould. 1984. A scheme of human hematopoietic differentiation based on the marker profiles of the cultured and fresh

leukemia–lymphomas: The result of workshop study. In: *Leucocyte typing*, A. Bernard, L. Boumsell, J. Dausset, C. Milstein, and S.F. Schlossman, eds. Springer-Verlag, Berlin, Heidelberg, pp. 519–527.

4. Perussia, B., E. Dayton, V. Fanning, P. Thiagarajan, J. Hoxie, and G. Trinchieri. 1983. Immune interferon and leucocyte conditioned medium induce normal and leukemic myeloid cells to differentiate along the monocytic pathway. *J. Exp. Med. 158:*2058.

5. Bodger, M.P., G.E. Francis, D. Delia, S.M. Granger, and G. Janossy. 1981. A monoclonal antibody specific for immature human hemopoietic cells and T lineage cells. *J. Immunol.* **6:**2269.

6. Mannoni, P., P. Dubreuil, B. Winkler-Lowen, D. Olive, L. Linklater, C. Mawas. Expression of myeloid and B cell associated antigens on T lineage cells. (2nd International Workshop, Boston, 1984).

7. Olive, D., P. Dubreuil, D. Charmot, C. Mawas, and P. Mannoni. 1985. T cell activation antigens: kinetics, tissue distribution, molecular weights and functions; induction on non T cell lines by lymphokines. 9th Leucocyte Culture Conference, Cambridge, England. A. Mitchison and M. Feldman, eds. Humana Press Cambridge. In Press.

8. Torok-Storb, B., J.A. Hansen, and P.J. Martin. 1981. Regulation of *in vitro* hemopoiesis by normal T cells—evidence for two T cell subsets with opposing function. *Blood* **58:**171.

CHAPTER 27

Phenotype of Hodgkin Cells. Expression of the Tac-Antigen and Other Determinants

Klaus Joachim Bross, Reinhard Andreesen,
Thomas Monnheimer, Juergen Osterholz, and
Georg-Wilhem Löhr

The nature and origin of Reed–Sternberg and Hodgkin cells (HD) are still obscure. Their origin in a normal counterpart has been attributed to most cells of the hematopoietic lineage. Evidence has been reported suggesting a descent from, for example, macrophages/histiocytes (1–5) T-lymphoid cells (6,7), B-lymphoid cells (8,9), myeloid progenitor cells (10), dendritic reticulum cells (11,12), interdigitating reticulum cells (13), and from a newly detected small-cell population, bearing the Ki-1 antigen (14). We have studied cell suspensions of different malignant lymphomas, obtained by needle aspiration or biopsy, with a panel of monoclonal antibodies (mAbs). Here we want to report the reaction pattern of five cases with histologically proven Hodgkin's disease.

Materials and Methods

Preparation of Cells

Cells from lymph nodes were obtained by needle aspiration with a 20-ml syringe containing 2-ml medium (Hepes buffered minimal essential medium, 0.2% bovine serum albumin, 0.1% EDTA). The cells were washed four times with the same medium. Ficoll–Hypaque density centrifugation was performed in some cases to eliminate excess erythrocytes. Finally the single cells were suspended in minimal essential medium. Lymph nodes obtained by surgery were minced to gain single cells and further processed as above. Viability of cells was proven by trypan blue exclusion. Dead cells were eliminated by DNase treatment.

Surface Marker Analysis

Cells were applied onto poly-L-lysine-coated glass slides for staining of surface antigens by the peroxidase–antiperoxidase (PAP) method (14,15) using a technique described earlier (16,17) with minor modification. Viable cells attached to the positively charged glass surface are fixed with 0.05% glutaraldehyde in Sørensen phosphate buffer pH 7,8 for 15 min at 4°C to block Fc receptors and preserve cell morphology. The glass slide contains 12 reaction areas with a diameter of 4 mm. The surrounding glass surface is coated with a polysiloxane-containing water repellant. A gelatin-containing medium is used for preincubation and dilution of antisera to avoid binding of immunoglobulins to the glass surface. The staining includes incubation with 1. monoclonal antibodies; 2. rabbit anti–mouse immunoglobulins (Dakopatts); 3. swine anti–rabbit immunoglobulins (Dakopatts); 4. peroxidase–antiperoxidase complex from rabbit (Dakopatts); 5. diaminobenzidine–H_2O_2, followed by postfixation with OsO_4. The slides are covered with glycerin and a cover glass. Controls were routinely performed with the different sandwich antisera and a panel of murine monoclonal antibodies of different Ig classes that did not react with the cells to be tested, serving as negative controls. The cell count on each reaction area was between 5000 and 50,000, depending on the cell yield.

The following monoclonal antibodies were used: OKT3, OKT4, OKT8, OKT9, OKT10, OKIa1 (Ortho Diagnostic Systems); anti-kappa, anti-lambda, LeuM1 (Becton Dickinson); anti-IgM, anti-IgD (Miles Laboratories); Clonab Tü 9 (Biotest Diagnostics); Coulter clone B-1 (Coulter Immunology); anti-human monocyte (Bethesda Research Lab.); anti-HLA, anti-common leukocyte antigen (Hybritech); Ki-1 (donated by Dr. Stein, Kiel); Vim-D5 (donated by Dr. Knap, Vienna); anti-Tac (donated by Dr. Waldman). Using a light microscope for evaluation, cells were counted positive when a dark brown cell membrane was seen, as indicated in Fig. 27.1.

Results

The reactivity with monoclonal antibodies of HD cells in cell suspension obtained by needle aspiration or minced lymph node is summarized in Table 27.1. Despite the low number of probes examined there seems to be a characteristic reaction pattern for HD cells. Surprisingly HD cells of 4/5 patients reacted strongly with the anti-Tac mAb (Fig. 27.1), which detects the receptor for interleukin-2 (IL-2) (18). To our knowledge the presence of IL-2 receptors on HD cells has not been described previously. HD cells of all patients reacted positively with the mAb OKIa1 (detecting HLA-DR related antigen), OKT9 (detecting the transferrin receptor), Ki-1 [detecting a HD associated antigen, probably an activation antigen (19,20)] and Vim-D5 (detecting a myeloid antigen). In three cases studied HD cells were stained with Tü 9 and LeuM1, also reacting with myeloid antigens. In two cases we saw a variable reaction of HD cells with OKT10 (binding to a possible proliferation antigen not yet exactly characterized). In one patient HD cells were stained by B-1 (detecting a pan B-lymphoid antigen). In three cases rosettes of HD cells with lymphocytes were noted.

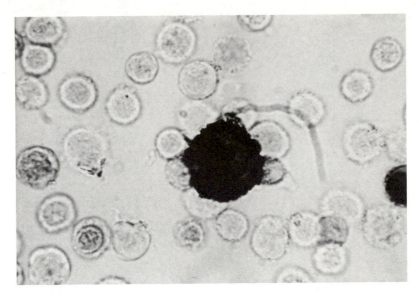

Fig. 27.1. Tac-positive Hodgkin cell forming a rosette with lymphocytes.

We never found T cell antigens or immunoglobulins M and D on the cell surface. Comparing this reaction pattern with HD-derived cell line L 428 (donated by Dr. Diehl) a good agreement can be noted, except the culture cells did not react with B-1 and OKT10.

Discussion

Using a panel of monoclonal antibodies to demonstrate cell membrane antigens on HD cells, a characteristic reaction pattern can be noted. HD cells of all patients were stained with the antibodies Ki-1, OKIa1, OKT9, anti-Tac, anti-HLA (A, B), and common leukocyte antigen. Rosette formation was seen in 3/5, reaction with OKT10 in 2/5, and with B-1 in 1/5 cases. Negative results were always seen with antibodies against immunoglobulins M and D, monocytes, and T-lymphoid antigens. This marker profile is not typical for a special cell lineage and cannot clarify the origin of the HD cells, perhaps with the exception of the reactivity with the antibody B-1, recognizing a pan B-lymphoid antigen, but only 1/5 HD cells expressed this antigen.

The Ki-1 antibody reacted in addition with few smaller cells that form rosettes and whose membrane were not ruffled, showing only some spikes. The identity of these cells is not known. The expression of myeloid antigens on HD cells (10) is to some extent characteristic, but does not prove the myeloid origin. We have demonstrated myeloid antigens on several cancer cells of carcinoma of the mamma and gastrointestinal tract (unpublished observation).

Table 27.1. Expression of membrane antigens on suspended lymph node cells obtained from patients with Hodgkin's disease.

Patient	Histology[a]	Material[b]	anti-Tac %	Ki-1 %	B1 %	OKIa1 %	VimD5 %	OKT9 %	OKT10 %	OKT3 %	OKT4 %	OKT8 %	anti-IgM-D %	Lymphocyte rosettes
									Monoclonal antibodies					
1 B.E.	MC[a]	A[b]	8[c]		48	52	3	11	15	43	26	19	41	
		HD	-/+[d]	(+)	-	+	+	(+)	-	-	-	-	-	(+)
2 S.F.	MC	A	7	6	56	63	1	14	26	42	31	10	52	
		HD	+	+	+	+	-	+	-/+	-	-	-	-	(+)
3 K.J.	NS	B	4	2	62	59	2	12	14	31	18	12	55	
		HD	+	+	-	+	-	+	+	-	-	-	-	-
4 S.F.	MC	A	2	2	21	23	2	8	12	59	44	14	19	
		HD	+	+	-	+	+	+	-	-	-	-	-	-
5 W.V.	MC	B	5	6	53	58	6	15	8	42	32	12	46	
		HD	+	+	-	+	+	+	-	-	-	-	-	+ +
L 428	HD-derived cell line[e]		3–11	94–100	-	>95	35–65	>95	-	-	-	-	-	+ +

[a] MC = mixed cellularity; NS = nodular sclerosis.
[b] B = Biopsy; A = aspirated.
[c] Percentage of total cells reacting.
[d] Positive and negative reactivity with Hodgkin cells.
[e] HD = Hodgkin cell.

Interleukin-2 receptors were primarily found on antigen- or mitogen-stimulated T cells. Using monoclonal antibodies against this receptor, a number of activated and transformed B cells have been found to display the IL-2 receptor, such as hairy cell leukemia (21) and certain EBV-transformed B cell lines (22). On the basis of this finding it is tempting to speculate that HD cells may be derived from activated T- or B-lymphoid cells by malignant transformation. IL 2-receptors are found on cells of two types of leukemia, adult T cell leukemia and hairy cell leukemia. This fact raises the possibility of an autocrine stimulation of proliferation. The same mechanism may occur in Hodgkin's disease. In addition, as noticed in other cell types, interleukin-2 may induce different factors and lymphokines which may explain the unusual appearance of this malignant lymphoma. Further studies are necessary to clarify the effect of interleukin-2 on HD cells.

Summary

The normal counterpart of the Hodgkin (HD) and Sternberg–Reed cell is still not identified. T cell, B cell, monocytic, and granulocytic origin has been discussed and recent data indicate a close relationship to antigen presenting dendritic cells. In an attempt to further investigate this question we have analyzed the phenotype of HD cells in needle aspirates of diseased lymph nodes. Cell suspensions were obtained by mechanical agitation and transferred to poly-L-lysine coated slides. Binding of monoclonal antibodies (mAbs) was detected by a modified, highly sensitive immunoperoxidase technique. Five lymph node aspirates contained enough HD cells for evaluation. HD cells were identified morphologically as well as by the fact that they frequently form rosettes with small lymphocytes and by their negative staining for monocyte-specific mAbs. In four cases all HD cells reacted strongly with the anti-Tac mAb which binds to the receptor for interleukin-2. They were also positive for Ki-1, OKT9, OKT10, OKIal and, in the case of a majority of them, for granulocytic markers (VIM-D5, LeuM1). This phenotype is identical to that of the permanent cell line L 428 which, however, constantly reacted only 2–8% with the anti-Tac mAb. The conclusion to be drawn is still uncertain as the Tac-antigen seems not to be T lymphocyte specific, as others have also shown on hairy cell leukemia of B cell type and some EBV-transformed B cell lines. However, these results make it tempting to speculate that HD cells may be derived from activated T cells or B cells by malignant transformation.

Acknowledgment. We gratefully acknowledge the excellent technical assistance of Vera Kresin and Uschi Habig-Buchwald. This work was supported in part by the Deutsche Forschungsgemeinschaft.

References

1. Kaplan, H.S., and S. Gartner. 1977. "Sternberg–Reed" giant cells of Hodgkin's disease: Cultivation *in vitro*, heterotransplantation and characterization as neoplastic macrophages. *Int. J. Cancer* **19**:511.
2. Kadin, M.E., D.P. Stites, R. Levy, and R. Warnke. 1978. Exogenous immunoglobulin and the macrophage origin of Reed–Sternberg cells in Hodgkin's disease. *New England J. Med.* **299**:1208.
3. Katz, D.R. 1981. The macrophage in Hodgkin's disease. *J. Pathol.* **133**:145.
4. Brook, J.S.J. 1979. Leukophagocytosis by Sternberg–Reed cells in Hodgkin's disease, *New England J. Med.* **300**:1115.
5. Resnick, G.D., and R.L. Nachman. 1981. Reed–Sternberg cells in Hodgkin's disease contain fibronectin. Blood **57**:339.
6. Order, S.E., and S. Hellman. 1972. Pathogenesis of Hodgkin's disease. *Lancet* **1972**(1):571.
7. De Vita, V.T. 1973. Lymphocyte reactivity in Hodgkin's disease: a lymphocyte civil war. *New England J. Med.* **289**:801.
8. Stuart, A.E., E. Jackson, and C.S. Morris. 1982. The reaction of xenogenetic and monoclonal antisera with Reed–Sternberg cells. *J. Pathol.* **137**:129.
9. Doreen, M.S., J.A. Habeshaw, A.G. Stansfeld, P.F.M. Wrigley, and T.A. Lister. 1984. Characteristics of Sternberg–Reed, and related cells in Hodgkin's disease: A immunohistological study. *Brit. J. Cancer* **49**:465.
10. Stein, H., B. Uchánska-Ziegler, J. Gerdes, A. Ziegler, and P. Wernet. 1982. Hodgkin and Sternberg–Reed cells contain antigens specific to late cells of granulopoiesis. *Int. J. Cancer* **29**:283.
11. Curran, R.C., and E.L. Jones. 1977. Dendritic cells and B lymphocytes in Hodgkin's disease. *Lancet* **1977**(2):349.
12. Curran, R.C., and E.C. Jones. 1978. Hodgkin's disease: an immunohistochemical and histological study. *J. Pathol.* **125**:39.
13. Kadin, M.E. 1982. Possible origin of the Reed–Sternberg cell from an interdigitating reticulum cell. *Cancer Treat. Rep.* **66**:601.
14. Stein, H., J. Gerdes, U. Schwab, H. Lemke, D.Y. Mason, A. Ziegler, W. Schienle, and V. Diehl. 1982. Identification of Hodgkin and Sternberg–Reed cells as an unique cell type derived from a newly-detected small-cell population. *Int. J. Cancer* **30**:445.
15. Sternberger, L.A. 1974. The unlabeled antibody enzyme method. *Immunocytochemistry foundation of immunology*. Prentice-Hall, Englewood Cliffs, New Jersey.
16. Bross, K.J., G.A. Pangalis, C.G. Staatz, and K.G. Blume. 1978. Demonstration of cell surface antigens and their antibodies by the peroxidase–antiperoxidase method. *Transplantation* **25**:331.
17. Bross, K.J., G.M. Schmidt, and K.G. Blume. 1979. Conformation of bone marrow engraftment by demonstration of blood group antigens on red cell ghosts. *Transplantation* **28**:257.
18. Leonhard, W.J., J.M. Depper, T. Uchiyama, K.A. Smith, T.A. Waldmann, and W.C. Greene. 1982. A monoclonal antibody that appears to recognize the receptor for human T-cell growth factor; partial characterization of the receptor. *Nature* **300**:267.
19. Diehl, V., H.H. Kirchner, H. Burrichter, H. Stein, C. Fonatsch, J. Gerdes,

M. Schaadt, W. Heit, B. Uchanska-Ziegler, A. Ziegler, F. Heintz, and K. Sueno. 1982. Characteristics of Hodgkin's disease-derived cell lines. *Cancer Treat. Rep.* **66:**625.

20. Andreesen, R., J. Osterholz, G.W. Löhr, and K.J. Bross. 1984. A Hodgkin cell-specific antigen is expressed on a subset of auto- and alloactivated T (helper) lymphoblasts. *Blood* **63:**1299.

21. Korsmeyer, S.J., W.C. Greene, J. Cossman, S.M. Hsu, J.P. Jensen, L.M. Neckers, S.L. Marshall, A. Bakhshi, J.M. Depper, W.J. Leonard, E.S. Jaffe, and Th.A. Waldmann. 1983. Rearrangement and expression of immunoglobulin genes and expression of Tac antigen in hairy cell leukemia. *Proc. Natl. Acad. Sci. U.S.A.* **80:**4522.

22. Robb, R.J. 1984. Interleukin 2: the molecule and its function. *Immunology Today* **5:**203.

CHAPTER 28

The Diversity of T Cell Activation Antigens. Serological Analysis Including Their Expression on Non-T Acute Lymphoblastic Leukemia Cells and B Cell Lines Derived from Adult T Cell Leukemia Patients

Yasuo Morishima, Tomoko Noumi, Ken-ichi Ohya, Saburo Mimami, Masao Okumura, Shin-ichi Mizuno, Ryuzo Ohno, and Kanji Miyamoto

Activated T cells display new cell surface antigens which are not expressed on resting T cells (1). Some of these T cell activation antigens have been shown to have important roles in immunological function of T cells. For example, the Tac antigen with a molecular weight (M.W.) of 55,000 on *in vitro* activated T cells (2,3) proved to be the interleukin-2 receptor (4). Tac antigen is also expressed on adult T cell leukemia (ATL) cells (5,6) which are infected with ATL virus (ATLV). (7). These combined observations imply a relationship between ATLV infection and expression of Tac antigen on ATL cells.

In order to investigate the tissue distribution of T cell activation antigens and their relation to ATLV, we attempted to find monoclonal antibodies (mAbs) detecting T cell activation antigens among the T cell protocol mAbs in the Second Workshop for Human Leucocyte Differentiation Antigens. Using these mAbs, we tested the expression of T cell activation antigens and other differentiation antigens on ATL cells, ATLV-infected T or B cell culture cell lines, and other leukemia cells.

Materials and Methods

One hundred and fifty-six mAbs included in the T cell protocol were serologically tested by indirect immunofluorescent (1.F.) assay using FITC-conjugated goat anti–mouse Ig, and analyzed by flow cytometry (EPICS-C). Complement-dependent micro-cytotoxicity test using baby rabbit complement was also employed in some analyses.

The following cells were used as panel cells for the serological assays. Peripheral blood T cells (PB-T cells) were separated from healthy donors' blood by Ficoll–Hypaque gradient centrifugation and elution from nylon-wool columns. PHA-stimulated PB-T cells (PHA-T cell) were obtained by culturing PB-T cells with PHA-M for 3 days. Four T cell-type ATL culture cell lines (KI, ATN, MT-1, KH-2) were derived from ATL patients without supplement of T cell growth factor. One T cell-type culture cell line (SA) was established by co-culturing cord blood cells with ATL culture cell line MT-2. Six B cell-type culture cell lines (BATL-1, BATL-2, BATL-3, BATL-6, BATL-7, KO) were established from ATL patients' PB cells as described elsewhere (8). EB virus-transformed B cell lines (KY, ER, SB), B or null cell culture cell lines (NALL-1, NKL-1, NKL-2), and T culture cell lines (MOLT-4, CCRF-CEM, JURKAT) were also used for analysis. KI, NKL-1, and NKL-2 were established in the First Department of Internal Medicine, Nagoya University, and SA, BATL-1, 2, 3, 6, 7, and KO were established in Okayama Red Cross Blood Center. MT-1 was supplied by Dr. I. Miyoshi and KH-2 by Dr. S. Maeda. Leukemia cells were collected from patients' peripheral blood or bone marrow. The following samples which contained more than 80% leukemia cells were used for analysis: four cases of T cell-type acute lymphoblastic leukemia (T-ALL), 4 cases of pre T-ALL, 36 cases of non-T ALL, 2 cases of B cell-type chronic lymphocytic leukemia (B-CLL), and 3 cases of acute nonlymphocytic leukemia (ANLL).

Results

Diversity of "T Cell Activation Antigens"

Thirteen out of 156 mAbs of the T cell protocol showed positive reactivity with PHA-T cells (more than 50%), but not with resting PB-T cells (less than 10%). As summarized in Tables 28.1 and 28.2, these 13 activated T mAbs were classified into five groups according to their reactivity against various hematopoietic cells.

Group 1 (anti-Tac): T135 (TIA), T140 (Tac/1HT4-4H3), T141 (B149.9), T159 (TAC), T143 (22A9.3), T145 (39C6.5), T146 (33B3.1)

These seven mAbs showed the same serological specificity against the panel of cells tested. That is, this group showed weak to strong reactivity against T-ATL cell lines, weak to moderate reactivity against B-ATL cell lines and ATL cases, and moderate reactivity against three non-T ALL cases. No reactivity was found with T-ALL, pre-T-ALL, B-CLL, B and T cell lines except ATL cell lines. Among the group 1 mAbs, four mAbs (T135, T140, T141, T159) had somewhat stronger reactivity with PHA-T

Table 28.1. Reactivity of T-activation mAbs to various lymphoid culture cell lines.[a]

Cells (No. of cells tested)	Group 1 T135 T140 T141 T159	T143 T145 T146	Group 2 T147	Group 3 T142	Group 4 T138	Group 5 T153
PBT (5)	−	−	−	−	−	−
PHA st. PBT (3)	+++	++/+++	+/++	+/++	++/+++	++/+++
ATL T cell line						
KI	+++	+/+++	±	+++	−	+
ATN	+++	+++	++	+++	++	+++
MT-1	+++	+++	+	+	−	−
KH-2	−/+	−	−	−	+	±
SAI	−/±	−	−	±	+	+++
ATL B cell line						
BATL-1	+	±	−	+	−	+
BATL-2	+	+	±	+	±	+
BATL-3	±/++	−/++	−	+	±	+
BATL-6	++	+/++	−	−	−	++
BATL-7	±/+	±	−	+	±	++
KO	+	±	−	−	−	++
EB virus-transformed						
B cell line (3)	−	−	−	−	−	−/+++
B, null cell line (4)	−	−	−	−/±	−	−/+
T cell line (3)	−	−	−	−/±	−/±	−/+++

[a] Tested by I.F. assay. +++ 100%–80%; ++ 80%–50%; + 50%–20%; ± 20%–10%; − 10%–0%.

Table 28.2. Reactivity of T-activation mAbs to various leukemia cells.[a]

Leukemia cells (No. of cells tested)	Group 1 T135 T140 T141 T159	T143 T145 T146	Group 2 T147	Group 3 T142	Group 4 T138	Group 5 T153
ATL						
#597	++	+	−	++	±	±
#2599	±	−	−	+	−	−
#1409	−	−	−	+	+	−
#1462	−	−	−	+	+	−
Non-T-ALL						
#2528	+	+/++	+	−	−	+
#376	±/+	±/+	−	−	−	−
#1441	+/++	+/++	−	−	−	−
Non-T-ALL (5 cases)	−	−	−	−	−	−
Pre-T-ALL (4 cases)	−	−	−	−	−/+	−
T-ALL (4 cases)	−	−	−	−	−/++	−
B-CLL (2 cases)	−	−	−	−	−	−
ANLL (3 cases)	−	−	−/++	−/++	−	−

[a] Tested by I.F. assay. +++ 100%–80%; ++ 80%–50%; + 50%–20%; ± 20%–10%; − 10%–0%.

cells, T-ATL cell lines, and ATL cases than the other mAbs (T143, T145, T146).

Group 2: T147 (38B7.3)

This mAb reacted moderately with PHA-T cells, and showed weak reactivity sporadically among T-ATL cell lines, B-ATL cell lines, other B cell lines, non-T ALL cases, and ANLL cases.

Group 3: T142 (B1.19.2)

This mAb reacted with PHA-T cells, T-ATL cell lines, B-ATL cell lines, and ATL cases. This pattern of reaction was similar to that of group 1 (anti-Tac) mAbs. However, T142 also reacted with one ANLL case, NALL-1, NKL-1 and MOLT-4, and failed to react with three non-T ALL cases that expressed group 1 antigen.

Group 4: T138 (1 MONO 2A6)

Although this mAb reacted weakly with some T-ATL cell lines, B-ATL cell lines, and ATL cases, the pattern of reaction was different from other groups of activated T mAbs. T138 also reacted with one T-ALL case and one pre-T-ALL case.

Group 5: T153 (AA3)

This mAb reacted not only with most T-ATL cell lines and B-ATL cell lines, but also with EB B cell lines (KY and ER) and other cell lines (MOLT-4, CCRF-CEM, NALL-1).

It is suggested from these serological data that five groups of activated T mAbs detect different antigenic determinants of T cell activation antigens, or detect different T cell activation molecules.

Expression of T Cell Activation Antigens and T Cell Antigens on ATL Cells

Analysis of cell surface antigens of 11 ATL cases was done by I.F. assay. As shown in Fig. 28.1, ATL had several distinct phenotypes of cell surface antigens. T cell antigens such as CD2, CD3, CD4, CD5, CD6, and 9.3 antigen were expressed on ATL cells tested, although a few cases which did not express CD3 and/or CD6 were found. CD7 could not be detected or was detected with only faint fluorescence by I.F. assay in all cases tested. This disappearance of CD7 on ATL cells contrasted with the strong expression of CD7 on T-ALL cells (data not shown). The antigens such as Tac antigen, transferrin receptor detected by 5E9, and Ia antigen, all of which are known to be expressed on PHA-T cells, have appeared on ATL cells. Additionally, ATL cells showed a variable amount of Tac

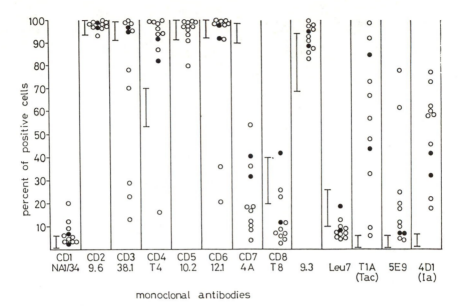

monoclonal antibodies

Fig. 28.1. Expression of cell surface antigens on ATL cells. Tested by I.F. assay. Smoldering ATL cases are indicated by (●). Mean ±1 SD of positive % in normal T cell (n = 15) is indicated as (——).

antigen (8–97%). The other T cell activation antigens detected by group 3 mAb T142 and group 4 mAb T138 were also preferentially expressed on ATL cells (Table 28.2).

The analysis of T cell subpopulation in smoldering ATL proposed by Yamaguchi *et al.* (9) were shown in Fig. 28.1 (marked as ●). These two smoldering cases had lymphocytes with convoluted nucleus in 20–30% of PB lymphocytes without any clinical signs and symptoms of ATL for more than one year. The phenotype of these two patients' T cells already showed the same pattern as ATL patients.

Expression of T Cell Activation Antigens on B Cell Lines Derived from ATL Patients

Six spontaneous B cell lines were established from ATL patients' PB cells without adding EB virus. As reported previously (7) all of six cell lines were EBNA-positive in more than 90% of cells. Most striking, however, was the observation that ATLV-associated antigen (6) was detected in four out of six cell lines in 0.1 to 2.0% of cells. Four out of five cell lines tested, turned out to contain proviral DNA of ATLV.

We attempted to analyze the cell surface antigens on these ATLV-infected B cell lines. Activated T mAbs and other well-characterized mAbs against hematopoietic antigens were used (Table 28.3). In spite of

Table 28.3. Characteristics of B cell line derived from ATL patients.

Cell line	% fluorescent cells		ATLV pro-viral DNA	Reactivity of mAb by I.F. test[a]						
	EBNA	ATLA		CD1–8[b]	T1A[c] (Tac)	B1	8B1[d]	BB-1[e]	NL-1[f] (CD10)	4D[g] (Ia)
BATL-1	>90	1–2	Present	−	+	+++	+	+++	+++	+++
BATL-2	>90	1–2	Present	−	+	+++	++	+	+	+++
BATL-3	>90	0	Absent	−	+	+++	+++	+++	+++	+++
BATL-6	>90	0	Present	−	++	++	++	+	−	+++
BATL-7	>90	0.1	Present	−	+	+++	+++	+++	+++	+++
KO	>90	0.1	N.T.	−	+	+++	+	+	+	+++

[a] Percent of positive cells by indirect immunofluorescent test; +++ 100%–80%, ++ 80%–50%, + 50%–20%, ± 20%–10%, − 10%–0%.
[b] These T cell antigens were tested with the following mAbs. CD1: T129, T130; CD2: T25, T26, T16; CD3: T124; CD4: T70, T71; CD5: T4; CD6: T46, T47; CD7: T30, T43; CD8: T83, T95.
[c] Anti-T cell activation antigen, T135.
[d] Anti-B cell activation antigen: B23.
[e] Anti-B cell activation antigen.
[f] Anti-common ALL antigen.
[g] Anti-HLA DR common.

the weak fluorescence and low percentage of positive cells, Tac antigen was detected on all of these cell lines. B cell-related antigens detected by B1 mAb, 8B1 mAb, BB-1 mAb, Ia antigen, and common ALL antigen (CALLA) were expressed on these cell lines, although no other T cell antigens were expressed on any of these cell lines.

Expression of T Cell Activation Antigens on Non-T ALL Cells

Unexpectedly, three out of 36 non-T ALL cases expressed Tac antigen by I.F. and C'-microcytotoxicity assay (Fig. 28.2). The phenotype of these three non-T ALL cases was almost identical. These cell surfaces expressed Ia antigen, CALLA, and B cell antigen 8B1, but not the other two B cell antigens (B1 and B2). None of the T cell antigens (CD1, CD2, CD3, CD4, CD5, CD6, CD7, and CD8) were present. Also, no intracytoplasmic Ig and ATL associated antigen were found.

Discussion

We demonstrated that some T cell protocol mAbs which detect antigens on PHA-activated T cells and not on resting PB-T cells could be classified into five groups according to their reactivity with various kinds of hemato-poietic cell lines and leukemia cells. Group 1 consists of 7 mAbs. The biochemical analysis of our group 1 mAb T135 (T1A) using T-ATL cell line KI showed that T135 recognized a cell surface antigen with M.W. 55,000 (data not shown). Other group 1 mAbs T159 (TAC) and T141 (B149.9) were also reported to detect the antigen with the same M.W.

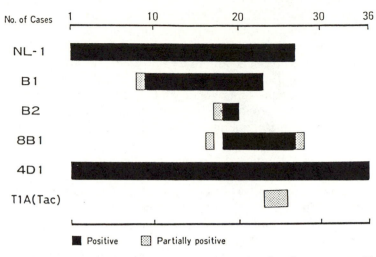

Fig. 28.2. Expression of Tac antigen and B cell-related antigens on non-T ALL cases. Tested by C′-micro cytotoxicity test. More than 50% killing is shown as positive, and 50–10% killing is shown as partially positive. mAb NL-1 detects CALLA, mAb B1, mAb B2, and mAb 8B1 detect B cell antigens, and mAb 4D1 detects Ia antigen.

Therefore, it is suspected that group 1 mAbs detect Tac antigen. Among these seven mAbs, there are two types of serological reactivity. That is, T135, T140, T141, and T159 showed more intense reactivity than other mAbs. This difference might be due merely to the difference of Ig class and/or titer of mAbs, or might reflect that each type of mAb detects different antigenic determinants of the same or different Tac antigens. Biochemical and functional studies are necessary to prove this hypothesis. Each of the other four groups of mAbs might also detect different molecules on PHA-activated T cells, or detect different antigenic determinants. Group 3 mAb T142 (B1.19.2) was reported to detect an antigen with M.W. 220,000. MAb 5E9 (anti-transferrin receptor), mAb 4F2, and mAb 4D1 (anti-Ia antigen), all of which appear on PHA-T cells, were also shown to have serologically different patterns of reaction against panel cells from any of group 1–5 activated T mAbs. Therefore, we could find at least seven kinds of mAbs detecting so called "T cell activation antigens," most of which are however known to be expressed not only on activated T cells but also on other types of hematopoietic cells and/or even non-hematopoietic cells.

Six culture cell lines derived from ATL patients were shown to have B cell surface antigens. Both EBNA- and ATL-associated antigen were present in the same cell lines, and ATLV was proven to be integrated into DNA. These cell lines have the same features as the cell lines reported by Yamamoto *et al.* (11). The fact that all of six B-ATL cell lines do express

Tac antigen on their cell surface provides serological evidence suggesting at least two mechanisms for the appearance of Tac antigen. Firstly, ATLV may have some role in the expression of Tac antigen, because most EB virus-transformed, not ATLV-infected cell lines from healthy donors did not show Tac antigen. ATLV gene integrated into the DNA of host B cells may activate other genes such as Tac gene, as suggested by Sodroski *et al.* (12). Secondary, Tac antigen may become a receptor of ATLV on the cell surface membrane, and the cell line with ATLV and Tac antigen may be established. Our demonstration that some non-T ALL cells express Tac antigen and Korsmeyer's finding (10) that hairy cell leukemia expresses Tac antigen suggest the possibility that at some stage during B cell maturation, pre-B cell expresses Tac antigen. Therefore, ATLV derived from ATL cells may infect patients' normal B cells which express Tac antigens during *in vitro* culture of patients' PB lymphocytes. The appearance of Tac antigen on non-T ALL or B-ATL cell lines also corresponds to the findings reported by Okubo *et al.*, (13) Yasuda *et al.*, (14) and Wano *et al.* (15) at the annual meeting of the Japan Hematology Society, 1984.

Weak or no expression of Tac antigen on some ATL cells and T-ATL cell lines suggests that the interleukin-2 receptor may have no role in autonomic proliferation of ATL cells *in vivo*.

In this paper, it was also demonstrated that mAbs against T cell surface antigens are useful to elucidate the stage of T cell maturation from which ATL arises, and to distinguish ATL from other types of leukemia in diagnosis. Expression of CD2, CD3, CD4, CD5, and CD6 antigens and lack of CD8 antigen on ATL cells suggest the preferential infectivity of ATLV of a distinct subset of mature T cells, as reported by Hattori *et al.* (5). Our previous preliminary data showing that weak or no expression of CD7 antigen detected by mAb 4A clearly discriminates ATL from immature T cell malignancy, T-ALL, was also confirmed (16).

Summary

1. Thirteen monoclonal antibodies which showed positive reactivity with PHA-T cells and not with PB-T cells were classified into five groups according to their reactivity with various leukemia cells and leukemia culture cell lines.
2. All of six cell-type culture cell lines derived from ATL patients expressed Tac antigen.
3. Three out of 36 non-T All cells expressed Tac antigens.
4. ATL cells had distinct phenotype of cell surface antigens: that is, CD2, CD3, CD4, CD5, CD6, 9.3 antigen, Tac antigen, Ia antigen, and transferrin receptor are expressed on most ATL cells, and CD1, CD7, and CD8 are not expressed, or weakly expressed on ATL cells.

Acknowledgment. We thank Dr. Ryuzo Ueda and Dr. Nancy H. Collins for critical review of the manuscript.

References

1. Cotner, T., J.M. Williams, L. Christenson, H.M. Shapiro, T.B. Strom, and J. Strominger. 1983. Simultaneous flow cytometric analysis of human T cell activation antigen expression and DNA content. *J. Exp. Med.* **157**:461.
2. Uchiyama, T., S. Broder, and T.A. Waldmann. 1981. A monoclonal antibody (anti-Tac) reactive with activated and functionally mature human T cells. *J. Immunol.* **126**:1393.
3. Wano, Y., T. Uchiyama, K. Fukui, M. Maeda, H. Uchino, and J. Yodoi. 1984. Characterization of human interleukin 2 receptor (Tac antigen) in normal and leukemic T cells: Co-expression of normal and aberrant receptors on HUT-102 cells. *J. Immunol.* **132**:3005.
4. Leonard, W.J., J.M. Depper, T. Uchiyama, K.A. Smith, T.A. Waldmann, and W.C. Creene. 1982. A monoclonal antibody that appears to recognize the receptor for human T-cell growth factor: partial characterization of the receptor. *Nature* **300**:267.
5. Hattori, T., T. Uchiyama, T. Toibana, K. Takatsuki, and H. Uchino. 1981. Surface phenotype of Japanese adult T-cell leukemia cells characterized by monoclonal antibodies. *Blood* **58**:645.
6. Hinuma, Y., K. Nagata, K. Hanaoka, M. Nakai, T. Matsumoto, K.I. Kinoshita, S. Shirakawa, and I. Miyoshi. 1981. Adult T-cell leukemia: antigen in an ATL cell line and detection of antibodies to the antigen in human sera. *Proc. Natl. Acad. Sci. U.S.A.* **78**:6476.
7. Yoshida, M., M. Seiki, K. Yamaguchi, and K. Takatsuki. 1984. Monoclonal integration of HTLV provirus in all primary tumors of adult T-cell leukemia suggests causative role of HTLV in the disease. *Proc. Natl. Acad. Sci. U.S.A.* **81**:2534.
8. Miyamoto, K., N. Tomita, A. Ishii, T. Nishizaki, and A. Togawa. 1984. Establishment and characterization of adult T cell leukemia virus containing B cell lines derived from peripheral blood with adult T cell leukemia patients. *Gann* **75**:655.
9. Yamaguchi, K., H. Nishimura, H. Kohrogi, M. Jono, Y. Miyamoto, and K. Takatsuki. 1983. A proposal for smoldering adult T-cell leukemia (Smoldering ATL): A clinicopathologic study of 5 cases. *Blood* **62**:758.
10. Korsmeyer, S.J., W.C. Greene, J. Cossman, S.M. Hsu, J.P. Jensen, L.M. Neckers, S.L. Marshall, A. Bakhshi, J.M. Deeper, W.J. Leonard, E.S. Jaffe, and T.A. Waldman. 1983. Rearrangement and expression of immunoglobulin genes and expression of Tac antigen in hairy cell leukemia. *Proc. Natl. Acad. Sci. U.S.A.* **80**:4522.
11. Yamamoto, N., T. Matsumoto, Y. Koyanagi, Y. Tanaka, and Y. Hinuma. 1982. Unique cell lines harbouring both Epstein-Barr virus and adult T-cell leukemia virus, established from leukemia patients. *Nature* **299**:367.
12. Sodroski, J.G., C.A. Roseu, and W.A. Haseltine. 1984. Trans-acting transcriptional activation of the lung terminal repeat of human T lymphotropic viruses in infected cells. *Science* **225**:381.

13. Ohkubo, K., K. Sagawa, Y. Matsuo, M. Yokoyama, Y. Sei, and H. Natori. 1984. Tac positive cells in a case at nonT nonB acute lymphoblastic leukemia. *Acta Haematol. Jap.* **47**:446 (abstract).
14. Wano, Y., H. Umadome, T. Uchiyama, H. Uchino, and K. Sagawa. Characterization of B cell-Tac antigen expressed on B-LCL derived from patients with ATL. *Acta Haematol. Jap.* **47**:447 (abstract).
15. Yasuda, K., K. Sagawa, and M. Yokoyama. 1984. Tac antigen expression on the established B cell lines derived from adult T cell leukemia patients. *Acta Haematol. Jap.* **47**:446 (abstract).
16. Morishima, Y., M. Kobayashi, S.Y. Yang, N.H. Collins, M.K. Hoffman, and B. Dupont. 1982. Functionally different T lymphocyte subpopulations determined by their sensitivity to complement-dependent cell lysis with the monoclonal antibody 4A. *J. Immunol.* **129**:1091.

CHAPTER 29

Expression Profiles of T Cell Associated Antigens on Adult T Cell Leukemia Cells: Results of a Workshop Study

Kimitaka Sagawa, Shizuo Hagiwara, Kaori Yasuda, and Mitchel Mitsuo Yokoyama

Adult T cell leukemia (ATL) is one of the T cell malignancies in man predominantly found in the Kyushu area in Southern Japan with characteristic clinical and hematologic features (1), and C-type retrovirus, isolated from the ATL cells, has recently been identified as the causative agent (2,3). Therefore, it has been of major interest to define leukemogenesis of mature T cells by ATL virus (ATLV). The Workshop presented an opportunity to study leukemia cells in ATL patients using its battery of monoclonal antibodies (mAbs) in a T cell protocol. Freshly obtained ATL cells can be used as a panel of cells possessing matured malignant T cell antigens on the cell surface (4) to evaluate the specific reaction of mAbs. Furthermore, the expression profile of T cell associated antigens on ATL cells could be well-characterized by the multiple sources of mAbs. A rarely observed subtype of ATL, with double markers (OKT4 and OKT8) present on the leukemic T cells, was also characterized phenotypically with the Workshop's battery of mAbs.

Materials and Methods

ATL Patients

Diagnosis of ATL was made by clinical manifestations, hematological features, and leukemia cell phenotyping at Kurume University Hospital and affiliated hospitals. The patients with ATL were all born on the island of Kyushu where ATL has been reported to be endemic (5).

Murine Monoclonal Antibodies

A total of 159 murine mAbs from the Workshop's antibody panel for T cell studies together with OKT11 (6), OKT4 (7,8), OKT8 (9), B1 (10),

Table 29.1. Surface marker phenotyping of the peripheral blood lymphoid cells of six ATL* cases and a double marker ATL** case.

ATL cases	Age	Sex	WBC ×10³/µl	% Lymphoid cells	% ATL cells	ATLA Ab	% Positive cells with						
							OKT11	OKT4	OKT8	B1	MCS-2	GIN-14	Tac
1*	34	M	76.0	97	90	+	99.1	97.4	1.4	0.8	0.4	0.2	57.8
2*	33	M	23.0	97	59	+	95.9	96.0	2.4	0.3	0.5	0.2	3.5
3*	60	F	15.0	58	43	+	96.9	94.5	3.4	3.1	1.7	1.1	19.6
4*	68	M	7.3	68	62	+	96.0	90.9	6.2	2.3	2.4	1.1	21.8
5*	73	M	100.0	94	82	+	96.3	95.2	2.0	0.6	0.7	0.4	36.0
6*	54	M	11.1	65	48	+	89.2	95.0	3.1	2.8	1.1	0.9	25.2
7**	46	M	72.8	94	90	+	94.9	90.8	90.8	2.4	1.9	2.2	32.4

MCS-2 (11), GIN-14 (12), and anti-Tac (13) were used for membrane marker analysis with ATL cells.

Indirect Membrane Immunofluorescence

An aliquot of heparinized peripheral venous blood was obtained containing 1×10^6 leukocytes from the patients with ATL, and first stained with the properly diluted mAb followed by incubation at 4°C for 30 min. After lysing the red cells with ammonium chloride solution, the leukocytes were washed twice and incubated at 4°C for 30 min with a mixture of appropriately standardized fluorescein-conjugated anti–mouse IgG and IgM antibodies (Cappel, Cockranville, PA). The cells were then washed twice in PBS and resuspended in 2-ml PBS containing 0.02% sodium azide. The fluorescein-positive cells among the lymphoid cell population of leukocytes were assessed by flow cytometry (Spectrum III, Ortho Diagnostic Systems, Raritan, NJ) and percent positive cells of 2000 cells counted were calculated.

Results and Discussion

As shown in Table 29.1, leukemic cells from six ATL patients presented a typical ATL phenotype as OKT11$^+$, OKT4$^+$, and OKT8$^-$, whereas one ATL case revealed an unusual ATL phenotype as a double marker phenotype with OKT11$^+$, OKT4$^+$, and OKT8$^+$. In the test panel cells, non-T cell contamination, representing B1$^+$ and MCS-2$^+$ cells, was very limited. Therefore, the ATL cells used in this study were considered to be highly purified leukemic T cells.

Serum samples from the ATL blood elicited the antibody activity against the ATL-associated antigen (ATLA) (14) found in all cases tested.

As shown in Table 29.2, 159 mAbs of the Workshop's T cell protocol were analyzed with the ATL cells. Classification of the mAbs submitted to the Workshop was made by specificity in reaction patterns according to the cluster of differentiation (CD) based on the information provided from the Workshop's headquarters.

As shown in Tables 29.2 and 29.3, the mAbs in categories CD2, CD3, and CD4 exhibited highly reactive patterns with ATL cells from six typical cases, whereas the mAbs in CD1 and CD8 showed lower reactivities. The mAbs clustered into CD5, CD6, CD7, pan T other or unknown, T cell subset other, T-activation, and leukemia specific exhibited a reactivity with ATL cells intermediate between those of the two groups above. All mAbs, except those in CD8 and CD7, reacted with double marker ATL cells in a manner similar to that with typical ATL cells. Those in CD8 and CD7 were highly reactive with double marker ATL cells.

The results suggest that the leukemic T cell of ATL is originally derived from the mature T cell population, whereas the double marker ATL cell is derived from a less mature T cell cluster.

ATLV-specific polypeptides p28 and p19, detected in the cytoplasm of ATLV-infected cell lines by GIN-14 mAb, could not be identified on the cell surface of fresh ATL cells in this study.

Summary

The present extensive surface marker analysis of leukemic T cells in seven ATL cases, using the Workshop's battery of mAbs, resulted in the surface antigen profiles of ATL cells. Typical ATL cells express a surface phenotype of CD1$^-$, CD2$^+$, CD3$^+$, CD4$^+$, CD5$^{+/-}$, CD6$^{+/-}$, CD7$^{-/+}$, CD8$^-$, pan T other or unknown$^{+/-}$, T cell subset other$^{+/-}$, T-activation$^{+/-}$, and leukemia specific$^{-/+}$. Double marker ATL cells express a surface phenotype of CD1$^-$, CD2$^+$, CD3$^+$, CD4$^+$, CD5$^{+/-}$, CD6$^+$, CD7$^{+/-}$, CD8$^+$, Pan T other or unknown$^{+/-}$, T cell subset other$^{+/-}$, T-activation$^{+/-}$, and Leukemia specific$^{-/+}$. A significant difference between the two types of ATL cells was observed only in the reactivity with CD8 and CD7.

Surface antigen profiles, generated according to the differentiation scheme of human T lymphocytes (15), suggest that the leukemic T cell of ATL is derived from the mature T cell population, whereas the double marker ATL cell has its origin in malignant transformation at the stage of a less differentiated T cell compared to the progenitor of the typical ATL cell.

Table 29.2. Reactivities of the workshop's battery of monoclonal antibodies with ATL cells.

Antibody group[a]	Code number	Antibody name	% Positive with ATL cells[b]	% Positive with double marker ATL cells[c]
NC	1	P3X63	0.8 ± 0.5	1.7
NC	2	PBS-BSA	0.7 ± 0.5	1.8
PC	3	A3D8	99.6 ± 0.3	97.6
CD5	4	H65	66.6 ± 33.6	88.6
	5	6-2	92.3 ± 5.6	91.3
	6	SJ10-2H10	22.5 ± 26.3	25.6
	7	L17F12/Leu 1	92.1 ± 6.8	90.3
	8	MT 61	92.7 ± 6.4	90.1
	9	MT 215	15.9 ± 25.3	91.7
	10	2H4	28.0 ± 35.0	28.6
	11	XIX102-3	16.9 ± 20.3	3.2
	12	BL-T2	23.3 ± 37.0	44.5
CD2	13	9-1	80.9 ± 12.3	93.4
	14	9-2	90.3 ± 6.1	94.6
	15	G19-3.1	70.3 ± 27.3	84.8

Table 29.2. *Continued*

Antibody group[a]	Code number	Antibody name	% Positive with ATL cells[b]	% Positive with double marker ATL cells[c]
	16	S2/Leu 5b	96.0 ± 3.4	95.2
	17	MT 26	94.3 ± 4.4	95.3
	18	MT 910	96.1 ± 4.0	96.1
	19	MT 1110	96.1 ± 3.4	96.6
	20	T11/3Pt2H9	96.9 ± 2.3	96.9
	21	T11/ROLD2-1H8	83.8 ± 9.3	93.2
	22	T11/3T4-8B5	96.0 ± 3.6	95.9
	23	T11/7T4-7A9	59.1 ± 15.2	83.5
	24	T11/7T4-7E10	95.2 ± 4.2	95.8
	25	9.6	96.7 ± 2.7	96.0
	26	35.1	96.2 ± 2.6	95.8
	27	T4IIB5	86.9 ± 8.7	94.7
	28	KOLT-2	82.0 ± 16.5	86.3
CD7	29	9-3	91.5 ± 1.9	81.6
	30	G3-7	17.9 ± 24.6	89.6
	31	4H9/Leu 9	15.8 ± 24.4	89.7
	32	BW264/50	40.7 ± 22.2	6.5
	33	BW264/217	79.2 ± 22.1	78.0
	34	BW264/215	13.2 ± 12.9	3.1
	35	PBS-BSA	0.9 ± 0.6	1.7
	36	A1	0.7 ± 0.3	1.8
	37	4D12.1	2.1 ± 1.3	8.3
	38	8H8.1	13.8 ± 24.9	87.9
	39	3A1A	17.0 ± 24.5	92.2
	40	3A1A(irrad.)	16.1 ± 24.6	92.8
	41	3A1B-4G6	8.7 ± 18.3	49.0
	42	3A1C-5A12	1.3 ± 0.9	1.7
	43	4A	13.9 ± 24.7	87.2
	44	1-3	14.8 ± 24.8	86.9
	45	I21	14.7 ± 24.0	88.0
CD6	46	T12/3Pt12B8	54.0 ± 47.6	88.9
	47	12.1.5	54.1 ± 47.1	88.2
Pan T	48	T10B9	62.4 ± 35.6	81.3
other	49	T12A10	46.9 ± 44.6	57.5
or	50	E9	98.4 ± 1.2	93.6
unknown	51	G3-5	51.6 ± 46.7	87.9
	52	G10-2.1	91.7 ± 11.1	96.9
	53	G19-1.2	94.8 ± 4.5	96.3
	54	T55	26.7 ± 35.9	88.4
	55	T56	8.8 ± 10.3	50.7
	56	T57	95.9 ± 2.5	94.4
	57	BW239/347	62.9 ± 35.7	80.1
	58	MT 211	43.7 ± 42.8	81.4
	59	MT 421	52.4 ± 47.6	87.4
	60	CRIS-3	97.2 ± 2.8	99.1
	61	CRIS-7	86.3 ± 15.5	89.3
	62	CRIS-8	95.7 ± 1.5	90.5
	63	K20	56.1 ± 36.9	83.5
	64	K50	0.8 ± 0.6	1.1

Table 29.2. *Continued*

Antibody group[a]	Code number	Antibody name	% Positive with ATL cells[b]	% Positive with double marker ATL cells[c]
	65	G144	8.9 ± 9.2	39.4
	66	D47	0.4 ± 0.2	1.5
CD4	67	T10C5	45.7 ± 43.7	54.2
	68	G19-2	94.9 ± 2.8	90.5
	69	91d6	94.9 ± 2.3	91.4
	70	94b1	94.5 ± 2.4	91.4
	71	BW264/123	89.5 ± 8.3	90.4
	72	MT 151	94.6 ± 2.2	92.4
	73	MT 321	93.9 ± 3.2	90.4
	74	T4/12T4D11	93.7 ± 2.7	91.8
	75	T4/18T3A9	94.4 ± 2.7	92.2
	76	MT 310	95.2 ± 1.4	92.2
	77	T4/19Thy 5D7	94.6 ± 2.6	92.1
	78	T4/7T4-6C1	94.1 ± 3.2	87.7
	79	66.1	93.7 ± 3.3	88.9
	80	TII19-4-7	3.9 ± 4.4	1.9
CD8	81	14	3.4 ± 2.3	89.4
	82	M236	5.4 ± 8.0	82.1
	83	G10-1.1	3.1 ± 2.0	87.9
	84	C12/D3	2.9 ± 2.7	92.0
	85	BW264/162	2.3 ± 1.7	50.0
	86	BW135/80	2.7 ± 2.0	85.2
	87	MT415	3.1 ± 1.9	90.8
	88	MT1014	2.7 ± 2.0	86.5
	89	MT122	4.1 ± 3.6	91.4
	90	T8/21thy2D3	3.0 ± 2.2	90.9
	91	T8/7Pt3F9	2.5 ± 1.8	87.2
	92	T8/2T8-1B5	3.0 ± 2.5	90.3
	93	T9-2T8-1C1	3.0 ± 2.0	87.1
	94	T8/2T8-2A1	2.7 ± 1.6	83.3
	95	T8/2ST8-5H7	2.3 ± 1.4	4.5
	96	66.2	4.2 ± 3.1	88.3
	97	51.1	3.3 ± 2.3	86.8
	98	T411E1	0.7 ± 0.5	2.1
	99	T41D8	3.7 ± 1.9	85.9
	100	BL-TS1	0.5 ± 0.3	1.8
T cell	101	BRC-T1	81.4 ± 24.7	86.5
subset	102	D44	19.0 ± 14.2	1.9
other	103	SK11/Leu 8	36.8 ± 29.9	24.2
	104	3AC5	21.1 ± 37.8	16.4
	105	CRIS-4	66.2 ± 27.1	78.5
	106	CRIS-5	69.9 ± 38.5	89.2
	107	EDU-2	94.8 ± 2.3	92.7
	108	TQ1/28T17G6	95.3 ± 3.1	94.2
	109	GM1	15.9 ± 29.3	9.2
	110	10B4.6	3.0 ± 2.1	86.6
	111	8E-1.7	2.2 ± 1.4	80.0
	112	6F10.3	61.4 ± 32.5	90.0
	113	13B8.2	94.4 ± 2.5	92.9

Table 29.2. *Continued*

Antibody group[a]	Code number	Antibody name	% Positive with ATL cells[b]	% Positive with double marker ATL cells[c]
	114	K51	12.6 ± 21.8	4.2
	115	BL-TS20	0.6 ± 0.3	1.5
	116	BL-TS14	0.5 ± 0.3	1.3
CD3	117	G19-4.1	87.1 ± 14.4	87.7
	118	SK7/Leu 4	85.5 ± 15.4	88.1
	119	89b1	90.0 ± 16.4	95.1
	120	BW264/56	86.3 ± 17.2	88.6
	121	BW242/55	27.7 ± 33.8	90.8
	122	T3/2Ad2A2	43.0 ± 34.7	77.2
	123	T3/2T8-2F4	51.0 ± 39.8	65.8
	124	T3/RW2-4B6	78.9 ± 25.1	89.4
	125	T3/RW2-8C8	78.1 ± 23.6	89.7
	126	X35-3	80.6 ± 20.7	89.2
	127	NU-T1	60.9 ± 26.6	82.3
CD1	128	M241	1.1 ± 0.5	4.5
	129	NA1/34	0.6 ± 0.3	2.3
	130	SK9/Leu 6	0.5 ± 0.3	1.5
	131	4A76	0.4 ± 0.2	1.9
	132	10D12.2	0.7 ± 0.4	1.4
	133	NU-T2	0.6 ± 0.3	2.5
	134	I19	0.5 ± 0.3	1.6
T-Act	135	T1A	29.9 ± 16.2	31.6
	136	TS145	2.5 ± 3.0	2.9
	137	100-1A5	69.7 ± 16.5	4.5
	138	1 MONO 2A6	1.1 ± 0.3	20.4
	139	4EL1C7	2.0 ± 1.7	2.7
	140	Tac/1HT4-4H3	32.6 ± 18.3	32.3
	141	B149.9	17.5 ± 13.7	21.4
	142	B1.19.2	26.1 ± 26.0	72.2
	143	23A9.3	6.5 ± 6.7	7.2
	144	39C1.5	88.4 ± 8.6	93.3
	145	39C6.5	5.1 ± 2.6	7.8
	146	33B3.1	12.9 ± 6.3	13.7
	147	33B7.3	0.9 ± 0.3	1.5
	148	39C8.18	32.0 ± 13.9	83.1
	149	39H7.3	39.0 ± 14.7	82.8
	150	41F2.1	70.2 ± 14.4	86.0
	151	KOLT-1	34.2 ± 23.7	65.8
LS	152	6-4	40.8 ± 23.1	91.2
T-Act	153	AA3	12.0 ± 14.5	7.3
LS	154	3-40	1.3 ± 0.5	3.7
LS	155	3-3	1.1 ± 0.5	3.0
PC	156	A3D8(irrad.)	98.4 ± 2.7	97.6
NC	157	P3(irrad.)	0.6 ± 0.2	2.0
NC	158	11G6(HTLV-8)	0.5 ± 0.3	1.7
T-Act	159	TAC	36.5 ± 17.9	41.1

[a] Abbreviations used: NC, negative control; PC, positive control; CD, cluster of differentiation; T-Act, T-activation; LS, leukemia specific.
[b] Mean ± standard deviation with leukemia cells of six ATL cases.
[c] Analysis with one double marker ATL case.

Table 29.3. Distribution of T cell associated antigens recognized by monoclonal antibodies on ATL cells and double marker ATL cells.

	ATL (6 cases)					Double marker ATL (1 case)				
		Distribution of antigens (%)[a]					Distribution of antigens (%)[a]			
Antibody group	Number of tests	3+	2+	1+	−	Number of tests	3+	2+	1+	−
CD1	42	0	0	0	100	7	0	0	0	100
CD2	96	90	8	2	0	16	100	0	0	0
CD3	66	64	14	15	8	11	91	9	0	0
CD4	84	88	1	1	10	14	86	7	0	7
CD5	54	44	6	22	28	9	56	11	22	11
CD6	12	50	0	33	17	2	100	0	0	0
CD7	96	11	15	8	66	16	63	6	0	31
CD8	120	0	0	2	98	20	80	5	0	15
Pan T other or unknown	114	53	7	12	28	19	74	11	5	11
T cell subset other	96	38	7	9	46	16	56	0	13	31
T-activation	114	11	19	30	39	19	26	11	26	37
Leukemia specific	18	6	17	6	72	3	33	0	0	67

[a] 3+: >70% positive cells; 2+: 70–40% positive cells; 1+: 40–10% positive cells; −: <10% positive cells.

References

1. Uchiyama, T., J. Yodoi, K. Sagawa, K. Takatsuki, and H. Uchino. 1977. Adult T-cell Leukemia: Clinical and hematologic features of 16 cases. *Blood* **50:**481.
2. Poiesz, B.J., F.W. Ruscetti, A.F. Gazdar, P.A. Bunn, J.D. Minna, and R.C. Gallo. 1980. Detection and isolation of type C retrovirus particles from fresh and cultured lymphocytes of a patient with cutaneous T-cell lymphoma. *Proc. Natl. Acad. Sci. U.S.A.* **77:**7415.
3. Yoshida, M., I. Miyoshi, and Y. Hinuma. 1982. Isolation and characterization of retrovirus from cell lines of human adult T-cell leukemia and its implication in the disease. *Proc. Natl. Acad. Sci. U.S.A.* **79:**2031.
4. Hattori, T., T. Uchiyama, T. Toibana, K. Takatsuki, and H. Uchino. 1981. Surface phenotype of Japanese adult T cell leukemia cells characterized by monoclonal antibodies. *Blood* **58:**645.
5. The T- and B-cell Malignancy Study Group. 1981. Statistical analysis of immunologic, clinical and histopathologic data on lymphoid malignancies in Japan. *Jpn. J. Clin. Oncol.* **11:**15.
6. Van Wauwe, J., J. Goossens, W. Decock, P. Kung, and G. Goldstein. 1981. Suppression of human T-cell mitogenesis and E-rosette formation by the monoclonal antibody OKT11A. *Immunology* **44:**865.
7. Reinherz, E.L., P.C. Kung, G. Goldstein, and S.F. Scholssman. 1979. Separation of functional subsets of human T cells by a monoclonal antibody. *Proc. Natl. Acad. Sci. U.S.A.* **76:**4061.

8. Kung, P.C., G. Goldstein, E.L. Reinherz, and S.F. Schlossman. 1979. Monoclonal antibodies defining distinctive human T cell surface antigens. *Science* **206**:347.

9. Thomas, Y., J. Sosman, O. Irigoyen, S.M. Friedman, P.C. Kung, G. Goldstein, and L. Chess. 1980. Functional analysis of human T cell subsets defined by monoclonal antibodies. I. Collaborative T-T interactions in the immunoregulation of B cell differentiation. *J. Immunol.* **125**:2402.

10. Stashenho, P., L.M. Nadler, R. Hardy, and S.F. Schlossman. 1980. Characterization of a human B lymphocyte-specific antigen. *J. Immunol.* **125**:1678.

11. Tatsumi, E., K. Sagawa, J. Mirro, C.I. Civin, H.D. Preisler, E.S. Henderson, and J. Minowada. 1981. Immunologic membrane phenotypes in human myeloid leukemia by monoclonal antibodies. *Cancer Res. (suppl).* **22**:181.

12. Tanaka, Y., Y. Koyanagi, T. Chosa, N. Yamamoto, and Y. Hinuma. 1983. Monoclonal antibody reactive with both p28 and p19 of adult T-cell leukemia virus-specific polypeptides. *Gann.* **74**:327.

13. Uchiyama, T., S. Broder, and T.A. Waldmann. 1981. A monoclonal antibody (anti-Tac) reactive with activated and functionally mature human T cells. I. Production of anti-Tac monoclonal antibody and distribution of Tac(+) cells. *J. Immunol.* **126**:1393.

14. Hinuma, Y., K. Nagata, M. Hanaoka, M. Nakai, T. Matsumoto, K. Kinoshita, S. Shirakawa, and I. Miyoshi. 1981. Adult T-cell leukemia: Antigen in an ATL cell line and detection of antibodies to the antigen in human sera. *Proc. Natl. Acad. Sci. U.S.A.* **78**:6476.

15. Reinherz, E.L., and S.F. Schlossman. 1980. The differentiation and function of human T lymphocytes. *Cell* **19**:821.

Part V. Phylogenetic Studies Using Anti–T Cell Antibodies

CHAPTER 30

The Phylogeny of T Cell Antigens

Margreet Jonker and Franciscus J.M. Nooij

Introduction

Human T cells express surface markers which can be identified by means of monoclonal antibodies (mAbs). It is possible to subdivide the T cells into functionally distinct subsets (1–5). Moreover, for some of these markers it is now known what role they play in the immune response. Thus, CD4 and CD8 are presumably involved in binding to the MHC class II or I antigens, respectively (6–8), of the target cells in the CML assay. The CD3 marker is involved in the lytic event of the CML after specific binding has taken place (9). The CD2 marker is also involved in the CML reaction, although its precise function is as yet unknown (10). Not all mAbs identifying these markers are able to block the above-mentioned functions, most likely because the epitopes recognized by the nonblocking antibodies are not involved in the immunological function of that molecule. It can be postulated that functional epitopes with a rather general function in the immune response not related to the specific immunological adaptation of one species will be preserved during evolution. On the other hand, functional epitopes which are responsible for immune functions related to the immunological adaptation of the species might be much less conserved throughout evolution.

It is of interest therefore to study these T cell markers in species other than man. Using subhuman primate species and a large panel of mAbs specific for T cell antigens, it is possible to define different epitopes for each T cell marker (11). It is also possible to define more or less conserved epitopes and correlate conservatism with the function of these epitopes. This knowledge will perhaps also be useful in the selection of mAbs as immunosuppressive agents to be used clinically for prevention of graft rejection or treatment of autoimmune diseases.

The panel of workshop T cell antibodies was tested on peripheral blood lymphocytes of nine primate species (including man).

Materials and Methods

Lymphocytes

Heparinized blood samples were obtained from the following primate species: man (*Homo sapiens*) (2), the chimpanzee (*Pan troglodytes*) (3); the gorilla (*Gorilla gorilla*) (1) and the orangutan (*Pongo pygmaeus*) (2) from the Hominoidae; the rhesus monkey (*Macaca mulatta*) (3), the stumptail monkey (*Macaca arctoides*) (2), the cynomolgus monkey (*Macaca fascicularis*) (3) and the African green monkey (*Cercopithecus aetiops*) (3) from the Cercopithecoidea or Old World monkeys; the common marmoset (*Callithrix jacchus*) (3) from the Ceboidea or New World monkeys. Lymphocyte suspensions were prepared by standard one-stage Ficoll–Hypaque gradient centrifugation. No further cell purification was done.

Immunofluorescence Assay

Lymphocyte pellets were incubated with the diluted antibodies for 30 min at 4°C. The cells were washed and then incubated with a fluorescence-labeled goat anti–mouse Ig antibody (CLB, Amsterdam) at 4°C for 30 min. The cells were washed and fixed overnight in 2% paraformaldehyde in PBS. They were then again washed and suspended in PBS for flow cytometric analysis using a modified FACS II (B and D) system. Electronic windows were set around the lymphocyte population using the forward and perpendicular light-scatter parameters. The fluorescence intensity of the lymphocytes was recorded using log amplification of the signal and a pulse height analyzer. For some antibodies, the specificity was determined on rhesus monkey cells using simultaneous staining with well-defined antibodies (12). Lymphocytes were then incubated with a Workshop antibody mixed with a reference antibody and with each of these two antibodies alone.

Data Analysis

The reactions were either complete (i.e., a distinct positive fluorescent peak was observed), incomplete (i.e., the fluorescence profile showed a positive shoulder) or negative. Examples of these reaction patterns are illustrated in Fig. 30.1(a), (b), and (c), respectively. For analysis of the data, a complete reaction was given a score of 1, an incomplete a score of ½, and a negative a score of 0. When two or more antibodies of the same putative CD group had identical scores in the nine primate species, these were considered to react with the same epitope of the CD molecule defined by the antibodies.

STUMPTAIL MACAQUE

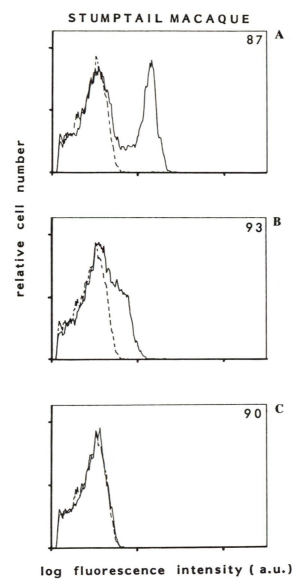

log fluorescence intensity (a.u.)

Fig. 30.1. Fluorescence profiles of three CD8 antibodies on lymphocytes of stumptail macaques. (A) a complete reaction, reactivity score 1; (B) an incomplete reaction, reactivity score of ½; and (C) a negative reaction, reactivity score of 0.

For each epitope, an (arbitrary) index of conservatism can be calculated. This index is defined by the number of species carrying the epitope divided by the total number of species tested. It gives only an indication of the evolutionary conservatism of the epitopes, since the evolutionary distance of the species is not taken into account.

Results

T Cell Antigen Phylogeny

Those antibodies classified in the Workshop panel into a particular CD group were analyzed. Antibodies which had reaction patterns in most species that suggested that they did not belong to that CD group were excluded from the analysis. Usually, the percentage of cells stained and the fluorescent profiles were similar in all species.

CD2

Thirteen epitopes could be defined (Table 30.1). Most of these were rather conservative. Nine had an index of conservatism of 0.67 or higher and were present in hominoids and macaques. The percent epitope sharing with man was correlated with the evolutionary distance of the species from man.

Table 30.1. Reactivity of CD2 antibodies on primates.

Epitope	mAbs	Hs[a]	Pt	Gg	Pp	Mm	Ma	Mf	Ca	Cj	Index of conservatism
a	18, 19, 20	1	1	1	1	1	1	1	½	1	0.94
b	16	1	1	1	1	1	1	½	½	1	0.89
c	25	1	1	1	1	1	1	1	0	½	0.83
d	27	1	1	1	1	1	1	1	½	0	0.83
e	28	1	1	1	1	1	1	½	1	0	0.83
f	17	1	1	1	½	1	1	½	½	0	0.72
g	21	1	1	1	1	½	1	½	½	0	0.72
h	22	1	1	½	1	1	1	½	0	0	0.67
i	14, 24	1	1	½	½	1	1	1	0	0	0.67
j	26	1	1	½	½	1	0	0	0	0	0.44
k	13	1	1	0	0	1	½	0	0	0	0.39
l	23	1	1	0	½	½	½	0	0	0	0.39
m	15	1	1	0	1	0	0	0	0	0	0.33
No. Epitopes present		13	13	8½	10	11	10	6½	3½	2½	
% Epitope sharing with man		100	100	65	77	85	77	50	27	19	

[a] Hs: *Homo sapiens*; Pt: *Pan troglodytes*; Gg: *Gorilla gorilla*; Pp: *Pongo pygmaeus*; Mm: *Macaca mulatta*; Ma: *Macaca arctoides*; Mf: *Macaca fascicularis*; Ca: *Cercopithecus aethiops*; Cj: *Callithrix jacchus*.

Table 30.2. Reactivity of CD3 antibodies on primates.

Epitope	mAbs	Reactivity score									Index of conservatism
		Hs[a]	Pt	Gg	Pp	Mm	Ma	Mf	Ca	Cj	
a	119	1	1	1	1	½	0	0	0	1	0.61
b	120	1	1	1	½	0	0	0	0	0	0.39
c	117, 118, 122, 123 124, 125, 126, 127	1	1	1	0	0	0	0	0	0	0.33
No. epitopes present		3	3	3	1½	½	0	0	0	1	
% Epitope sharing with man		100	100	100	50	17	0	0	0	33	

[a] For definition of abbreviations, see footnote to Table 30.1.

CD3

Three epitopes could be defined (Table 30.2). Only one occurred outside the hominoids and was present in the marmoset, while Old World monkeys were virtually negative with all antibodies. Thus, the percent epitope sharing with man was not completely related to the evolutionary distance of the species from man.

CD5

Nine epitopes could be defined (Table 30.3). Only four of these occurred outside the hominoids. The percent epitope sharing with man was correlated with the evolutionary distance of the species from man.

Table 30.3. Reactivity of CD5 antibodies on primates.

Epitope	mAbs	Reactivity score									Index of conservatism
		Hs[a]	Pt	Gg	Pp	Mm	Ma	Mf	Ca	Cj	
a	10	1	1	1	1	1	1	1	1	1	1.0
b	8	1	1	1	1	1	1	1	1	0	0.89
c	9	1	1	1	½	1	1	½	0	0	0.67
d	7	1	1	1	1	0	½	0	0	0	0.50
e	5	1	1	1	1	0	0	0	0	0	0.44
f	4	1	1	1	0	0	0	0	0	0	0.33
g	11	1	½	1	0	0	0	0	0	0	0.28
h	12	1	0	1	½	0	0	0	0	0	0.28
i	6	1	0	½	0	0	0	0	0	0	0.17
No. epitopes present		9	6½	8½	5	3	3½	2½	2	1	
% Epitope sharing with man		100	72	94	56	33	39	28	22	11	

[a] For definition of abbreviations, see footnote to Table 30.1.

Table 30.4. Reactivity of CD7 antibodies on primates.

Epitope	mAbs	Reactivity score									Index of conservatism
		Hs[a]	Pt	Gg	Pp	Mm	Ma	Mf	Ca	Cj	
a	29	1	1	0	½	1	½	½	½	0	0.56
b	39	1	1	1	1	0	0	0	0	0	0.44
c	32, 38, 40, 41, 43	1	1	1	½	0	0	0	0	0	0.39
d	33, 34, 44	1	1	½	½	0	0	0	0	0	0.33
e	30, 31	1	1	1	0	0	0	0	0	0	0.33
f	45	1	0	0	½	0	0	0	0	0	0.17
No. epitopes present		6	5	3½	3	1	½	½	½	0	
% Epitope sharing with man		100	83	58	50	17	8	8	8	0	

[a] For definition of abbreviations, see footnote to Table 30.1.

CD6

The two antibodies defined two different epitopes. Antibody T46 was reactive with all primate species. Antibody T47 reacted with hominoids and the marmoset.

CD7

Six epitopes could be defined (Table 30.4). Only one occurred in Old World monkeys, while none could be detected in the marmoset. Again, the percent epitope sharing with man was correlated with the evolutionary distance of the species from man.

Table 30.5. Reactivity of CD4 antibodies on primates.

Epitope	mAbs	Reactivity score									Index of conservatism
		Hs[a]	Pt	Gg	Pp	Mm	Ma	Mf	Ca	Cj	
a	76	1	1	1	1	1	1	1	1	1	1.0
b	69, 70	1	1	0	1	1	1	1	1	1	0.89
c	77	1	1	1	1	1	1	1	0	½	0.83
d	75	1	1	1	1	1	1	0	0	½	0.72
e	79	1	1	0	1	1	1	0	0	½	0.61
f	71	1	1	1	1	0	0	0	0	0	0.44
g	78	1	0	0	0	1	1	0	0	0	0.33
h	68, 72, 73, 74	1	1	0	1	0	0	0	0	0	0.33
i	80	1	½	0	0	0	0	0	0	0	0.17
No. epitopes present		9	7½	4	7	6	6	3	2	3½	
% Epitope sharing with man		100	83	44	78	67	67	33	22	39	

[a] For definition of abbreviations, see footnote to Table 30.1.

CD4

Nine epitopes could be defined (Table 30.5). Most occurred both in some of the hominoids and in some of the Old World monkeys. Surprisingly, the gorilla shared fewer epitopes with man than did two of the three macaque species, indicating either the loss of certain epitopes during evolution in the gorilla or the independent acquisition of these in some hominoids and some Old World monkeys.

CD8

Sixteen epitopes could be identified (Table 30.6). Most of these were rather conservative. Again the gorilla lacked epitopes present in Old World monkeys and the marmoset. Also some epitopes were present in the marmoset but absent in most Old World monkeys.

Overall Results

The data for all the antibodies analyzed are summarized in Fig. 30.2, where the percentages epitope sharing with man are depicted in histograms for each CD group in the nine primate species. It is clear that CD8, CD2, and CD4 are the most conservative molecules, while CD7 and CD3 are the least conservative ones. The assumed phylogenetic relationships

Table 30.6. Reactivity of CD8 antibodies on primates.

Epitope	mAbs	Hs[a]	Pt	Gg	Pp	Mm	Ma	Mf	Ca	Cj	Index of conservatism
a	83, 96	1	1	1	1	1	1	1	1	1	1.0
b	82, 84	1	1	1	1	1	1	1	1	0	0.89
c	88	1	1	0	1	1	1	1	1	1	0.89
d	95	1	1	1	1	1	1	1	1	0	0.89
e	81, 91	1	1	1	1	1	1	1	½	0	0.83
f	94	1	1	1	1	1	1	½	1	0	0.83
g	97	1	1	1	1	1	1	½	½	0	0.78
h	86, 89	1	1	0	1	1	1	1	1	0	0.78
i	87	1	1	0	0	1	1	1	1	1	0.78
j	99	1	1	1	½	1	1	½	½	0	0.72
k	85	1	1	0	1	1	1	½	½	0	0.67
l	93	1	1	1	1	1	1	0	0	0	0.67
m	92	1	1	1	1	1	0	0	0	1	0.67
n	90	1	1	0	1	1	0	0	1	1	0.67
o	98	1	½	1	1	1	0	0	0	0	0.50
p	100	1	0	1	1	0	0	0	0	0	0.33
No. epitopes present		16	14½	11	14½	15	12	9	10	5	
% Epitope sharing with man		100	91	69	91	94	75	56	63	31	

[a] For definition of abbreviations, see footnote to Table 30.1.

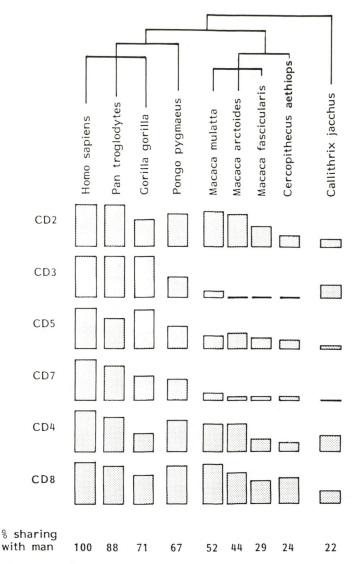

Fig. 30.2. Percent epitope sharing with man of T cell antigens among primate species. The phylogenetic relationships are indicated at the top of the figure. The bars represent the percent sharing (man, *Homo sapiens* is 100% for all CD groups). The percent sharing of all epitopes of these six CD antigens is given at the bottom of the figure.

of the species are indicated at the top of the figure. When all CD groups are considered together, the percent sharing with man is correlated with the phylogenetic distances of the species from man.

Specificity of T Cell Antibodies

The specificity of some antibodies was determined in rhesus monkeys using antibodies reactive with CD4, CD8, all T cells, and all B cells as reference antibodies.

This analysis revealed that some antibodies reacted with different subsets than did the other antibodies of the same putative CD group. Examples of these were: antibody T37 which was classified as CD7, but reacted with a CD8-like subset; antibody T121 which was classified as CD3, but was also reactive with a CD8-like subset in rhesus monkeys. These antibodies also reacted with a smaller percentage of cells in most other primate species than would be expected for a CD7 or CD3 antibody (see Table 30.7) and were therefore excluded from the evolutionary analysis described above. For other antibodies with aberrant reaction patterns such as listed in Table 30.7, the specificities were determined by use of rhesus monkey cells. Antibody T9 was reactive with a subset of T cells and also stained a smaller percentage of cells in other primate species than did other antibodies classified as CD5. Antibody T27 was reactive with all T cells in some monkeys, but with a subset of T cells in others. This antibody also stained a smaller percentage of cells in some other primate species. Antibody T95 was reactive with a subset of CD8 positive cells, ranging from 25 to 80% of the CD8 positive cells. The results for this

Table 30.7. Reactivity patterns of aberrant antibodies.

Antibody	CD group	% of Cells stained ($\times 10^{-1}$)								
		Hs[a]	Pt	Gg	Pp	Mm	Ma	Mf	Ca	Cj
T9	CD5	7	5	3	1	2	4	4	3	0
T10	CD5	9	7	9	8	8	8	9	9	5
T27	CD2	8	5	7	6	5	6	4	0	6
T18	CD2	8	8	8	6	7	8	6	2	0
T37	CD7	2	5	3	2	5	5	4	5	0
T29	CD7	8	4	0	0	8	3	0	0	0
T39	CD7	9	6	4	5	0	0	0	0	0
T95	CD8	2	2	2	1	4	2	2	3	0
T96	CD8	2	5	2	1	5	4	5	5	3
T121	CD3	6	8	7	3	5	4	5	4	0
T119	CD3	7	6	7	2	3	1	0	0	5

[a] For definition of abbreviations, see footnote to Table 30.1.

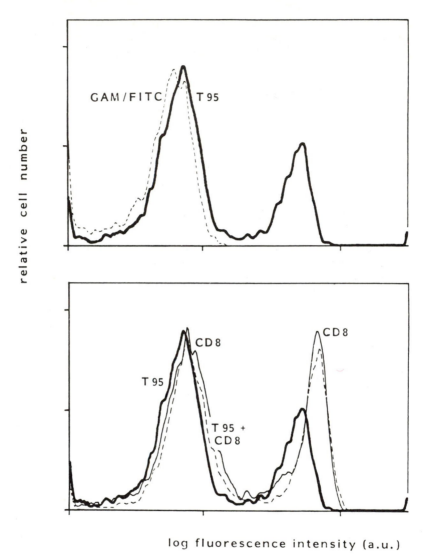

Fig. 30.3. Fluorescence profiles of rhesus monkey cells stained with antibody T95 (top panel), with a CD8-like reference antibody, and with a mixture of these two antibodies (bottom panel). T95: thick drawn line; goat anti-mouse/FITC control: dotted line in top panel; CD8: thin drawn line; T95 + CD8: dotted line in bottom panel.

antibody are depicted in Fig. 30.3. T95 stained 28% of the lymphocytes, a local rhesus specific CD8 antibody GM9 (12) stained 37% of them, and the mixture stained 39%, indicating that the T95 positive population is included in the CD8 positive population. When T95 was mixed with a CD4 or a B cell specific antibody, the percent of lymphocytes stained was additive. When T95 was mixed with a pan T cell antibody, no additional staining was observed. Again, in other primate species such as the chimpanzee and the other Old World monkeys, a smaller percentage of cells was stained by T95 than by the other CD8 antibodies.

Some of the unclassified antibodies could be classified in this manner as CD4 (T107), CD8 (T110 and T111), pan T (T108), and as a subset of CD8 (T115) in the rhesus monkey.

To determine whether the antibodies reacted with all T cells or with a subset thereof without using antibody mixtures, the percentage of cells stained was related to one pan T cell antibody used as a reference for all species: MT 910, a CD2 antibody which was also included in the Workshop panel (T18). Since cells of the African green monkey reacted poorly with this antibody, antibody T8 (CD5) was used as a reference for this species.

The CD2 and CD5 antibodies usually stained all T cells in all species. The CD3 antibodies stained 70 to 80% of the T cells in the chimpanzee, the gorilla, and the marmoset. Only 30 to 50% of the T cells were stained in the orangutan and rhesus monkey.

The CD7 antibodies stained only 50 to 70% of the chimpanzee and gorilla T cells, while the only antibodies reactive with orangutan and rhesus monkey stained 90% of the T cells.

The CD4 and CD8 antibodies reacted with T cell subsets in all species. However, the 4/8 ratios varied among the species. The ratios were higher than the 1.0 in hominoids and in the marmoset, but lower than the 1.0 in Old World monkeys. The percentages of the CD4 and CD8 positive cells when added together never exceeded 100% in any of the tested species.

One of the CD1 antibodies (T128) was clearly positive with a small subset in the orangutan, the rhesus monkey, and the stumptail macaque. Using antibody mixtures, it was shown that the cells stained by T128 were B cells in the rhesus monkeys.

Polymorphism of T Cell Antigens

Some antibodies appeared to detect polymorphisms in some of the primate species. Since only a limited number of individuals was tested in each species, it is to be expected that more polymorphisms exist. Table 30.8 summarizes the antibodies which were found to be polymorphic. The observed polymorphisms of the CD8 antibodies were confirmed in rhesus monkeys by repeatedly testing these antibodies in the same animals. Also, more rhesus monkeys were tested with these antibodies, including two sets of MHC identical siblings. Table 30.9 summarizes the results for the polymorphic CD8 antibodies in macaques. Most of the animals reacted with antibodies 93 and 37 only, while some showed different reaction patterns. Since antibodies 90 and 98 reacted differently with the cells of one set of MHC identical siblings, it is unlikely that the CD8 polymorphism is linked to the MHC.

Table 30.8. Polymorphic antibodies.[a]

mAb	CD group	Pt[b]	Mm	Ma	Mf	Ca	Cj
14	CD2		+		+		
17	CD2		+		+		
25	CD2						+
50	pan T						+
55	pan T		+		+	+	
56	pan T				+	+	
60	pan T				+		
67	CD4	+					
37	CD8		+				
85	CD8					+	
90	CD8					+	
92	CD8		+				
93	CD8		+		+		
98	CD8		+		+		+
102	T subset						+
114	T subset	+	+		+		
115	T subset		+		+		

[a] + Indicates polymorphism found.
[b] For definition of abbreviations, see Table 30.1.

Discussion

The phylogenetic relationships of the nine primate species used in this study as depicted in Fig. 30.2 are based on amino acid homologies of several proteins (13). The combined data for the T cell specific mAbs are in accord with these relationships, indicating that T cell surface markers are subject to the same evolutionary mechanisms as are other proteins in general.

When considering individual epitopes of the identified proteins, it was sometimes observed that an epitope occurred in hominoids and in the marmoset (as a representative of New World monkeys), but was almost absent in Old World monkeys. Similar findings were reported by Clark *et*

Table 30.9. Polymorphism of CD8 antibodies on macaques.

CD8 antibody	Reactivity scores									
	Rhesus							Stumptail	Cynomolgus	
	1[a]	1	2	1	1	1	11	2	1	2
93	1	0	½	1	1	1	1	1	½	0
37	1	0	1	1	1	0	1	1	1	1
98	1	1	½	½	0	0	0	0	½	0
90	0	1	0	½	½	0	0	0	0	0
92	0	1	½	0	0	0	0	0	0	0

[a] Number of monkeys with a particular reaction pattern.

al. (11). It is possible that these epitopes were lost in Old World monkeys and conserved in hominoids and marmosets (divergent evolution) or that they were acquired independently by the hominoids and marmosets (convergent evolution). Since two such epitopes belonged to CD8 (epitopes m and n, Table 30.6) and the antibodies defining them could block the CML reaction in man (this volume, Chapter 16), it can be speculated that similar forces were involved in selecting for these epitopes. Also, the more conservative CD8 epitopes were generally identified by antibodies which blocked the CML reaction (this volume, Chapter 16). This indicated that, at least for CD8, evolutionary conservatism is related to the function of the molecule. However, it should be tested whether the same antibodies block the CML reaction in lower primates as do so in man to confirm this. No such relationship between function and epitope conservatism was seen for CD2, CD3, or CD4 (this volume, Chapter 16).

The reaction patterns of the antibodies tested in subhuman primates were usually similar to those observed in man, indicating that the same structures were identified. A few exceptions were found. Some antibodies stained a smaller percentage of cells than did other antibodies classified into the same CD group in some or all primate species (see Table 30.7). When it is evident that an antibody has stained a subset of T cells rather than all T cells in some species or individuals, it can be concluded that such antibodies must react with a different structure than do the other antibodies of the same putative CD group. This means that, although perhaps in human studies no evidence is found for different molecular structures identified by, for instance, T9 and T10 (CD5), T27 or T18 (CD2), and T95 or T96 (CD8), the primate studies clearly indicate that this must be so.

It is possible that the antigens identified by these antibodies have a different cell distribution in some primates than in man, as was also the case with antibody T128 (CD1), which was expressed on a small subset in some primate species that could be identified as B cells in the rhesus monkey. Similar findings were reported for other antigens which were absent on human peripheral lymphocytes but present on peripheral cells of other primate species (11, 14). Since the precise functions of these molecules are not known, it is impossible to speculate on the reason for the different cellular expressions of T cell antigens.

As was observed in other studies (11, 15), it was found that epitopes which appear to be monomorphic in man are polymorphic in subhuman primate species. These findings may indicate that although polymorphic epitopes are rarely found in man (16), they do exist. It is perhaps due to the manner in which the mAbs are selected that not many polymorphic epitopes are found.

In conclusion, it can be stated that testing anti-human mAbs in subhuman primates can help to further analyze the molecular structures they identify. Also, the knowledge that antigens are expressed on subhuman primates in a similar fashion as in man may be useful when these antibodies are considered as immunosuppressive agents, as has already been done in the past (17, 18, 19).

Summary

The panel of T cell antibodies was tested against peripheral blood lymphocytes of eight primate species belonging to the families of Hominoidae and Cercopithecoidea (both Anthropoidea) and Ceboidea. For analysis of the data, the tentative CD group specifities were used unless we found clear evidence that an antibody did not belong to a certain CD group. Both the percent reactivity and fluorescent profiles of the FACS analysis were taken into account. Each CD group could be divided into antibodies with identical reactivity patterns in all eight primate species, presumably reacting with the same epitope of a particular CD molecule. Thus, a minimum number of epitopes could be determined for each CD group. The number of epitopes shared between man and subhuman primate species in each CD group was determined. It was found that CD8 was the most conservative group. CD7 and CD3 were the least conservative and were virtually only demonstrable in Homonioidae. Interestingly, some antibodies belonging to the CD8 group, all defining different epitopes, showed polymorphism in macaques.

Acknowledgments. The authors wish to thank Dr. J. Kreeftenberg, Dr. H.M. McClure, and Dr. M.T. Frankenhuis for providing non-human primate blood samples. The technical assistance of G. van Meurs and A. Kok is greatly acknowledged. We thank D. de Keizer and J. de Kler for their help in preparing the manuscript and Dr. A.C. Ford for his critical reading This work was supported in part by the Dutch ZWO-FUNGO Organization and the Nierstichting Nederland.

References

1. Meuer, S.C., S.F. Schlossman, and E.L. Reinherz. 1982. Clonal analysis of human cytotoxic T lymphocytes T4$^+$ and T8$^+$ effector T cells recognize products of different major histocompatibility complex regions. *Proc. Natl. Acad. Sci. U.S.A.* **79:**4395.
2. Spits, H., H. Yssel, A. Thompson, and J.E. deVries. 1983. Human T4$^+$ and T8$^+$ cytotoxic T lymphocyte clones directed at products of different class II major histocompatibility complex loci. *J. Immunol.* **131:**678.
3. Reinherz, E.L., P.C. Kun, G. Goldstein, and S.F. Schlossman. 1979. Separation of functional subsets of human T cells by a monoclonal antibody. *Proc. Natl. Acad. Sci. U.S.A.* **76:**4061.
4. Reinherz, E.L., S. Meuer, K.A. Fitzgerald, R.E. Hussey, H. Levine, and S.F. Schlossman. 1982. Antigen recognition by human T lymphocytes is linked to surface expression of the T3 molecular complex. Cell 30: 735.

5. Reinherz, E.L., R.E. Hussey, K.A. Fitzgerald, P. Snow, C. Terhorst, and S.F. Schlossman. 1981. Antibody directed at a surface structure inhibits cytolytic but not suppressor function of human T lymphocytes. *Nature* **299**:168.

6. Meuer, S., R.E. Hussay, J.C. Hodgdon, S.F. Schlossman, and E.L. Reinherz 1982. Surface structures involved in target recognition by human cytotoxic T lymphocytes. Science **218**:471.

7. Biddison, W.E., P.E. Rao, M.A. Talk., C.M. Boselli, and G. Goldstein. 1984. Distinct epitopes on the T8 moleculare are differentially involved in cytotoxic T cell function. *Hum. Immunol.* **9**:117.

8. Biddison, W.E., P.E. Rao, M.A. Talk, G. Goldstein, and S. Shaw. 1982. Possible involvement of the OKT4 molecule in T cell recognition of class II HLA antigens. *J. Exp. Med.* **156**:1065.

9. Landegren, U., U. Ramstedt, I. Axberg, M. Ullberg, M. Jondal, and H. Wigzell. 1982. Selective inhibition of human T cell cytotoxicity at levels of target recognition or initiation of lysis by monoclonal OKT3 and Leu-2a antibodies. *J. Exp. Med.* **155**:1579.

10. Martin, P., G. Longtong, J.A. Ledbetter, W. Newman, M.P. Braun, P.G. Beatty and J.A. Hansen. 1983. Identification and functional characterization of two distinct epitopes on the human T cell surface protein Tp50. *J. Immunol.* **131**:180.

11. Clark, E.A., P.J. Martin, J-A. Hansen, and J.A. Ledbetter. 1983. Evolution of epitopes on human and nonhuman primate lymphocyte cell surface antigens. *Immunogen.* **18**:599.

12. Jonker, M., and G. van Meurs. 1984. Monoclonal antibodies specific for B cells, cytotoxic/suppressor T cells and a subset of cytotoxic/suppressor T cells in the rhesus monkey. In: *Leukocyte typing,* A. Bernard, L. Boumsell, J. Dausset, C. Milstein, and S. Schlossman, eds. Springer-Verlag, Berlin, Heidelberg, pp. 328–336.

13. Goodman, M. 1975. Protein sequence and immunological specificity: their role in phylogenetic studies of primates. In: *The phylogeny of primates,* W. Luckett and F. Szalay, eds. Plenum Press, New York, London, pp. 219–248.

14. McKenzie, J.L., and J. Fabre. 1981. Human Thy-1: unusual localization and possible functional significance in lymphoid tissues. *J. Immunol.* **126**:843.

15. Parham, P., P.K. Seghal, and F.M. Brodsky. 1979. Anti HLA-A, -B, -C monoclonal antibodies with no alloantigenic specificity in humans defined polymorphisms in other primate species. Nature **279**:639.

16. Fuller, T.C., J.E. Trevithick, A.A. Fuller, R.B. Colvin, A.B. Cosimi, and P.C. Kung (1984). Antigenic polymorphism of the T4 differentiation antigen expressed on human T helper/inducer lymphocytes. *Hum. Immunol.* **9**:89.

17. Cosimi, A.B., R.C. Burton, R.C. Kung, R. Colvin, G. Goldstein, J. Lifter, W. Rhodes, and P.S. Russell. (1981) Evaluation in primate renal allograft recipients of monoclonal antibody to human T-cell subclasses. *Transplant. Proc.* **13**:499.

18. Jonker, M., G. Goldstein, and H. Balner. 1983. Effects of *in vivo* administration of monoclonal antibodies specific for human T cell subpopulations on the immune system in a rhesus monkey model. *Transplantation 35:*521.

19. Jonker, M., P. Neuhaus, C. Zurcher, A. Fuccello, and G. Goldstein. 1985. OKT4 and OKT4A antibody treatment as immunosuppression for kidney transplantation in rhesus monkeys. *Transplantation,* **39**:247.

CHAPTER 31

Conserved T Lymphocyte-Specific Antigens in Primates

Norman L. Letvin

Recent studies utilizing limited numbers of monoclonal antibodies (mAbs) reactive with subsets of human leukocytes have suggested that the phylogenetic relationship of primate species to man is reflected in the degree to which they share granulocyte and lymphocyte membrane antigenic structures (1–4). Because the extent of this antigenic conservation is so great among primate species, the expression of leukocyte surface antigens has proved to be a useful criterion for taxonomic classification of certain species (5). We have now confirmed and extended this observation of antigenic conservation utilizing a large panel of mAbs reactive with human T lymphocytes. T cell binding of 11 anti-T3, 14 anti-T4, and 20 anti-T8 reagents with peripheral blood lymphocytes (PBLs) of seven different primate species has been assessed. These studies suggest that the structure of T3 is not phylogenetically conserved to as great an extent as the structure of T4 and T8.

Materials and Methods

Animals

The family and representative species of the primates used in these studies include: Hominidae : man (2); Cercopithecidae : Guinea baboon (*Papio papio*) (1), rhesus monkey (*Macaca mulatta*) (4); Cebidae : owl monkey (*Aotus trivirgatus*) (4); Callitrichidae : common marmoset (*Callithrix jacchus*) (2), cotton-top tamarin (*Saguinus oedipus*) (4); Lemuridae : ring-tailed lemur (*Lemur fulvus*) (2). The numbers shown in parentheses indicate the number of animals of each species from which PBLs were examined.

Staining and Analysis of Peripheral Blood Lymphocytes

PBLs were prepared from heparinized venous blood of the primate species by density gradient centrifugation using a 9% Ficoll (Sigma, St. Louis, MO)/34% sodium diatrizoate (Sterling Drug, New York) solution having a specific gravity of 1.076 g/ml. The cells were treated with 0.15 M NH_4Cl to lyse erythrocytes and washed with Hanks' balanced salt solution containing 2.5% newborn calf serum. Aliquots of 1×10^6 cells were incubated with monoclonal antibodies at 4°C for 30 min. These cells were then washed twice with Hanks' balanced salt solution/2.5% pooled human AB serum and incubated with fluorescein isothiocyanate-conjugated goat anti–mouse Ig (TAGO, Burlingame, CA) for 30 min at 4°C. Each sample was washed twice with PBS and the cells were then analyzed on a fluorescence-activated cell sorter (FACS I; Becton Dickinson, Mountain View, CA).

Results and Discussion

The data shown in Tables 31.1 and 31.2 illustrate an impressive conservation of epitopes of the T4 and T8 structures in phylogenetically distant primate species. The extent of conservation of some of these epitopes—for example, those regions of T4 bound by mAbs 69 and 70 and of T8 bound by mAbs 83 and 89—is quite striking. In general, however, these data reinforce the observation that species that have recently diverged in

Table 31.1 The phylogenetic relationship of a primate species to man is reflected in the degree of their sharing of T4 epitopes.[a]

CD4 series	Man	Baboon	Rhesus monkey	Owl monkey	Common marmoset	Cotton-top tamarin	Ring-tailed lemur
67	53	—	—	17 ± 2	24 ± 10	13 ± 5	—
68	7	—	—	—	—	—	—
69	47	35	38 ± 4	30 ± 6	37 ± 6	17 ± 13	—
70	48	30	31 ± 2	17 ± 12	46 ± 1	18 ± 3	—
71	41	—	—	—	—	—	—
72	33	—	—	—	—	—	—
73	—	—	—	—	—	—	—
74	41	27	—	30 ± 15	—	—	—
75	48	—	21 ± 10	—	17 ± 7	—	—
76	34	—	18 ± 8	—	—	—	—
77	—	—	—	—	—	—	—
78	25	9	—	—	—	—	—
79	45	29	37 ± 10	—	—	—	—
80	10	—	—	—	—	—	—

[a] The data are expressed as the percent of PBLs staining positive ± SD. The symbol "—" denotes that <5% of the PBLs stained positively.

Table 31.2. T8 epitopes are conserved in distantly related primate species.[a]

CD8 series	Man	Baboon	Rhesus monkey	Owl monkey	Common marmoset	Cotton-top tamarin	Ring-tailed lemur
81	19 ± 7	26	17 ± 2	16 ± 3	—	—	—
82	16 ± 7	27	20 ± 3	—	—	—	—
83	16 ± 7	27	22 ± 4	33 ± 9	28 ± 1	16 ± 9	—
84	10 ± 4	24	16 ± 4	—	—	—	—
85	—	—	—	—	—	—	—
86	17 ± 7	23	25 ± 2	6 ± 3	—	—	—
87	12 ± 4	31	23 ± 2	—	—	—	—
88	10 ± 5	26	25 ± 1	—	32 ± 3	27 ± 14	—
89	22 ± 5	39	27 ± 1	31 ± 5	27 ± 7	22 ± 13	—
90	12 ± 1	—	—	—	—	—	—
91	24 ± 7	29	23 ± 3	21 ± 12	—	—	—
92	13 ± 7	—	—	—	—	—	—
93	7 ± 3	20	—	—	—	—	—
94	14 ± 5	24	16 ± 2	33 ± 8	—	—	—
95	16 ± 6	23	15 ± 2	—	—	—	—
96	11 ± 4	16	—	9 ± 4	23 ± 8	—	—
97	12 ± 2	25	17 ± 1	—	—	—	—
98	—	—	—	—	—	—	—
99	—	—	—	—	—	—	—
100	—	—	—	—	—	—	—

[a] The data are expressed as the percent of PBLs staining positive ± SD. The symbol "—" denotes that <5% of the PBLs stained positively.

evolution from man share more epitopes of T4 and T8 with man than those whose divergence occurred more remotely in time.

The data shown in Table 31.3 are therefore surprising. Very few of the antibodies in this panel which recognize the human T3 structure bind to T lymphocytes of non-human primates. This suggests that the structure of

Table 31.3. Little conservation of T3 epitopes exists in primate species.[a]

CD3 series	Man	Baboon	Rhesus monkey	Owl monkey	Common marmoset	Cotton-top tamarin	Ring-tailed lemur
117	41	—	—	—	—	—	—
118	64 ± 6	—	—	—	—	—	—
119	64 ± 3	—	12 ± 6	30 ± 9	50 ± 10	—	—
120	70	—	—	—	—	—	—
121	46	39	44 ± 12	41 ± 1	—	—	—
122	68 ± 5	—	—	—	—	—	—
123	67 ± 6	—	—	—	—	—	—
124	53 ± 3	—	—	—	—	—	—
125	69 ± 7	25	—	—	—	—	—
126	67 ± 3	—	—	—	—	—	—
127	33 ± 11	—	—	—	—	—	—

[a] The data are expressed as the percent of PBLs staining positive ± SD. The symbol "—" denotes that <10% of the PBLs stained positively.

T3 is not phylogenetically conserved to as great an extent as the structure of T4 and T8.

These mAbs should prove to be powerful tools in the study of spontaneous diseases in monkeys. For example, studies can now be done to define the abnormalities of lymphocytes seen in animals with the newly described macaque immunodeficiency syndrome (6). Also, spontaneous lymphomas and lymphoproliferative abnormalities occuring in macaques (7) can be characterized with these reagents. In addition, the experimentally induced lymphomas and lymphoproliferative disorders produced by *Herpes saimiri* and *Herpes ateles* in New World monkeys (8) can be more precisely defined. We have recently shown that monoclonal antibodies which recognize specific surface antigens on human lymphocytes can be used with an avidin–biotin immunoperoxidase technique to stain lymph nodes from non-human primates (9). The data presented in Tables 30.1, 30.2, and 30.3 should be useful for selecting the appropriate mAbs for such studies.

Finally, comparisons of the reactivity pattern of various mAbs with a series of PBLs from primate species may allow a convenient means of assessing whether particular mAbs recognize the same or different epitopes of a cell-surface molecule. For example, mAbs 82, 84, 87, 95, and 97, anti-T8 mAbs which react with baboon and rhesus PBL but not PBL of other primate species, may be recognizing the same epitope of T8.

Summary

Recent studies utilizing limited numbers of mAbs reactive with subsets of human leukocytes have suggested that the phylogenetic relationship of primate species to man is reflected in the degree to which they share granulocyte and lymphocyte membrane antigenic structures. We have confirmed this observation in assessing the reactivity of 11 anti-T3, 14 anti-T4, and 20 anti-T8 reagents with PBL of seven different primate species. These studies also demonstrate that significantly fewer of the anti-T3 antibodies react with various non-human primate PBL populations than do the anti-T4 and anti-T8 reagents. This suggests that the structure of T3 is not phylogenetically conserved to as great an extent as the structure of T4 and T8. Finally, only some epitopes of these T cell-specific antigenic structures are conserved between man and individual non-human primate species. Thus, for example, PBL of *Callithrix jacchus* reacted with five of the 14 anti–human T4 mAbs tested. Comparisons of the reactivity pattern of various mAbs with a series of PBL from primate species therefore allows a convenient means of assessing whether particular mAbs recognize the same or different epitopes of a cell-surface molecule. Anti-T8 which react with baboon and rhesus PBL but not PBL of other primate species may therefore be recognizing the same epitope of T8.

Acknowledgments. The technical assistance of Wayne R. Aldrich, Mary Kornacki, and David Leslie, and the assistance of Bettye-Jean Roy in the preparation of this manuscript are gratefully acknowledged. This work was supported by NIH grant AI 20729.

References

1. Haynes, B.F., B.L. Dowell, L.L. Hensley, I. Gore, and R.S. Metzgar. 1982. Human T cell antigen expression by primate T cells. *Science* **215**:298.
2. Letvin, N.L., R.F. Todd, L.S. Palley, S.F. Schlossman, and J.D. Griffin. 1983. Conservation of myeloid surface antigens on primate granulocytes. *Blood* **61**:408.
3. Letvin, N.L., N.W. King, E.L. Reinherz, R.D. Hunt, H. Lane, and S.F. Schlossman. 1983. T lymphocyte surface antigens in primates. *Eur. J. Immunol.* **13**:345.
4. Letvin, N.L., W.R. Aldrich, D.A. Thorley-Lawson, S.F. Schlossman, and L.M. Nadler. 1984. Surface antigen changes during B lymphocyte activation in primates. *Cell. Immunol.* **84**:163.
5. Palley, L.S., S.F. Schlossman, and N.L. Letvin. 1984. Common tree shrews and primates share leukocyte membrane antigens. *J. Med. Primatol.* **13**:67.
6. Letvin, N.L., K.A. Eaton, W.R. Aldrich, P.K. Sehgal, B.J. Blake, S.F. Schlossman, N.W. King, and R.D. Hunt. 1983. Acquired immunodeficiency syndrome in a colony of macaque monkeys. *Proc. Natl. Acad. Sci. U.S.A.* **80**:2718.
7. Hunt, R.D., B.J. Blake, L.V. Chalifoux, P.K. Sehgal, N.W. King, and N.L. Letvin. 1983. Transmission of naturally occurring lymphoma in macaque monkeys. *Proc. Natl. Acad. Sci. U.S.A.* **80**:5085.
8. Hunt, R.D., L.V. Melendez, N.W. King, C.E. Gilmore, M.D. Daniel, M.E. Williamson, and T.C. Jones. 1970. Morphology of a disease with features of malignant lymphoma in marmosets and owl monkeys inoculated with *Herpesvirus saimiri*. *J. Natl. Cancer Inst.* **44**:447.
9. Chalifoux, L.V., S.F. Schlossman, and N.L. Letvin. 1984. Delineation of lymphocyte subsets in lymph nodes of non-human primates. *Clin. Immunol. Immunopathol.* **31**:96.

Part VI. Study of Anti–T Cell Antibodies on Frozen Tissue Sections of Human Tissue

CHAPTER 32

Ontogeny of Human T Cell Antigens

David F. Lobach, Lucinda L. Hensley, Winifred Ho, and
Barton F. Haynes

Introduction

During early fetal ontogeny, the thymic rudiment is formed by a combination of mesodermal, endodermal, and ectodermal elements (1–4). Between 9 and 10 weeks of fetal gestation, the human epithelial thymus is colonized by blood-borne T cell precursors (3–6). Cortical-medullary partitioning of the thymus occurs at 14–15 weeks of gestation and Hassall's bodies, keratinized epithelial swirls in the medulla, first appear at 15–16 weeks of gestation (3–6). Thus by 16 weeks of gestation, thymic architecture resembles the morphology of postnatal thymus (3–6).

Monoclonal antibodies have been described which characterize both lymphocyte and T cell subsets. These reagents have been used to define antigenically maturation pathways of postnatal human thymocytes (7,8). It has been postulated that prothymocytes enter the thymus in the subcapsular cortex where they express antigen 3A1 and the sheep erythrocyte rosette receptor (9). Following migration from the subcapsular cortex to the cortex, thymocytes acquire the T6, T4, and T8 antigens. In the medulla and in scattered foci of the inner cortex, the T6 antigen is lost and the A1G3 (p80) antigen (10) and the T3 antigen are acquired (7,8). Medullary thymocytes reciprocally express T4 and T8 antigens (11,12). While pathways of thymocyte maturation are inferred from intra-thymic phenotypic studies on postnatal thymus (7,8,12), the order of appearance of human T cell antigens during ontogeny on T cell precursors and on mature thymocytes is not known.

In this study, we evaluated the reactivity patterns of a panel of anti–T cell antibodies on frozen thymus tissue sections from 7 weeks of gestation through birth using indirect immunofluorescence (IF). Our results revealed that all of the anti–T cell antibodies evaluated in this investigation (Table 32.1) reacted with human thymus by 12 weeks of fetal gestation. Of particular interest was the reactivity of anti-T3 monoclonal antibodies

Table 32.1. Monoclonal antibody specificity.

Antibody	Antigen/specificity
L17F12/Leu 1	T1/pan T cell
SK7/Leu 4	T3/pan T cell, T3 antigen associated with T cell antigen receptor.
T4/19Thy 5D7	T4/inducer T cell
NA1/34	T6/cortical thymocytes
T8/2T8-1C1	T8/suppressor T cells
F10-89-4	T200/pan leukocyte
3A1$_A$	3A1/pan T cell
35.1	Sheep erythrocyte rosette receptor
A1G3	p80, mature T cells
5E9	Transferrin receptor
DU-HL60-3	DU-HL60-3/monocytes, granulocytes, tissue macrophages
3F10	Nonpolymorphic determinant on Class I MHC molecule[a]
L243	Nonpolymorphic determinant on Class II MHC molecule
AE1	Low-molecular weight keratins

[a] MHC = Major histocompatibility complex.

with both thymocytes and thymic epithelial cells in fetal and postnatal thymus. Our findings suggest that a critical period for establishment of normal T cell maturation in human thymus occurs between 7 and 12 weeks of fetal gestation.

Methods

Tissue and Fixation

Human thymus tissue was obtained at the time of postmortem examination from 7 fetuses. Gestational age as determined by crown–rump length (13) or menstrual records ranged from 7 to 24 weeks. Full-term neonatal thymus and postnatal thymus (age 2 mo–12 yr) were also evaluated in this study. In addition to thymus tissue, the thorax and abdomen of a 7-week fetus (crown–rump length = 17 mm) were serially sectioned at 4-micron intervals from the liver through the oral cavity as described elsewhere (2,14–16).

Thymus specimens were divided into 5-mm cubes, snap frozen in a dry ice/ethanol slurry, and stored in liquid nitrogen. Tissue cubes were embedded in OCT compound (Lab Tek Products, Naperville, IL), cut into 4-μm sections, air dried, and fixed in cold (−20°C) acetone for 5 min. Sections were either used immediately in IF assays or stored at −70°C.

Monoclonal Antibodies

The specificities of the monoclonal antibodies used in this study are listed in Table 32.1 (10,17–27). Each antibody was used at an optimal saturating concentration as determined from titration experiments.

Antibodies 3A1 and AE1 were directly fluoresceinated using fluorescein isothiocyanate (Research Organics, Inc., Cleveland, OH) (fluorescence to protein ratio for 3A1 was 6.7 and for AE1 8.7; saturating titer for 3A1 was 1:50 and for AE1 1:100) as previously described in detail (28) for use in double IF assays.

Immunofluorescence Assays

Indirect IF was performed on acetone-fixed, 4-μm tissue sections as previously described (29). Stained sections were viewed on a Nikon optiphot microscope.

Double IF studies, as previously described in detail (28), were carried out using fluorescein-conjugated antibody 3A1 and antibody T200 on 7-week fetal thymus sections. Double immunofluorescence studies were also performed on postnatal thymus using fluorescein-conjugated antibodies AE1 and 3A1 with anti-T3 reagents.

Results

Reactivities of Monoclonal Reagents with the 7-Week Fetus

Evaluation of antibody reactivity with fetal tissue at 7 weeks of gestation afforded the opportunity to characterize both the thymic epithelial rudiment and T cell antigen expression on fetal lymphoid cells in perithymic mesenchyme, large vessels, and fetal liver prior to lymphoid colonization of the thymus. We have previously reported that the 7-week thymic epithelial rudiment reacted with antibody TE-4, a marker of keratinized, endocrine thymic epithelium in the subcapsular cortex and medulla, and with antibody A2B5, a marker of complex gangliosides found in neuroendocrine tissues (2). In the present study, we found that the 7-week thymic epithelial rudiment also reacted with anti-keratin antibody AE1 and anti-Ia antibody L243. It is important to note that thymic epithelium in the 7-week fetus did not react with antibody 3A1 or antibody T200, confirming that no lymphoid cells were present in the thymic rudiment.

With regard to T cell antigens, only antibodies T200 and 3A1 were found to react with single cells throughout the perithymic mesenchyme. Using double IF assays, the 3A1+ cells were shown to be a subset of the

T200+ cells. Antibody T4 reacted with scattered reticular (non-lymphoid appearing) cells in the mesenchyme surrounding fetal liver. Antibodies T1, T3, T6, T8, and 35.1 all failed to react with any tissues in the 7-week fetus.

Antibody A1G3 (anti-p80) reacted with epithelium and cells surrounding a subset of fetal gut segments; and antibody DU-HL60-3 reacted with single reticular cells (tissue macrophages) scattered throughout fetal tissue and also reacted with skin and spinal cord. Varying intensities of reactivity with antibody 5E9 (anti–transferrin receptor) were observed on >80% of the cells in the 7-week fetus.

In addition to reacting with the thymic rudiment, antibody AE1 (anti-keratin) reacted with thyroid, gut epithelium, notocord, and skin; and antibody L243 (anti-Class II MHC antigen) reacted with thyroid, skin, cartilage, spinal cord, notocord, spinal ganglia, and rim-positive single cells in fetal mesenchyme. While absent on the fetal thymus, tissue reactivity with antibody 3F10 (anti-Class I MHC antigen) was observed with fetal thyroid, skin, notocord, trachea, gut and esophageal epithelia, and single cells throughout fetal mesenchyme.

Reactivity of Monoclonal Reagents Following Lymphocyte Colonization of the Thymus (10 weeks of fetal gestation through birth)

Antibody reactivity was evaluated on fetal thymic tissue at 10, 12, 15, 16, 18, and 24 weeks of gestation (Fig. 32.1). Additionally, reactivity was assayed with fetal spleen and liver at 16 weeks of gestation. As expected from their presence at 7 weeks of gestation, antibodies T200 and 3A1 reacted with thymocytes from 10 weeks of gestation through birth. Furthermore, antibody 5E9 reactivity was present on 1 to 5% of thymocytes in the subcapsular cortex, inner cortex, and interlobular septae from 10 weeks of gestation through birth.

Antibodies T1, T4, and T8, which failed to react with 7-week fetal lymphoid tissue, all reacted with fetal thymocytes from 10 weeks of gestation through birth. Antibodies T3 and T6 first reacted with fetal thymus at 12 weeks of gestation; initially, antibodies T6 and T3 reacted with thymocytes throughout the thymus. Antibody T6 reactivity changed to the cortical thymocyte staining pattern characteristic of postnatal thymus by 15 weeks of gestation after cortico-medullary partitioning of the thymus occurred. Antibody T3 reactivity, on the other hand, was maintained throughout the thymus through birth.

Evaluation of four postnatal thymuses (age 2 mo, 6 mo, 11 mo, and 12 yr) with five anti-T3 reagents (SK7/Leu 4, T3/2Ad2A2, T3/2T8-2F4, T3/RW2-4B6, and T3/RW2-8C8) also revealed pan-thymic reactivity in a pattern suggestive of both anti-thymocyte and anti–epithelial cell reactiv-

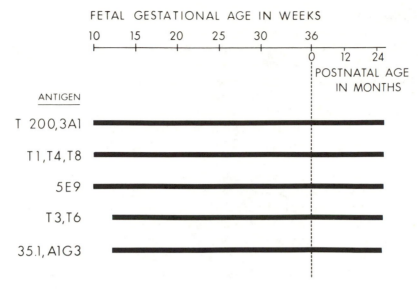

Fig. 32.1. Acquisition of T cell antigens during ontogeny. Cells reacting with antibodies T200, 3A1, T1, T4, T8, and 5E9 were present at 10 weeks of gestation in the fetal thymus. By 12 weeks of gestation, cells reacting with antibodies T3, T6, 35.1, and A1G3 were identified in fetal thymus.

ity. Double IF assays comparing two anti-T3 antibodies (SK7/Leu 4 and T3/2T8-2F4) with anti-keratin antibody AE1 and anti-thymocyte antibody 3A1 confirmed the reactivity of both thymocytes and thymic epithelial cells with anti-T3 antibodies in thymic tissue frozen sections.

Thymocyte reactivity with antibodies 35.1 (anti–E-rosette receptor), and A1G3 also first appeared at 12 weeks gestation. After 15 weeks gestation, all anti-thymocyte reagents tested reacted in patterns characteristic of postnatal thymus. Finally, anti-HLA (3F10) and anti-Ia (L243) antibodies reacted with thymocytes and/or thymic epithelium in patterns similar to their reactivity with postnatal thymus.

While all of the anti-T-cell reagents evaluated reacted with thymus by 16 weeks of gestation, not all of these reagents reacted with lymphoid cells in 16-week fetal liver or spleen. Antibodies T1, T4, 3A1, and A1G3 reacted with cells in 16-week fetal liver, while antibodies T3, T6, T8, and 35.1 were non-reactive. In 16-week fetal spleen, only antibodies T6 and 35.1 were non-reactive while T1, T3, T4, T8, 3A1, and A1G3 antibodies reacted with lymphoid cells.

Discussion

In this study we used a panel of monoclonal reagents against T cell antigens, cell activation antigens, and MHC-encoded antigens to map the ontogeny of human T cell and MHC-encoded antigens. Additionally, we evaluated the reactivity of these reagents with tissue from a 7-week fetus at a time prior to lymphoid colonization of the thymus. Finally, we have investigated the reactivities of anti-keratin monoclonal antibody AE1 and anti-macrophage monoclonal antibody DU-HL60-3 with these same tissues.

We found that a subset of single cells which reacted with the pan-leukocyte marker T200 also reacted with antibody 3A1 at a time prior to lymphocyte colonization of the thymus. Moreover, antigens reacting with antibodies T1, T4, and T8 were present on thymocytes by 10 weeks of gestation, and antigens reacting with antibodies T3, T6, 35.1, and A1G3 were present on thymocytes by 12 weeks of gestation.

While our study is limited by the amount of tissue available from prenatal thymuses such that only indirect immunofluorescence can be performed on frozen tissue sections, several important points can be made.

First, the appearance of antigens 3A1 and T200 on lymphoid cells in perithymic mesenchyme strongly suggests that these antigens do not require passage through the thymus for expression, whereas intra-thymic passage may be required for T4, T8, T3, T6, and p80 expression on lymphoid cells. Several lines of evidence have accrued to suggest that 3A1 is an early marker of the human T cell lineage. Prothymocytes present in the subcapsular cortex of postnatal thymus express the 3A1 antigen which is preserved throughout T cell development (9). These 3A1+ subcapsular cortical thymocytes are postulated to represent T cells at the earliest stage of intra-thymic maturation (9). Phenotypic analysis of T cells in acute lymphoblastic leukemia (ALL) using anti–T cell antibodies revealed heterogeneity of T cell antigen expression with 3A1 the only T cell-specific antigen detected on most T-ALL leukemic cells (30,31). From this analysis of T-ALL, antibody 3A1 serves as the best marker of immature malignant T cells, and, if one assumes that the phenotype of malignant T cells mirrors stages of normal T cell maturation, the 3A1 antigen likely is acquired at an early stage of T cell differentiation.

Recent evidence suggests some 3A1+ ALL cells are leukemic multipotent stem cells (32). In support of the suggestion that the 3A1 antigen may be expressed on a lymphoid–myeloid stem cell, cases of acute myelogenous leukemia have been reported in which malignant cells bear both characteristic myeloid differentiation antigens and the 3A1 antigen (33). The appearance of cells reacting with antibody 3A1 prior to lymphoid colonization of the fetal thymus is consistent with the designation of 3A1 as an early T cell lineage differentiation antigen.

The monomorphic 20- to 25-Kd T3 molecule and the 90-Kd Ti (T cell antigen receptor) form a complex on the T cell surface (34) and appear to be concomitantly expressed intra-thymically by T-cells. Additionally, re-arrangement of the Ti gene has been detected in thymocytes (35). The association of Ti with the T3 molecule suggests that Ti may also be expressed by 12 weeks of fetal gestation. Since intra-thymic rearrangement is a prerequisite for Ti surface expression, development of the T cell antigen receptor repertoire likely is initiated between 10 and 12 weeks in fetal thymus. Interestingly, monoclonal anti-T3 reagents reacted not only with thymocytes but also with thymic epithelial cells. The T3–Ti complex or related antigens on thymic epithelial cells may serve as receptors for the obligatory thymocyte–thymic epithelial contact required during intra-thymic T cell maturation. Alternatively, the presence of anti-T3 reactivity on keratin-containing thymic epithelial cells might reflect either passive absorption *in vivo* of T3 antigen to a surface receptor for T3 antigen on thymic epithelium or antigenically cross-reactive determinants expressed in thymocytes and thymic epithelial cells.

The development of the T cell repertoire during early ontogeny is consistent with the early detection of lymphoid cell function including NK cell activity, mitogen-induced T cell proliferation, and antibody production (36,37). Furthermore, B cell differentiation, which is a T cell-dependent process, occurs between 12 and 20 weeks of gestation in the human, at a time after the T cell repertoire presumably has been established (38).

Therefore, in man the critical period for the development of the thymus and presumably diversification of the T cell repertoire appears to be between 7 and 12 weeks of fetal gestation. Biochemical, molecular, and functional studies of human T cells should focus on this critical window of time in thymic development.

Summary

Human thymus tissue was examined from 7 weeks of gestation through birth for the expression of antigens reacting with a panel of anti–T cell monoclonal antibodies. Additionally, the reactivity of reagents against the transferrin receptor, leukocytes, low-molecular weight keratins, and major histocompatibility complex (MHC) antigens was studied on human fetal thymic tissue. Frozen tissue sections were evaluated using single and double immunofluorescence assays. At 7 weeks of gestation, no lymphoid cells were identified in the thymus; however, scattered cells reacting with both antibody 3A1, a pan T cell marker, and antibody T200, a pan leukocyte reagent, were identified in perithymic mesenchyme. Following lymphoid colonization of the thymic rudiment at 10 weeks of fetal gestation, fetal thymic tissue reacted with antibodies T1, T4, and T8. At 12 weeks of gestation, antibodies T3, T6, A1G3 (anti-p80, a marker of mature thymocytes), and 35.1 (anti–E-rosette receptor) all reacted with thymic tissue. Our results show that the 3A1 antigen is acquired very early in ontogeny and that passage through the thymus may not be required for the expression of the 3A1 antigen by T cell precursors. Furthermore, anti-T3 monoclonal antibodies reacted with both thymocytes and thymic epithelial cells in indirect immunofluorescence assays on fetal and postnatal thymus. Finally, by 16 weeks of fetal gestation, human thymic architecture and thymocyte antigen expression resembled the morphology and antigenic reactivity of normal postnatal thymus.

Acknowledgments. This work was supported by a Basic Research Grant from the National March of Dimes Foundation. Portions of this chapter have been published (*J. Immunol.* **135:**1752–1759, 1985) and are used here with permission.

References

1. Haynes, B.F. 1984. The human thymic microenvironment. *Adv. Immunol.* **36:**87.
2. Haynes, B.F., R.M. Scearce, D.F. Lobach, and L.L. Hensley. 1984. Phenotypic characterization and ontogeny of mesodermal-derived and endocrine epithelial components of the human thymic microenvironment. *J. Exp. Med.* **159:**1149.
3. Weller, G.L. 1933. Development of the thyroid, parathyroid and thymus glands in man. *Contrib. Embryol. Carnegie Inst.* **22:**95.
4. Norris, E.H. 1938. The morphogenesis and histogenesis of the thymus gland in man: In which the origin of the Hassall's corpuscles of the human thymus is discovered. *Contrib. Embryol. Carnegie Inst.* **27:**193.
5. Haar, J.L. 1974. Light and electron microscopy of the human fetal thymus. *Anat. Rec.* **179:**463.
6. vonGaudecker, B., and H.K. Muller-Hermelink. 1978. Ontogenetic differentiation of epithelial and non-epithelial cells in the human thymus. *Adv. Exp. Med. Biol.* **114:**19.
7. Reinherz, E.L., P.C. Kung, G. Goldstein, R.H. Levey, and S.F. Schlossman. 1980. Discrete stages of human intrathymic differentiation: Analysis of normal thymocytes and leukemic lymphoblasts of T-cell lineage. *Proc. Natl. Acad. Sci. U.S.A.* **77:**1588.
8. Reinherz, E.L., and S.F. Schlossman. 1980. The differentiation and function of human T lymphocytes. *Cell* **19:**821.
9. Haynes, B. F. 1984. Phenotypic characterization and ontogeny of the human thymic microenvironment. *Clin. Res.* **32:**500.
10. Haynes, B.F., E.A. Harden, M.J. Telen, M.E. Hemler, J.L. Strominger, T.J. Palker, R.M. Scearce, and G.S. Eisenbarth. 1983. Differentiation of human T lymphocytes I. Acquisition of a novel human cell surface protein (p80) during normal intrathymic T cell maturation. *J. Immunol.* **131:**1195.

11. Reinherz, E.L., P.C. Kung, G. Goldstein, and S.F. Schlossman. 1979. Further characterization of the human inducer T-cell subset defined by monoclonal antibody. *J. Immunol.* **123:**2894.

12. Bhan, A.K., E.L. Reinherz, S. Poppema, R.T. McCluskey, and S.F. Schlossman. 1980. Location of T cell and major histocompatibility complex antigens in the human thymus. *J. Exp. Med.* **152:**771.

13. Hamilton, W.J., J.D. Boyd, and H.W. Mossman. 1962. *Human embryology*. The Williams and Wilkins Company, Baltimore, pp. 119–134.

14. Patten, B.M. 1968. *Human embryology*. McGraw-Hill, New York, pp. 427–448.

15. Gasser, R.F. 1975. *Atlas of human embryos*. Harper and Row, Hagerstown, Maryland, pp. 163–240.

16. Hamilton, W.J., J.D. Boyd, and H.W. Mossman. 1962. *Human embryology*. The Williams and Wilkins Company, Baltimore, pp. 223–224.

17. Haynes, B.F. 1981. Human T lymphocyte antigens as defined by monoclonal antibodies. *Immunol. Rev.* **57:**127.

18. Kung, P.C., G. Goldstein, E.L. Reinherz, and S.F. Schlossman. 1979. Monoclonal antibodies defining distinctive human T cell surface antigens. *Science* **206:**347.

19. Reinherz, E.L., P.C. Kung, G. Goldstein, and S.F. Schlossman. 1979. A monoclonal antibody with selective reactivity with functionally mature human thymocytes and all peripheral human T cells. *J. Immunol.* **123:**131.

20. Reinherz, E.L., P.C. Kung, G. Goldstein, and S.F. Schlossman. 1979. Further characterization of the human inducer T cell subset defined by monoclonal antibody. *J. Immunol.* **123:**2894.

21. McMichael, A.J., J.R. Pilch, G. Galfre, D.Y. Mason, J.W. Fabre, and Cesar Milstein. 1979. A human thymocyte antigen defined by a hybrid myeloma monoclonal antibody. *Eur. J. Immunol.* **9:**205.

22. Dalchau, R., J. Kirkley, and J.W. Fabre. 1980. Monoclonal antibody to a human leukocyte specific membrane glycoprotein probably homologous to the leukocyte common (LC) antigen of the rat. *Eur. J. Immunol.* **10:**737.

23. Haynes, B.F., G.S. Eisenbarth, and A.S. Fauci. 1979. Human lymphocyte antigens: Production of a monoclonal antibody that defines functional thymus-derived lymphocyte subsets. *Proc. Natl. Acad. Sci. U.S.A.* **76:**5829.

24. McKolanis, J.R., M.J. Borowitz, F.L. Tuck, and R.S. Metzgar. 1984. Membrane antigens of human myeloid cells defined by monoclonal antibodies. In: *Leucocyte typing*, A. Bernard, L. Boumsell, J. Dausset, C. Milstein, and S. Schlossman, eds. p 387–394. Springer-Verlag, Berlin, Heidelberg.

25. Haynes, B.F., E.G. Reisner, M.E. Hemler, J.L. Strominger, and G.S. Eisenbarth. 1982. Description of a monoclonal antibody defining an HLA allotypic determinant that includes specificities within the B5 cross reacting group. *Hum. Immunol.* **4:**273.

26. Lampson, L., and R. Levy. 1980. Two populations of Ia-like molecules on a human B cell line. *J. Immunol.* **125:**293.

27. Woodcock-Mitchell, J., R. Eichner, W.G. Nelson, and T.-T. Sun. 1982. Immunolocalization of keratin polypeptides in human epidermis using monoclonal antibodies. *J. Cell Biol.* **95:**580.

28. Haynes, B.F., D.L. Mann, M.E. Hemler, J.A. Schroer, J.A. Shelhamer, G.S.

Eisenbarth, C.A. Thomas, H.S. Mostowski, J.L. Strominger, and A.S. Fauci. 1980. Characterization of a monoclonal antibody which defines an immunoregulatory T cell subset for immunoglobulin synthesis in man. *Proc. Natl. Acad. Sci. U.S.A.* **77**:2914.

29. Haynes, B.F., L.L. Hensley, and B.V. Jegasothy. 1982. Differentiation of human T lymphocytes II. Phenotypic difference in skin and blood malignant T cells in cutaneous T cell lymphoma. *J. Invest. Dermatol.* **78**:323.

30. Mann, D.L., B.F. Haynes, C. Thomas, D. Cole, A.S. Fauci, and D.G. Poplack. 1983. Heterogeneity of acute lymphocytic leukemia cell surface markers as detected by monoclonal antibodies. *J. Natl. Cancer Inst.* **71**:11.

31. Haynes, B.F., R.S. Metzgar, J.D. Minna, and P.A. Bunn. 1981. Phenotypic characterization of cutaneous T-cell lymphoma. Use of monoclonal antibodies to compare with other malignant T cells. *New England J. Med.* **304**:1319.

32. Hershfield, M.S., J. Kurtzberg, E. Harden, J.O. Moore, J. Whang-Peng, and B.F. Haynes. 1984. Conversion of a stem cell leukemia from a T-lymphoid to a myeloid phenotype induced by the adenosine deaminase inhibitor 2'-deoxycoformcin. *Proc. Natl. Acad. Sci. U.S.A.* **81**:253.

33. Sutherland, D.R., C.E. Rudd, and M.F. Greaves. 1984. Isolation and characterization of a human T lymphocyte associated glycoprotein (gp40). *J. Immunol.* **133**:327.

34. Meuer, S.C., D.A. Cooper, J.C. Hodgdon, R.E. Hussey, K.A. Fitzgerald, S.F. Schlossman, and E.L. Reinherz. 1983. Identification of the receptor for antigen and major histocompatibility complex on human inducer T-lymphocytes. *Science* **222**:1240.

35. Toyonaga, B., Y. Yanagi, N. Sucui-Foca, M. Minden, and T.W. Mak. 1984. Rearrangements of T-cell receptor gene YT35 in human DNA from thymic leukemia T-cell lines and functional T-cell clones. *Nature* **311**:385.

36. Hayward, A.R. 1981. Development of lymphocyte responses and interactions in the human fetus and newborn. *Immunol. Rev.* **57**:39.

37. Torvanen, P., J. Uksila, A. Leino, O. Lassila, T. Hirvonen, and O. Ruuskanen. 1981. Ontogeny of B cell markers in the human fetal liver. *Immunol. Rev.* **57**:89.

38. Hofman, F.M., J. Danilovs, L. Husmann, and C.R. Taylor. 1984. Development of mitogen responding T cells and natural killer cells in the human fetus. *J. Immunol.* **133**:1197.

CHAPTER 33

Cross-reactivity of Anti-lymphocyte Monoclonal Antibodies on Human Skin Components

Jean Brochier and Daniel Schmitt

Monoclonal antibodies have become extraordinary specific tools for identifying cell subpopulations such as, for example, lymphocytes. In utilizing them in such a manner, it has become clear that due to their specificity for a given epitope, they can also give apparent loss of specificity when reacting with one epitope shared by two different unrelated antigens. We have prepared monoclonal antibodies against human lymphoid cells with the aim of selecting antibodies specific for antigens defining lymphocyte subpopulations. In the course of the selection process, we screened hybridoma supernatants on normal human skin as a non-lymphoid organ. We found unexpected and interesting staining patterns (1) which led us to generalize these control screenings and to select monoclonal antibodies recognizing most human skin cells. The 159 monoclonal antibodies of the panel for T cell studies were screened on human skin sections in the same manner; 21 of them were found to react on skin components. The possible biological significances of these cross-reactivities will be discussed.

Materials and Methods

Monoclonal antibodies were prepared by fusing SP2/0 myeloma cells with splenocytes from BALB/c mice immunized with various human lymphoid cells according to the technique of Köhler and Milstein (2). The antibodies most typically used in this study are listed in Table 33.1. In addition, two anti-keratin monoclonal antibodies, KL1 (3) and KL3 (4), were used, as well as the 159 monoclonal antibodies of the panel for T cell studies from the Second International Workshop on Human Leukocyte Differentiation Antigens (Boston, 1984).

Normal human skin was obtained as discarded material from surgical operations. Indirect immunofluorescence was performed on 4-μm frozen sections using a fluoresceinated goat anti–mouse immunoglobulin antiserum (Meloy, Springfield, VA).

Table 33.1. Characteristics of mouse monoclonal antibodies prepared against human lymphoid cells cross-reacting with normal human skin components.

Name of antibody	Isotype	Immunogen	Lymphoid specificity
BL2	IgG2b	B-CLL	HLA-class II
BL6	IgG1	Thymocytes	CD1
BL7	IgM	Thymocytes	Thymic epithelial cells
BL9	IgG3	Raji cell line	All leukocytes
HB8	IgG1	Thoracic duct lymphocytes	All leukocytes
HB10	IgM	U266 cell line	Still unknown
HB11	IgM	U266 cell line	Still unknown
HB12	IgM	U266 cell line	Still unknown

Results

Specificity of BL, HB, and KL Antibodies on Skin

As shown in Table 33.2, the major types of skin cells were stained by the various antibodies. All keratinocytes were stained by BL9 [Fig. 33.1(a)] and KL3 [Fig. 33.1(b)] antibodies. The density of the antigen revealed by BL9 decreased from the basal layer to the stratum granulosum, whereas the opposite was seen with KL3. Only basal keratinocytes were stained by BL7 [Fig. 33.1(c)], whereas suprabasal keratinocytes reacted with HB10 [Fig. 33.1(D)] and with KL1 specific for 55–57-Kd keratin polypeptides (3). The epidermal granular layer was stained by HB12 [Fig. 33.1(e)] and the dermal–epidermal junction was decorated by HB11 [Fig. 33.1(f)].

In the epidermis, Langerhans cells appeared to bear HLA-class II antigens and the 49-Kd antigens characteristics of the CD1 group, which confirms previous observations (5–7). Various cells or fibrous compo-

Table 33.2. Specificity of BL, HB, and KL antibodies on skin.

Skin components	C/M[a]	Antibody	Isotype	Immunogen or specificity
Epidermis				
Epidermal granular layer	C	HB12	IgM	Plasma cell
Suprabasal keratinocytes	C	HB10	IgM	Plasma cell
	C	KL1	IgG1	55–57-Kd keratin
Basal keratinocytes	C	BL7	IgM	Epithelial thymic cells
Total keratinocytes	M	BL9	IgG3	All leukocytes
	M	KL3	IgM	?
Langerhans cells	M	BL2	IgG2b	HLA-class II
	M	BL6	IgG1	CD1 (49 Kd)
Dermo–epidermal junction		HB11	IgM	Plasma cell
Dermis				
Elastic fiber glycoproteins		HB8	IgG1	All leukocytes
Oxytalan fiber glycoproteins				
Histiocytes	M	BL2	IgG2b	HLA-class II

[a] C: cytoplasmic, M: membrane immunofluorescence staining.

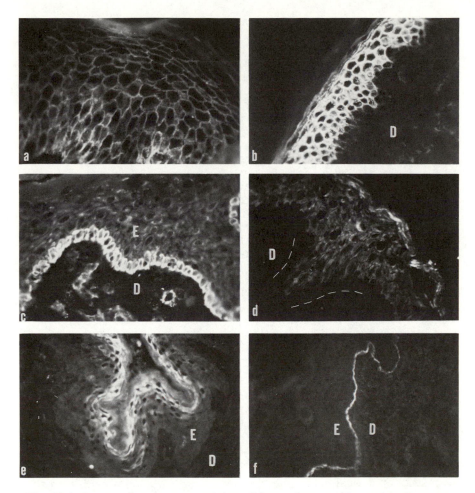

Fig. 33.1. Immunofluorescence staining of frozen human skin sections by mono-clonal antibodies BL9 (a), KL3 (b), BL7 (c), HB10 (d), HB12 (e), and HB11 (f). D = dermis; E = epidermis.

nents could be identified in the dermis—for example, elastic fibers by HB8 antibody (8), or histiocytes which express HLA-class II antigens revealed by BL2.

Cross-reactivity of the 159 Antibodies of the T Cell Panel on Skin

Among the 159 monoclonal antibodies expected to be specific for T cells, 21 reacted with skin components (Table 33.3).

Five of the seven anti-CD1 antibodies stained Langerhans cells. The isotype was identified in three cases and was found to be IgG. M241 and 4A76 antibodies did not stain any skin component.

Table 33.3. Cross-reactivity of the 159 antibodies of the T cell panel.

Antibody	Original cluster group[a]	Isotype	C/M[b]	Skin specificity
NA1/34	CD1	NK[c]	M	Langerhans cells
SK9/Leu 6	CD1	IgG2b	M	Langerhans cells
10D12.2	CD1	IgG1	M	Langerhans cells
NU-T2	CD1	IgG1	M	Langerhans cells
I19	CD1	NK	M	Langerhans cells
BW264/217	CD7	IgM	C	Epidermal granular layer
T4/7T4-6Cl	CD4	IgM	C	Epidermal granular layer
CRIS-5	T Subset	IgM	C	Basal keratinocytes
T10B9	Pan T	IgM	C	Suprabasal keratinocytes
CRIS-8	Pan T	IgG	C	Suprabasal keratinocytes
100-1A5	T-activ.	NK	C	Suprabasal keratinocytes
66-1	CD4	IgM	C	All epidermal cells
A3D8	Positive control	IgG	M	All epidermal cells
T3/2T8-F4	CD3	IgG1	C	Dermal fibroblasts
3-40	Leukemia	IgM	C	Dermal fibroblasts
TQ1/28T17G6	T subset	IgG1	M	Vascular endothelium
GM1	T subset	IgG1	M	Vascular endothelium
T3/2Ad2A2	CD3	IgM	M	Vascular endothelium
K20	Pan T	NK	C	Smooth muscles ?
T8/2T8-2A1	CD8	IgG2b	C	Nervous fibers ?
BW264/56	CD3	IgG2a	C	Unidentified dermal cells

[a] See Chapter 1 for final antibody cluster group.
[b] C: cytoplasmic, M: membrane fluorescence staining.
[c] NK: not known.

Eight antibodies reacted against epidermal cells, two against the epidermal granular layer (HB12-like), one against the basal keratinocytes (BL7-like), three against the suprabasal keratinocytes (HB10-like), and two against all epidermal cells, one binding to surface determinants and the other to cytoplasmic structures. Five of the seven identified isotypes were IgM.

Eight antibodies were directed to dermal components. Two stained the dermal fibroblasts and three the vascular endothelium. The three others recognized cells or structures which cannot be definitely identified by immunofluorescence techniques. Five of the antibodies were IgG and two were IgM.

Discussion

These results confirm and extend our previous observation, reported at the First International Workshop on Human Leucocyte Differentiation Antigens (9), that anti-lymphocyte antibodies may cross-react with various skin components.

It is well-established that certain anti-CD1 antibodies such as OKT6 (6) and BL6 (7) recognize human Langerhans cells. It was recently demonstrated that the antigens immunoprecipitated from thymocytes and Langerhans cells by these antibodies possessed the same 49 + 12 Kd apparent molecular weight (10). This means that they recognize the same antigen expressed on the membrane of cells belonging to two very different lineages. All anti-CD1 antibodies do not react with Langerhans cells. During the First International Workshop some heterogeneity of the anti-CD1 antibodies was evidenced since NA1/34 and T6, D47, and M241 could be distinguished on biochemical and serological bases (11). A similar heterogeneity is found on skin since these antibodies identify, respectively, Langerhans cells, eccrine sweat glands, and no structure in the epidermis (9). Langerhans cells have been reported to bind anti-CD4 antibodies (12). No fluorescent staining of these cells was seen with the 14 anti-CD4 antibodies of the panel; this is in agreement with the very small number of antigenic sites detected by the OKT4 antibody on Langerhans cells by a semiquantitative ultrastructural immunogold method (13).

In the absence of biochemical studies, no evident biological significance can be attached to the cross-reactivity of the other anti–T lymphocyte antibodies on skin cells. The absence of cross-reactivity for a particular type of skin cell of antibodies defining a particular CD argues against the existence of common antigens shared by different unrelated cells, as was the case with anti-CD1 antibodies reacting with Langerhans cells. Different antigens can share common epitopes; this is not so frequent within protein antigens. It is interesting to note that whereas no IgM isotype is found among anti-CD1 antibodies cross-reacting with Langerhans cells, seven are found among the 14 identified isotypes cross-reacting with other skin components, and five among the seven which detect epidermal cells. Since anti-osidic antigens are often IgM, it is tempting to hypothesize that most of them detect glucidic epitopes, these being particularly rich on epidermal cells. Whether these antibodies were synthesized by hybridomas selected from clones directly induced by immunogens or from clones of the natural repertoire of the mice is not known. Natural antibodies of wide specificity have been found in mouse and human sera (14); we have ourselves selected from mice immunized against lymphocytes other hybridomas secreting antibodies of similar activity, such as an anti–ds-DNA (15).

The biological significance of the high number of cross-reactivities of anti–T lymphocyte antibodies to skin cells remains unknown. It would be first interesting to know whether they are restricted to skin components or present in any non-lymphoid tissue. We can say that this phenomenon is not a property of anti–T lymphocyte antibodies since in our experience a similar number of anti-B cell monoclonal antibodies (Raji and plasma cells) showed an identical pattern of cross-reactivity.

From a practical point of view, these results emphasize the utility of exhaustive distribution studies on non-lymphoid tissues of anti-lympho-cyte antibodies. Obviously such cross-reactivities complicate the use of the antibodies for immunohistological studies. Accordingly, therapists should refrain from using antibodies *in vivo* before having done such distribution studies, particularly when toxins will be coupled to the anti-bodies. On the other hand, these cross-reacting antibodies have provided dermatologists with very useful tools which appear to be nicely specific among skin cells. They have already revealed the heterogeneity of Langerhans cells; they may well be useful for studying normal and malig-nant keratinocyte differentiation.

Summary

By screening on frozen skin sections the supernatants of hybridomas prepared against human lymphoid cells, the authors have selected a series of monoclonal antibodies cross-reacting with most of the skin cells, pro-viding useful tools for dermatological studies. The 159 antibodies of the panel for T cell studies were screened on skin in the same manner. Twenty-one of them exhibited cross-reactivity against various skin com-ponents. Five anti-CD1 antibodies stained epidermal Langerhans cells. Eight antibodies reacted on different epidermal keratinocytes and eight on various dermal components. No evident biological significance could be attached to this observation. Of interest is the presence among the cross-reacting antibodies of a high number of IgM isotypes, which could indi-cate that they are directed to osidic determinants.

Acknowledgments. The authors would like to thank Martine Blanc, Véronique Buisson, and Michèle Jeannin for their help in preparing the monoclonal antibodies, Christiane Ohrt for immunofluorescence tests, and Caroline Boujeon for typing the manuscript. This work was sup-ported by grants from the MIR (No. 81 MO 833), the INSERM (CRL No. 81 10 28) and the U.E.R. de Biologie Humaine, Université Lyon I.

Note added in proof. In a new series of experiments we have found that CD1, Nu-T$_2$ antibody did not recognize Langerhans cells on tissue sec-tions, whereas CD1, M241 was slightly positive.

References

1. Thivolet, J., D. Schmitt, J. Viac, and J. Brochier. 1983. Les antigènes recon-nus par les anticorps monoclonaux antilymphocytes peuvent avoir une locali-sation tissulaire inattendue. *C.R. Acad. Sci. Paris* **296**:203.
2. Kohler, G., and C. Milstein. 1975. Continuous cultures of fused cells secreting antibody of predefined specificity. *Nature* **256**:495.

3. Viac, J., A. Reano, J. Brochier, M.J. Staquet, and J. Thivolet. 1983. Reactivity pattern of a monoclonal antikeratin antibody (KL1). *J. Invest. Dermatol.* **81:**351.

4. Viac, J., M. Haftek, M. J. Staquet, A. Reano, J. Brochier, and J. Thivolet. 1984. A monoclonal antibody labelling the keratinocyte membrane: a marker of epidermal differentiation. *Acta Dermatovener* (Stockholm) in press.

5. Klareskog, L., U.M. Tjernlund, and M. Fosum. 1977. Epidermal Langerhans cells express Ia antigen. Nature **26:**248.

6. Fithian, E., P. Kung, G. Goldstein, M. Rubenfeld, C. Fenoglio, and R. Edelson. 1981. Reactivity of Langerhans cells with hybridoma antibody. *Proc. Natl. Acad. Sci. U.S.A.* **78:**3858.

7. Yonish-Rouach, E., D. Schmitt, J. Viac, R. Knowles, G. Cordier, and J. Brochier. 1984. Monoclonal anti-thymic cell antibodies detecting epidermal cells. *Thymus* **6:**67.

8. Brochier, J., S. Saeland, G. Cordier, and D. Schmitt. 1984. An antilymphocyte monoclonal antibody (HB8) which cross reacts with human dermal elastic fibers. *Immunol. Lett.* **7:**279.

9. Brochier, J., D. Schmitt, E. Yonish-Rouach, G. Cordier, and J. Viac. 1984. Use of tissue distribution studies to determine the specificity of monoclonal antilymphocyte antibodies. In: *Leucocyte typing,* A. Bernard, L. Boumsell, J. Dausset, C. Milstein, and S. Schlossman, eds. Springer-Verlag, Berlin, Heidelberg, p. 465.

10. Takesaki, S., S.L. Morrison, C.L. Berger, G. Goldstein, A.C. Chu, and R.L. Edelson. 1982. Biochemical characterization of a differentiation antigen shared by human epidermal Langerhans cells and cortical thymocytes. *J. Clin. Immunol.* **2:**1285.

11. Bernard, A., L. Boumsell, J. Dausset, C. Milstein, and S. Schlossman, eds. 1984. *Leucocyte typing.* Springer-Verlag, Berlin, Heidelberg.

12. Wood, G.S., N.L. Warner, and R.A. Warnke. 1983. Anti-Leu-3/T4 antibodies react with cells of monocyte/macrophage and Langerhans lineage. *J. Immunol.* **131:**212.

13. Schmitt, D., M. Faure, C. Dambuyant-Dezutter, and J. Thivolet. 1984. The semi-quantitative distribution of T4 and T6 surface antigens on human Langerhans cells. *Brit. J. Dermatol.* **111:**655.

14. Guilbert, B., G. Dighiero, and S. Avrameas. 1982. Naturally occurring antibodies against nine common antigens in human sera. I. Detection, isolation and characterization. *J. Immunol.* **128:**2779.

15. Monier, J.C., J. Brochier, A. Moreira, C. Sault, and B. Roux. 1984. Generation of hybridoma antibodies to double-stranded DNA from non autoimmune Balb/c strain. Studies on anti-idiotype. *Immunol. Lett.* **8:**61.

Part VII. Study of Antibodies Reactive with Antigens of Activated T Cells

CHAPTER 34

Flow Cytometric Analysis of the Antigens Expressed by Peripheral Blood Lymphocytes Stimulated by Phytohemagglutinin Using the Workshop T Cell Panel and Selected B and M Cell Panel Monoclonal Antibodies

Daniel Olive, Patrice Dubreuil, Claude Mawas, and Patrice Mannoni

Flow cytometric analysis was performed on peripheral blood lymphocytes (PBLs) following mitogen-dependent activation using the lectin phytohemagglutinin (PHA), with the complete T cell set of monoclonal antibodies (mAbs) submitted to the Workshop and a selection of mAbs from the B and M cell set. This study has allowed us to classify the mAbs submitted as activation antigens and to explore some of the changes occurring in the fluorescence patterns with activation of the various mAbs defining the clusters of differentiation (CD).

Materials and Methods

PBLs were Ficoll–Hypaque separated from the buffy costs of three unrelated healthy blood donors, and subsequently pooled. 5×10^6 PBLs, without further separation, were stimulated with the lectin PHA (PHA, M, Gibco, Biocult, Grand Island, NY) at a final concentration of 1/100 in Falcon flasks in a total volume of 10 ml RPMI 1640–10% fetal calf serum.

Day 0, 1, 4, and 7 cells were then collected and 1×10^6 (day 0 and day 1) and 5×10^5 (day 4 and 7) cells were labeled at 4°C with the Workshop mAbs for 1 hr, washed twice with ice-cold PBS–BSA–azide, and incubated 30 min with fluorescein-conjugated $F(ab')_2$ fragments of a mixture of goat anti–mouse and goat anti–rat IgG (Cappel Laboratories, Westchester, PA).

The cytometric analysis was performed with an EPICS V cell sorter (Coultronics, Hialeah, FL). Prior to analysis, all samples were fixed using 2% paraformaldehyde in PBS.

Results

Temporal Appearance of Activation Antigens on Mitogen-stimulated T Cells

The time course of the appearance of the interleukin-2 (IL-2) receptor mAbs submitted to the workshop is shown in Table 34.1. mAbs 144, 148, 149, and 150 are not recognized activation antigens but rather could belong to the CD2 subset. mAbs 138 and 142 are both late activation antigens. Figure 34.1 shows that the fluorescent patterns for the six selected mAbs are very homogeneous.

CD2 Fluorescence Patterns on Mitogen-stimulated T Cells

The variation of the percent of labeled cells with time is indicated in Table 34.2.

Table 34.1. Kinetics: Anti-IL-2 receptor in the T-activation group.

	Day 0	Day 1	Day 4	Day 7
T135 T1A	8	37	82	28
T140 Tac/1HT4-H3	12	34	80	26
T141 B149.9	12	52	78	22
T143 18 E6.4	4	27	73	22.5
T145 39C6.5	8	27	68	36
T146 33B3.1	6	44	72.5	18
T147 33B7.3	10	28	40	8
T159 TAC	16	61	84	29

Table 34.2. Kinetics: CD2.

	Day 0	Day 1	Day 4	Day 7
T13	42	42	95	96
T14	20	26	68.5	86
T15	54	26	88.5	93
T16	48	55	96	99
T17	50	53	95	97
T18	36	53	97	96
T19	70	57	98	97
T20	52	66	97	98
T21	25	45	88.5	98
T22	51	80	95	97
T23	53	30	61	68
T24	45	52	93	95
T25	56	62	96	98
T26	52	23	6	68
T27	39	54	94	99
T28	35	20	50	92

T activation:

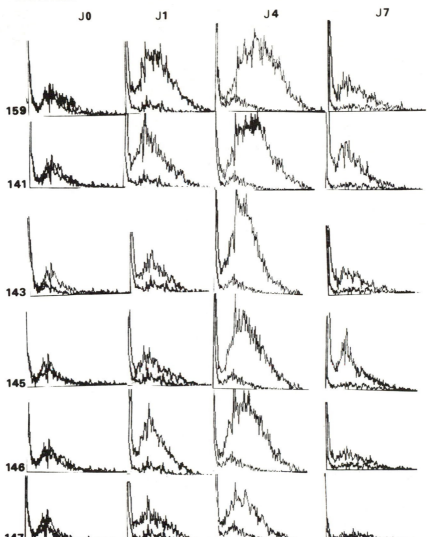

Fig. 34.1. Time course of the appearance of the IL-2 receptor. From left to right, each panel stands for a time course kinetic point: day 0, 1, 4, and 7. From top to bottom, each line corresponds to a given workshop mAb: T159, 141, 143, 145, 146, and 147. For each panel, horizontal axis: intensity of fluorescence (logarithmic scale); vertical axis: cell number.

Many mAbs labeled on day 0 a percent of cells inferior to the standard used as control: 9.6 of John Hansen, ascites used at a dilution of 1/100. With the latter, 67.5% of cells were labeled (against 56% with its Workshop equivalent, mAb T25). With time, most mAbs react as pan T mAbs. However, on close scrutiny, mAbs fall into various fluorescence patterns as shown in Fig. 34.2: two patterns on day 0, three on day 4, and two on day 7.

CD4 Fluorescence Patterns on Mitogen-stimulated T Cells

The percent of labeled cells is indicated in Table 34.3. In most cases, the percent of labeled cells on day 1 is inferior to that on day 0 and on day 4.

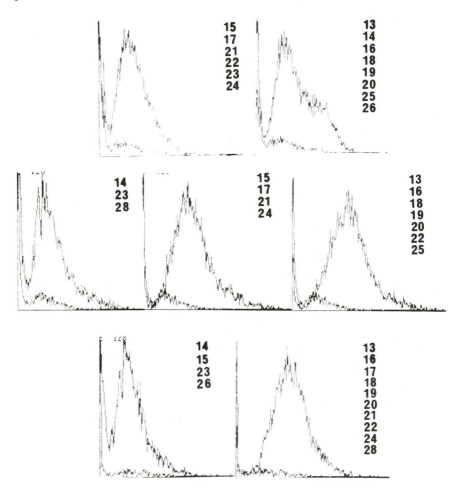

Fig. 34.2. Fluorescence patterns of CD2 mAbs. From left to right, various patterns of fluorescence for the mAbs tested in the Workshop. From top to bottom, day 0, day 4 and day 7. Horizontal and vertical axes as in Fig. 34.1.

Table 34.3. Kinetics: CD4.

	Day 0	Day 1	Day 4	Day 7
T67	18	14	40	34
T68	47	22	65	56
T69	53	23	94.5	81
T70	53	25	93	78
T71	52	18	88	83
T72	50	20	80	95
T73	49	16	52	96
T74	60	16	60	64
T75	70	24	60	77
T76	47	20	95	64
T77	46	19	92.5	92
T78	17	18	90	60
T79	52	27	84.5	48
T80	34	20	72	58

This has been a consistent finding following PHA activation and was found only for CD4 and CD3, as shown later.

The fluorescence patterns of the mAbs used fall into two subgroups for each day tested (Fig. 34.3).

The percent of cells labeled on day 4 and 7 would suggest, if confirmed, that many cells could express both CD4 and CD8 antigenic markers.

Table 34.4. Kinetics: CD8.

	Day 0	Day 1	Day 4	Day 7
T81	40	24	92	37
T82	25	26	86	89
T83	24	33	48	38
T84	22	22	65.5	42.5
T85	46	22	28.5	42.5
T86	46	22	40	36
T87	60	32	40	74
T88	48	29	40	90
T89	50	27	93	32
T90	40	24	75	40
T91	25	20	73	32
T92	26	26	51	34
T93	25	27	93	32.5
T94	24.5	28	44	32
T95	27	21	49	38
T96	25	31	45	35
T97	17	30	40	34
T98	21	30.5	4	4
T99	20	25	29	23

CD8 Fluorescence Patterns on Mitogen-stimulated T Cells

Table 34.4 shows the percent of labeled cells with time: the peak is clearly around day 4, with here again percents suggesting the existence of cells expressing both CD4 and CD8 markers.

This group of mAbs is the most heterogeneous, as far as fluorescence patterns are considered. As shown in Fig. 34.4, at least four patterns are seen with the CD8 mAbs and the mAbs belonging to each pattern are indicated in each panel of the figure.

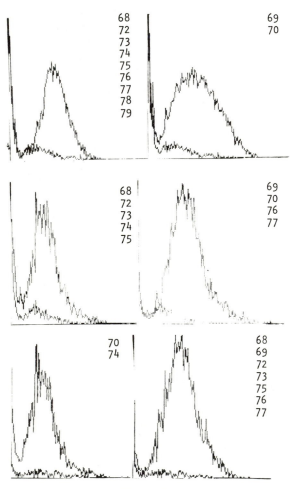

Fig. 34.3. Fluorescence patterns of CD4 mAbs. Legend as in Fig. 34.2.

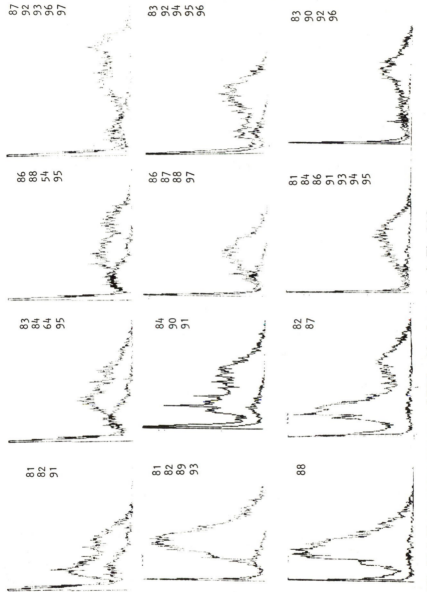

Fig. 34.4. Fluorescence patterns of CD8 mAbs. Legend as in Fig. 34.2.

Table 34.5. Kinetics: CD3.

	Day 0	Day 1	Day 4	Day 7
T117	42	9	52	83
T118	35	22	48	82.5
T119	48.5	35	80	96
T120	36	26	74.5	98
T121	18	44.5	43	70
T122	23	44	17	80
T123	12	30	35	54.5
T124	36	26	50	66
T125	25	20	24	69
T126	28	18	27	71
T127	17	57	62	92

CD3 Fluorescence Patterns on Mitogen-stimulated T Cells

This group of mAbs, within the conditions of the Workshop, and with
PHA as an activator, did not label all T cells on day 0 but by day 7 appears
to be a good pan T marker. In four cases a clear drop in labeled cells is
observed between day 0 and day 1 (Table 34.5). Fluorescence patterns are
unremarkable.

Selective Patterns of Reactivity from the B and M Cell Panel of mAbs Tested on Mitogen-stimulated T Cells

As will be shown more extensively in an accompanying paper (Vol. III,
Chapter 29, Mannoni, Dubrevil, Winkler-Lowen, Olive, Linklater, and
Mawas), mAbs either submitted to the B or M cell studies are in many
cases expressed early in the course of T cell activation by mitogens. It is
worth noting that very few of them were negative on T cells (Table 34.6).

Conclusions

The study of the time course of the appearance of antigens is crucial for
the definition of intermediate- or late-onset activation antigen, using days
as time scale. The time required for the appearance of early activation
antigens is of the order of hours as suggested by the peak in the appearance of many antigens defined by the B and M set of mAbs.

Fluorescence patterns can vary for one point in the kinetic studies with
various mAbs, and the patterns can change with time for a given mAb, as
best shown for CD8 mAbs, thus allowing further classification of various
mAbs belonging to the same cluster.

mAbs against so-called B or myeloid antigens are in many cases expressed by T cells during mitogen activation, a reverse image of the T cell
antigens expressed by activated B or some non-T cell tumor lines.

Table 34.6. Time course of appearance of antigens defined by selected mAbs from the B and M workshop set.

mAbs used	Day 0	Day 1	Day 4	Day 7
9.6	67	63	84	98
T3	54	16	90	79
T4	52	20	60	89
T8	26	29	35	31
TC1	52	60	82.5	
TC2	26	40	24	
TC3	26.5	20	9	
TC4	91	89	87	
B14	14	31	8.5	6
B38	58.5	74	32	30
B49	14	66	9	14
B59	46	77	8	22
B62	21	29	12	7
B70	17	33	17	11
B74	—	50	13	12
M2	10	50	4	11
M11	47	84	95	85
M12	34	84.5	73	77
M18	18	44	13	92
M49	33	48	8	12
M61	22.5	28	9.5	6
M62	22	26	7	5.5
M63	54.5	48	28	71
M64	45	49	13	21
M65	23	30	23	56
M66	50.5	31	12	20
M69	90	76	35	56
M71	41	31	9	23
M73	52.5	54	32	81
M77	49	53	19	20
M78	52	55	14	31
M79	37	32	12	15
10G3.3 (monocyte)	13	14	4	6
50H19 (B cell)	18	14	6	3

Finally, these systematic studies, although raising more questions than they can solve, have the merit of suggesting new approaches for studying differentiation and/or cell activation.

Acknowledgments. This work was supported by INSERM and CNRS. P. Dubreuil was supported as a visiting scientist by the Alberta Heritage Foundation for Medical Research.

CHAPTER 35

Regulation of Activation and Proliferation in T Cells

Peter C.L. Beverley, Kieran O'Flynn, Diana L. Wallace,
Jonathan R. Lamb, Arthur W. Boylston, and
David C. Linch

Introduction

The emphasis in studies of lymphocyte function has shifted in recent years from the definition of functionally distinct subsets, using phenotypic markers for cell separation, to studies of the function of cell surface molecules. This change has been brought about by the development of monoclonal antibodies (mAbs) and monoclonal cell sources. The former have provided reagents for identifying and characterizing molecules and the latter, cell populations which can be manipulated *in vitro* under relatively defined conditions. Nevertheless, since it is a feature of the immune system that no cell type functions in isolation, results obtained with interleukin-2 (IL-2)-dependent clones or tumors need to be confirmed with polyclonal populations. Further, the requirements for activation of resting cells may not be identical to those for restimulation of *in vitro* grown and already activated cells.

In this paper, therefore, we shall illustrate features of the control of the control of initial activation and maintenance of proliferation of T lymphocytes with examples which use both IL-2-dependent T cell clones and uncloned populations taken from blood or lymphoid tissue. In the case of the T cell clones, accessory cells and antigen or IL-2 are used as stimuli while for peripheral blood lymphocytes we have used monoclonal antibodies against the CD3 antigen present on all mature functional T cells. It is the thesis of this paper that there are alternative mechanisms for the initial activation and for the maintenance of T cell proliferation which can be partially separated using monoclonal antibodies. The functional consequences in terms of the spectrum of effector cells generated by activation in different ways are not yet clear.

Methods

Isolation of Cell Populations

Peripheral blood mononuclear cells (PBMs) were isolated from heparinized venous blood by centrifugation over Ficoll–Hypaque. Sheep red blood cell rosette-forming cells (E^+) were separated from PBMs by centrifugation over Ficoll–Hypaque following rosette formation for 1 hr on ice with AET-treated sheep red cells (1). The sheep red cells were lysed with hemolytic gelatin Gey's solution (2). Depletion of accessory cells was performed by passing the cells over a Sephadex G10 column (3). Thymocytes were obtained from specimens obtained at cardiac surgery by teasing the tissue with needles and allowing clumps to sediment for 5 min at room temperature.

Cell Cultures

Cell cultures were carried out in an atmosphere of 5% CO_2 in air in RPMI 1640 medium with 2 g/liter of sodium bicarbonate and 10mM Hepes buffer supplemented with 10% heat-inactivated fetal calf serum. For mitogen responses 1.5 or 2×10^5 cells were cultured in flat-bottomed 96-well microtiter plates in a final volume of 0.2 ml. Mitogens were added at optimal stimulatory concentration. Cultures were pulsed overnight at an appropriate time with either 0.5 μCi/well of iododeoxyuridine or 1 μCi/well of tritiated thymidine.

Measurement of Intracellular Free Calcium Ion Concentration

Quin 2 acetoxymethyl ester (Lancaster Synthetics) dissolved in dimethyl sulfoxide was added to cells suspended at 10^7/ml in RPMI 1640 with 1% bovine serum albumin to a final concentration of 25 μM. The cells were incubated at 37°C for 20 min, diluted fivefold with RPMI/albumin, and incubated for a further 40 min. The cells were then washed once and resuspended in RPMI/albumin.

Immediately before fluorescence measurements, aliquots of $2-3 \times 10^6$ cells were centrifuged and resuspended in 1 ml of a buffered salt solution containing 145 mM NaC1, 5 mM KC1, 0.5 mM Na$_2$HPO$_4$, 5 mM glucose, and 10 mM Hepes at pH 7.4. The cells were then incubated in quartz tubes for 10–15 min before fluorescence measurement in an Aminco-Bowman spectrofluorimeter. Absolute values for intracellular $(Ca^{2+})_i$ were calculated as described previously (4).

Immunocytochemical Staining

A modification of the method of Cordell *et al.* (5) was used. $2-4 \times 10^4$ cells were cytocentrifuged onto clean glass slides. Slides were air dried overnight and stored in sealed containers at −20°C. Prior to use, slides were air dried for 10 min, fixed in acetone for 10 min, and allowed to dry.

Prepared slides were dipped in phosphate-buffered saline (PBS) and then incubated in a moist chamber with monoclonal antibody for 30 min. After a PBS wash, the slides were again incubated for 30 min with human immunoglobulin-absorbed polyspecific rabbit anti–mouse immunoglobulin antibody (RaMIg). After a further wash preformed complexes of mouse monoclonal alkaline phosphatase–anti-alkaline phosphatase were added for a further 30 min. The slides were again washed and a further three layers of RaMIg and alkaline phosphatase–anti-alkaline phosphatase were applied with washes between. Each incubation with these additional layers was for 10 min only. After the last PBS wash the slides were incubated in fast red substrate solution for 30 min, washed in distilled water, and counterstained with haematoxylin for 3 min. Finally the slides were blued in tap water and mounted in a water-based mountant.

Monoclonal Antibodies

UCHT1 is an IgG1 anti-CD3 antibody (6). WT32 is an IgG2a anti-CD3 antibody (7). It was a gift of Dr. W. Tax. Anti-idiotypic antibodies to HPB-ALL, 3D6, 2D4, and 1C2 have been described elsewhere (8). Anti-Tac (9) was kindly provided by Dr. T.A. Waldmann and DMS2 anti-IL-2 (10) by Dr K. Smith.

Results and Discussion

Initial Activation Events

Physiological activation of T lymphocytes requires presentation of antigen by accessory cells, which are presumed to provide a second signal, such as interluekin-1 (IL-1) (11). However, binding of a variety of ligands to T cell surfaces in the absence of accessory cells is known to initiate metabolic changes. One of the early accessory cell-independent processes which is thought to be important in lymphocyte activation is an increase in intracellular free calcium concentration, $(Ca^{2+})_i$ (12,13) which can be measured using the fluorescent calcium indicator, Quin 2 (4).

Both the T cell mitogens PHA and Con A are capable of inducing this effect in human T lymphocytes (4). However, these ligands bind to many cell surface molecules and it is therefore difficult to define which cell surface molecules are important in transmitting the activation signals. Monoclonal antibodies to cell surface antigens provide better defined probes for investigating which molecules are important and we have used Quin 2 to show that the anti-CD3 mAb UCHT1 (4) and other anti-CD3 antibodies (14) can mobilize Ca^{2+} in human peripheral blood T cells.

Since a proportion of normal individuals fail to respond significantly to

IgG1 anti-CD3 antibodies as mitogens, a defect shown to be due to an accessory cell polymorphism (7,15,16), it was of interest to examine the effect on "nonresponder" T cells of stimulation with anti-CD3. Our results show as expected that both nonresponder and responder T cells show a similar rise in $(Ca^{2+})_i$ confirming that non-response is indeed an accessory cell effect (14). A further example of the dissociation of the calcium response and initiation of proliferation is seen in thymocytes (Fig. 35.1 and Table 35.1). While anti-CD3, PHA, and Con A can all increase $(Ca^{2+})_i$, anti-CD3 antibodies do not initiate a proliferative response. It is not yet clear why thymocytes fail to respond although the use of cross-linked anti-CD3 in the form of UCHT1–Sepharose beads does not reconstitute the thymocyte response as it does the response of nonresponder peripheral blood T cells. This result may therefore provide further evidence indicating that even medullary cells show functional immaturity, as well as phenotypic differences, with respect to peripheral T cells.

We have suggested (17) that CD3 may act as a signal transducer for the T cell receptor (Ti). In any event while no natural ligand has been demonstrated for CD3, it is clear that it is functionally closely associated with Ti. It was therefore of interest to determine whether ligand binding to Ti can induce an increase in $(Ca^{2+})_i$. We have previously shown that a soluble peptide antigen of influenza hemagglutinin (P20) does not mobilize $(Ca^{2+})_i$ in the influenza virus-specific clone HA1.7 (14). However, this may be because it must be presented in association with HLA-D region antigen. We therefore examined the effect on $(Ca^{2+})_i$ of anti-idiotypic antibodies to the T cell tumor line HPA-ALL (8). Figure 35.2 shows that such antibodies as well as anti-CD3 can induce a rise in intracellular Ca^{2+}. In our hands

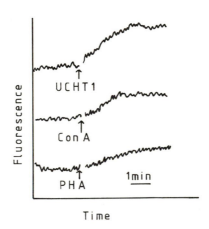

Fig. 35.1. Fluorescence traces obtained from human infant thymocytes loaded with the Ca^{2+} indicator Quin 2 and treated with PHA (10 μg/ml) UCHT1 (5 μg/ml), or Con A (10 μg/ml).

Table 35.1. Proliferative response of human infant thymocytes to mitogens.

Mitogen	^{3}H-Tdr[a] (cpm)	Stimulation index
—	957	—
PHA, 5 μg/ml	370,293	387
Con A, 10 μg/ml	165,881	173
UCHT1 10 μg/ml	2024	2.1
WT32 5 μg/ml	1533	1.6

[a] Mean cpm of triplicate wells containing 10^6 thymocytes in flat-bottomed microtiter plates, pulsed with 1 μCi/well of ^{3}H-TdR for the final 6 hr of a 3-day culture. S.E. of the mean less than $\pm 10\%$.

a variety of other antibodies to T cell surface antigens have been unable to induce a change in $(Ca^{2+})_i$. These antibodies include anti-HLA Class I, anti-CD1, anti-CD4, anti-CD8, and anti-CD2 (4).

In contrast to these negative data both Con A and PHA readily mobilize (Ca^{2+}) (Fig. 35.1). However, the mitogenic response, particularly to PHA, differs from the response to anti-CD3 in various aspects including kinetics magnitude of peak response and sensitivity to accessory cell depletion (unpublished results). Furthermore, PHA probably does not bind to CD3 (Crumpton and Kanellopoulos, personal communication) so that the mechanism of activation of PHA may differ from that of anti-CD3. We

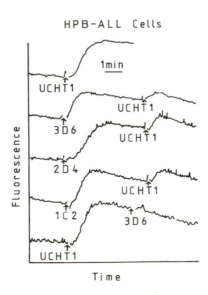

Fig. 35.2. Fluorescence traces obtained from HPB-ALL T cell line loaded with the Ca^{2+} indicator Quin 2 and treated with UCHT1 (5 μg/ml) or a 1 : 100 dilution of ascites of the anti-idiotypic mAbs 3D6, 2D4, and 1C2.

have sought to confirm this by examining the inhibition of PHA-induced mobilization of $(Ca^{2+})_i$ by monoclonal antibodies and have shown recently that preincubation with anti-CD2 monoclonal antibodies can prevent a subsequent response to PHA whereas the response to anti-CD3 is unaffected (18). These results imply that the sheep red blood cell receptor may be a receptor for the mitogenic signal delivered by PHA.

A number of authors have shown that anti-CD2 antibodies can inhibit mitogenic responses to PHA, Con A, anti-CD3, and antigens (19–21). This has led to the view that ligand binding to CD2 delivers an "off" signal to the cell (19–21). More recently it has been shown that a combination of two monoclonal antibodies directed against different epitopes of the CD2 antigen is strongly mitogenic (22). The epitope recognized by one of these antibodies T11$_3$ is only exposed following binding of the first antibody. Thus binding of many conventional anti-CD2 antibodies cannot trigger a mitogenic response and may interfere in the response to PHA by direct inhibition of binding to mitogenic sites. Inhibitory effects of anti-CD2 on other responses may be due to effects at the accessory cell level. Whether anti-CD2 can indeed mediate a direct inhibitory effect on T cell responses remains to be determined. Our data however are in agreement with the view (22) that there may be at least two pathways for the initial activation of T cells.

The published report on anti-CD2-induced proliferation indicates that this process is accessory cell independent (22). In the same report the response to PHA is shown to require accessory cells, indicating that these responses may differ in their mode of triggering T cells. Alternatively anti-CD2 and PHA may trigger by the same pathway but anti-CD2 may be a much more effective cross-linking ligand, perhaps minimizing the requirement for accessory cells. Our own data show that Sepharose-bound UCHT1 can stimulate a proliferative response in both nonresponder and responder T cells (Table 35.2) depleted of accessory cells by E-rosette formation and passage over G10 while soluble IgG1 or IgG2 anti-CD3 antibodies fail to stimulate. While these data suggest that large-scale cross-linking of the Ti–CD3 complex can override the requirement for accessory cells even in resting T cells, it does not prove it since the antibody-coated Sepharose beads may be a more potent stimulus to IL-1 production by a very small number of remaining accessory cells. Resolution of this question will require yet more rigorous depletion experiments combined with limiting dilution analysis or the use of accessory cell poisons (23).

Maintenance of Proliferation

Current dogma has it that initiation of proliferation in resting T cells requires contact with antigen in the context of MHC antigen and a second signal, interleukin-1, usually provided by accessory cells. Cells activated

Table 35.2. Response of accessory cell-depleted T cells to UCHT1–sepharose beads.

Source of T cells	Number of beads per well	^{3}H-Tdr[a] (cpm)
E$^+$ G10 nonadherent, nonresponder	300	5419
E$^+$ G10 nonadherent, nonresponder	600	17,092
E$^+$ G10 nonadherent, nonresponder	1200	26,045
E$^+$ G10 nonadherent, nonresponder	0	1425
E$^+$ G10 nonadherent, responder	300	5666
E$^+$ G10 nonadherent, responder	600	10,853
E$^+$ G10 nonadherent, responder	1200	13,516
E$^+$ G10 nonadherent, responder	0	1447

[a] Mean cpm of triplicate wells of flat-bottomed microtiter plates containing 1.5×10^5 accessory cell-depleted T cells pulsed for the last 6 hr of a 3-day culture with 1 μCi/well of ^{3}H-Tdr.

in this way express IL-2 receptors and proliferate in response to binding of IL-2. The proliferation may be via an autocrine mechanism in which the cell both secretes and accepts IL-2. Some recent data however, challenge this view and raise the possibility that, for some T cells at least, proliferation by an IL-2-independent pathway may be possible. Evidence for an IL-2-independent pathway has been obtained with the calcium ionophore A 23187 (24) and more recently investigations using the anti-CD3 monoclonal antibodies UCHT1 (IgG1) and WT32 (IgG2a) have suggested that these antibodies of differing isotype may maintain proliferation by different mechanisms (25). The results of this study are summarized in Table 35.3(a). The essential difference between stimulation with IgG1 and IgG2a anti-CD3 is that while both lead to expression of IL-2 receptors and proliferation, in the case of IgG1-stimulated T cells it is difficult to detect secreted IL-2 and proliferation cannot be inhibited by anti-Tac antibody to the IL-2 receptor.

We have obtained exactly analogous data using influenza virus-specific IL-2-dependent T cell clones (26). One helper clone does not secrete detectable IL-2 and its response to antigen plus accessory cells cannot be inhibited by anti-Tac while a second clone produces readily detectable IL-2 and the proliferative response to antigen plus accessory cells is readily inhibited. When exogenous IL-2 is used as a stimulus, the proliferative response of both clones is readily inhibited [Table 35.3(b)]. Both these clones are of the CD4 (helper/inducer) phenotype and might therefore be

Table 35.3. Comparison of "IL-2-dependent" and "IL-2-independent" pathways of response for fresh PBMs and T cell clones.

	IL-2 dependent	IL-2 independent
(a) PBMs		
Blasts express IL-2 receptor	Yes	Yes
Produce IL-2	Yes	No
Blocked by anti-Tac	Yes	No
(b) IL-2-dependent T cell clones		
Blasts express IL-2 receptor	Yes	Yes
Response to IL-2 blocked by anti-Tac	Yes	Yes
Response to antigen + accessory cells blocked by anti-Tac	Yes	No
Produce IL-2	Yes	No

expected to produce inducing lymphokines such as IL-2. It is a common observation in line with the results in Table 35.3 that many clones even of helper/inducer phenotype do not produce detectable IL-2 (27).

While the data discussed above indicate the possibility that some T cells may proliferate by an IL-2-independent pathway we were concerned to eliminate other possibilities: for example, that when IL-2 secretion is not detectable this is because the cells secrete only low amounts of IL-2 which is rapidly absorbed by high-affinity IL-2 receptors (autocrine stimulation). In addition, in our laboratory the amount of IL-2 detected in the supernatants of anti-CD3-stimulated T cells is low compared to PHA supernatants and the difference between supernatants of IgG1- and IgG2-stimulated cells has not always been convincing (unpublished data). We therefore turned to a more direct method, the use of immunocytochemical staining by the alkaline phosphatase–anti-alkaline phosphatase method (5) to detect IL-2 in T cell blasts. An example of our preliminary results is shown in Fig. 35.3. Cells stimulated with UCHT1 or WT32 were harvested at 48 hr and cytocentrifuge preparations stained using anti-Tac or the antibody DMS 2 against IL-2 (10). The results with anti-Tac confirm the earlier data using cell surface staining since both UCHT1-stimulated [Fig. 35.3(B)] and WT32-stimulated (not shown) T cells express readily detectable Tac antigen. In addition however staining with DMS 2 is clearly seen both in UCHT1- (IgG1) and WT32- (IgG2a) stimulated blasts. The data indicate therefore that IL-2 may be involved in both responses and weaken the arguments given above in favor of an IL-2-independent pathway of T cell proliferation. Nevertheless there appear to be differences in the way in which T cells respond to IL-2, exemplified by the insensitivity of some T cell clones and of IgG1 anti-CD3-stimulated T cells to inhibition by anti-Tac (Table 35.3). Additional weight is added to this argument by the results we have obtained using the Workshop panel of

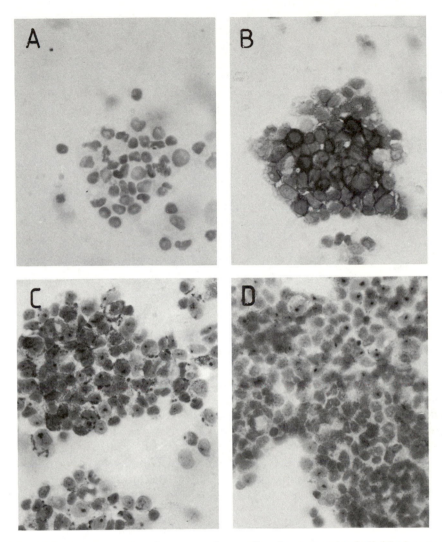

Fig. 35.3. Peripheral blood mononuclear cells of a responder individual were stimulated for 48 hr with an optimal dose of UCHT1 or WT32 anti-CD3 antibodies. Cytocentrifuge preparations of these were stained by the alkaline phosphatase–anti-alkaline phosphatase method (5). (A) UCHT1-stimulated cells, omitting monoclonal antibody; (B) UCHT1-stimulated cells, anti-Tac stained; (C) UCHT1-stimulated cells, DMS2 (anti-IL-2) stained; (D) WT32-stimulated cells, DMS2 stained.

Table 35.4. Inhibition of proliferative responses to UCHT1 or WT32 monoclonal antibodies by selected workshop antibodies

Workshop number	% Inhibition of control response[a]	
	UCHT1 (IgG1)	WT32 (IgG2a)
135 (IgG2)	10	8
139 (IgG1)	51	10
149 (NK)[b]	69	74
150 (NK)	76	50
151 (IgG1)	56	74
156 (IgM)	94	33

[a] Responder PBMs were stimulated by an optimal mitogenic dose of UCHT1 or WT32 with a 1 : 100 dilution of Workshop antibody for 3 days. % Inhibition was calculated by the formula

$$100 - \left(\frac{\text{cpm in presence of inhibitor} - \text{background cpm}}{\text{cpm with no inhibitor} - \text{background cpm}} \times 100 \right)$$

Figures are means of three experiments.
[b] Not known.

antibodies to activation and other antigens. Table 35.4 shows results obtained when Workshop antibodies were added at a fixed final concentration to PBMs stimulated with UCHT1 or WT32. Some antibodies block one response more than the other, some both, and some neither. There is no obvious relationship of blocking to antibody isotype, an important point since anti-Tac is IgG2a and blocks the response to IgG2a anti-CD3, an effect which could perhaps be mediated by competition for accessory cell Fc receptors. The results suggest therefore differences in the mechanisms of proliferation of IgG1- and IgG2a-stimulated cells. Clearly more exhaustive blocking experiments with adequate titration of antibodies and the use of F(ab)$_2$ fragments will be required for a proper analysis of these effects.

Conclusion

Our results using the calcium-sensitive indicator Quin 2 show that ligand binding to the CD3–Ti complex can provide a signal leading to an increase in $(Ca^{2+})_i$. This signal in itself is not sufficient to trigger proliferation of T cells. When accessory cells are depleted the response to soluble anti-CD3 is lost before that to Sepharose bead-bound (multimeric) anti-CD3, suggesting that more extensive cross-linking of receptors on the T cell surface can compensate for accessory cell depletion. The level at which the signals from CD3–Ti and accessory cell monokines are integrated remains to be determined. Inhibition studies suggest that PHA may activate cells via CD2, a finding in line with other data (22) showing that antibodies to CD2 can activate T cells by a second pathway.

The evidence regarding an IL-2-independent pathway of proliferation is equivocal but the detection of IL-2 by immunocytochemical staining in T cell blasts whose proliferation cannot be inhibited by anti-Tac suggests a high-affinity interaction of IL-2 with its receptor. Whether the proportion of high-affinity and low-affinity IL-2 receptors (28) varies on different T cell types is not known. It is also possible that anti-Tac does not detect all IL-2 receptors. Irrespective of the mechanisms the data suggest that there are two classes of T cells which differ in terms of IL-2 production and sensitivity to inhibition by anti-Tac. What significance this has and whether these represent functionally distinct populations remains to be determined.

Summary

We have used monoclonal antibodies to human lymphocyte surface antigens to investigate the mechanisms of activation and regulation of proliferation in human T cells. Antibodies to CD3 and to idiotypic determinants of Ti cause a rise in intracellular free Ca^{2+} concentration. This calcium mobilization is dissociated from initiation of proliferation in thymocytes and peripheral blood T cells of individuals unable to respond to IgG1 anti-CD3 antibodies (nonresponders). The proliferative response can be restored by using Sepharose bead-coupled anti-CD3, suggesting that extensive cross-linking reduces the requirement for accessory cells. PHA can also induce a rise in intracellular free Ca^{2+} which can be inhibited by prior incubation with anti-CD2 antibodies implying that PHA may deliver an activation signal via CD2.

Data on T cell clones and fresh lymphocytes stimulated with IgG1 or IgG2a anti-CD3 suggests that some T cells may proliferate by an IL-2-independent pathway. However, T cells stimulated by anti-CD3 antibodies of these two subclasses both show immunocytochemical staining with anti-IL-2 monoclonal antibodies. Nevertheless the use of a panel of Workshop antibodies to inhibit proliferative responses to IgG1 or IgG2a anti-CD3 suggests differences in the mechanism of proliferation.

References

1. Kaplan, M.E., and C. Clark. 1974. An improved rosetting assay for detection of human T lymphocytes. *J. Immunol. Methods* **5**:131.
2. Dresser, D.W. 1978. In: *Handbook of experimental immunology*, 3rd Ed., D.M. Weir, ed. Blackwell Scientific Publications, Oxford, Chapter 28, p. 22.
3. Jerells, T.R., J.H. Dean, G.L. Richardson, and R.B. Herberman. 1980. Depletion of monocytes from human peripheral blood mononuclear leucocytes:

Comparison of the Sephadex G_{10} column method with other commonly used techniques. *J. Immunol. Methods* **32:**11.

4. O'Flynn, K., D.C. Linch, and E.R. Tatham. 1984. The effect of mitogenic lectins and monoclonal antibodies on intracellular free calcium concentration in human T-lymphocytes. *Biochem. J.* **219:**661.

5. Cordell, J.L., B. Falini, W.N. Erber, A.K. Ghosh, Z. Abdulaziz, S. Mac-Donald, K.A. Pulford, H. Stein, and D.Y. Mason. 1984. Immunoenzymatic labelling of monoclonal antibodies using immune complexes of alkaline phosphatase and monoclonal anti-alkaline phosphatase (A PAAP complexes). *J. Histochem. Cytochem.* **32:**219.

6. Beverley, P.C.L., and R.E. Callard. 1981. Distinctive functional characteristics of human "T" lymphocytes defined by E rosetting or a monoclonal anti-T cell antibody. *Eur. J. Immunol.* **11:**329.

7. Tax, W.J.M., H.W. Willems, P.P.M. Reekers, P.J.A. Capel, and R.A.P. Koene. 1983. Polymorphism in mitogenic effects of IgG1 monoclonal antibodies against T3 antigen on human T cells. *Nature* **304:**445.

8. Boylston, A.W., R.D. Goldin, and C.S. Moore. 1984. A human T cell tumour which expresses the putative T cell antigen receptor. *Eur. J. Immunol.* **14:**273.

9. Leonard, W.J., J.M., Depper, T. Uchimaya, K.A. Smith, T.A. Waldmann, and W.C. Greene. 1982. A monoclonal antibody that appears to recognise the receptor for human T-cell growth factor: partial characterisation of the receptor. *Nature* **300:**267.

10. Smith, K.A., M.F. Favata, and S. Oroszlan. 1983. Production and characterisation of monoclonal antibodies to human interleukin-2: strategy and tactics. *J. Immunol.* **131:**1808.

11. Mizel, S.B. 1982. Interleukin 1 and T cell activation. *Immunol. Rev.* **63:**51.

12. Lichtman, A.H., G.B. Segel, and M.A. Lichtman. 1983. The role of calcium in lymphocyte proliferation—(An interpretive review). *Blood* **61:**413.

13. Metcalfe, J.C., T. Pozzan, G.A. Smith, and T.R. Hesketh. 1980. A calcium hypothesis for the control of cell growth. *Biochem. Soc. Symp.* **45:**1.

14. O'Flynn, K., E.D. Zanders, J.R. Lamb, P.C.L. Beverley, D.L. Wallace, P.E.R. Tatham, W.J.M. Tax, and D.C. Linch. 1985. Investigation of early T-cell activation: analysis of the effect of specific antigen, IL-2 and monoclonal antibodies on intracellular free calcium concentration. *Eur. J. Immunol.* **15:**7.

15. Van Wauwe, J.P., and J.G. Goossens. 1983. The mitogenic activity of OKT3 and anti-Leu-4 monoclonal antibodies: a comparative study. *Cell. Immunol.* **77:**23.

16. Kaneoka, H., G. Perez-Rojas, T. Sasasuki, C.J. Benike, and E.G. Engleman. 1983. Human T lymphocyte proliferation induced by a pan-T monoclonal antibody (anti-Leu-4): heterogeneity of response is a function of monocytes. *J. Immunol.* **131:**158.

17. Beverley, P.C.L. 1983. The importance of T3 in the activation of T lymphocytes. *Nature* **304:**398.

18. O'Flynn, K., A.M. Krensky, P.C.L. Beverley, S.J. Burakoff, and D.C. Linch. 1985. Phytohaemagglutinin activation of T cells through the sheep red blood cell receptor. *Nature.* **313:**686.

19. Palacios, R., and O. Martinez-Maza. 1982. Is the E receptor on human T lymphocytes a "negative signal receptor?" *J. Immunol.* **129:**2479.

20. Martin, P.J., G. Longton, J.A. Ledbetter, W. Newman, M.P. Bruan, P.A. Beatty, and J.A. Hansen. 1983. Identification and functional characterisation of two distinct epitopes on the human T cell surface protein Tp50. *J. Immunol.* **131**:180.
21. Kensky, A.M., F. Sanchez-Madrid, E. Robbins, J.A. Nagy, T. Springer, and S. Burakoff. 1983. The functional significance, distribution and structure of LFA-1, LFA-2, and LFA-3: cell surface antigen associated with CTL target interactions. *J. Immunol.* **131**:611.
22. Meuer, S.C., R.E. Hussey, M. Fabbi, D. Fox, O. Acuto, K.A. Fitzgerald, J.C. Hodgdon, J.P. Protentis, S.F. Schlossman, and E.L. Reinherz. 1984. An alternative pathway of T-cell activation: A functional role for the 50 kd T11 sheep erythrocyte receptor protein. *Cell* **36**:897.
23. Thiele, D.L., M. Kurosaka, and P.E. Lipsky. 1983. Phenotype of the accessory cell necessary for mitogen-stimulated T and B cell responses in human peripheral blood: delincation by its sensitivity to the lysozomotropic agent, L-leucine methyl ester. *J. Immunol.* **131**:2282.
24. Koretzky, G.A., R.P. Daniele, W.C. Greene, and P.C. Nowell. 1983. Evidence for an interleukin-independent pathway for human lymphocyte activation. *Proc. Natl. Acad. Sci. U.S.A.* **80**:3444.
25. Van Wauwe, J.P., J.G. Goossens, and P.C.L. Beverley. 1984. Human T lymphocyte activation by monoclonal antibodies: OKT3, but not UCHT1, triggers mitogenesis via an interleukin-2 dependent mechanism. *J. Immunol.* **133**:129.
26. Lamb, J.R., E.D. Zanders, M. Feldman, D.D., Eckels, J.N. Wood, P. Lake, and P.C.L. Beverley. 1983. The dissociation of interleukin-2 production and antigen specific helper activity by clonal analysis. *Immunol.* **50**:397.
27. Kelso, A. and H.R. MacDonald. 1982. Precursor frequency analysis of lymphokine secreting alloreactive T lymphocytes. Dissociation of subsets producing interleukin-2, macrophage activating factor and granulocyte-macrophage colony stimulating factor on the basis of Lyt-2 phenotype. *J. Exp. Med.* **156**:1366.
28. Smith, K.A. 1984. Interleukin 2. *Ann. Rev. Immunol.* **2**:319.

CHAPTER 36

Phenotypic Analysis of Activation Antigens on Mitogen-stimulated T Cells Utilizing Monoclonal Antibodies

Tehila Umiel and Ellen Saltz-Tal

Introduction

The development of hybridoma technology (1) coupled with the analytical and separation capabilities of fluorescence-activated cell sorting and *in vitro* techniques, to discriminate functional properties and interactions of isolated T cell subsets, led to an extensive classification of human lymphocytes into defined subsets (2–6). Studies directed toward dissecting and characterizing human T cells by cell surface determinants have identified functionally distinct T cell subsets (3,4). Antigen expression on these T cell subsets has been correlated with functional properties and the differentiation state of cells (3). Moreover, surface molecules have themselves a function as recognition elements in the cellular interaction. Indeed, the 20,000 mol. wt. T3 surface molecule was found recently to be associated with the T cell receptor structure for antigen on all T cells (7,8). In addition, T cells activated by mitogens, soluble antigens, and alloantigen express new activation surface antigens linked to the specific stimulus and the genetic program of the cells responding to this stimulus (9–16). Although in most cases the actual physiological role of these cell products is as yet unknown, they may be important as part of a network through which cell–cell signals are conveyed by activated subsets of T cells. Recently a functionally distinct surface antigen defined by anti-Tac antibody was demonstrated exclusively on activated and terminally differentiated T cells (16–18). This antigen has functional importance as the specific interleukin-2 (IL-2) receptor on activated T cells (17,18). Further development, production, and characterization of more mAbs directed at activation antigens may eventually provide a useful probe with which it will be possible to further analyze the nature of immunologic activation of human T lymphocytes.

In the present study we analyzed a new panel of 19 mAbs directed at T cell activation antigens. We found that the highest reactivity of all antibodies was obtained with 3-day mitogen-stimulated T cells. However, the pattern of reactivity differed with various antibodies. Some antibodies reacted with the majority of activated T cells, whereas others reacted with restricted subsets only. These results suggest that subsets of functionally distinct activated T cells may also express distinct surface antigens related to their stimulus and specific function.

Materials and Methods

Isolation of Lymphocytes

Peripheral blood mononuclear cells from healthy donors were isolated from heparinized venous blood by Ficoll–Hypaque gradient density centrifugation (Pharmacia Fine Chemicals, Sweden), using a standard technique.

Monoclonal Antibodies

A panel of 19 mAbs directed at T cell activation antigens were utilized. These antibodies were submitted to the Second International Workshop on Human Leukocyte Differentiation Antigens by several laboratories for further characterization. We employed two additional monoclonal antibodies against activated antigens in this study, as positive controls for reactivity. One was the anti-Tac, termed Tac[a] in this study, and the other is anti-Ia. (Tac[a] was a gift of T.A. Waldmann from the NIH, Bethesda, MD, and the Ia was a gift from L. Nadler, Dana-Farber Cancer Institute, Boston, MA.)

Phenotypic Analysis of Activation Antigens on T Cells

Flow cytofluorographic analysis of activated T cells was performed by indirect immunofluorescence (2). Samples of 1×10^6 T cells cultured for 1–5 days with mitogens in 100 μl of RPMI 1640 medium, containing 10% heat-inactivated human serum, were incubated with 100 μl of mAbs (final dilution 1/400) at 4°C for 30 min. After two washings the cells were incubated with 25-μl (of 1/10 dilution) medium containing fluorescein isothiocyanate (FITC)-conjugated goat anti–mouse IgG (Bio-Yeda, Rehovot, Israel). Control samples were incubated with the FITC-coupled agent only. After 30 min incubation at 4°C cell samples were washed twice and analyzed on a flow cytometer (FACS II; Becton Dickinson & Co., Sunnyvale, CA).

Lymphocyte Transformation Studies

Isolated mononuclear cells were suspended in RPMI 1640 containing 10% heat-inactivated human AB serum at 1×10^6 cells/ml. 100-μl cell suspension was distributed in triplicate in microtiter plates with 100-μl optimal concentration of mitogens; (PHA, 2 μg/ml; Con A, 4 μg/ml and PWM; 5 μg/ml). Control cultures were stimulated by media alone. Cultures were incubated for 3 days, labeled for the last 4 hr with 2-μCi of tritiated thymidine (^{3}H-TdR, specific activity 2 mCi/mM; Amersham, England), and harvested on an automated microtiter harvester. Radioactivity was determined in a liquid scintillation counter. Stimulation was expressed as mean $\pm$ S.E. of ^{3}H-TdR incorporation of triplicate cultures.

Results

The aim of this study was to analyze expression of activation antigens on T cells stimulated by mitogens, utilizing a panel of 19 mAbs. Table 36.1 summarizes some of the properties of these antibodies. As shown in the table, not all antibodies were fully characterized. From those antibodies

Table 36.1. Properties of mAbs reactive with activation antigens on T cells.[a]

Antibody	Binds SPA[b]	Fixes complement	Ig subclass
T1A	NK[c]	Yes	IgG2
TS145	Yes	NK	IgG1
100-1A5	NK	NK	NK
1-MONO-2A6	Yes	Yes	IgG3
4EL1C7	Yes	No	IgG1
Tac/1HT4-4H3	NK	NK	NK
B149.9	Yes	Yes	IgG2a
B1.19.2	Yes	Yes	IgG2a
23A9.3	NK	NK	NK
39C1.5	NK	NK	NK
39C6.5	NK	NK	NK
33B3.1	NK	NK	NK
33B7.3	NK	NK	NK
39C8.18	NK	NK	NK
39H7.3	NK	NK	NK
41F2.1	NK	NK	NK
KOLT-1	NK	No	IgG1
AA3	NK	NK	IgG1
TAC	Yes	Yes	IgG2a

[a] The data presented here were obtained from those antibodies submitted by the individual laboratories.
[b] SPA: Staph protein A.
[c] NK: Not known.

characterized, all bound Staph A protein; 1 MONO 2A6, B149.9, B1.19.2, and TAC fix complement while KOLT-1 does not. Antibodies Tac, T1A, B149.9, B1.19.2 are of the IgG2a subclass of immunoglobulin, KOLT-1, AA3, 4EL1C7, and TS145 are of IgG1 class, and 1 MONO 2A6 is of the IgG3 subclass.

To establish the proportion of cells bearing a variety of surface activation antigens after mitogenic stimulation, antibodies were reacted with T cells activated with mitogens for 3 days. Table 36.2 summarizes the results of these experiments. T cells induced with either PHA, Con A, or PWM consistently expressed activation antigens detectable by the entire panel of antibodies. Activation antigens detectable by antibodies T1A, Tac/1TH4-4H3, 39C1.5, 39C6.5, 33B3.1, and 33B7.3 were expressed on a high percentage of T cells (30–60%), whereas antigens detectable by antibodies TS145, 1 MONO 2A6, 4EL1C7, AA3, B1.19.2, 23A9.3, and 39C8.18 were expressed on 15–20% of the cells. Moreover, antibodies

Table 36.2. Comparison of activation antigen expression on T cells activated with various T cell mitogens detected by mAbs.

Antibody	Stimulus		
	PHA	Con A	PWM
	% Reactivity		
T1A	36 ± 5[a]	46.3 ± 11.9	63 ± 3
TS145	23 ± 2.1	3.3 ± 2.9	29.5 ± 2.5
100-1A5	11.5 ± 4.5	15.6 ± 3.8	10 ± 1.2
1 MONO 2A6	28 ± 4	30 ± 3	14 ± 2
4EL1C7	21.5 ± 3.5	27 ± 4	28 ± 9
Tac/1HT4-4H3	60 ± 9	50.6 ± 10	72 ± 7
B149.9	21.5 ± 8.5	28.3 ± 6.3	22.5 ± 4.5
B1.19.2	17.5 ± 5.5	26.6 ± 4.3	13 ± 2.3
23A9.3	15 ± 6.2	14 ± 3	10 ± 2.1
39C1.5	14.5 ± 5.1	43 ± 6.1	71 ± 3.4
39C6.5	44.5 ± 9.5	52 ± 7.1	71 ± 5
33B3.1	44 ± 12	46 ± 15	71 ± 11
33B7.3	45 ± 10.1	16.6 ± 3.9	14 ± 2.5
39C8.18	18 ± 2.5	24.5 ± 8.2	10 ± 2.8
39H7.3	12.5 ± 5.5	21 ± 5	12 ± 2
41F2.1	11 ± 5	17 ± 3	9 ± 3
KOLT-1	11 ± 5	20 ± 4.5	7 ± 2
AA3	18 ± 2	20 ± 5	11 ± 1.2
TAC	50 ± 5	59 ± 12	75 ± 5.5
Ia[b]	54 ± 2.0	50 ± 5.0	88 ± 9.0
Tac[a][b]	54 ± 7.0	56 ± 3.0	80 ± 5.5

[a] Mean ± S.E.
[b] TAC[a] and Ia antibodies were not included in the panel of antibodies tested for the Workshop and were used here as positive controls for the detection of activation antigen on T cells (as described in Materials and Methods).

39C1.5, 39C6.5, 33B3.1, and T1A reacted with a larger proportion of cells stimulated by PWM (71–80%) than with those stimulated by PHA or Con A (40–60%). Anti-Tac[a] (16) and anti-Ia (9) antibodies, which served as positive controls in these experiments, reacted with 50–80% of the cells stimulated by either mitogen. No evidence of reactivity with mAbs could be observed on T cells cultured *in vitro* without mitogens (data not shown), suggesting that these antibodies indeed detect only antigens expressed as a consequence of activation by mitogen. The fluorescence patterns of cells reacting with the various antibodies are summarized in Fig. 36.1, where the antibodies are classified according to their intensity of their staining into four major groups represented by antibodies (A) T1A, 39C1.5, 39C6.5 33B3.1; (B) Tac/1HT4-4H3, TAC; (C) TS145, 1 MONO 2A6, 4EL1C7, 39H7.3, B149.9, B1.19.2, 33B7.3, AA3; (D) 100-1A5, 39C8.18, 41F2.1, KOLT-1.

To study the kinetics of activation antigen expression on mitogen-activated T cells, cultures stimulated with mitogens were harvested and stained with antibodies on each of days 1, 2, 3, 4, and 5 after stimulation. As summarized in Tables 36.3, 36.4, and 36.5, no activation antigens could be detected on T cells by any of the antibodies tested on 1-day stimulated cells. The peak expression of activation antigens was noted on T cells cultured for 3 days, and declined on day 5. Antigens detectable by antibodies T1A, 1 MONO 2A6, Tac/1HT4-4H3, 33B3.1, 39C1.5, and 39C.5, TAC, Ia, and Tac[a] were still found on 5-day cultured cells stimulated by Con A and PHA. In addition, antigens reactive with antibodies 100-1A5, 4EL1C7, TS145, and B149.9 were still expressed on 4- and 5-day PWM stimulated cells. In the next experiment we tried to directly corre-

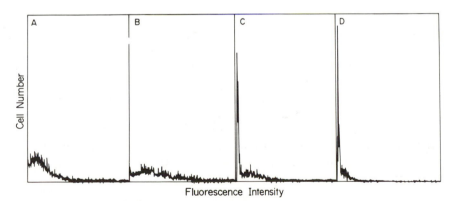

Fig. 36.1. Fluorescence intensity histograms for distribution of activation antigens on T cells activated by mitogens and stained with mAbs. Histograms for antigens reactive with antibodies: (A) T1A, 39C1.5, 39C6.5, 33B3.1; (B) Tac/1HT4-4H3, TAC, 140, 159; (C) TS145, 1 MONO 2A6, 4EL1C7, 39H7.3, B149.9, B1.19.2, 23A9.3, 33B7.3, AA3; (D) 100-1A5, 39C8.18, 41F2.1, KOLT-1.

Table 36.3. Reactivity of mAbs with activation antigens on PHA-stimulated T cells.

Antibody	Days in culture[a]				
	1	2	3	4	5
	% Reactivity				
T1A	3	18	36	40	27
TS145	5	8	23	16	14
100-1A5	5	4	16	5	4
1 MONO 2A6	5	10	28	5	9
4EL1C7	3	4	21	10	16
Tac/1HT4-4H3	6	24	60	61	38
B149.9	4	4	22	10	5
B1.19.2	4	6	17	10	3
23A9.3	3	6	22	7	3
39C1.5	8	30	21	61	30
39C6.5	6	25	26	63	45
33B3.1	5	15	44	56	23
33B7.3	3	33	45	16	10
39C8.18	3	5	18	6	5
39H7.3	3	5	18	6	6
41F2.1	3	6	16	4	4
KOLT-1	4	3	16	3	4
AA3	4	3	18	7	4
TAC	3	16	50	75	53
Ia	10	15	54	40	27
Tac[a]	4	30	54	72	30

[a] Cultures were stimulated with PHA (2 μg/ml). A group of cultures were stained each day with the entire panel of mAbs and analyzed by flow cytofluorometry.

late the time and extent of activated cell proliferative capacities with the expression of surface activation antigens. The kinetic pattern of lymphocyte transformation after PHA, Con A, and PWM stimulation is shown in Fig. 36.2. Responses to the three types of stimulus, applying both ^{3}H-TdR incorporation and blast transformation assays, did not differ markedly—peak responses appeared on days 2 and 3 and declined on day 5. The peak response of lymphocyte transformation correlated with the maximal expression of surface activation antigen. These results indicate that activated cells which actively synthesize DNA, also strongly express surface activation antigens.

Discussion

Evidence has been accumulated to support the concept that activation of T cells by antigens or mitogens requires at least two signals. One signal is provided by the antigen and the second signal is provided by soluble

Table 36.4. Reactivity of mAbs with activation antigens on Con A-stimulated T cells.

Antibody	Days in culture				
	1	2	3	4	5
	% Reactivity				
T1A	3	18	46	10	8
TS145	5	8	31	10	6
100-1A5	5	5	19	6	3
1 MONO 2A6	4	3	30	30	6
4EL1C7	3	5	40	27	6
Tac/1HT4-4H3	7	24	50	18	14
B149.9	5	4	28	10	6
B1.19.2	5	10	26	7	6
23A9.3	4	3	17	3	3
39C1.5	10	31	43	15	25
39C6.5	7	20	52	15	11
33B3.1	8	15	46	10	8
33B7.3	3	10	20	6	5
39C8.18	5	5	24	5	4
39H7.3	5	3	21	13	3
41F2.1	5	3	21	8	5
KOLT-1	5	6	20	6	5
AA3	5	8	26	7	4
TAC	4	10	59	21	16
Ia	10	15	45	18	9
Tac[a]	11	30	60	26	15

Table 36.5. Reactivity of mAbs with activation antigens on PWM-stimulated T cells.

Antibody[a]	Days in culture[a]				
	1	2	3	4	5
	% Reactivity				
T1A	6	8	63	25	38
TS145	8	7	29	10	12
100-1A5	5	5	19	6	3
1 MONO 2A6	3	4	14	12	10
4EL1C7	3	4	28	15	37
Tac/1HT4-4H3	7	10	71	29	3
B149.9	3	3	22	14	19
B1.91.2	5	3	13	5	3
39C1.5	6	18	71	17	23
39C6.5	4	10	70	29	23
33B3.1	5	8	71	27	20
33B7.3	3	3	14	3	4
TAC	3	14	75	14	27
Ia	nd	15	88	30	27
Tac[a]	nd	12	80	56	25

[a] mAbs 39C8.18, 39H7.3, 41F2.1, KOLT-1, 23A9.3 and AA3 reacted with 10% or less of PWM activated cells.

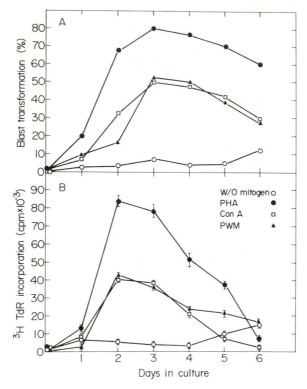

Fig. 36.2. Kinetics of T cell transformation responses following stimulation with PHA (2 μg/ml), Con A (4 μg/ml), and PWM (5 μg/ml) detected by blast cell transformation (A) and thymidine incorporation (B). Values are expressed as % for (A) and as mean ± S.E. for (B).

mediators, i.e., lymphokines, liberated by accessory cells and T cells (19–21). The interaction of T cells with both signals induces their activation and clonal expansion. Moreover, new surface determinants are also expressed on T cells in the process of activation (10,11–17,22). Although the actual physiological role of the various activation antigens is as yet unknown, they may be a part of the network through which cell–cell signals are conveyed by functional subsets of T cells. Indeed the functional role of one such activation antigen named Tac, which is expressed exclusively on activated T cells, has been recently proven to be associated with the human IL-2 receptor on activated cells (18,19,22–23). The anti-Tac antibody was found to interact with the IL-2 receptor and to block IL-2-dependent proliferation of activated cells (22,23).

In the present study we examined a panel of new mAbs all directed against T cell surface antigens. Cells which were activated with either PHA, Con A, or PWM mitogens for 3 days were all reactive with this panel; cells cultured in the absence of mitogens did not express detectable surface antigens. This suggests that surface antigens detected by the above mAbs are directed only against antigens expressed as a result of T cell activation.

The strength of reactivity of T cells with the different antibodies varied from intensive reactivity with antibodies T1A, Tac/1HT4-4H3, TAC, 39C6.5, 33B3.1, 33B7.3 (30–60%) to moderate reactivity with mAbs TS145, 1 MONO 2A6, 4EL1C7, AA3, B1.19.2, 39C1.5, and 39C8.8 (20–25%) to weak reactivity (20% or less) for the rest of the mAbs in the panel. To test the possibility that maximal expression of the various activation antigens detectable by mAbs follows a different kinetics, cultures were stimulated with mitogens for various time intervals, and then reacted with the mAbs panel. Activation antigens detected on 3-day stimulated cells represent the maximal amounts of expression of activation determinants. Moreover, kinetic studies of blast transformation following mitogenic stimulation indicated peaked DNA synthesis on days 2 and 3 after stimulation, thus further supporting cell surface studies. The variability of reactivity of mAbs with their target cells resulted from either the reactivity of some mAbs with only a small subset of activated T cells and others with a major subset of activated T cells, or from the nature of the stimulus which triggered some cell subsets but not others. Since our studies were not performed on separated T cell subsets, we cannot distinguish between these possibilities. Further characterization of activation antigen functions will come from extensive analysis of mAbs reactive with the restricted region of molecules displayed on restricted subsets of activated T cells.

Summary

A panel of 19 monoclonal antibodies (mAbs) against T cell activation antigens was employed on mitogen PHA, Con A, and PWM-stimulated cells utilizing flow cytofluorometry analysis. Positive reactivity (20–60%) with activation antigens on 3-day mitogen-stimulated T cells was detected by the entire panel of antibodies tested. Highest reactivity (>30%) was observed by antibodies T1A, Tac/1HT4-4H3, 33B3.1, 33B7.3, 39C6.5, and TAC on Con A- and PHA-stimulated cells and TS145, 1 MONO 2A6, 39C1.5, 39C6.5, 33B3.1 on Con A- and PWM-stimulated cells. Other antibodies reacted either moderately (20–25%) or with a low percentage of T cells (<20%). Generally, antibodies T1A, TS145, Tac/1HT4-4H3, 39C1.5, 39C6.5, 33B3.1, and TAC reacted both more intensively and with a higher percentage of activated cells. Kinetic studies directed at determining the time of appearance of activation antigens recorded antigen expression detectable by antibodies T1A, 39C1.5, Tac/1HT4-4H3, 39C6.5, 33B3.1, and TAC already on day 2 following mitogenic stimulation. The maximal expression of activation antigen could be detected by the entire panel of antibodies on 3-day activated cells and a decline in expression was recorded on days 4 and 5 after stimulation. Antigens detected by antibodies T1A, TS145, Tac/1HT4-4H3, 39C1.5, 39C6.5, 33B3.1, 4EL1C7, and TAC were still expressed, even on 5-day PHA-, Con A-, and PWM-activated cells. In addition, antigens reactive with antibodies 1 MONO 2A6, 100-1A5, and 4EL1C7 were still expressed on 4- and 5-day PWM-activated cells. DNA synthesis and blast transformation kinetics correlated with the phenotypic expression of activation antigens.

Acknowledgments. The authors wish to acknowledge the generous gifts of monoclonal antibodies from Drs. T.A. Waldmann of N.I.H. (anti-TAC[a]) and L.M. Nadler of the Dana-Farber Institute (α-Ia). Ms. Pamela Rubinstein edited and typed this manuscript.

References

1. Kohler, G., and C. Milstein. 1975. Continuous cultures of fused cells secreting antibody of predefined specificity. *Nature* **256**:495.
2. Reinherz, E.L., P.C. Kung, G. Goldstein, and S.F. Schlossman. 1979. A monoclonal antibody with selective reactivity with functionally mature human thymocytes and all peripheral human T cells. *J. Immunol.* **123**:1312.
3. Reinherz, E.L., P.C. Kung, G. Goldstein, and S.F. Schlossman. 1979. Further characterization of T human inducer T cell subset defined by monoclonal antibody. *J. Immunol.* **123**:2894.
4. Reinherz, E.L., P.C. Kung, G. Goldstein, and S.F. Schlossman. 1980. A monoclonal antibody reactive with the human cytotoxic/suppressor T cell subset previously defined by a hetero-antiserum termed TH2. *J. Immunol.* **124**:1301.
5. Engleman, E.G., C. Benike, B. Osborne, and R. Goldsby. 1980. Functional characterization of human T cell subpopulations distinguished by a monoclonal antibody. *J. Immunol.* **77**:1607.
6. Reinherz, E.L., and S.F. Schlossman. 1980. The differentiation and function of human T lymphocytes. *Cell* **19**:821.
7. Meuer, S.C., R.E. Hussey, J.C. Hodgen, T. Herced, S.F. Schlossman, and E.L. Reinherz. 1982. Surface structure involved in target recognition of human cytotoxic T lymphocytes. *Science* **218**:471.
8. Meuer, S.C., K.A. Fitzgerald, R.E. Hussey, J.C. Hodgdon, S.F. Schlossman, and E.L. Reinherz. 1983. Clonotypic structure involved in antigen specific human T cell function. Relationship to the T3 molecular complex. *J. Exp. Med.* **157**:705.
9. Reinherz, E.L., P.C. Kung, J.M. Pesando, J. Ritz, G. Goldstein, and S.F. Schlossman. 1979. Ia determinants on human T cell subsets defined by monoclonal antibody: activation stimuli required for expression. *J. Exp. Med.* **150**:1472.
10. Ko, H.S., S.M., Fu, R.J. Winchester, D.T.Y. Yu, and H.G. Kunkel. 1979. Ia determinants on stimulated human T lymphocytes. Occurrence on mitogen and antigen stimulated T cells. *J. Exp. Med.* **150**:246.

11. Evans, R.L., T.J. Faldetta, R.E. Hymphreys, D.M. Pratt, E.J. Yunis, and S.F. Schlossman. 1978. Peripheral human T cells sensitized in mixed leukocyte culture synthesize and express Ia-like antigens. *J. Exp. Med.* **148**:1440.

12. Omery, M.B., I.S. Trowbridge, and J. Minowada. 1980. Human cell surface glycoprotein with unusual properties. *Nature* **286**:888.

13. Corte, G., L. Moretta, G. Damiani, M.C. Ming, and A. Bargelles. 1981. Surface antigens specifically expressed by activated T cells in humans. *Eur. J. Immunol.* **11**:162.

14. Terhorst, C., A. van Agthoven, K. Le Clair, P. Snow, E. Reinherz, and S.F. Schlossman. 1981. Biochemical studies of the human thymocyte cell surface antigen T6, T9, T10. *Cell* **23**:771.

15. Haynes, B.F., M.E. Hember, D.L. Mann et al. 1981. Characterization of a monoclonal antibody (4F2) that binds to human monocytes and to a subset of activated lymphocytes. *J. Immunol.* **126**:1409.

16. Uchiyama, T., S. Broder, and T.A. Waldmann. 1981. A monoclonal antibody (anti-Tac) reactive with activated and functionally mature human T cell. I. Production of anti-Tac monoclonal antibody and distribution of Tac (+) cells. *J. Immunol.* **126**:1393.

17. Uchiyama, T., D.L. Nelson, T.A. Fleisher, and T.A. Waldmann. 1981. A monoclonal antibody (anti-Tac) reactive with activated and functionally mature human T cells. II. Expression of Tac antigen on activated cytotoxic T cells, suppressor cells and one of two types of helper T cells. *J. Immunol.* **126**:1398.

18. Smith, K.A., T.A. Waldmann, and W.C. Greene. 1982. A monoclonal antibody that appears to recognize the receptor from human T cell growth factor: partial characterization of the receptor. *Nature* **300**:267.

19. Larsson, E., A. Coutinho, and C. Martinez. 1980. A suggested mechanism for T lymphocyte activation: Implication on the acquisition of functional reactivities. *Immunol. Rev.* **51**:61.

20. Palacios, R. 1982. Mechanism of T cell activation: Role of functional relationship of HLA-DR antigens and interleukins. *Immunol. Rev.* **63**:73.

21. Mizel, S.B. 1982. Interleukin 1 and T cell activation. *Immunol. Rev.* **63**:51.

22. Miyawaki, T., A. Yachie, N. Uwadana, S. Ohzeki, T. Nagaoki, and N. Taniguchi. 1982. Functional significance of Tac antigen expressed on activated human T lymphocytes: Tac antigen interacts with T cell growth factor in cellular proliferation. *J. Immunol.* **129**:2474.

23. Depper, J.M., W.J. Leonard, R.J. Robb, T.A. Waldmann, and C. Greene. 1983. Blockade of the interleukin 2 receptor by ant-Tac antibody. Inhibition of human lymphocyte activation. *J. Immunol.* **131**:690.

CHAPTER 37

T-Activation Antigens: Kinetics of Appearance and Effect on Cell Proliferation Studied with Monoclonal Antibodies

Luigi Del Vecchio, Mario De Felice, Maria Caterina Turco, Michele Maio, Emilio Pace, Catia Lo Pardo, Clemente Vacca, Salvatore Venuta, and Serafino Zappacosta

The immunological detection of T surface antigens has been successfully applied to the study of molecules that regulate T cell physiology. In particular, investigations of activation antigens led to the recognition of growth factor receptors, such as those for interleukin-2 (1,2) and transferrin (3,4), thus providing critical information for biochemical and functional studies of membrane molecules regulating T cell proliferation.

We have studied 19 monoclonal antibodies (mAbs) directed against T-activated cells and have identified a set of molecules involved in T cell proliferation.

Materials and Methods

Peripheral Blood Mononuclear Cells (PBMC) Isolation and Culture Conditions

PBMC were isolated from peripheral blood of healthy volunteers by centrifugation on Ficoll–Hypaque density gradient. Viability was assessed by Trypan blue exclusion. PBMC were seeded at 2×10^6/ml in RPMI 1640 medium (Flow Laboratories, Helsinki, Finland) supplemented with 5% heat-inactivated fetal calf serum (FCS), 1% PHA (Pharmacia, Uppsala, Sweden), and 5 ng/ml of mAb OKT3 (Ortho Diagnostic Systems, Raritan, NJ, USA)

Indirect Immunofluorescence (IIF)

IIF was performed with cytofluorograph Spectrum III, Ortho Diagnostic Systems, Raritan, NJ, USA. For each test, 1×10^6 cells were incubated in

50 μl phosphate-buffered saline (PBS) and 50 μl mAb (1 : 200 dilution) were added. After 30-min incubation at 4°C, cells were washed twice with PBS and 50 μl of fluorescein isothiocyanate-conjugated rabbit anti–mouse IgG (Miles Laboratories Inc., Elkhart, IN, USA) were added. After 30 min at 4°C, cells were washed twice with PBS and examined by cyto-fluorograph.

Nineteen mAbs, code numbers 1, 135–151, 153, and 159, directed against T-activated cell specificities, were provided by Dr. B.F. Haynes on behalf of the Organizing Committee of the Second International Workshop on Human Leukocyte Differentiation Antigens. The mAb anti-Tac was a gift from Dr. T. Waldmann, National Institutes of Health, Bethesda, MD, USA. mAbs OKT9, OKT10, and OKIa1 were obtained from Ortho Diagnostic Systems, Raritan, NJ, USA. The anti-β_2 microglobulin mAb (used as a positive control) was obtained from Becton & Dickinson Laboratories, Oxnard, CA, USA.

Functional Studies

In order to test cell proliferation, or inhibition of proliferation, PBMC were seeded in microtiter plates at 4×10^5 cells/well, in RPMI 1640 supplemented with 5% FCS, and with or without OKT3 (5 ng/ml) or PHA (1%). mAbs were added 12 hr after plating; 0.5 μCi/well [^{3}H]thymidine (47 Ci/mM, Amersham International plc, UK) was added 68 hr after plating, and cells were harvested 4 hr later. Thymidine incorporation was measured in a β-counter.

Results

IIF Analysis

The binding of 19 mAbs directed against T-activated cell specificities was first tested on cells other than lymphocytes. Monocytes and granulocytes were used and only one mAb (142) was found to react with 95% of granulocytes. The reactivity of the mAbs with resting lymphocytes ranged from 2 to 66% of the cells. The distribution of the reactivity appeared to be bimodal, so that two distinct subsets of mAbs could be identified (Table 37.1): (a) a group of 13 mAbs recognizing 2–16% of the cells ($\bar{x} = 6$; SD = ± 5); (b) a group of 5 mAbs, staining 33–49% of the cells ($\bar{x} = 41$; SD = ± 7). mAb 144 detected 66% of the cells.

We found a variability of about 30% in the expression of the same antigen in our population of 13 healthy individuals. However, individual variation did not affect the comparative analysis of the reactivity of the mAbs. Results obtained with anti-Tac, OKT9, OKT10, and OKIa1 were comparable to those reported by others (1,4–6) at the start of the cultures (T_0) as well as throughout the study (Table 37.1).

Table 37.1. Binding of 19 "T-activation" mAbs on stimulated PBMC from 13 normal donors.

mAb	T_0	T_{44}	T_{72}	T_{190}	T_{20}/T_0
135	5 (3)[a]	44 (10)[a]	55 (11)[a]	28 (15)[a]	4.4[b]
136	15 (6)	27 (12)	28 (9)	19 (8)	1.2
137	11 (7)	20 (5)	26 (11)	9 (6)	1.4
138	33 (11)	63 (20)	64 (13)	56 (17)	1.6
139	16 (6)	33 (20)	34 (14)	26 (10)	1.5
140	5 (2)	43 (19)	52 (11)	24 (16)	4.3
141	3 (1)	35 (14)	38 (12)	15 (8)	4.6
142	10 (4)	43 (17)	58 (10)	25 (15)	2.0
143	2 (1)	30 (7)	41 (9)	17 (11)	6.9
144	66 (13)	77 (11)	74 (10)	83 (4)	1.1
145	3 (2)	32 (16)	35 (9)	12 (8)	4.0
146	2 (1)	32 (10)	37 (9)	17 (13)	7.3
147	2 (1)	14 (13)	20 (11)	9 (3)	2.2
148	45 (11)	65 (9)	65 (16)	48 (20)	1.3
149	45 (11)	73 (12)	61 (16)	54 (13)	1.3
150	49 (22)	64 (14)	56 (11)	49 (7)	1.1
151	33 (13)	32 (8)	35 (10)	31 (12)	0.5
153	4 (1)	41 (5)	29 (14)	9 (6)	2.3
159	6 (2)	40 (16)	54 (14)	31 (15)	4.0
anti-Tac	4 (1)	40 (9)	55 (8)	28 (20)	3.7
OKIa1	12 (2)	38 (16)	39 (19)	21 (13)	2.1
OKT9	6 (6)	29 (9)	40 (12)	5 (3)	2.3
OKT10	16 (5)	38 (8)	48 (13)	36 (17)	1.3
1	2 (1)	6 (3)	9 (2)	10 (6)	1.7
anti-β_2m	97 (1)	97 (1)	97 (1)	88 (4)	1.0

[a] % of IIF stained positive cells: mean (SD).
[b] T_{20}/T_0 ratio of IIF stained positive cells.

Although the antigenic pattern did not appear to be modified 10 hr after mitogen addition to cells, increase in the expression of some antigens could be detected at 20 hr following stimulation (T_{20}). The ratio between the proportion of positive cells at T_{20} and that at T_0 (T_{20}/T_0) was determined for each antigen (Table 37.1). (This ratio can be used to identify a subset of antigens expressed early in the activation process.) Seven mAbs recognized antigens with a T_{20}/T_0 ratio of at least 4, and two of the mAbs, 143 and 146, showed a 7-fold increase in their reactivity with cells during the first 20 hr of the culture. This group of mAbs appears to be a useful marker of T-activation.

The reactivity of the mAbs was maximal after 72 hr of culture and ranged from 22 to 66% positive cells. The analysis performed at 190 hr did not reveal any further increase and often showed a decrease in the fraction of positive cells. In conclusion, according to the IIF pattern, the identified antigens can be classified as follows (Fig. 37.1):

1. "early" (characterized by a high T_{20}/T_0 ratio, >4, and recognized by mAbs 135, 140, 141, 143, 145, 146, 159)

2. "constitutive low" (expressed in a low fraction of the cells, $\bar{x} = 16\%$, throughout the mitogenic stimulation and recognized by mAbs 136, 137, 147, 153)
3. "constitutive high" (expressed in a high fraction of the cells, $\bar{x} = 59\%$, throughout the stimulation and recognized by mAbs 138, 144, 148, 149, 150)

Data for mAbs 139, 142, and 151, which do not fit with our classification, are given in Table 37.1 (and above).

To evaluate if the antigens recognized by the Workshop mAbs were related to known activation antigens, i.e., Tac, T9, T10, and DR, a test of the correlation between the expression of these antigens was performed.

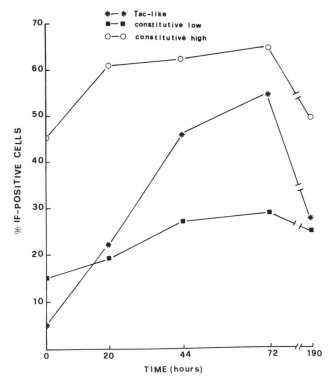

Fig. 37.1. Kinetics of the expression of membrane antigens on OKT3-stimulated PBMC as recognized by mAbs belonging to different subsets (see text). Symbols represent the mean values of antigen expression on 13 normal cell preparations stained with a representative mAb for each subset (∗135, ■136, ○148). SD did not exceed 20% of the mean values.

The correlation coefficient (r) was significant ($r > 0.90$) when mAbs 135, 140, 143, or 159 were compared to anti-Tac and mAb 147 to OKT9.

Functional Studies

To study whether the T-activation antigens recognized by the Workshop mAbs were involved in triggering or regulating cell activation, we tested their ability to induce T cell proliferation or to inhibit the proliferation of OKT3- (or PHA-) stimulated lymphocytes. In the latter case, mAbs were added 12 hr after mitogen stimulation. As shown in Table 37.2, 11 of these mAbs inhibited T cell proliferation by more than 35% (average value 75%).

The ascite of mAb 137 was found to be strongly mitogenic for PBMC (titration of the mitogenic activity is shown in Table 37.3) and to induce interleukin-2 production in the stimulated cultures (not shown). This result was surprising since only 10% of the cells were stained by the mAb in IIF at T_0 (Table 37.1). The mitogenic capacity of mAb 137 has been confirmed by using a partially purified preparation of the antibody.

Table 37.2. Inhibition of OKT3-induced proliferation in PBMC by 17 mAbs Recognizing "T-activation antigens".

mAb	% Inhibition	
	Donor 1	Donor 2
135	61	86
136	5	16
138	91	94
139	50	68
140	83	91
141	53	66
142	NT[a]	NT[a]
143	18	26
144	28	32
145	77	83
146	16	36
147	11	30
148	87	91
149	81	92
150	39	41
151	49	73
153	31	38
159	78	85

[a] NT, Not tested; the mAb preparation contained sodium azide.

Table 37.3. Mitogenic effect of mAb 137 on PBMC.

mAb added	^{3}H-Tdr incorporation
None	905 (233)[a]
OKT3, 5 ng/ml	38,050 (3535)
136, 1 : 100[b]	1314 (155)
137, 1 : 100	31,055 (2072)
137, 1 : 1000	29,705 (700)
137, 1 : 5000	12,882 (293)
137, 1 : 20,000	2300 (205)

[a] cpm (SD).
[b] mAb dilution.

Discussion

Immunological detection of T surface structures has led to identification of molecules functionally involved in the mechanism of T cell proliferation, e.g., T3 (7), T11 (8,9), Tac (1,2), and T9 (3,4). In this study, PBMC from 13 healthy individuals were stimulated with OKT3 (or PHA) and analyzed in IIF for their expression of antigens recognized by 19 mAbs characterized as reacting with activated T cell specificities.

Comparative analysis of mAbs binding to T cells, kinetics of appearance of the recognized antigens, and correlations to Tac, T9, T10, and DR expression, as well as functional studies allowed us to identify mAb subsets that recognize definite molecular structures. The first subset consists of mAbs 135, 140, and 159. The three mAbs inhibited OKT3-induced proliferation over 75% and recognized an antigen present on 5% of the resting lymphocytes, and on over 50% of proliferating T cells. The kinetics of expression of this antigen closely resembles that of Tac, as confirmed by the correlation test, high ($r > 0.90$) for Tac and low for DR, T9, and T10. Because of the poor representation, at least as shown by IIF, of this antigen on T lymphocytes at T_0, it is unlikely that it corresponds to the T3 or T11 molecules. Therefore, mAbs 135, 140, and 159 appear to recognize a Tac-like molecule. The interference of these mAbs with the binding of interleukin-2 or anti-Tac to activated T cells should be tested in order to support this conclusion.

mAb 143 appears to react with Tac, but at a different epitope from that bound by anti-Tac. In fact, the expression of the 143 antigen correlates well with Tac ($r > 0.90$); however, mAb 143 is only slightly inhibitory for proliferating T cells. This mAb will contribute to the definition of a functional domain on Tac molecules.

One subset of "early" mAbs (146, 145, 141) defines a molecular structure different from Tac (Fig. 37.2), as there is no correlation between the expression of Tac and that of the structure recognized by these mAbs. This subset appears to be heterogeneous. In particular, mAb 146 has a very low inhibitory capacity and a T_{20}/T_0 ratio of 7.3 (Table 37.1 and Fig. 37.2), while mAb 145 inhibits 80% of T cell proliferation with a T_{20}/T_0 ratio of 4.0. On the basis of our data we cannot discriminate whether different epitopes or different molecules are recognized by these mAbs.

Another group of mAbs (138, 148, 149, and 150) recognized an antigen present on 43% of cells at T_0 and on 55% of cells at T_{72}. The expression of this antigen is therefore constitutively high; however, its increase is not significant (Fig. 37.1). As expected, a high correlation could not be found with the expression of any of the classical activation antigens considered. These mAbs were found to interfere with T cell proliferation and, in particular, mAbs 138, 148, and 149 inhibited proliferation by about 90%. This subset of mAbs appears to identify a molecule constitutively present on the lymphocyte membrane and involved in T cell proliferation. These

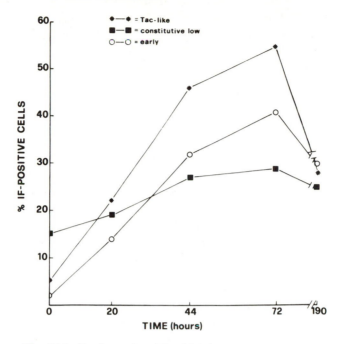

EXPRESSION OF MEMBRANE ANTIGENS DURING T CELL ACTIVATION

Fig. 37.2. See legend to Fig. 37.1 (*135, ■136, ○146).

data do not exclude the possibility that this antigen, the "constitutive high" antigen of Fig. 37.1, is analogous to T11 (9).

The antigens recognized by mAbs 136, 153, and 144 do not appear to participate in mitogen-induced T cell proliferation since their membrane expression is not altered by OKT3 or PHA and/or these mAbs do not affect T cell activation by mitogens.

Finally, of all the Workshop mAbs, only 137 turned out to be mitogenic for lymphocytes. This mAb was active up to a 1:5000 dilution of the ascite and induced interleukin-2 secretion in the culture medium. A preparation of DEAE-purified 137 also activates PBMC proliferation. If these data are confirmed, it could be interesting to determine the identity of the structure recognized by 137, since the antigen reacting with this mAb is detected by IIF only on 11% of resting and 25% of OKT3-stimulated cells. Even though IIF is less sensitive than the mitogenic assay in antigen detection, the possibility remains that the 137 molecule does not correspond to T3 or T11 (or the antigen receptor).

In conclusion, our study led to the identification of subsets of mAbs that recognize T surface antigens. A functional role in the regulation of T cell proliferation can be hypothesized for some of these antigens. It would be of interest to verify these data under different experimental conditions, such as antigenic or allogeneic stimulation, in order to establish whether different T surface molecular patterns are displayed under different stimuli. This approach could be helpful also to distinguish between early, stimulus-specific and late, more general regulatory steps of T cell proliferation.

Summary

Monoclonal antibodies designated by the Second International Workshop on Human Leukocyte Differentiation Antigens as "T-activation antigens" were tested by direct immunofluorescence on peripheral blood mononuclear cells obtained from 13 healthy donors and stimulated with OKT3 (or PHA). The test was performed at various times of culture, parallel to determination of anti-Tac-, OKT9-, OKT10-, and OKIa1-stained positive cells. The mAbs were also tested for their ability to stimulate PBMC or to inhibit OKT3-activated cells in proliferation assays.

A comparative analysis of all the data obtained revealed groups of mAbs with homogeneous characteristics. Each mAb subset appeared to recognize a specific T surface molecule. The study of these molecules could yield valuable information on the mechanisms regulating T cell activation.

Acknowledgments. We thank Mrs. J. Gilder for carefully reviewing the manuscript. This work was supported in part by CNR grants (Progetto Finalizzato "Oncologia" and Progetto Finalizzato "Ingegneria Genetica e Basi Molecolari della Malattie Ereditarie").

References

1. Uchiyama, T., D.L. Nelson, T.A. Fleisher, and T.A. Waldmann. 1981. A monoclonal antibody (anti-Tac) reactive with activated and functionally mature human T cells. *J. Immunol.* **126**:1398.
2. Miyawaki, T., A. Yachie, N. Uwadana, S. Ohzeki, T. Nagaoki, and N. Taniguchi. 1982. Functional significance of Tac antigen expressed on activated human T lymphocytes: Tac antigen interacts with T cell growth factor in cellular proliferation. *J. Immunol.* **129**:2474.
3. Sutherland, R., D. Delia, C. Schneider, R. Newman, J. Kemshead, and M. Greaves. 1981. Ubiquitous cell-surface glycoprotein on tumor cells is proliferation-associated receptor for transferrin. *Proc. Natl. Acad. Sci. U.S.A.* **78**:4515.
4. Terhorst, C., A. van Agthoven, K. LeClair, P. Snow, E. Reinherz, and S. Schlossman. 1981. Biochemical studies of the human thymocyte cell surface antigens T6, T9 and T10. *Cell* **23**:771.

5. Reinherz, E.L., P.C. Kung, J.M. Pesando, J. Ritz, J. Goldstein, and S.F. Schlossman. 1979. Ia determinants on human T-cell subsets defined by monoclonal antibody. *J. Exp. Med.* **150**:1472.
6. Yu, D.T.Y., R.J. Winchester, S.M. Fu, A. Gibofsky, H.S. Ko, and H.G. Kunkel. 1980. Peripheral blood Ia-positive T cells. *J. Exp. Med.* **151**:91.
7. Van Wauwe, J.P., J.R. De Mey and J.G. Goossens. 1979. OKT3: a monoclonal anti-human T lymphocyte antibody with potent mitogenic properties. *J. Immunol.* **124**:2708.
8. Meuer, S.C., R.E. Hussey, M. Fabbi, D. Fox, O. Acuto, K.A. Fitzgerald, J.C. Hodgdon, J.P. Protentis, S.F. Schlossman, and E.L. Reinherz. 1984. An alternative pathway of T-cell activation: a functional role for the 50 kd T11 sheep erythrocyte receptor protein. *Cell* **36**:897.
9. Palacios, R., and O. Martinez-Maza. 1982. Is the E receptor on human T lymphocytes a "negative signal receptor"? *J. Immunol.* **126**:2479.

Part VIII. Study of T Cell Leukemia-Associated Antigens

CHAPTER 38

Antibody 3-40 Binds to Keratin and Vimentin Intermediate Filaments

Andrew J. Laster, Thomas J. Palker, Elizabeth A. Harden,
Winifred Ho, Kazuyuki Naito, Bo DuPont, and
Barton F. Haynes

Introduction

In 1983, Naito *et al.* reported the production of the murine monoclonal
antibody 3-40, produced by immunizing mice with the human T-ALL cell
line MOLT-4 (1). By cytotoxicity, absorption, and indirect immunofluorescence assays, antibody 3-40 reacted with a 35–40-Kd surface protein
on most T-ALL cell lines, but not with surface molecules of normal
hematopoietic cells, including thymocytes (1).

While studying normal thymocyte and thymic epithelial cell maturation
in our laboratory, we noted that antibody 3-40 bound not only to the
surface of T-ALL cells, but also reacted in indirect immunofluorescent
(IF) assays with the cytoskeleton of T-ALL cells, normal thymocytes,
epithelial cells, and fibroblasts. In this report, we show that antibody 3-40
binds to keratin and vimentin intermediate filaments (IMF), as well as to a
39-Kd intermediate filament-associated protein in epithelial cells and fibroblasts.

Methods

Cell Lines

Five cell lines were utilized to examine in detail the reactivity pattern of
antibody 3-40. Rat thymic epithelial cells (IT26R21) and rat fibroblasts
(IT45R91) were kindly provided by Dr. Tsunetoshi Itoh of the Dana-
Farber Cancer Institute, Boston, MA, and human foreskin fibroblasts by
Dr. Kay Singer at Duke University, Durham, NC. HEp-2 is an epithelial
cell line derived from a human laryngeal carcinoma, and HSB-2 is a
T-ALL cell line.

Other Monoclonal Antibodies

Monoclonal antibodies AE-1 and AE-3 against human keratins (2) were the generous gift of Dr. Tung-Tien Sun, New York University School of Medicine, New York, NY. Antibody 43βE8 was kindly provided by Dr. Arthur Vogel, University of Washington, Seattle, WA, and reacts with vimentin and glial fibrillary acidic protein (3). A2B5 is an IgM monoclonal antibody that recognizes complex gangliosides on endocrine thymic epithelial cells (4). Rabbit polyclonal antisera to tubulin and actin were purchased from Miles Laboratories, Inc., Naperville, IL. Rabbit anti-thymosin α_1 was the gift of Dr. Allan Goldstein, George Washington University, Washington, DC and was absorbed and used as described (4). P3X63-Ag8, a murine myeloma cell line that secretes IgG, and DMH 1.3.3.5, an IgM antibody to human Ia-like antigen (kindly provided by Dr. Bernard Amos at Duke University, Durham, NC) were used as immunoglobulin isotype controls.

Immunofluorescence Assays

Indirect and direct immunofluorescent staining of viable cells in suspension and 4-micron acetone-fixed tissue sections were performed as previously described in detail (5). Monoclonal antibody 3-40 was directly fluoresceinated (F/P = 7.3) as previously described (6). Double immunofluorescence assays with directly fluoresceinated antibody 3-40 and either A2B5 or rabbit anti-thymosin α_1 were performed as described (4,7).

IT26R21 and IT45R91 cell lines were also plated on Lab-tek slides and one of the following cytoskeletal inhibitors was then added for the specified remainder of a 24-hr growth period: (a) colcemid, 20 μg/ml (Gibco Laboratories, Grand Island, NY) in RPMI $\times$ 16 hr; (b) cytochalasin B, 10 μg/ml (Sigma Chemicals, St. Louis, MO) $\times$ 2 hr; (c) vinblastine sulfate, 5×10^{-5} M for 2 hr—prepared as a stock solution of 1×10^{-2} M in spectral grade DMSO (Mallinckrodt, Paris, KY) as previously described (8). Slides were then washed in RPMI 1640 + 15% HIFCS, fixed in acetone ($-20°C$) for 10 min, and indirect immunofluorescence was performed.

Preparations of Cytoskeletal Extracts

Cytoskeletal extracts of IT45R91, IT26R21, HSB-2 T-ALL cells, and human epidermal skin were isolated as described by Pruss *et al.* (9).

Immunoblot Analysis

Western blot analysis of cell/tissue cytoskeletal preparations and Triton-X-soluble fractions were performed according to the techniques of Towbin *et al.* (10), with modifications of Palker *et al.* (11).

Results

Components of Normal Tissues Reactive with Antibody 3-40

As previously reported, antibody 3-40 reacted with a variety of normal human tissues tested (Table 38.1). It was of particular interest to characterize the 3-40$^+$ cell types present in thymus. Morphologically, it could be seen that 3-40 reacted with mesodermal-derived thymic capsule and interlobular septae and vessels, as well as with epithelial cells within the thymic cortex and medulla (not shown). Double immunofluorescence stains were performed using directly fluoresceinated 3-40 with either antibody A2B5 that identifies endocrine thymic epithelium or with rabbit thymosin α_1 antibody (4). We found that all cortical and medullary thymic epithelial cells that were 3-40$^+$ were A2B5$^+$ and contained thymosin α_1.

Reactivity of Antibody 3-40 with Rodent and Human Cell Lines

To further characterize the reactivity of antibody 3-40 with specific cell types within thymus, we assayed 3-40 reactivity in rodent and human fibroblast and epithelial cell lines.

In indirect immunofluorescent assays, antibody 3-40 identified a Triton-X-resistant cytoskeletal antigen in both rodent and human epithelial cells and fibroblasts [Fig. 38.1(A), (B), (C), (D)]. We have previously shown that the IT26R21 cell line reacts by immunofluorescence with antibodies

Table 38.1. Components of normal human tissues reactive with 3-40 monoclonal antibody.[a]

Tissue	Components reactive with 3-40
Postnatal thymus	Neuroendocrine thymic epithelium, vessel endothelium, capsule, interlobular septae, and Hassall's bodies
Skin	Langerhan's cells in epidermis, reticular cells in dermis, epidermal keratinocytes (faintly reactive), vessel endothelium
Adenoid	Basal epidermis, scattered reticular cells in adenoid stroma
Tonsil	Basal epidermis, scattered reticular cells in tonsillar stroma
Lymph node	Vessel endothelium, numerous large reticular cells, subset of lymphocytes
Postnatal spleen	Reticular cells distributed throughout spleen
Postnatal liver	Large reticular cells scattered among negative hepatocytes
Pancreas	Islets and subset of acinar cells, vessel endothelium
Fetal thymus	Same as postnatal thymus
Fetal liver	Reticular cells scattered throughout liver
Fetal spleen	Vessel endothelium and stroma
Pituitary	Pituicytes
Brain cortex	Filamentous pattern
Medulla	Filamentous pattern

[a] Reactivity determined by indirect immunofluorescence as described in Materials and Methods.

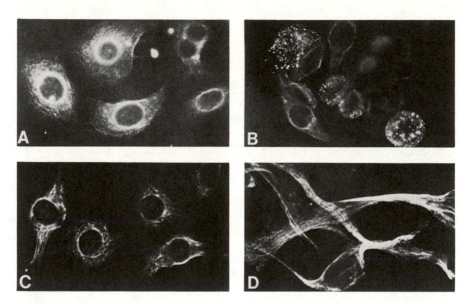

Fig. 38.1. Reactivity of antibody 3-40 on human and rodent cell lines. Antibody 3-40 reacted with keratin intermediate filaments in the IT26R21 rat thymic epithelial cell line (A) and HEp-2 cells (B). [The reactivity with spheroid granules seen in mitotic HEp-2 cells has been previously reported for other anti-keratin antibodies and was also demonstrated using antibody AE-1.] Antibody 3-40 also reacted with vimentin in the IT45R91 rat fibroblast cell line (C) and in human foreskin fibroblasts (D) (400×).

AE-1 and AE-3 (anti-keratin) but not 43βE8 (anti-vimentin) (12). Similarly the IT45R91 line is 43βE8 positive, but AE1 and AE3 negative.

When rat fibroblasts were treated with vinblastine or colcemid followed by incubation with antibody 3-40, perinuclear coils characteristic of vimentin were observed on fluorescent analysis (Fig. 38.2). Similar changes were noted with the anti-vimentin antibody. Cytochalasin B had no effect on the pattern of antibody 3-40 reactivity by immunuofluorescence assay. Antibodies to tubulin decorated a crystal-like formation in IT45R91 cells treated with vinblastine, and anti-actin demonstrated retraction-like processes in cytochalasin B-treated IT45R91 cells. In contrast, in the rat thymic epithelial line, colcemid, vinblastine, or cytochalasin B had no effect on the pattern of 3-40 immunofluorescence, a reactivity pattern characteristic of keratin intermediate filaments.

Cytoplasmic immunofluorescence was also observed in cytopreps of HSB-2 cells, normal thymocytes and a subset of peripheral blood mononuclear cells (Table 38.2) after staining with antibody 3-40. However, as expected from the work of Naito *et al.* (1), cell surface immunofluorescence was positive only on HSB-2 cells and not on normal thymocytes, normal peripheral lymphocytes, rodent epithelial cells, or fibroblasts (Table 38.2).

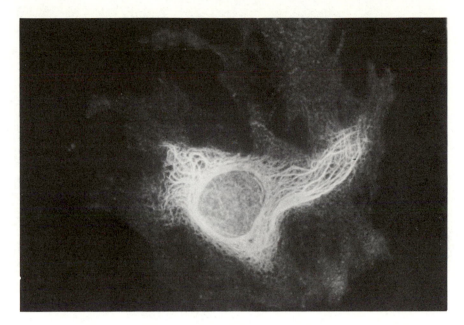

Fig. 38.2. Indirect immunofluorescent reactivity of antibody 3-40 on rat fibroblasts treated with vinblastine. When rat fibroblasts were incubated with vinblastine ($5 \times 10^{-5} M \times 2$ hr) and reacted with antibody 3-40, each cell demonstrated a perinuclear coil. Similar reactivity was seen with colcemid (20 μg/ml $\times$ 16 hr) or when a control antibody to vimentin (43βE8) was used (400$\times$).

Biochemical Characterization of the 3-40-Reactive Intracellular Antigen

To determine whether antibody 3-40 identified intermediate filaments or an intermediate filament-associated protein, we performed immunoblots using the insoluble cytoskeletal pellets derived from the human and rodent cell lines, HSB-2 T cells, and human skin. Western blots of HSB-2

Table 38.2. Summary of reactivity of antibody 3-40 to normal and malignant cell types.

Cell type	Surface reactivity[a] by IF (% of cells positive)	Intracytoplasmic[b] reactivity by IF
PB mononuclear cells	−	+
Thymocytes	−	+
IT26R21 Rat thymic epithelial cells	−	+
IT45R91 Rat fibroblasts	−	+
T-ALL (#1) fresh leukemic cells	+ (20)	+
T-ALL (#2) fresh leukemic cells	+ (7)	+
HSB-2 T-ALL cell line	+ (98)	+

[a] Surface reactivity assayed by indirect immunofluorescence (IF) on viable cells.
[b] Intracytoplasmic reactivity determined by indirect IF on acetone-fixed cells.

cytoskeletal preparations demonstrated that antibody 3-40 identified a 55-Kd protein that co-migrated with the protein recognized by a known monoclonal antibody to vimentin, and as well a 39-Kd protein [Fig. 38.3(A)]. Similar results were also obtained using the rat fibroblast line [Fig. 38.3(B)].

In the rat epithelial cell line, antibody 3-40 reacted with a family of cytoskeletal proteins between 43 and 56 Kd that were recognized by known anti-keratin antibodies (Fig. 38.4). In addition, 3-40 recognized a 39-Kd protein (Fig. 38.4). In human skin, antibody 3-40 identified two keratin bands of 56.5 and 50 Kd.

Because Naito *et al.* reported that antibody 3-40 identified a 35–40-Kd membrane-associated NP-40 soluble antigen in MOLT-4 cells, immunoblots were performed on the 6 M KCl Triton-X-soluble fraction of HSB-2 cells; we observed a band of 37 Kd–39 Kd. Immunoprecipitation of ^{125}I surface-labeled HSB-2 cells with antibody 3-40 demonstrated a 60–63-Kd antigen.

Discussion

Using indirect immunofluorescence and immunoblot analysis, we have shown that antibody 3-40 recognizes cytoplasmic intermediate filaments in both normal and malignant cells. Antibody 3-40 identified a family of cytokeratins found in a rodent epithelial cell line and in human skin and bound to vimentin in fibroblasts, T-ALL cells, and thymocytes. Antibody 3-40 also identified a 39-Kd cytoskeletal-associated protein in normal cells and HSB-2 T-ALL cells. Furthermore, in HSB-2 T-ALL cells, antibody 3-40 recognized a 37–39-Kd soluble antigen and a 63-Kd surface antigen. Naito *et al.* have previously shown (1) that antibody 3-40 recognized a 35–40-Kd surface protein in MOLT-4 T-ALL cells. Cell surface reactivity was not seen in nonmalignant cells (1).

Monoclonal antibodies reacting with more than one class of intermediate filament have been previously described (9,13). The binding of antibody 3-40 with keratin and vimentin is demonstrated in this report. Moreover, indirect immunofluorescence of antibody 3-40 on brain shows a pattern similar to glial fibrillary acidic protein (unpublished observations); cross-reactivity with other intermediate filaments remains to be demonstrated biochemically.

The ability to recognize keratin or vimentin intermediate filaments therefore explains the prior report of Naito *et al.* (1), who noted antibody 3-40 reactivity on frozen sections of thymus, pancreatic islets, skin, ovarian stroma, fetal testis, and in some melanomas, ovarian, breast, and colonic cancers. In the present report, we have also noted antibody 3-40 reactivity with both keratin-containing epithelial organs (thymus, skin, pancreas) and vimentin-containing mesenchymal derived tissue (vessels, connective tissue stroma, macrophages) (Table 38.1).

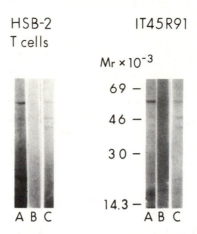

HSB-2
T cells

IT45R91

Mr × 10⁻³

69 —

46 —

30 —

14.3 —

A B C   A B C

Fig. 38.3. Immunoblot analysis of antibody 3-40 reactivity with proteins from the HSB-2 and IT45R91 cell lines. Cytoskeletal proteins were extracted from the HSB-2 T-cell line (left panel) or IT45R91 rat thymic fibroblasts (right panel) as previously described (9). Samples were reduced in 5% 2-ME with sample buffer, separated by 10% SDS–PAGE, and electrophoretically transferred to nitrocellulose. Molecular weight markers are indicated in the center. Lane A = antibody 43βE8 (anti-vimentin), Lane B = P3X63 (negative control), Lane C = antibody 3-40. Antibody 3-40 identified a 55-Kd protein in both HSB-2 and IT45R91 cells that co-migrated with a protein recognized by the antibody to vimentin; antibody 3-40 also recognized a 39-Kd protein in both cell lines as well as a 46-Kd protein also recognized by 43βE8.

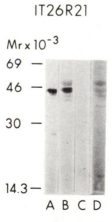

IT26R21

Mr × 10⁻³
69 —

46 —

30 —

14.3 —

A B C D

Fig. 38.4. Immunoblot analysis of antibody 3-40 reactivity with keratins from the IT26R21 cell line. Cytoskeletal proteins were extracted from the IT26R21 cell line, reduced in 5% 2-ME with sample buffer, separated by 10% SDS–PAGE, and electrophoretically transferred to nitrocellulose. Molecular weight markers are indicated on the left. Lane A = antibody AE-1 (anti-keratin), Lane B = antibody AE-3 (anti-keratin), Lane C = P3X63 negative control, Lane D = antibody 3-40. Antibody 3-40 identified rodent keratins of 56 Kd, 45 Kd, and 43 Kd, and as well identified a 39-Kd protein not recognized by the other anti-keratin antibodies.

472   A.J. Laster *et al.*

Monoclonal antibodies to double-stranded DNA (14), measles virus phosphoprotein (15), herpes simplex virus protein (15), and the Thy-1 surface antigen (16) have been shown to cross-react with vimentin intermediate filaments. We now extend this list of cross-reacting antigens to the 3-40 surface antigen found on T-ALL cells. Using a monoclonal antibody to vimentin (43βE8), we have recently shown positive surface immunofluorescence of viable T-ALL cells from one of three patients (A. Laster *et al.,* unpublished observations). Whether vimentin intermediate filaments exist on the surface of T-ALL cells or antibodies 3-40 and 43βE8 recognize determinants common to both vimentin and surface antigens on T-ALL cells is currently being investigated.

Furthermore, whether the 39-Kd cytoskeletal-associated protein in normal and HSB-2 cells, the 37–39-Kd HSB-2 soluble antigen, and the 35–40-Kd MOLT-4 membrane-associated antigen all identified by antibody 3-40 are identical remains to be determined. It is possible that this 3-40 antigen found in normal cells may be selectively expressed on the surface of human T cells during malignant transformation.

Acknowledgment. This work was supported by grants CA28936 and K0400695 from the NCI, NIH.

References

1. Naito, K., R.W. Knowles, F.X. Real, Y. Morishima, K. Kawashima, and B. Dupont. 1983. Analysis of two new leukemia-associated antigens detected on human T-cell acute lymphoblastic leukemia using monoclonal antibodies. *Blood* **62:**852.
2. Woodcock-Mitchell, J., R. Eichner, W.G. Nelson, and T-T. Sun. 1982. Immunolocalization of keratin polypeptides in human epidermis using monoclonal antibodies. *J. Cell Biol.* **95:**580.
3. Gown, A.M., and A.M. Vogel. 1984. Monoclonal antibodies to human intermediate filament proteins. II. Distribution of filament proteins in normal human tissues. *Am. J. Pathol.* **114:**309.
4. Haynes, B.F., K. Shimizu, and G.S. Eisenbarth. 1983. Identification of human and rodent thymic epithelium using tetanus toxin and monoclonal antibody A2B5. *J. Clin. Invest.* **71:**9.
5. Haynes, B.F., L.L. Hensley, and B.V. Jegasothy. 1982. Differentiation of human T lymphocytes. II. Phenotypic difference in skin and blood malignant T cells in cutaneous T cell lymphoma. *J. Invest. Dermatol.* **78:**323.
6. Haynes, B.F., D.L. Mann, M.E. Hemler, J.A. Schroer, J.A. Shelhamer, G.S. Eisenbarth, C.A. Thomas, H.S. Mostowski, J.L. Straminger, and A.S. Fauci. 1980. Characterization of a monoclonal antibody which defines an immunoregulatory T-cell subset for immunoglobulin synthesis in man. *Proc. Natl. Acad. Sci. U.S.A.* **77:**2914.
7. Haynes, B.F., R.M. Scearce, D.F. Lobach, and L.L. Hensley. 1984. Phenotypic characterization and ontogeny of mesodermal-derived and endocrine epithelial components of the human thymus microenvironment. *J. Exp. Med.* **159:**1149.

8. Weber, K., T. Bibring, and M. Osborn. 1975. Specific visualization of tubulin-containing structures in tissue culture cells by immunofluorescence. Cytoplasmic microtubules, vinblastine-induced paracrystals and mitotic figures. *Exp. Cell Res.* **95**:111.

9. Pruss, R.M., R. Mirsky, and M.C. Raff. 1981. All classes of intermediate filaments share a common antigenic determinant defined by a monoclonal antibody. *Cell* **27**:419.

10. Towbin, H., T. Staehelin, and J. Gordon. 1979. Electrophoretic transfer of proteins from polyacrylamide gels to nitrocellulose sheets. Procedures and some complications. *Proc. Natl. Acad. Sci. U.S.A.* **76**:4350.

11. Palker, T.J., R.M. Scearce, S.E. Miller, M. Popovic, D.P. Bolognesi, R.M. Gallo, and B.F. Haynes. 1984. Monoclonal antibodies against human T-cell leukemia–lymphoma virus (HTLV) p24 interval core protein. *J. Exp. Med.* **159**:1117.

12. Laster, A.J., and B.F. Haynes. 1985. Human thymic epithelial cells contain keratins of differentiated cornified epithelium. *Clin. Res.* **33**:381A.

13. Dellagi, K., J.C. Brouet, J. Perrcau, and D. Paulin. 1982. Human monoclonal IgM with autoantibody activity against intermediate filaments. *Proc. Natl. Acad. Sci. U.S.A.* **79**:446.

14. Andrè-Schwartz, J., S.K. Datta, Y. Shoenfeld, D.A. Isenbery, D. Stollar, and R.S. Schwartz. 1984. Finding of cytoskeletal proteins by monoclonal anti-DNA lupus autoantibodies. *Clin. Immunol. Immunopathol.* **31**:261.

15. Fujinami, R.S., M.B.A. Ostone, Z. Wroblewska, M.E. Frankel, and H. Koprowski. 1983. Molecular mimicry in virus infection: Cross-reaction of measles virus phosphoprotein or of herpes simplex virus protein with human intermediate filaments. *Proc. Natl. Acad. Sci. U.S.A.* **80**:2346.

16. Dulbecco, R., M. Unger, M. Bologna, H. Battifora, P. Syka, and S. Okada. 1981. Cross reactivity between Thy 1 and a component of intermediate filaments demonstrated using a monoclonal antibody. *Nature* **292**:772.

Part IX. Other Types of Studies and Description of New T Cell Markers

CHAPTER 39

Screening of Monoclonal Antibodies against T Cell Differentiation Antigens Using Transfectants or Somatic Cell Hybrids

Ryuzo Ueda, Nobuhiko Emi, Ikuya Tsuge,
Keiko Nishida, Kazuhiko R. Utsumi, Shigeru Takamoto,
Takashi Maruyama, Kazuo Ota, and Toshitada Takahashi

Introduction

With the development of hybridoma techniques, a large number of mono-clonal antibodies have been produced against cell surface antigens of human hematopoietic cells. In order to compare the specificity of these antibodies produced by various investigators, the ideal target cells are those which express only one or a few antigens on the cell surface. In our laboratories, as a first step to study the genes coding T cell differentiation antigens, transfection of mouse L cells with high molecular weight DNA from human T cells has been carried out and a stable transfectant expressing 41-Kd pan T antigen detected by the Tp40 antibody (1) was established. In addition, to study the chromosomal regulation of T cell differentiation antigens, human–mouse T cell hybrids have been produced and two clones retaining a few human chromosomes were found to be positive with Tp120 antibody (1), detecting the 120-Kd pan T antigen.

In this paper, we report the analysis of 159 T cell-related monoclonal antibodies (mAbs) registered in this Second International Workshop by testing against the transfectant and hybrid cells established in our laboratories.

Materials and Methods

Monoclonal Antibodies (mAbs) and Serological Assays

Tp40 and Tp120 antibodies detecting 40-Kd and 120-Kd pan T antigens, respectively, were produced and characterized in our laboratories (1). For screening of T cell-related mAbs registered in this Workshop against transfectant or somatic cell hybrids, mouse mixed hemadsorption (M-MHA) and immune adherence (IA) assays were carried out on Terasaki microplates (2,3). Radioimmunoprecipitation was carried out as described elsewhere (1,4).

Transfectants (Fig. 39.1)

Establishment and characterization of a mouse L cell transfectant expressing 41-Kd pan T antigen and HLA class 1 antigen will be described elsewhere. Briefly, mouse L cells lacking thymidine kinase gene (*tk*) (Ltk⁻) were co-transfected with cellular DNA from HPB-ALL human T cell line and the herpes simplex virus *tk* (5). The *tk* positive colonies were screened with monoclonal antibodies against human membrane antigens by M-MHA and positive clones were selected. One clone, 27B-T1, was found to express both 41-Kd pan T (Tp40) antigen and HLA-class 1 antigen. The expression of both antigens on 27B-T1 cells was confirmed by cytofluorometric analysis and also by the immunoprecipitation experiments. The Tp40 molecule on the transfectant was found to be slightly smaller than that on HPB-ALL cells.

Human–Mouse Hybrids (Fig. 39.2)

Isolation and characterization of two human–mouse hybrids expressing 120-Kd pan T antigen will be described elsewhere. Briefly, two hybrid clones reactive with Tp120 antibody were established from the fusion between concanavalin A-stimulated human peripheral blood lymphocytes and hypoxanthine-guanine phosphoribosyl transferase negative mouse T cell leukemia, BW5147 (6). The expression of the 120-Kd pan T antigen was confirmed by cytofluorometric analysis and immunoprecipitation experiments. Karyotype analysis showed that one clone retained human chromosome nos. 6, 7, and 11 and the other had nos. 11 and 21. As soon as the latter clone lost chromosome 11, the expression of Tp120 became negative, indicating that the presence of chromosome 11 was essential for the expression of the 120-Kd pan T antigen. The presence of human chromosome 11 was confirmed by the isozyme analysis of lactate dehydrogenase.

Results and Discussion

Reactivity of T Cell-Related mAbs with 27B-T1 Transfectant Cells Assayed by M-MHA and IA

27B-T1 transfectant cells expressing both 41-Kd pan T antigen and HLA-class I antigen were screened with 159 T cell-related mAbs registered in this Workshop by M-MHA or IA assays on Terasaki microplates and the

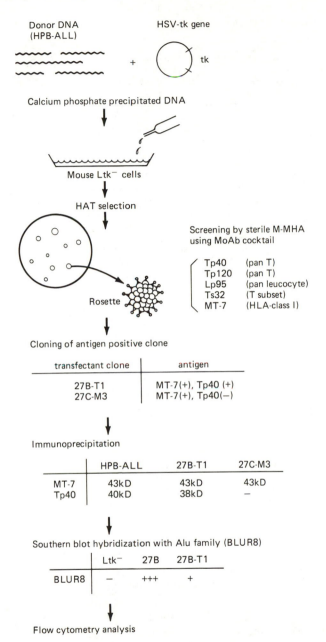

Fig. 39.1. Establishment of a mouse L cell transfectant expressing the 41-Kd pan T antigen, Tp40.

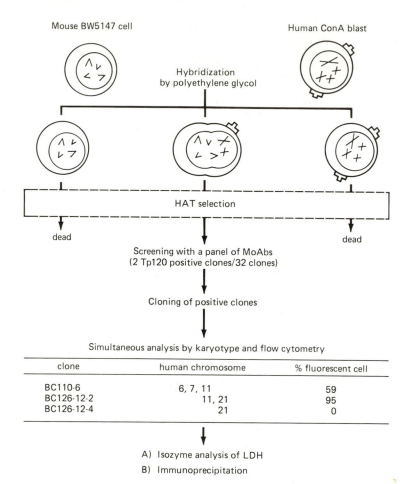

Fig. 39.2. Establishment of two human–mouse hybrids expressing the 120-Kd pan T antigen, Tp120.

results are summarized in Table 39.1. Interestingly, all mAbs which showed positive reactions were found to belong to the CD7 group [T, p41], with one exception, i.e., antibody no. 17 of the CD2 group [T, p50]. Among the CD7 group, one-half of the antibodies showed positive reactions. Testing of CD7 group antibodies against Tp40-positive HPB-ALL cell line demonstrated that only these antibodies reactive with 27B-T1 cells were positive, indicating that the rest of the mAbs cannot be detected by the assays employed or the antibody activity was not strong enough to give positive reactions. Next, Nonidet P-40 (NP-40) lysates were prepared from Tp40-positive Jurkat cell line, and immunoprecipitation experiments were carried out with nine mAbs among the CD7 group. As shown in Fig. 39.3, immunoprecipitates with a molecular weight of

Table 39.1. Reactivity of T cell-related mAbs with 27B-T1 transfectant cells assayed by M-MHA and IA.

Positive	Negative
CD7[a] [T, p41]: 9 Abs (30[b], 31, 38, 39, 40, 41, 43, 44, 45), Tp40[c]	CD7 [T, p41]: 8/17 Abs (29, 32, 33, 34, 35, 36, 37, 42)
CD2 [T, p50]: 1 Ab (17)	CD1 [Thy, p45, 12]: all 7 Abs
	CD2 [T, p50]: 15/16 Abs
	CD3 [T, p19-29]: all 11 Abs
	CD4 [T, p55]: all 14 Abs
	CD5 [T, p67]: all 9 Abs
	CD6 [T, p120]: all 2 Abs
	CD8 [T, p32-33]: all 20 Abs
	Pan T, others: all 19 Abs
	T subset, others: all 16 Abs
	T-activated: all 18 Abs

[a] Workshop cluster.
[b] Workshop code number.
[c] Made by Aichi Cancer Center.

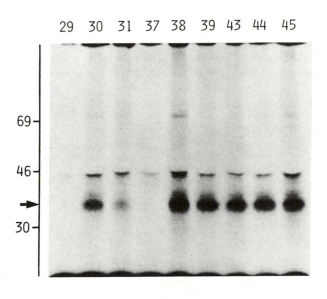

Jurkat

Fig. 39.3. Autoradiogram of ^{125}I-labeled proteins from NP-40 lysates of Jurkat cell lines immunoprecipitated by mAbs in the CD7 [T, p41] group and analyzed by sodium dodecyl sulfate–polyacrylamide gel electrophoresis (reduced samples).

approximately 38-Kd were obtained with seven out of nine mAbs tested, which was in good correspondence with the serological reactivity against the transfectant cells (Table 39.2).

mAb no. 17 was the one exceptional antibody which was positive with the 27B-T1 cells. To confirm the specificity, sheep erythrocyte (E) rosette inhibition assay was carried out. As shown in Fig. 39.4, this antibody showed significant inhibition up to a dilution of $1/10^4$ similar to the 9.6 antibody (7), indicating that this antibody belongs to the CD2 group. Since 27B-T1 transfectant cells were shown to express both Tp40 and HLA-class 1 antigens, it is possible that genes coding other cell surface antigens including the E-rosette receptor-associated pan T antigen were transfected as well. However, the rest of the antibodies (15 mAbs) in the CD2 group were found to be negative with the transfectant cells, which suggested that the positive reaction to 27B-T1 cells may not be directly related to antibody activity against the E-rosette receptor. Further experiments, such as immunoprecipitation of the transfectant cells with this antibody, are necessary to determine this interesting reactivity of antibody no. 17.

Reactivity of T Cell-Related mAbs with BC110 and BC126 Human–Mouse Hybrid Cells

The serological reactivity against BC110 and BC126 hybrid cells, both of which were positive with Tp120 antibody, is summarized in Tables 39.3

Table 39.2. Reactivity of CD7 [T, p41] group mAbs against 27B-T1 transfectant cells.

Code number	Antibody name	SPA binding	C fixing	Ig subclass	Serological reactivity[a]	Immunoprecipitation with [^{125}I] Jurkat
29	9-3	NK	+	G2b	−	−
30	G3-7	−	−	G1	+	+
31	4H9/Leu 9	+	NK	G2a	+	+
32	BW264/50	−	+	M	−	
33	BW264/217	−	+	M	−	
34	BW264/215	−	+	M	−	
35	PBS/BSA	−	−	—	−	
36	A1	+	NK	G2a	−	
37	4D12.1	NK	NK	G1	−	−
38	8H8.1	+	NK	G2a	+	+
39	3A1A	+	+	G1	+	+
40	3A1A (irrad.)	+	+	G1	+	
41	3A1B-4G6	+	+	G2	+	
42	3A1C-5A12	−	+	M	−	
43	4A	+	+	G2	+	+
44	1-3	+	+	G2a	+	+
45	I21	+	NK	G	+	+

[a] Mouse-MHA reactivity against HPB-ALL target cells.

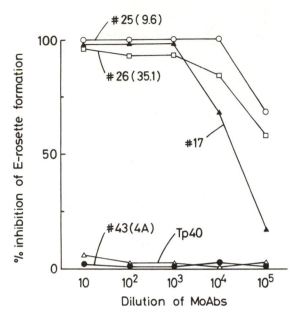

Fig. 39.4. E-rosette inhibition assays by antibody no. 17 in the CD2 [T, p50] group.

and 39.4, respectively. Karyotype analysis demonstrated that BC110 and BC126 clones maintained human chromosome nos. 6, 7, and 11 and nos. 19 and 21, respectively, at the time of serological assays. Both hybrid cells were found to be reactive with two mAbs in CD6 [T, p120] similar to the Tp120 antibody. Besides these, three mAbs, nos. 51, 59, and 142, reacted with both hybrids. Two mAbs, nos. 49 and 67, were, however, reactive only with BC126 cells.

The provisional assignment of the antigens recognized by these mono-clonal antibodies is summarized in Table 39.5. The expression of the antigens detected by the mAbs reactive with both hybrid cells was esti-mated to be associated with chromosome 11, i.e., the presence of chro-mosome 11 is necessary for the expression of the 120-Kd pan T antigen and also for that of the antigens detected by three other mAbs (nos. 51, 59, and 142). Serological study of these three mAbs against a panel of T cell lines demonstrated that both nos. 51 and 59 showed reactivity quite similar to that of Tp120, indicating that these two belong to the CD6 group. However, antibody no. 142 showed different specificity, which suggested that the antigen detected by this antibody was also associated with the presence of chromosome 11.

Two other mAbs, nos. 49 and 67, showed reactivity only against BC126. The serological reactivity against various cell lines revealed that

Table 39.3. Reactivity of T cell-related mAbs with BC110 human–mouse hybrid cells (with human chromosomes nos. 6, 7, 11) assayed by M-MHA and IA.

Positive	Negative
CD6[a] [T, p120]: both Abs (46[b], 47), Tp120[c]	CD1 [Thy, p45, 12]: all 7 Abs CD2 [T, p50]: all 16 Abs CD3 [T, p19-29]: all 11 Abs CD4 [T, p55]: all 14 Abs CD5 [T, p67]: all 9 Abs CD7 [T, p40]: all 17 Abs CD8 [T, p32-33]: all 20 Abs
Pan T, others: 2 Abs (51,59)	Pan T, others: 17/19 Abs T subset, others: all 16 Abs
T-activated: 1 Ab (142)	T-activated: 17/18 Abs

[a] Workshop cluster.
[b] Workshop code number.
[c] Made by Aichi Cancer Center.

Table 39.4. Reactivity of T cell-related mAbs with BC126 human–mouse hybrid cells (with human chromosomes nos. 11, 21) assayed by M-MHA and IA.

Positive	Negative
CD6[a] [T, p120]: both Abs (46[b], 47), Tp120[c] CD4[T, p55]: 1 Ab (67)	CD1 [Thy, p45, 12]: all 7 Abs CD2 [T, p50]: all 16 Abs CD3 [T, p19-29]: all 11 Abs CD4 [T, p55]: all 13/14 Abs CD5 [T, p67]: all 9 Abs CD7 [T, p40]: all 17 Abs CD8 [T, p32-33]: all 20 Abs
Pan T, others: 3 Abs (49,51,59)	Pan T, others: 16/19 Abs T subset, others: all 16 Abs
T-activated: 1 Ab (142)	T-activated: 17/18 Abs

[a] Workshop cluster.
[b] Workshop code number.
[c] Made by Aichi Cancer Center.

Table 39.5. Reactivity of T cell-related mAbs with two human–mouse hybrid cells.

| mAb | Hybrid (human chromosomes present) | | Assignment to human chromosome |
	BC110 (6,7,11)	BC126 (11,21)	
Tp120 [T, p120]	+	+	Chromosome 11
CD6 [T, p120]			
(46, 47)	+	+	Chromosome 11
CD4 [T, p55]			
(67)	−	+	Chromosome 21[a]
Pan T, others			
(49)	−	+	Chromosome 21[a]
(51, 59)	+	+	Chromosome 11
T-activated			
(142)	+	+	Chromosome 11

[a] The possibility of assignment to chromosome 11 remains.

the specificities of these two mAbs are quite similar but are different from that of the Tp120 antibody. Thus, the antigen detected by either antibody no. 49 or 67 is probably associated with the presence of chromosome 21, although the possibility for the assignment to chromosome 11 still remains.

In this study, we demonstrated that a mouse L cell transfectant expressing Tp40 antigen is very useful for selecting a group of antibodies detecting the 41-Kd pan T antigen from 159 mAbs in this Workshop. Just recently, transfectants expressing either Leu-1 (67-Kd pan T antigen) or Leu-2 (32-Kd T subset antigen) were established by Kavathas and Herzenberg (8), but no other reports describing experiments on transfection of genes coding for T cell or B cell differentiation antigens have appeared yet. A panel of transfectants expressing various surface antigens will provide us valuable target cells for analysis of monoclonal antibodies. The other type of target cells used in this study was human–mouse hybrid cells. Typing of T cell-related mAbs with two hybrid cells reactive with Tp120 antibody suggested that the antigen detected by antibody no. 142, which has a quite different specificity from Tp120, is also associated with the presence of chromosome 11 and that the expression of the antigen detected by either antibody no. 49 or 67 is related to chromosome 21. Thus, such hybrid cells are useful not only for clustering of mAbs, but also for estimating the chromosomal regulation of the antigen detected.

Summary

Mouse L cell transfectants or human–mouse hybrids were used to analyze monoclonal antibodies (mAbs) against T cell differentiation antigens. 27B-T1 transfectant cells expressing Tp40 antigen [T, p41] were screened with 159 mAbs registered in this Workshop by mouse mixed hemadsorption and immune adherence assays. One-half of the mAbs in the CD7 group [T, p41] were positive, indicating that these mAbs detect the 41-Kd pan T antigen as originally described by the producers of the antibodies. Unexpectedly, one antibody (no. 17) in CD2 [T, p50] was positive, but the rest of the CD2 mAbs were negative, which suggested that the 50-Kd pan T antigen was not expressed in this 27B-T1 transfectant. The nature of the antigen detected by antibody no. 17 remains to be elucidated.

Two human–mouse T cell hybrids expressing Tp120 antigen [T, p120] were established. BC110 and BC126 hybrids were found to retain human chromosome nos. 6, 7, and 11 and nos. 11 and 21, respectively, suggesting that the presence of chromosome 11 is essential for the expression of the Tp120 antigen. Besides two mAbs in CD6 [T, p120], three mAbs in other CD groups were reactive with both hybrid clones. Among these, two showed a specificity quite similar to that of the Tp120 antibody, but the third antibody, no. 142, had different reactivity, which indicated that the antigen detected by this antibody is also associated with the presence of chromosome 11. Two mAbs, nos. 49 and 67, which showed quite similar specificities, were positive only with BC126 hybrids, suggesting that the antigen detected by either antibody is associated with the presence of chromosome 21. Thus, these transfectants and hybrid cells were found to be useful for the analysis of mAbs.

Acknowledgments. This work was supported in part by a Grant-in-Aid for Comprehensive Ten-Year Strategy for Cancer Control from the Ministry of Health and Welfare; a Grant-in-Aid for Cancer Research from the Ministries of Education, Science and Culture, and Health and Welfare in Japan; and by the Cancer Research Institute Inc., New York, U.S.A.

References

1. Tsuge, I., R. Ueda, K. Nishida, R. Namikawa, M. Seto, T. Maruyama, S. Takamoto, H. Matsuoka, S. Torii, K. Ota, and T. Takahashi. 1984. Five antigens on human T cells detected by mouse monoclonal antibodies. *Clin. Exp. Immunol.*, **58**:444.
2. Carey, T.E., T. Takahashi, L.A. Resnick, H.F. Oettgen, and L.J. Old. 1976. Cell surface antigens of human malignant melanoma: Mixed hemadsorption assays for humoral immunity to cultured autologous melanoma cells. *Proc. Natl. Acad. Sci. U.S.A* **73**:3278.
3. Ueda, R., M. Tanimoto, T. Takahashi, S. Ogata, K. Nishida, R. Namikawa, Y. Nishizuka, and K. Ota. 1982. Serological analysis of cell surface antigens of null cell acute lymphocytic leukemia by mouse monoclonal antibodies. *Proc. Natl. Acad. Sci. U.S.A* **79**:4386.
4. Ueda, R., S. Ogata, D.M. Morrissey, C.L. Finstad, J. Szkudlarek, W.F. Whitmore, H.F. Oettgen, K.O. Lloyd, and L.J. Old. 1981. Cell surface antigens of

human renal cancer defined by mouse monoclonal antibodies: Identification of tissue specific kidney glycoproteins. *Proc. Natl. Acad. Sci. U.S.A* **78:**5122.

5. Wigler, M., R. Sweet, G.K. Sim, B. Wold, A. Pellicer, E. Lacy, T. Maniatis, S. Silverstein, and R. Axel. 1979. Transformation of mammalian cells with genes from procaryotes and eucaryotes. *Cell* **16:**777.

6. Weiss, M.C., and H. Green. 1967. Human–mouse hybrid lines containing partial complements of human chromosomes and functioning human genes. *Proc. Natl. Acad. Sci. U.S.A.* **58:**1104.

7. Kamoun, M., P.J. Martin, J.A. Hansen, M.A. Brown, A.W. Siadak, R.C. Nowinski. 1981. Identification of a human T lymphocyte surface protein associated with the E-rosette receptor. *J. Exp. Med.* **153:**207.

8. Kavathas, P., and L.A. Herzenberg. 1983. Stable transformation of mouse L cells for human membrane T cell differentiation antigens, HLA and β_2-microglobulin. *Proc. Natl. Acad. Sci. U.S.A.* **80:**524.

CHAPTER 40

Association of IL-2 Production with the Expression of Dipeptidyl Peptidase IV (DPIV) on Human T Lymphocytes

Wolfgang Scholz, Alfred C. Feller, Artur J. Ulmer, and Hans-Dieter Flad

Introduction

T cell-derived interleukin-2 (IL-2) has been functionally and biochemically characterized. It plays a central role in the growth and differentiation of T lymphocytes (1–4). Studies have been undertaken to reveal the IL-2-producing subset (5, 6), but subsets defined by the established markers (7, 8) T4 (helper/inducer) and T8 (cytotoxic/suppressor) could not discriminate between IL-2-producing and nonproducing T cells (9, 10). As an additional cell surface marker we introduced recently the enzyme dipeptidyl peptidase IV (DPIV), which has been reported as a T cell marker (11, 12) and could be detected on the cell surface by monoclonal anti-DPIV antibodies (13). First experiments with rabbit anti-DPIV antiserum indicated a relationship between IL-2 production and DPIV expression (14). Therefore, we decided to isolate DPIV$^+$ cells by cell sorting and to test their capacity to produce IL-2. In further experiments we intended to study the co-expression of DPIV with Leu-3, Leu-2, and Leu-1, by using flow cytometry and the two-color immunofluorescence technique with phycoerythrin (PE) as the second dye in a single laser system (15, 16). In addition, it was of interest to study the IL-2 production and proliferation of selected subsets after stimulation with PHA and their differentiation during culture.

Materials and Methods

Isolation and Subfractionation of Cells

Peripheral blood mononuclear cells (PBMC) were isolated by discontinuous density gradient centrifugation on Percoll-Hank's as described previously (17). PBMC were depleted of phagocytes by incubation with carbonyl-iron as described (17). In indicated cases PBMC were incubated for 2 hr at 37°C in AB serum-pretreated culture flasks. The nonadherent cells were further depleted of phagocytes by the carbonyl-iron method. Adherent and nonadherent phagocyte-depleted cells (NPC) were incubated overnight in RPMI 1640 + 10% fetal calf serum (FCS) supplemented with 100 U/ml penicillin, 100 μg/ml streptomycin, and 2 mM L-glutamine. The following day NPC were processed for immunofluorescence staining and cell sorting, while the adherent cells were collected and kept on ice until use. The viability exceeded 90% and the purity of adherent cells was >95%, while the purity of NPC was <1% alpha-napthylacetate esterase-positive monocytes as evaluated in cytospins.

Production of IL-2-containing Supernatants and Determination of IL-2 Activity

Briefly, the respective cell population was adjusted to 5×10^5 cells per ml in RPMI 1640 + 2% FCS + 8 μl PHA, and 250 μl of this suspension were distributed to each of three wells in a microtiter plate (flat bottom) and incubated at 37°C in a humidified atmosphere of 5% CO_2. Supernatants (100 μl/well) were harvested under sterile conditions after 48 hr and subjected to an IL-2 assay. The remaining cells were supplemented with 100-μl RPMI 1640 medium + 22.5% FCS (resulting in a final concentration of 10% FCS) and cultured for one further day before their proliferative capacity was measured by ^{3}H-dT incorporation. IL-2 activity was determined using 50-μl/well thawed cultured human T lymphocytes suspended in RPMI 1640 medium + 20% AB serum at a concentration of 4×10^5/ml. These cells were mixed with 50-μl undiluted or diluted culture supernatant and incubated in microtiter plates (round bottom) for 3 days at 37°C in 5% CO_2 in air. The ^{3}H-dT incorporation of the cells was determined after a pulse of 0.2 μCi/culture during the last 5 hr of the culture period, as described previously (17). IL-2 units were determined as described by Gillis et al. (18).

Antibodies

The monoclonal antibodies were purchased as follows: phycoerythrin (PE)-conjugated Leu-1, Leu-2a, Leu-3a, and Leu-11a–FITC and avidin–PE from Becton Dickinson (Heidelberg, FRG); OKT4, OKT8, and OKT9 from Ortho (Heidelberg, FRG); coulterclone T11-FITC from Coulter Electronics (Krefeld, FRG); biotinylated F(ab')$_2$ fragment of goat anti–mouse IgG from Medac (Hamburg, FRG); and FITC-conjugated avidin from Vector Laboratories (Burlingame, CA, USA).

Anti-Tac was a gift of Dr. Waldmann (NIH, Bethesda, MD, USA). Clonab T8 is similar to Leu-2a and was a kind gift of Biotest (Offenbach,

FRG). A monoclonal anti-DPIV antibody was prepared by immunization of mice with purified human placental DPIV (19) and hybridomas secreting DPIV antibodies were selected. Specificity has been tested in an ELISA system using purified human placental DPIV.

Immunofluorescence and Flow Cytometry

Immunofluorescence was performed as indicated by the distributors of the antibodies. Anti-DPIV ascites was used in a final dilution of 1 : 200. All steps were performed on ice in ice-cold PBS.

For flow cytometry usually 5000–10,000 cells were monitored with a cytofluorograph (System 50H, Ortho Diagnostic Systems Inc., Raritan, NJ, USA). The raw data of narrow-angle light scatter, green (FITC) and red (PE or ethidium bromide) fluorescence or, in single fluorescence analysis, 90°-angle light scatter were stored in list mode on a 2150 computer system. In double fluorescence analyses electronic compensation (16) corrected for fluorescein spillover into the red channel and for phycoerythrin spillover into the green channel. Hereby we used an offset of 100 channels from the origin in the linear scale, and these corrected signals were referred to as green and red fluorescence. All single parameter data were displayed as histograms of scatter-gated cells with the fluorescence channel on the x-axis (linear scale) and the relative number of cells on the y-axis. Sorting of double-labeled cells was achieved by setting the appropriate regions in the histograms for green and red fluorescence. The purity of the isolated population was evaluated by reanalyzing part of the sorted cells without further treatment.

Results

IL-2 Production of Single Fluorescence Labeled DPIV[+] Cells after Enrichment by Cell Sorting

PBMC or phagocyte-depleted PBMC were labeled with anti-DPIV or OKT4 monoclonal antibodies and kept on ice until and during sorting. Controls were treated with the second antibody only and left unseparated. Figure 40.1 shows the data for the DPIV-labeled starting population (53% DPIV[+] cells) and the reanalyses of the appropriate sorted cells in a typical experiment. Both populations consisted of >95% positive or negative cells after sorting. The data obtained with OKT4-stained cells were comparable.

Two typical examples of PHA-induced IL-2 production and proliferation of the separated cells are given in Table 40.1. Highest amounts of IL-2 activity were found in the DPIV[+] population, whereas DPIV[−] cells

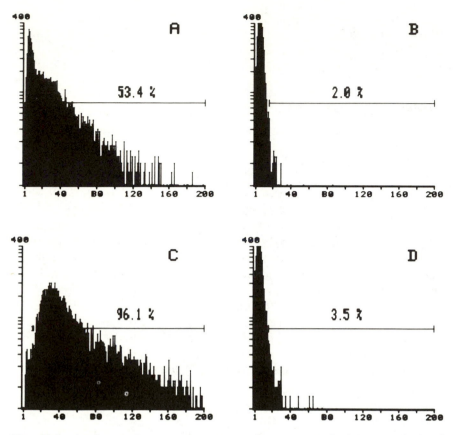

Fig. 40.1. Analyses of pre- and post-sorted scatter-gated phagocyte-depleted PBMC. (A) Unseparated cells with DPIV positive cells in region 1. (B) Related control with goat anti–mouse–FITC. (C) The positive enriched population within region 1. (D) Reanalysis of the negative population; region 1 shows few residual positive cells.

produced no IL-2 or only small amounts of it. OKT4$^+$ cells were also good IL-2 producers, but OKT4$^-$ cells were producers, too. It should be mentioned that OKT4$^+$ and OKT4$^-$ cells are easy to distinguish by cytofluorimetry, whereas the distinction between DPIV$^+$ and DPIV$^-$ cells is much more difficult. Since DPIV is an enzyme, only a few molecules could be expected on the cell surface, and this could explain the low fluorescence intensity observed in DPIV-stained populations. Unseparated PBMC showed less IL-2 production than unseparated phagocyte-depleted PBMC, but higher DNA synthesis. We interpret this as the influence of factors produced by monocytes, such as IL-1 and prostaglandins, and the resulting balance in the culture system. OKT4$^+$ cells showed optimal proliferation.

Table 40.1. DNA synthesis and IL-2 production of T cell subsets highly purified by cell sorting.[a]

Cell source	DNA synthesis[b] (cpm/culture)	IL-2 production[c] (units)
Exp. 1:		
Unselected	11,253 ± 867	26
DPIV⁺	8,169 ± 406	44
DPIV⁻	5,656 ± 266	7
OKT4⁺	11,053 ± 700	45
OKT4⁻	5,973 ± 634	66
Exp. 2:		
Unselected	4,763 ± 331	35
DPIV⁺	9,251 ± 482	52
DPIV⁻	1,664 ± 112	0
OKT4⁺	9,880 ± 643	18
OKT4⁻	1,508 ± 704	11

[a] Fresh mononuclear cells were used in experiment 1 and phagocyte-depleted PBMC in experiment 2. [b] DNA synthesis of the cells (measured on day 3) is given as cpm/culture; each value represents the mean ± SD of three independent cultures. [c] IL-2 production is expressed as IL-2 units/ml.

Double Labeling of Cells with Anti-DPIV and Leu-3

Further experiments should reveal the relationship between DPIV and Leu 3 expression. Therefore, DPIV⁺ cells were labeled with FITC as usual and Leu-3⁺ cells were monitored directly with anti-Leu-3a–PE [Fig. 40.2(A)]. In nine experiments with cells from different healthy blood donors we detected 38 ± 6% DPIV⁺/Leu-3⁺ cells. Three other subsets comprised 20 ± 4% DPIV⁺/Leu-3⁻, 32 ± 7% DPIV⁻/Leu-3⁻, and 10 ± 5% DPIV⁻/Leu-3⁺ cells. From these data we calculated that 58% of the cells were DPIV⁺ and 48% were Leu-3⁺. Positive enrichment resulted in the four subsets as shown in Fig. 40.2(B) with a purity of >95% of the appropriate subset.

Functional studies with these subsets isolated from phagocyte-depleted cells led to the result that the cells no longer produced IL-2, but some of them gave a proliferative response. We interpreted this finding as a proof of the high degree of purification of lymphoid cells and as an indication of differential minimal requirements for accessory cells in proliferative and IL-2- producing responses. Therefore we changed our protocol for isolation of cells in such a way that adherent cells were used for restoration of responsiveness.

As shown in Table 40.2, the addition of 10% adherent cells (>95% esterase-positive monocytes) enhanced the proliferative capacity and re-

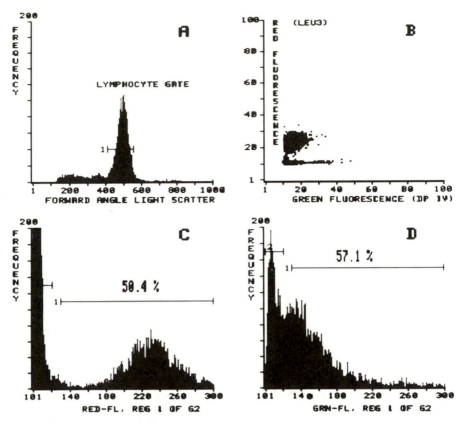

Fig. 40.2A. Double labeling of phagocyte-depleted nonadherent cells with anti-DPIV and Leu-3a and analysis in a cell sorter. Histogram A monitors the distribution of forward-angle light scatter and region 1 shows the lymphocyte gate. Cytogram B shows Leu-3a (red) on the *y*-axis and DPIV (green) on the *x*-axis. The distributions of DPIV and Leu-3a are given in histograms D and C, respectively, where we used an electronic offset of 100 channels.

vealed the highest level of IL-2 production in the DPIV⁺/Leu-3⁺ population. DPIV⁻/Leu-3⁻ cells showed neither substantial proliferation nor IL-2 production. Both DPIV⁺/Leu-3⁻ and DPIV⁻/Leu-3⁺ cells produced intermediate levels of IL-2 activity and proliferated normally in the presence of adherent cells. It is of interest to note the proliferation of DPIV⁺/Leu-3⁻ cells in the absence of additional adherent cells.

Relationship between Expression of DPIV and Leu-2a

The next experiments were performed to demonstrate the co-expression of DPIV and Leu 2. In three experiments we detected 14 ± 2% DPIV⁺/

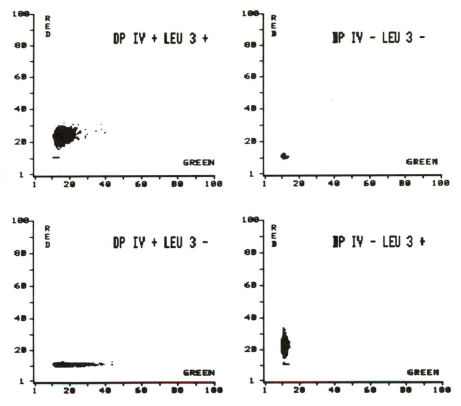

Fig. 40.2B. Reanalysis of double-labeled and sorted lymphocytes. All cytograms show red fluorescence (Leu-3a) on the *y*-axis and green fluorescence (DPIV) on the *x*-axis. Within the DPIV$^-$/Leu-3a$^+$ population the purity of DPIV$^-$ was 90%; in all other cases the purity of the selected subset exceeded 95–97%.

Table 40.2. DNA synthesis and IL-2 production of double fluorescence labeled lymphocytes highly purified by cell sorting.[a]

	DNA synthesis[b]		IL-2 production[c]	
	Addition of adherent cells		Addition of adherent cells	
Cell source	0%	10%	0%	10%
DPIV$^+$Leu-3a$^+$	7.4 ± 0.3	41.2 ± 3.3	ND[d]	157
DPIV$^+$Leu-3a$^-$	17.4 ± 2.2	27.7 ± 0.9	4	106
DPIV$^-$Leu-3a$^+$	0.6 ± 0.0	26.6 ± 2.4	ND	67
DPIV$^-$Leu-3a$^-$	3.1 ± 1.2	4.3 ± 1.4	6	29
Unseparated	27.0 ± 1.0	29.4 ± 2.3	52	123

[a] Phagocyte-depleted nonadherent lymphocytes were stained with anti-DPIV and Leu-3a and the resulting subpopulations were sorted. The purity of the sorted cells was greater than 95% as shown in reanalyses and the adherent cells consisted of 97% esterase-positive monocytes. [b] ^{3}H-dT incorporation given as cpm × 10^3; each value represents the mean ± SD of three independent cultures. [c] IL-2 units/ml compared with a standard preparation containing 100 units. [d] ND = Not detectable.

Table 40.3. DNA synthesis and IL-2 production of lymphocytes highly purified by cell sorting after double labeling with anti-DPIV and Leu-2A.[a]

Cell source	DNA synthesis[b]		IL-2 production[c]	
	Addition of adherent cells		Addition of adherent cells	
	0%	10%	0%	10%
DPIV⁺Leu-2a⁺	11.2 ± 1.1	16.7 ± 2.0	<1	142
DPIV⁺Leu-2a⁻	17.0 ± 2.1	26.3 ± 1.7	<1	205
DPIV⁻Leu-2a⁺	—[d]	—	—	—
DPIV⁻Leu-2a⁻	2.0 ± 0.2	8.4 ± 0.6	<1	79
Unseparated	12.1 ± 0.4	18.9 ± 3.9	31	184

[a] Phagocyte-depleted nonadherent lymphocytes were stained with anti-DPIV and Leu-2a and the resulting subpopulations were sorted. The purity of the sorted cells was greater than 95% as shown in reanalyses and the adherent cells consisted of 97% esterase-positive monocytes. [b] ^{3}H-dT incorporation given as cpm × 10³; each value represents the mean ± SD of three independent cultures. [c] IL-2 units/ml compared with a standard preparation containing 100 units. [d] — = Not tested.

Leu-2⁺, 51 ± 6% DPIV⁺/Leu-2⁻, 9 ± 3% DPIV⁻/Leu-2⁺, and 27 ± 5% DPIV⁻/Leu-2⁻. Similar percentages were obtained using clonab T8–FITC and PE-labeled DPIV.

The proliferation and IL-2 production of the resulting subsets in a typical experiment are given in Table 40.3. Again we found that DPIV⁺ cells proliferated without additional adherent cells but produced no detectable IL-2. DPIV⁺/Leu-2a⁻ cells were expected to produce the highest amounts of IL-2, since they correspond to DPIV⁺/Leu-3a⁺ cells, and this was confirmed after addition of adherent cells. DPIV⁻/Leu-2a⁻ cells should be similar but *not* identical to DPIV⁻/Leu-3a⁺ cells, and here, too, we obtained comparable results inasmuch as they produced some IL-2 and proliferated much less than control cells.

DPIV⁻/Leu-2a⁺ cells have not been tested, since they correspond in part to DPIV⁻/Leu-3a⁻ cells (shown to be nonproducers) and occur only in low frequency.

Relationship between Expression of DPIV and Leu-2 + Leu-3, Leu-1, T11, and Leu-11a

Double-labeling experiments with DPIV/Leu-3 and DPIV/Leu-2 indicated a subset of DPIV⁺/Leu-2⁻Leu-3⁻ cells. Therefore we stained phagocyte-depleted cells by DPIV (green) and Leu-2a–PE + Leu-3a–PE. The result is given in Fig. 40.3(A). It is obvious that DPIV⁺/Leu-2⁻Leu-3⁻ cells exist, but in low frequency (3%). Their expected capacity to produce IL-2 has not been tested so far. Furthermore, the bulk of DPIV⁺ cells (96%) expresses the Leu-1 antigen, as seen in Fig. 40.3(B).

Further experiments using PE-labeled anti-DPIV, anti-Leu-11a–FITC, and anti-T11–FITC demonstrated that only few DPIV⁺ cells seem to

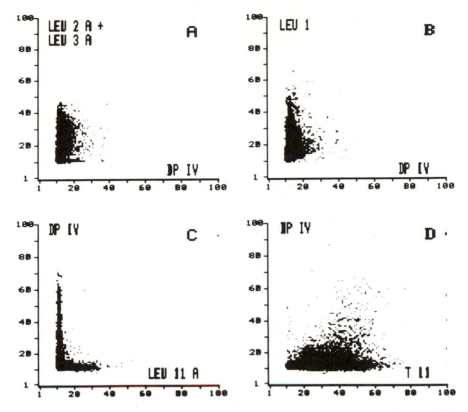

Fig. 40.3. Double labeling with DPIV and Leu-2a–PE + Leu-3a–PE, Leu-1–PE, Leu-11a–FITC, and T11–FITC. All cytograms show red fluorescence on the y-axis and green fluorescence on the x-axis, each with an offset of 100 channels. DPIV was labeled either with goat anti–mouse F(ab')₂–FITC (A,B) or with biotinylated goat anti–mouse F(ab')₂ and avidin–PE (C,D).

express Leu-11a [Fig. 40.3(C)]; however, the bulk of them were positive for T11 [Fig. 40.3(D)] as expected. Since in our hands T11⁺ cells were not HLA-DR⁺ (data not shown), we assume that the majority of DPIV⁺ cells are also HLA-DR⁻.

Reappearance of DPIV in DPIV⁻ Selected Populations During Culture

Since DPIV⁻ cells proliferated to some extent, we investigated the phenotype of the cells at the end of the culture period. Therefore, nonadherent, phagocyte-depleted cells were labeled, and DPIV⁻/Leu-2a⁻ and DPIV⁺/Leu-2a⁻ cells were sorted and cultured with PHA as usual. On day 3 the cells of 10–20 wells in a microtiter plate were harvested, pooled, and

Table 40.4. Expression of surface markers after stimulation by PHA.

Surface marker[a]	% Positive cells selected as	
	DPIV$^+$/Leu-2a^{-b}	DPIV$^-$/Leu-2a^{-c}
DPIV	76	25
OKT4	94	54
OKT8	7	13
T11	98	85
OKT9	74	49
Tac	83	55
—[d]	7	1

[a] Cells were sorted and stimulated with PHA as indicated. After 3 days the cells were harvested, and viable cells were analyzed for surface markers using a cytofluorograph.
[b] Viability 70%.
[c] Viability 55%.
[d] Control incubated with PBS instead of antibodies.

labeled with the surface markers given in Table 40.4. Only viable cells were analyzed using ethidium bromide staining for the exclusion of dead cells. Although DPIV$^-$/Leu-2a$^-$ cells were 92% pure on the day they had been selected, 25% DPIV$^+$ cells and 13% OKT8$^+$ cells were detected on day 3 after culture (viability 55%). Furthermore, most cells were T11$^+$ (83%) and OKT4$^+$ (54%), and a considerable proportion bore the transferrin receptor (49% OKT9$^+$) and the receptor for IL-2 (55% Tac$^+$). The selected DPIV$^+$/Leu-2a$^-$ cells showed higher viability (70%), the expected phenotype T11$^+$, DPIV$^+$, OKT4$^+$, OKT8$^-$, and high percentages of OKT9 and anti-Tac positive cells, indicating that the cells were proliferating.

Discussion

The data presented here show that monoclonal antibodies directed against DPIV bind to T cells which produce IL-2 upon stimulation by PHA. In DPIV-negative selected cell populations we detected only minor proliferation and negligible IL-2 production. Probably the IL-2 production can be attributed to small amounts of contaminating monocytes (<1%) which are required for IL-2 production (5). Since the discrimination between DPIV$^+$ and DPIV$^-$ cells is difficult [Fig. 40.1(A)], a few cells considered as DPIV$^-$ might express low amounts of DPIV$^+$. In contrast, the discrimination between OKT4$^+$ and OKT4$^-$ cells is easy to achieve, but IL-2 production is found not to be restricted to OKT4$^+$ cells, in agreement with previous reports (9, 10). Since further experiments showed that DPIV$^+$ cells as well as DPIV$^-$ cells consisted of T4$^+$ and T8$^+$ cells (data not shown), we dissected these populations by double fluorescence labeling and cell sorting.

We expected the IL-2 production to segregate with the DPIV marker in all possible combinations of surface markers. However, first experiments indicated that DPIV$^+$ cells containing subsets proliferated fairly well but did not produce significant IL-2. We attributed this finding to the absence of monocytes or monocyte-derived IL-1. Therefore, we changed our protocol for the isolation of cells by introducing an additional step to recover adherent cells of high purity for reconstitution experiments. Next, the proliferative and IL-2-producing capacity of the four resulting subsets obtained in DPIV/Leu-3-stained populations [Fig. 40.2(B)] were investigated in the presence or absence of additional adherent cells. If adherent cells are present in such cultures, our findings obtained with single fluorescence (DPIV) labeled cells could be confirmed. Thus, DPIV$^+$/Leu-3a$^+$ cells produced maximal amounts of IL-2, and considerable amounts were also produced by DPIV$^+$/Leu-3a$^-$ cells. In spite of the fact that no IL-2 was found in the supernatant when the cells were cultured in the absence of additional adherent cells, both populations were able to proliferate under these conditions. Since the cells proliferate and it is known that IL-2 is produced in the late G1-phase of the cell cycle (3), one might expect that IL-2 has been produced. Therefore, we assume that these DPIV$^+$ cells produce minimal amounts of IL-2 which are consumed during direct cell to cell interaction so that no free IL-2 activity is detectable in the supernatant. In contrast, DPIV$^-$/Leu-3a$^-$ cells neither proliferated nor produced IL-2 in a substantial amount, independent of whether or not adherent cells were present. Thus we conclude that, at least in the PHA-driven system, these cell are mainly nonreactive.

In the presence of adherent cells DPIV$^-$/Leu-3a$^+$ cells produced intermediate amounts of IL-2, which appears to contradict our hypothesis that DPIV is a marker for IL-2-producing cells. Furthermore, when the correspondent subset DPIV$^-$/Leu-2a$^-$ was isolated by sorting we found comparable proliferation and IL-2 production (Table 40.3). However, the proliferating capacity of these cells was far below control levels of unseparated cells.

These findings could be explained by further experiments which demonstrated that after 3 days of culture and stimulation by PHA a significant amount of DPIV$^+$ cells (IL-2 producers?) is detectable in DPIV$^-$/Leu-2a$^-$ sorted populations (Table 40.4). It has not been established whether these DPIV$^+$ cells were growing from contaminating DPIV$^+$ cells or whether DPIV$^+$ cells with only low amounts of surface DPIV (not detected on day 0) differentiate into cells strongly expressing DPIV. Obviously, more cells express OKT4, OKT9, and Tac antigen than DPIV. These findings could be explained by the assumption that DPIV$^-$ cells proliferate due to IL-2 produced by DPIV$^+$ cells. DPIV$^+$/Leu-2a$^-$ cells showed a better viability than DPIV$^-$/Leu-2a$^-$ cells and more cells expressed the OKT9 and Tac antigen as expected.

In our hands, all double labeling experiments with DPIV/Leu-3, DPIV/

Leu-2, and, in non-reported experiments, with DPIV/Leu-1, led to comparable results inasmuch as DPIV$^+$-containing subsets were IL-2-producing cells. Therefore, this finding supports our hypothesis that IL-2-producing cells express DPIV on their surfaces.

Since it has been reported (20) that cells with the phenotype T11$^+$/T3$^-$ [large granular lymphocytes (LGL)] were also capable of producing IL-2, we examined further the phenotype of DPIV$^+$ cells. Our results indicate the existence of subpopulations with the phenotypes DPIV$^+$/T4$^-$/T8$^-$ [Fig. 40.3(A)] and DPIV$^+$/Leu-11a$^+$ [Fig. 40.3(C)], although most Leu-11a$^+$ cells were DPIV$^-$. Further experiments must be undertaken to demonstrate directly the presence of DPIV$^+$ cells within LGL enriched populations. Furthermore, we could show that most DPIV$^+$ cells were Leu-1$^+$ and T11$^+$, but DPIV$^-$/Leu-1$^+$ and DPIV$^-$/T11$^+$ cells do also exist. Thus, DPIV seems to represent a surface marker overlapping most subpopulations so far known as IL-2 producers.

Several important questions concerning DPIV are so far unanswered. Is DPIV involved in regulatory processes *in vivo*? Is DPIV a "functional requirement" of IL-2-producing cells or just co-expressed on these cells? Can DPIV process IL-2 or other "factors" and what is the naturally occurring substrate of this enzyme? Further experiments using different cell lines, cells of patients with various immunodeficiencies, monoclonal antibodies against IL-2, as well as the search for specific inhibitors of DPIV, should help us to answer these questions.

Acknowledgments. The technical assistance of Mrs. F. Klützke and Mrs. R. Bergmann is gratefully acknowledged. We thank Dr. T.A. Waldmann for providing us with the monoclonal anti-Tac antibody. This work was supported by a grant of Deutsche Forschungsgemeinschaft Fl 104/4-2.

References

1. Gillis, S., K.A. Smith, and J. Watson. 1980. Biochemical characterisation of lymphocyte regulatory molecules. *J. Immunol.* **124:**1954.
2. Miyawaki, T., A. Yachie, N. Uwadana, S. Ohzeki, T. Nagaoki, and N. Taniguchi. 1982. Functional significance of Tac antigen expressed on activated human T lymphocytes: Tac antigen interacts with T cell growth factor in cellular proliferation. *J. Immunol.* **129:**2474.
3. Stadler, B.M., and J.J. Oppenheim. 1982. Human interleukin 2: Biological studies using purified IL-2 and monoclonal anti-IL-2 antibodies. In: S.B. Mizel (Ed.) *Lymphokines,* Vol. 6. Academic Press, New York, p. 117.
4. Taniguchi, T., H. Matsui, T. Fujita, C. Takaoka, N. Kashima, R. Yoshimito, and J. Hamuro. 1983. Structure and expression of a cloned cDNA for human interleukin 2. *Nature* **302:**305.
5. Solbach, W., S. Barth, M. Röllinghoff, and H. Wagner. 1982. Interactions of human T cell subsets during the induction of cytotoxic T lymphocytes: The role of interleukins. *Clin. Exp. Immunol.* **49:**167.

6. Silva A.G., J.M. Alvarez, G.D. Bonnard, and M.O. de Landazuri. 1981. Human interleukin 2: Production by both T$_g$ cells and other T cells. *Scand. J. Immunol.* **14**:315.
7. Reinherz, E.L., P.C. Kung, G. Goldstein, and S.F. Schlossman. 1979. Separation of functional subsets of human T cells by a monoclonal antibody. *Proc. Natl. Acad. Sci. U.S.A.* **76**:4061.
8. Reinherz, E.L., P.C. Kung, G. Goldstein, and S.F. Schlossman. 1980. A monoclonal antibody reactive with the human cytotoxic/suppressor T cell subset previously defined by a heteroantiserum termed TH$_2$. *J. Immunol.* **124**:1301.
9. Luger, T.A., J.S. Smolen, T.M. Chused, A.D. Steinberg, and J.J. Oppenheim. 1982. Human lymphocytes with either the OKT4 or OKT8 phenotype produce interleukin 2 in culture. *J. Clin. Invest.* **70**:470.
10. Meuer, S.C., R.E. Hussey, A.C. Penta, K.A. Fitzgerald, B.M. Stadler, S.F. Schlossman, and E.L. Reinherz. 1982. Cellular origin of interleukin 2 (IL-2) in man: Evidence for stimulus restricted IL-2 production by T4+ and T8+ lymphocytes. *J. Immunol.* **129**:1076.
11. Lojda, Z. 1977. Studies on glycyl-proline naphthylamidase. I. Lymphocytes. *Histochemistry* **54**:299.
12. Feller, A.C., C.J. Heijnen, R.E. Ballieux, and M.R. Parwaresch. 1982. Enzyme histochemical staining of Tμ lymphocytes for glycyl-proline-4-methoxy-beta-naphthylamide-peptidase (DAP IV). *Brit. J. Haematol.* **51**:227.
13. Mentlein, R., E. Heymann, W. Scholz, A.C. Feller, and H.-D. Flad. 1984. Dipeptidylpeptidase IV as a new surface marker for a subpopulation of human T lymphocytes. *Cell. Immunol.,* **89**:11.
14. Scholz, W., E. Heymann, R. Mentlein, A.C. Feller, and H.-D. Flad. 1983. Dipeptidylaminopeptidase IV (DAP IV) as a new surface marker for a human T cell subpopulation associated with the production of interleukin 2 (IL-2). *Immunobiol.* **165**:355.
15. Loken, M.R., D.R. Parks, and L.A. Herzenberg. 1977. Two-color immunofluorescence using a fluorescence-activated cell sorter. *J. Histochem. Cytochem.* **25**:899.
16. Oi, V.T., A.N. Glazer, and L. Stryer. 1982. Fluorescent phycobili-protein conjugates for analysis of cells and molecules. *J. Cell Biol.* **93**:981.
17. Ulmer, A.J., W. Scholz, M. Ernst, E. Brandt, and H.-D. Flad. 1984. Isolation and subfractionation of human peripheral blood mononuclear cells (PBMC) by density gradient centrifugation on Percoll. *Immunobiol.* **166**:238.
18. Gillis, S., M.M. Ferm, W. Qu, and K.A. Smith. 1978. T-cell growth factor: Parameters of production and a quantitative microassay for activity. *J. Immunol.* **120**:2027.
19. Püschel, G., R. Mentlein, and E. Heymann. 1982. Isolation and characterization of dipeptidyl peptidase IV from human placenta. *Eur. J. Biochem.* **126**:35.
20. Kasahara, T., J.Y. Djeu, S.F. Dougherty, and J.J. Oppenheim. 1983. Capacity of human large granular lymphocytes (LGL) to produce multiple lymphokines: Interleukin 2, interferon, and colony stimulating factor. *J. Immunol.* **131**:2379.

CHAPTER 41

A Novel Disulfide-Linked Cell Surface Molecule Present on Resting and Activated Human T Lymphocytes

Robert D. Bigler and Nicholas Chiorazzi

Introduction

Human T cell leukemias provide an excellent source of homogeneous material to study T cell surface molecules. The monoclonal nature of these malignant cells provides a convenient means to dissect the functional and structural basis of surface antigens present on T cell subpopulations. Using the leukemic OKT4-positive T cells of a patient with Sezary syndrome, we have developed a monoclonal antibody (mAb), termed S152, that reacts with the leukemic cells and a subpopulation of circulating T cells. The antigen recognized by this mAb is detected at a low intensity on circulating T cells and not on T cell lines. When cells are stimulated with mitogens, the intensity of staining by S152 increases several fold over that seen on resting T cells. The initial characterization of the antigen detected by this mAb reveals it to be a disulfide-linked dimer with two chains of similar or identical molecular weight. Disulfide-linked molecules on the T cell surface have been shown to be limited to very few molecules (1). These molecules, such as the T cell receptor (2,3), transferrin receptor (4,5), and 4F2 (6), all appear to be involved in early T cell activation (7). Thus not only is the molecule defined by S152 a member of a rare molecular species but also its relationship to activation suggests that this molecule may play a functional role in T cell proliferation.

Materials and Methods

Monoclonal Antibody

BALB/c mice were immunized with cells from a patient with Sezary syndrome as described previously (2). The mAb S152 was selected from one of the fusions, cloned in soft agar two times, and injected into pristane-primed mice. The ascites obtained was precipitated with 45% ammonium sulfate and eluted from DEAE-cellulose by a 0–0.2 M NaCl gradient. Either culture supernatants from the cloned line or purified antibody were used in saturating amounts for indirect immunofluorescence using flow cytometry as described (2).

Cells for Specificity Screening

The preparation and analysis of different cell types for specificity screening of the mAb have been described previously (2). Briefly, peripheral blood mononuclear cells were isolated by standard Ficoll–Hypaque separation and further separated by sheep erythrocyte rosetting. Rosetting and non-rosetting populations plus granulocytes, erythrocytes, platelets, and cryopreserved thymocytes were used to determine the reactivity of the cloned antibody. The T cell, B cell, and myeloid lines used have been described. To obtain activated lymphocytes, peripheral blood mononuclear cells were stimulated with the mitogens concanavalin A (Con A) at 10 μg/ml (Sigma Chemical Co., St. Louis, MO), phytohemagglutinin (PHA) 1 : 100, and pokeweed mitogen (PWM) 1 : 100 (Gibco Laboratories, Grand Island, NY) in RPMI 1640 plus 10% fetal calf serum. Cells from these cultures and cells cultured concurrently in media alone were removed daily during the 6-day culture period, washed, and stained for immunofluorescent analysis.

Immunoprecipitation

Cells were surface-labeled with ^{125}I using the lactoperoxidase method and analyzed by sodium dodecyl sulfate–polyacrylamide gel electrophoresis (SDS–PAGE) on a 15% discontinuous vertical gel system as described elsewhere (2).

Results

Isolation of mAb and Screening

Murine hybridomas were developed by immunization with leukemic T cells and were screened for reactivity against the immunizing cells. The hybrids secreting antibody reactive with the leukemic cells were expanded and cloned in soft agar. The mAb described, termed S152, was shown to be an IgG1k antibody by double immunodiffusion. By flow cytometric analysis this antibody was found to react with all of the leukemic T cells (Fig. 41.1A). The fluorescence histogram showed a reactive population of more than 80%, which corresponds to the amount of leukemic cells present in the sample as determined by visual differential

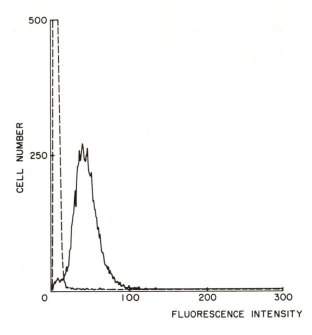

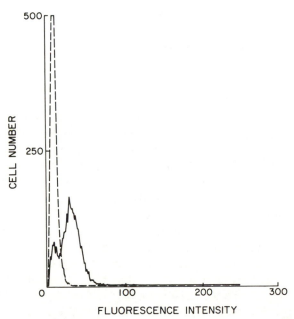

Fig. 41.1. Fluorescence histograms of peripheral blood cells stained by indirect immunofluorescence using mAb S152. (A) Staining of the mononuclear cells of the immunizing leukemia. (B) Staining of normal T cells. Both histograms compare 10,000 cells stained without (---) or with (——) mAb S152 plus fluoresceinated goat anti–mouse IgG.

Table 41.1. Percentage of cells stained by S152.

	Immunizing leukemia S	Normal cell preparations					Cell lines			
		T	Non-T	PMN	RBC	Thymo-cytes	T	T-T hybrids	B	Myeloid
Number[a]	—	10	9	6	4	3	7	16	4	3
Percent reactive[b]	>80	63	2.5	<0.5	<0.5	3.5	<0.5	<0.5	1.3	<0.5

[a] Number of different preparations of normal cells or cell lines.
[b] Mean value.

counts, as well as a small nonreactive population. This observation was confirmed by fluorescence microscopy where small lymphocytes were unstained and large leukemic cells were stained.

Staining of normal peripheral blood T lymphocytes revealed a mean of 63% of T cells reactive with the antibody (Table 41.1). The density of staining by this antibody was consistently low when analyzed by flow cytometry (Fig. 41.1B). Fluorescence microscopy confirmed this observation since the stained cells were barely detectable above background. Mononuclear cells depleted of T cells by a single sheep erythrocyte rosetting showed a mean of 2.5% of the cells reacted with S152. Whether this represents a few residual T cells in these preparations or a small population of reactive non-T cells is unclear. Additional peripheral blood cells including erythrocytes, granulocytes, and platelets were not reactive (Table 41.1).

Screening of Activated Cells

Cell lines were studied to further define the reactivity of this antibody on proliferating cells (Table 41.1). T cell lines, and multiple T-T hybridomas (courtesy of Dr. Lloyd Mayer), were studied and found to be nonreactive with this antibody. Three different myeloid cell lines were also found to be unreactive. Four B cell lines were studied, of which three were unreactive and the fourth had 5% of the cells reactive with the mAb. Thus the antigen does not appear to be expressed on a variety of lymphoid and myeloid cell lines; however, as mentioned above, the possibility of a small reactive B cell population cannot be excluded.

This observation was extended by stimulating normal mononuclear cells with mitogens to evaluate the presence of the antigen on normal activated cells. The change in antigen distribution on the cell surface was analyzed daily. The data displayed represent day 4 of PHA, Con A, and PWM stimulation. Normal cells cultured in media alone showed no change in staining intensity and had the same percentage of reactive cells, 50%, as on day 0 (Fig. 41.2A). When stimulated with PHA and Con A, the intensity of staining on the cells increased approximately fivefold during the period of maximal blastogenesis (Fig. 41.2B,C). In addition,

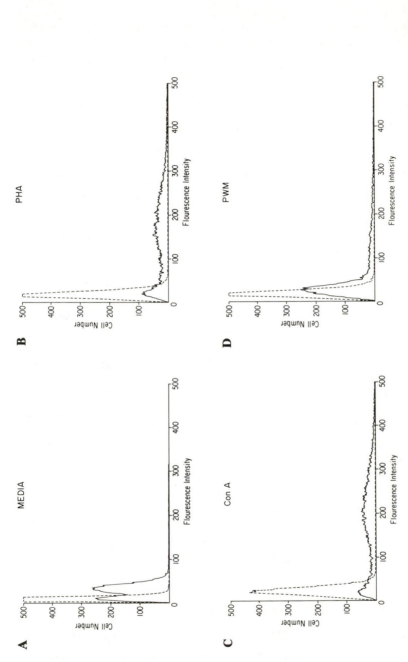

Fig. 41.2. Fluorescence histograms of normal peripheral blood cells stained by indirect immunofluorescence after four days of culture. The histogram of cells cultured in media alone (A) is com-pared with the histograms of cells cultured in media plus PHA (B), Con A (C), or PWM (D). Histograms compare 10,000 cells counted after staining without (---) or with (——) mAb S152.

the percentage of reactive cells increased from 34% to 79% in the PHA cultures and from 48% to 82% in the Con A cultures. In contrast to this increase after activation by PHA and Con A, there is a less pronounced change in the antigen expression during PWM mitogenesis during the first two or three days of the response when T cells are activated. When evaluated between days 4 to 6 there is evidence of expression of this antigen on a population of cells in the pokeweed culture, as seen in Fig. 41.2(D). From day 1 when the PWM cultures contained 52% S152 reactive cells, the reactive population decreased to 36% on day 4 and 43% on day 6. Staining with the anti-Tac mAb on day 4 showed 28% reactive cells and 43% on day 6 which correlates with the S152 reactivity. This suggests, but does not confirm, that the reactive cells are T cells.

Initial Characterization of the S152 Antigen

The leukemic cells used as immunogen and the T cell line KE-37 were surface-iodinated using the lactoperoxidase method. The surface-labeled proteins were extracted, immunoprecipitated with S152, and analyzed by autoradiography after SDS–PAGE electrophoresis. The mobility of the unreduced S152 antigen is shown to correspond to a mol. wt. of approximately 123 Kd when compared to molecules of previously defined mol. wt. that were analyzed on the same gel (Fig. 41.3, lane a). Upon reduction this protein displays a decreased mobility corresponding to a mol. wt. of approximately 65 Kd (lane c). Whether this molecule is composed of two identical chains or two chains of very similar molecular mobility cannot be ascertained in this experiment. The T cell line KE 37 serves as a negative control (lanes b,d) and confirms that this molecule is not present on the T cell line as indicated by the immunofluorescence data. The molecular weight and cell surface distribution distinguish this molecule from two other disulfide-linked surface antigens, the T cell receptor and the transferrin receptor. The heterodimeric structure of the T cell receptor on this same leukemic cell is shown in lane e. Similarly, immunoprecipitation studies using the mAb 5E9 (kindly provided by Dr. Barton Haynes), which reacts with the transferrin receptor, have shown that the mobility of these two proteins, as determined by SDS–PAGE analysis, are different (data not shown).

Discussion

This study describes a mAb, termed S152, which was produced by somatic cell hybridization after priming mice with T4-positive T cells from a patient with Sezary syndrome. The antigen defined by mAb S152 appears to be expressed primarily on a subpopulation of normal T cells. The molecule was not detected on various cultured T cell and myeloid cell

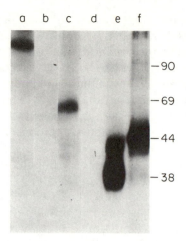

Fig. 41.3. SDS–PAGE analysis of the immunoprecipitation of ^{125}I-labeled surface molecules on the immunizing leukemia and the T cell line KE 37. Immunoprecipitation of the molecules on the leukemic cells using S152 is compared before reduction (lane a) and after reduction (lane c). Immunoprecipitation of the molecules on the cell line KE 37 using S152 is shown before (lane b) and after (lane d) reduction. These results are compared with the T cell antigen receptor that was immunoprecipitated with a previously described anti-idiotypic mAb and reduced prior to gel analysis (lane e). The HLA molecule present on KE 37 is precipitated in lane f. Molecular weight markers include the unreduced T cell antigen receptor (90 Kd), bovine albumin (69 Kd), HLA heavy chain (44 Kd), and the lower-weight chain of the antigen receptor (38 Kd).

lines or circulating granulocytes, erythrocytes, and platelets. The antibody did react with a small percentage of the T-depleted population of peripheral blood mononuclear cells and 5% of the cells in one B cell line. Thus, although it is primarily expressed on T cells, the antigen may also be expressed on a small B cell population. To investigate the T cell reactivity, peripheral blood cells were stimulated with different mitogens. Both PHA and Con A were shown to cause a progressive increase in the intensity of staining by the S152 mAb. During stimulation with these mitogens the percentage of cells reactive with the mAb also was noted to increase from about 50% to 80%, consistent with an expansion of the S152 reactive population. Stimulation with PWM revealed an increase in the mAb staining intensity but at a lower level than seen with PHA and Con A. The percentage of reactive cells in the PWM culture did not increase, and actually decreased from 52% to 36%, during days 4 through 6 when B cell proliferation is most pronounced. The parallel reactivity that was observed with anti-Tac, showing a comparable percentage of reactive cells, suggests that the S152 reactive cells are T cells but B cell reactivity cannot be completely excluded. The initial characterization of this molecule by immunoprecipitation revealed it to be a disulfide-bound dimer. Analysis by SDS–PAGE indicated a mobility of approximately 123 Kd unreduced and 65 Kd reduced. The resolution of this system did not permit the distinction of whether this molecule is composed of two identical chains or two different chains of similar mobility.

The lymphoid cell distribution of the S152 antigen is somewhat similar to other structures on the T cell surface; however, the combination of its disulfide-linked dimeric structure and activation characteristics suggest that it is a previously undescribed antigen. One similar marker, the murine Ly-1, exists on most T cells and on a population of B cells (8). The human homologue of Ly-1, Leu-1, also is expressed on a population of T cells as well as certain leukemic B cells (9). LFA-1, a noncovalently associated dimer, has been shown to be present on T cells but also on a wide range of activated T cells, B cells, monocytes, and other non-lymphoid cells (10). Similarly the mAb TA-1 reacts with a large percentage of circulating T cells plus monocytes and about 10% of B cells (11). The antigens detected in these systems as well as the population reactivities clearly distinguish these molecules from that detected by S152.

The disulfide-linked nature of the S152 molecule relates it to a small number of similar species detected on the T cell surface. The Ly-2/3 molecule in the mouse is a tetramer composed of a covalently bound homodimer associated noncovalently with two other proteins (1). Likewise the insulin receptor is composed of two different covalently bound chains (12). The Ia molecule also has been shown to exist on activated T cells as well as on circulating B cells and monocytes (13). Several activation antigens expressed primarily on T lymphocytes have been described. The transferrin receptor, a disulfide-linked homodimer, although absent from resting cells, is expressed within 4–8 hr after T cell activation (7). Another early activation antigen expressed on >90% of monocytes and at a low level on T and B cells is 4F2. The 4F2 molecule, a heterodimer composed of 40-Kd and 80-Kd peptide chains, when detected by immunofluorescence on activated cells increases in staining intensity within 4 hr of activation (6,7). The human T cell antigen receptor is a heterodimer expressed on nonactivated cells. This molecule, present on circulating normal cells and on antigen-specific clones, has been shown to play a role in the initiation of T cell activation (2,3). The only disulfide-bound molecule in this group that is comparable to the S152 molecule is the transferrin receptor. The existence of S152 on resting cells and its molecular weight distinguish it from the transferrin receptor. Thus it appears that the molecule detected by S152 on normal and activated T cells is unique within this group of surface antigens.

Many of the lymphocyte surface structures that are involved in cellular recognition and activation are disulfide-linked molecules. The occurrence and importance of dimeric structures in this regard has been discussed previously and a functional role based on cross-linking of this type of structure has been postulated (1). Of those molecules on T cells involved in the recognition of antigen, such as the T cell antigen receptor, or expressed shortly after activation, such as the transferrin receptor and the 4F2 molecule, the predominant structure is disulfide-linked. Similarly, the major structure of antigen recognition on B cells, the immunoglobulin molecule, is also disulfide-linked. When considering the rare occurrence of such molecular species on the surface of T cells, the prominence that these molecules have in activation is striking. Although the function of the S152 molecule has not been determined at present, its structure and expression during activation would suggest that this molecule may be of similar importance during early activation. Experiments are currently in progress to investigate the role that this molecule may play during mitogenic or antigenic activation.

Acknowledgments. This research was funded in part by PHS grants AI 19080 and AI 10811. R.D. Bigler was supported in part by a fellowship from the National Leukemia Association.

References

1. Goding, J.W., and A.W. Harris. 1981. Subunit structure of cell surface proteins: Disulfide bonding in antigen receptors, Ly-2/3 antigens, and transferrin receptors of murine T and B lymphocytes. *Proc. Natl. Acad. Sci. U.S.A.* **78**:4530.
2. Bigler, R.D., D.E. Fisher, C.Y. Wang, E.A. Rinnooy-Kan, and H.G. Kunkel. 1983. Idiotype-like molecules on cells of a human T cell leukemia. *J. Exp. Med.* **158**:1000.
3. Meuer, S.C., K.A. Fitzgerald, R.E. Hussey, J.C. Hodgdon, S.F. Schlossman, and E.L. Reinherz. 1983. Clonotypic structures involved in antigen specific human T cell function: Relationship to the T3 molecular complex. *J. Exp. Med.* **157**:705.
4. Haynes, B.F., M. Hemler, T. Cotner, D.L. Mann, G.S. Eisenbarth, J.L. Strominger, and A.S. Fauci. 1981. Characterization of a monoclonal antibody (5E9) that defines a human cell surface antigen of cell activation. *J. Immunol.* **127**:347.
5. Trowbridge, I.S., and M.B. Omary. 1981. Human cell surface glycoprotein related to cell proliferation is the receptor for transferrin. *Proc. Natl. Acad. Sci. U.S.A.* **78**:3039.
6. Haynes, B.F., M.E. Hemler, D.L. Mann, G.S. Eisenbarth, J. Shelhamer, H.S. Mostowski, C.A. Thomas, J.L. Strominger, and A.S. Fauci. 1981. Characterization of a monoclonal antibody (4F2) that binds to human monocytes and to a subset of activated lymphocytes. *J. Immunol.* **126**:1409.
7. Cotner, T., J.M. Williams, L. Christenson, H.M. Shapiro, T.B. Strom, and J. Strominger. 1983. Simultaneous flow cytometric analysis of human T cell activation antigen expression and DNA content. *J. Exp. Med.* **157**:461.
8. Lanier, L.L., N.L. Warner, J.A. Ledbetter, and L.A. Herzenberg. 1981. Expression of Lyt-1 antigen on certain murine B cell lymphomas. *J. Exp. Med.* **153**:998.

9. Wang, C.Y., R.A. Good, P. Ammirati, G. Dymbort, and R.L. Evans. 1980. Identification of a p69,71 complex expressed on human T cells sharing determinants with B-type chronic lymphatic leukemic cells. *J. Exp. Med.* **151**:1539.
10. Krensky, A.M., F. Sanchez-Madrid, E. Robbins, J.A. Nagy, R.A. Springer, and S.J. Burakoff. 1983. The functional significance, distribution, and structure of LFA-1, LFA-2, and LFA-3: Cell surface antigens associated with CTL-target interactions. *J. Immunol.* **131**:611.
11. LeBien, T.W., J.G. Bradley, and B. Koller. 1983. Preliminary structural characterization of the leukocyte cell surface molecule recognized by monoclonal TA-1. *J. Immunol.* **130**:1833.
12. Lang, U., C.R. Kahn, and L.C. Harrison. 1980. Subunit structure of the insulin receptor of the human lymphocyte. *Biochemistry* **19**:64.
13. Ko, H., S.M. Fu, R.J. Winchester, D.T.Y. Yu, and H.G. Kunkel. 1979. Ia determinants on stimulated human T lymphocytes. *J. Exp. Med.* **150**:246.

CHAPTER 42

T14, A Non-modulating 150-Kd T Cell Surface Antigen

Hannes Stockinger, Otto Majdic, Kristof Liszka,
Ursula Köller, Wolfgang Holter, Christian Peschel,
Peter Bettelheim, Heinz Gisslinger, and Walter Knapp

Introduction

Monoclonal antibodies to human T lymphocyte surface structures have essentially contributed to a better understanding of cellular mechanisms and interactions involved in the generation of human T cell responses (1). Such antibodies have also proven useful in recent years in the diagnosis of autoimmune, immunodeficiency, and malignant diseases (2). Not surprisingly, monoclonal antibodies to human T lymphocytes are also increasingly used in the treatment of malignant diseases and for selective T cell elimination in bone marrow (3–5) and kidney transplantation (6–8).

One of the main problems so far encountered in most attempts to eliminate certain cell types by *in vivo* application of monoclonal antibodies has been antigen modulation (9–12). We therefore tried to avoid this problem when we began our attempts to raise a monoclonal T cell antibody for therapeutic purposes. The antibody obtained (VIT14) detects a novel 150-Kd T cell antigen which is not modulated in the presence of antibody.

Materials and Methods

Monoclonal Antibodies

The hybridoma cell line producing the VIT14 antibody is derived from a fusion experiment after Köhler and Milstein (13) in which spleen cells previously immunized with E-receptor-positive peripheral blood lymphocytes were hybridized with X63-Ag8.653 myeloma cells. The hybrids were cloned twice by limiting dilution and then further propagated *in vitro* and *in vivo*. The immunization, fusion, and cloning protocols were essentially the same as described previously (14). The VIT14 antibody is of the IgG2b class.

Table 42.1. Monoclonal antibodies used in this study.

Antibody designation	Ig class	Cluster designation[a]	Reactive membrane protein	Main specificity
VIT3b	IgG1	CD3	p19 − 29	Pan T lymphocytes
VIT4	IgG2a	CD4	p55	Helper/inducer T lymphocytes
VIT8	IgG1	CD8	p32 − 33	Suppressor/cytotoxic T lymphocytes
VIT12	IgG1	CD6	p120	Pan T lymphocytes
OKT1[b]	IgG1	CD5	p67	Pan T lymphocytes
VIM12	IgG1	CD11	p94 + 155	C3bi receptor on monocytes, granulocytes, and LGLs
VIBC5	IgM			B lymphocytes and precursors
Leu-3a–PE[c]	IgG1	CD4	p55	Helper/inducer T lymphocytes
Leu-2a–PE[c]	IgG1	CD8	p32 − 33	Suppressor/cytotoxic T lymphocytes

[a] As proposed by the IUIS/WHO Nomenclature Subcommittee for Leukocyte Antigens.
[b] Kindly provided by Dr. P. Kung.
[c] Phycoerythrin-labeled antibodies from Becton Dickinson, Sunnyvale, CA.

The other antibodies used in our study for comparative purposes and for the characterization of the investigated lymphoid cell preparations are summarized in Table 42.1.

Normal and Malignant Hematopoietic Cells

Mononuclear cells (MNC), lymphocytes, granulocytes, monocytes, and thrombocytes were isolated as described previously (14).

T cells were enriched by rosetting MNC with neuraminidase-treated sheep red blood cells (E) followed by density gradient centrifugation. The non-T fraction (E⁻) was isolated from the interphase; the T-enriched fraction (E⁺ cells) was obtained from the pellet after distilled water lysis of rosetted E's.

Table 42.2. Characterization of the human hematopoietic cell lines used in this study.

Cell line	Cell type	References
HL60	Promyelocytic	Collins *et al.*, 1977 (15)
KG1	Myeloblastoid	Koeffler and Golde, 1978 (16)
U937	Monoblastoid	Sundström and Nilsson, 1976 (17)
THP1	Monoblastoid	Tsuchiya *et al.*, 1980 (18)
K562	Erythroid/myeloid	Lozzio and Lozzio, 1975 (19)
HEL	Erythroid	Martin and Papayannopoulou, 1982 (20)
Reh-6	Non-B non-T	Rosenfeld *et al.*, 1977 (21)
Raji	B-lymphoid	Pulvertaft, 1964 (22)
MOLT-4	T-lymphoid	Minowada *et al.*, 1973 (23)
Jurkat	T-lymphoid	Schneider *et al.*, 1977 (24)

The diagnosis of leukemia was made using standard clinical, morphological, and cytochemical criteria. All neoplastic preparations selected for this study showed >75% abnormal cells.

Human Hematopoietic Cell Lines

The cell lines HL60, KG1, U937, THP1, K562, HEL, Reh6, Raji, MOLT-4, and Jurkat were used in the present study. Their characteristics, as well as references describing these lines, are outlined in Table 42.2.

Immunofluorescence

The binding of mouse monoclonal antibodies was assessed by indirect immunofluorescence with fluoresceinated goat F(ab')$_2$ anti–mouse IgG + IgM antibodies.

For double staining, fluoresceinated VIT14 and phycoerythrin-labeled Leu-3a and Leu-2a antibodies (Becton Dickinson, Sunnyvale, CA) were used.

Fluorescence of cells was evaluated using a Leitz Ortholux microscope (Leitz, Wetzlar, FRG) or a fluorescence-activated cell sorter (FACS 440, Becton Dickinson, Sunnyvale, CA).

Immunoperoxidase Staining

Frozen 7-μm tissue sections of human lymph node and tonsil were fixed in chloroform and acetone and then incubated with monoclonal antibodies. Bound antibodies were demonstrated with a double antibody technique, using peroxidase-conjugated rabbit anti–mouse immunoglobulins and peroxidase-conjugated swine anti–rabbit immunoglobulins.

Cytotoxicity Testing

Complement-dependent cytotoxicity of the VIT14 antibody was tested in a standard two-stage cytotoxicity assay with a 30-min incubation at 4°C with antibody followed by a further 30-min incubation at 37°C with rabbit complement.

Antigen Modulation Experiments

The antibody-induced modulation of cell surface antigens was assessed by incubating cells for 12 hr at 37°C in the presence and absence of the respective antibody (10 μg/ml) and then evaluating the antigenic profile of these cells.

Evaluation of Progenitor Cell Reactivity

Complement-dependent cytotoxicity assays were used to determine the reactivity of granulocytic, erythroid, and megakaryocytic progenitor cells with the VIT14 antibody. For this purpose, equal volumes of bone marrow mononuclear cells (2×10^6/ml culture medium) obtained from healthy volunteers and monoclonal antibody (final dilution 1:100) were incubated for 30 min at 4°C, followed by a further incubation for 60 min at 37°C with rabbit complement. Afterwards cells were washed and suspended in the original volume of culture medium.

In vitro cultures of these cells were performed according to methods previously described for stimulation of committed granulocytic (25), erythropoietic (26), and megakaryocytic (27) progenitor cells.

Radiolabeling and Immunoprecipitation

Freshly isolated T lymphocytes were surface labeled with $Na^{125}I$ (New England Nuclear, Boston, MA) as described by Meuer *et al.* (28). Ten μl glucose (0.5 mol/liter), 100 μl lactoperoxidase (1 mg/ml), 2 mCi $Na^{125}I$, and 20 μl glucose oxidase (10 mU/ml) were added to 2×10^7 cells suspended in PBS. After 20 min the reaction was stopped by washing 3 times with PBS–1% BSA–10 mM KJ.

Radiolabeled cells were suspended and lysed in 0.5 ml lysis buffer (20 mM Tris-HCl, 150 mM NaCl, 1% Nonidet P-40 (NP-40), 2 mM phenylmethylsulfonylfluoride, 1% deoxycholate sodium salt, pH 7.2).

Cell lysates were then incubated with monoclonal antibody immunosorbents for 2 hr at 4°C. Bound material was eluted by boiling in gel buffer (0.1 mol/liter Tris-HCl, 40% glycerol, 2% SDS, pH 6.8) for 5 min. To obtain reducing conditions 5% 2-mercaptoethanol was added.

Immunosorbents were prepared by incubating 100 μl hybridoma ascites with 100 μl protein-A-Sepharose (Pharmacia Fine Chemicals, Uppsala, Sweden) for 2 hr at 4°C.

Samples were analyzed by SDS in a discontinuous buffer system on 12% acrylamide slab gels. Dried gels were fluorographed at −70°C on Kodak XS-5 films.

Results

VIT14 Reactivity with Normal Human Leukocytes

Blood Cells

Among human peripheral blood cells, VIT14 exclusively recognizes lymphoid cells. Monocytes, granulocytes, thrombocytes, and erythrocytes are completely negative. Within the mononuclear cell population 43 to 50% (mean 47%) of cells are VIT14 positive [Fig. 42.1(A)]. The major-

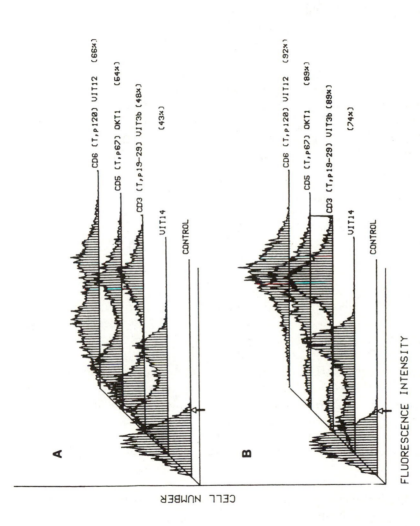

Fig. 42.1. Reaction pattern of the monoclonal antibody VIT14 in comparison to antibodies of the CD3, CD5, and CD6 type with unseparated mononuclear cells (MNC) (A) and with a T cell-enriched E$^+$ MNC fraction from peripheral blood (B).

ity, if not all, of these cells seem to be T lymphocytes. This is shown by the fact that 74% to 90% (mean 82%) of the cells in T cell-enriched (E$^+$) fractions of mononuclear cell samples are T14$^+$ [Fig. 42.1(B)] and in double-staining experiments with antibodies of the CD4 and CD8 type (Fig. 42.2). Whether the reactivity with a low proportion of cells (3–12%) in the non-T (E$^-$) fraction indicates a reactivity with another so far undefined lymphocyte subset remains to be seen.

It is evident from our experiments that the proportion of VIT14-positive cells is always somewhat lower than the proportion of cells reactive with T cell antibodies of the CD2, CD3, CD5, and CD6 type. A typical example of this relation is shown in Fig. 42.1(A), (B).

For a further characterization of the nature of VIT14$^-$E$^+$ (CD2$^+$) lymphocytes, E$^+$ cells were treated with VIT14 antibody and complement, and then submitted to Ficoll–Hypaque separation in order to remove dead cells. After this procedure 9×10^7 (11%) of the initial 8.5×10^8 cells were recovered. The immunological phenotype of these cells is shown in Table 42.3.

Lymphoid Organs

Typical reaction patterns of the VIT14 antibody with mononuclear cell suspensions from lymph node, thymus, and tonsil (E$^+$ and E$^-$ fraction) are shown in Fig. 42.3.

In the lymph node roughly 70% of the cells are VIT14 positive [Fig. 42.3(A)], a proportion which approximately correlates to that seen with other T cell antibodies. In the thymus VIT14 only reacts with a small (<15%) proportion of cells [Fig. 42.3(B)]. These VIT14$^+$ cells are all small and probably represent mature thymocytes. In T cell-enriched preparations (E$^+$) of tonsil cells approximately 85 to 95% of the cells are VIT14 positive as expected [Fig. 42.3(C)]. Surprisingly, however, one also finds small proportions (15–25%) of weakly reactive cells in E$^-$ fractions of tonsil cells [Fig. 42.3(D)], which do not or only minimally (<10%) react with other T cell antibodies.

These weakly reactive cells in the non-T fraction cannot be localized in peroxidase stainings of tonsils and lymph nodes, however. The VIT14

Table 42.3. Effect of complement-mediated lysis of VIT14 monoclonal antibody on lymphocytes of peripheral blood.

Total cell number	VIT14	VIT3b (CD3)	VIT4 (CD4)	VIT8 (CD8)	VIT12 (CD6)	OKT1 (CD5)	VIBC5	VIM12 (CD11)
Before lysis								
8.5×10^8	79	87	64	29	89	86	5	6
After lysis								
9.0×10^7	<1	60	40	16	63	60	15	20

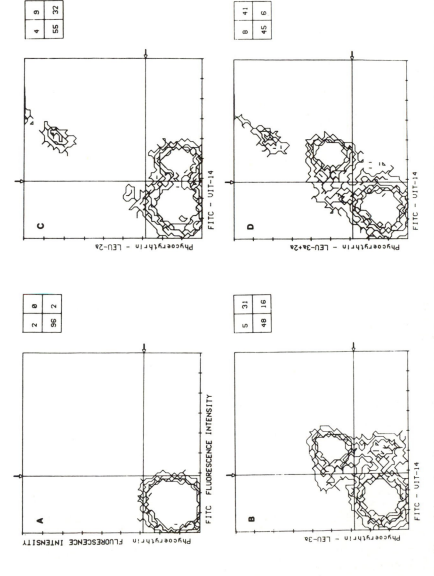

Fig. 42.2. Double staining of peripheral blood mononuclear cells using FITC-labeled VIT14 and phycoerythrin-labeled Leu-3a and Leu-2a. (A) Negative control; (B) double staining with VIT14 and Leu-3a; (C) double staining with VIT14 and Leu-2a; (D) double staining with VIT14 and Leu-3a + Leu-2a. Numbers in squares give the percentage of cells in the corresponding sector.

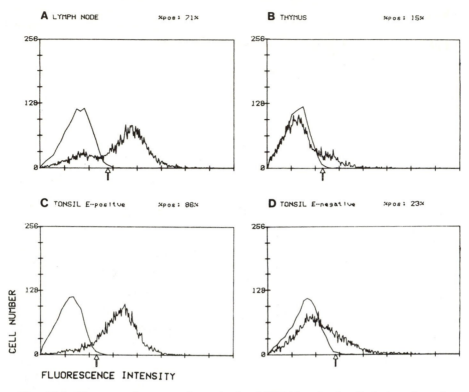

Fig. 42.3. Flow cytofluorometric analysis of VIT14-stained cells in lymph node (A) and thymus (B) (cell suspensions), and in T cell-enriched E⁺ (C) and T cell-depleted E⁻ (D) fractions of tonsil mononuclear cells.

antibody predominantly stains the paracortical T cell area. Lymphoid follicles are negative except for a few cells scattered in germinal centers. This staining pattern is not significantly different from that observed with other T cell antibodies.

Bone Marrow

Reactivity of the VIT14 antibody with bone marrow cells is restricted to cells with the morphological appearance of lymphoid cells. No reactivity with morphologically recognizable cells of other cell lineages can be detected. Potential reactions with hematopoietic progenitor cells were evaluated in complement-dependent cytotoxicity assays. CFU-GM day 7, CFU-GM day 14, CFU-e, BFU-e, and CFU-Mega were not diminished after VIT14 and complement treatment.

VIT14 Reactivity with Leukemic Cells

T14 Expression on Human Hematopoietic Cell Lines

To further delineate the cell type specificity of the T14 antigen, we tested 10 different human hematopoietic cell lines. The results of this study are illustrated in Fig. 42.4.

Except for a very weak reaction with the Burkitt-line Raji, none of the cell lines show any reactivity.

T14 Expression on Leukemic Cells

Typical reaction patterns of the VIT14 antibody with human leukemia cells are summarized in Fig. 42.5.

Samples from patients with T-CLL [Fig. 42.5(A)] or Sezary syndrome [Fig. 42.5(B)], representing mature T cells, are positive. Within the CLLs of B cell type we observed a heterogeneous reaction pattern. From samples of 15 patients tested, two react under 10% with VIT14 and are classified as negative [Table 42.4, Fig. 42.5(D)]. Within the other 13 samples, all staining intensities ranging from weak binding of a few cells [Fig. 42.5(E)] to strong staining of all cells [Fig. 42.5(F)] can be observed. Immature T cells of patients with T-ALL [Fig. 42.5(C)] are completely T14 negative. The same was observed for B-ALL, cALL, AML, and CML cells (Table 42.4).

Modulation Experiments

One of the main problems so far encountered in all attempts to eliminate certain cell types *in vivo* with monoclonal antibodies was antigen modulation (9–12). We therefore were very pleased to find that the VIT14 anti-

Table 42.4. Reactivity of the VIT14 antibody with leukemia/lymphoma cells.

Diagnosis	Number of patients tested	Number of cases VIT14 positive[a]
AML	17	0
cALL	10	0
B-ALL	3	0
T-ALL	3	0
B-CLL	15	13
T-CLL	2	2
Sezary syndrome	3	3

[a] Positive = >10% leukemic cells reactive.

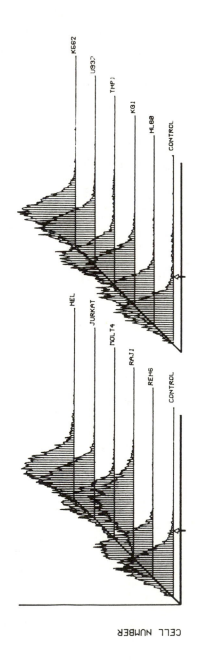

Fig. 42.4. T14 antigen expression on human hematopoietic cell lines. (The characteristics of the cell lines and references describing them are summarized in Table 42.2.)

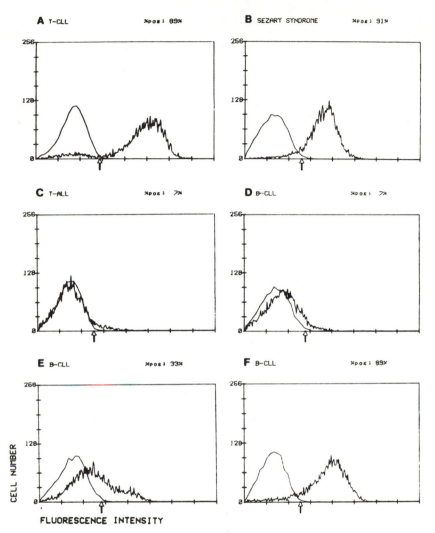

Fig. 42.5. Typical FACS profiles of VIT14-stained leukemic cells from patients with T-CLL (A), Sezary syndrome (B), T-ALL (C), and B-CLL (D–F). The reaction patterns in D–F show the heterogeneity of T14 expression in B-CLL.

body does not seem to induce antigen modulation (Fig. 42.6). Incubation of lymphocytes for 12 hr at 37°C with the VIT14 antibody does not remove the T14 antigen from their surfaces. In comparison, the CD3 and CD5 antigens disappear completely after incubation with the VIT3b and OKT1 antibodies, respectively. The T14 structure thus seems to be even more stable in this respect than the CD6 structure detected by the VIT12 antibody. VIT12, an antibody which immunoprecipitates the same 120-Kd

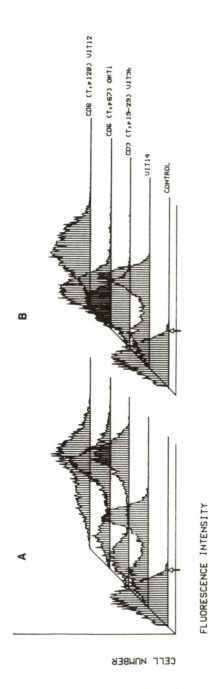

Fig. 42.6. Antigen modulation experiments with VIT14 and anti-bodies of the CD3, CD5, and CD6 type on peripheral blood lymphocytes. Cells were incubated for 12 hr at 37°C in the absence (A) or presence (B) of the respective antibody. Then the cells were stained again with the same antibody and analyzed with the cell sorter for residual antigen expression.

protein as the anti-T12 antibody (3,29), but recognizes a different epitope, gives a slightly weaker staining after 12-hr preincubation (Fig. 42.6).

Molecular Weight of T14

From NP-40 lysates of ^{125}I-labeled E$^+$ blood lymphocytes the VIT14 antibody immunoprecipitates a plasma membrane protein with a molecular weight of 150 Kd (Fig. 42.7). Under reducing conditions the protein migrates at 60 Kd. This may indicate that the T14 antigen is composed of two or three identical disulfide-bridged subunits. As control an IgG2b monoclonal antibody, which does not react with peripheral blood MNC, was used.

Discussion

Monoclonal antibodies to cell surface glycoproteins on human T lymphocytes, either alone or in combination with pharmacologic or toxic agents, may provide major therapeutic agents which allow the selective elimination or functional inhibition of human T cells or T cell subsets.

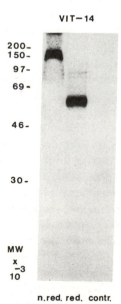

Fig. 42.7. SDS–PAGE of ^{125}I-labeled VIT14 immune precipitates from peripheral blood T cells. n.red. = non-reduced, red. = reduced, contr. = control IgG2b antibody under reducing conditions.

One of the major problems so far encountered in serotherapy with monoclonal antibodies is antigenic modulation (9–12). It was observed in several instances that the respective cell surface antigen, but not necessarily the cells themselves, disappeared after *in vivo* administration of monoclonal antibody (9–12). Such a behavior of surface antigens in response to antibody addition can also be observed under *in vitro* conditions and is termed antigenic modulation (9,10,29,30). It may either be due to antigen release after antibody binding or due to endocytosis of the antigen–antibody complex.

The degree of antigenic modulation seems to be influenced by both the nature of the antibody (30) and the nature of the cell surface antigen (29). The exact conditions are poorly understood so that a non-modulating antibody to a cell surface antigen can, at least for the time being, only be found by trial and error. In our attempt to obtain a monoclonal T cell antibody for therapeutic purposes, we have, therefore, right from the beginning selected an antibody to a T cell surface antigen which is not modulated in the presence of this antibody.

The results of this approach are described in this paper. We have obtained an antibody (VIT14) which defines a novel T lymphocyte surface antigen termed by us T14. The VIT14 antibody is of the IgG2b class, does not modulate T14, and is highly cytotoxic in the presence of rabbit complement.

The T14 antigen is of protein nature with a molecular weight of 150 Kd. Under reducing conditions it migrates at 60 Kd. Apart from the molecular weight, the T14 antigen differs also in several other aspects from all T cell surface antigens of the CD2 [T, p50], CD3 [T, p19-29], CD5 [T, p67], CD6 [T, p120] and CD7 [T, p44] clusters described thus far.

The distribution of T14 within the human hematopoietic system seems to be restricted to T cells and to a small, not as yet very well-defined subset of B cells. All other hematopoietic cells are negative.

Within the T cell lineage T14 is only expressed by the more mature T lymphocytes. The majority of thymocytes are negative. The same holds true for T cell malignancies with immature lymphoblast-like appearance as, for instance, acute lymphoblastic leukemias of T cell type.

Most of the T cells in peripheral blood and lymphoid organs and the corresponding T cell malignancies, such as the Sezary syndrome, are T14 positive. A small subset of peripheral blood lymphocytes with otherwise the normal phenotypic surface characteristics of human T cells is constantly T14⁻, however. The functional characteristics of these T14⁻ cells have not as yet been studied.

Surprisingly, T14, like other previously described pan T lymphocyte surface structures such as CD5 (31) and CD6 (29), can occasionally be found on leukemic cells of B cell type from patients with chronic lymphocytic leukemia. Studies on non-T cell fractions of human tonsils have shown T14 also on certain normal cells of the B lineage. The exact stage of differentiation at which T14 is expressed in normal and malignant B cell differentiation is not as yet defined, however.

Of major importance from the therapeutic point of view is the fact that—besides the stability of the antigen in the presence of antibody—hematopoietic progenitor cells do not seem to express this surface structure and that VIT14, in contrast to other T cell antibodies (32), is also not mitogenic. We therefore believe that the VIT14 antibody might prove to be a useful addition to the presently available armamentarium of immunosuppressive agents and possibly superior to other previously used antibodies. Since recent studies showed that T14 is also expressed on T lymphocytes from rhesus monkeys, it should be possible to validate our assumption.

Summary

In this report we describe a novel T lymphocyte surface antigen. This antigen, termed by us T14, is defined by the monoclonal antibody VIT14, which is of the IgG2b class and highly cytotoxic in the presence of rabbit complement. The T14 antigen is of protein nature with a molecular weight of 150 Kd. Under reducing conditions it migrates at 60 Kd.

The specificity of the T14 antigen within the hematopoietic system seems to be restricted to mature T cells and to a small subset of B cells which probably includes the normal counterpart cell of CLL cells.

Of particular importance is the observation that the T14 antigen is not modulated in the presence of the VIT14 antibody.

This and the observation that VIT14 does not react with hematopoietic precursor cells and is not mitogenic for human T cells makes it an attractive candidate for therapeutic applications.

Acknowledgments. We wish to thank Mrs. Tina Boeckhold, Mrs. Brigitte Fischer-Colbrie, Mrs. Dagmar Mandl, and Mrs. Elisabeth Gschwandtler for their skillful technical assistance.

References

1. Reinherz, E.L., and S.F. Schlossman. 1980. The differentiation and function of human T lymphocytes. *Cell* **19**:821.
2. Schlossman, S.F., and E.L. Reinherz. 1984. Human T-cell subsets in health and disease. *Springer Semin. Immunopathol.* **7**:9.
3. Reinherz, E.L., R. Geha, J.M. Rappeport, M. Wilson, A.C. Penta, R.E. Hussey, K.A. Fitzgerald, J.F. Daley, H. Levine, F.S. Rosen, and S.F. Schlossman. 1982. Reconstitution after transplantation with T-lymphocyte-depleted HLA haplotype-mismatched bone marrow for severe combined immunodeficiency. *Proc. Natl. Acad. Sci. U.S.A.* **79**:6047.

4. Blacklock, H.A., H.G. Prentice, and M.J.M.L. Gilmore. 1983. Attempts at T-cell depletion using OKT3 and rabbit complement to prevent a GvHD in allogeneic BMT. *Exp. Hematol.* **11**(suppl. 13):37.
5. Prentice, H.G., G. Janossy, L. Price-Jones, L.K. Trejdosiewicz, D. Panjwani, S. Graphakos, K. Ivory, H.A. Blacklock, M.J.M.L. Gilmore, N. Tidman, D.B.L. Skeggs, S. Ball, J. Patterson, and A.V. Hoffbrand. 1984. Depletion of T lymphocytes in donor marrow prevents significant graft-versus-host disease in matched allogeneic leukemic marrow transplant recipients. *Lancet* **1984**(1):472.
6. Cosimi, A.B., R.C. Burton, R.B. Colvin, G. Goldstein, F.L. Delmonico, M.P. LaQuaglia, N. Toilkoff-Rubin, R.H. Rubin, J.T. Herrin, and P.S. Russell. 1981. Treatment of acute renal allograft rejection with OKT3 monoclonal antibody. *Transplantation* **32**:535.
7. Cosimi, A.B., R.B. Colvin, F.L. Delmonico, and P.S. Russell. 1981. Use of monoclonal antibodies to T cell subsets for immunologic monitoring and treatment in recipients of renal allografts. *New England J. Med.* **305**:308.
8. Carpenter, C.B., and T.B. Strom. 1984. Immunosuppressive therapy for renal transplantation. *Springer Semin. Immunopathol.* **7**:43.
9. Miller, R.A., D.G. Maloney, J. McKillop, and R. Levy. 1981. *In vivo* effects of a murine hybridoma monoclonal antibody in a patient with T cell leukemia. *Blood* **58**:78.
10. Ritz, J., J.M. Pesandro, S.E. Sallan, L.A. Clavell, J. Notis-McConorty, P. Rosenthal, and S. Schlossman. 1981. Serotherapy of acute lymphoblastic leukemia with monoclonal antibody. *Blood* **58**:141.
11. Miller, R.A., and R. Levy. 1981. Response of cutaneous T cell lymphoma to therapy with hybridoma monoclonal antibody. *Lancet* **1981**(2):226.
12. Miller, R.A., A.R. Oseroff, R.T. Stratte, and R. Levy. 1983. Monoclonal antibody therapeutic trials in seven patients with T-cell lymphoma. *Blood* **62**:988.
13. Köhler, G., and C. Milstein. 1975. Continuous cultures of fused cells secreting antibody of predefined specificity. *Nature* **256**:495.
14. Majdic, O., K. Liszka, D. Lutz, and W. Knapp. 1981. Myeloid differentiation antigen defined by a monoclonal antibody. *Blood* **58**:1127.
15. Collins, S.J., R.C. Gallo, and R.E. Gallagher. 1977. Continuous growth and differentiation of human myeloid leukaemic cells in suspension culture. *Nature* **270**:347.
16. Koeffler, H.P., and D.W. Golde. 1978. Acute myelogenous leukemia: a human cell line responsive to colony-stimulating activity. *Science* **200**:1153.
17. Sundström, C., and K. Nilsson. 1976. Establishment and characterization of a human histiocytic lymphoma cell line (U-937). *Int. J. Cancer* **17**:565.
18. Tsuchiya, S., Y. Yamaguchi, Y. Kobayashi, T. Konno, and K. Tada. 1980. Establishment and characterization of a human acute monocytic leukemia cell line (THP-1). *Int. J. Cancer* **26**:171.
19. Lozzio, C.B., and B.B. Lozzio. 1975. Human chronic myelogenous leukemia cell line with positive Philadelphia chromosome. *Blood* **45**:321.
20. Martin, P., and T. Papayannopoulou. 1982. HEL cells: A new human erythroleukemia cell line with spontaneous and induced globin expression. *Science* **216**:1233.

21. Rosenfeld, C., A. Goutner, A.M. Venuat, C. Choquet, J.L. Pico, J.F. Dore, A. Liabeuf, A. Durandy, C. Desgrange, and G. De-The. 1977. An effective human leukaemic cell line, Reh. *Eur. J. Cancer* **13**:377.
22. Pulvertaft, R.J.V. 1964. Cytology of Burkitt's tumour. *Lancet* **1964**(1):238.
23. Minowada, J., T. Olinuma, and G.E. Moore. 1973. Rosette-forming human lymphoid cell line. Establishment and evidence for origin of thymus derived lymphocytes. *J. Natl. Cancer Inst.* **49**:891.
24. Schneider, U., H.U. Schwenk, and G. Bornkamm. 1977. Characterization of EBV-genome negative "null" and "T"-cell lines derived from children with acute lymphoblastic leukemia and leukemic transformed non-Hodgkin lymphoma. *Int. J. Cancer* **19**:621.
25. Konwalinka, G., Ch. Peschel, D. Geissler, B. Tomaschek, J. Boyd, R. Odavic, and H. Braunsteiner. 1983. Myelopoiesis of human bone marrow cells in a micro-agar culture system: comparison of two sources of colony stimulating activity (CSA). *Int. J. Cell Cloning* **1**:401.
26. Konwalinka, G., Ch. Peschel, J. Boyd, D. Geissler, M. Ogriseg, R. Odavic, and H. Braunsteiner. 1984. A miniaturized agar culture system for cloning human erythropoietic progenitor cells. *Exp. Haemat.* **12**:75.
27. Geissler, D., G. Konwalinka, Ch. Peschel, J. Boyd, R. Odavic, and H. Braunsteiner. 1983. Clonal growth of human megakaryocytic progenitor cells in a micro agar culture system: simultaneous proliferation of megakaryocytic, granulocytic and erythroid progenitor cells (CFU-M, CFU-C, BFU-E) and T-lymphocytic colonies (CFU-TL). *Int. J. Cell Cloning* **1**:377.
28. Meuer, S.C., K.A. Fitzgerald, R.E. Hussey, J.C. Hodgolon, S.F. Schlossmann, and E.L. Reinherz. 1983. Clonotypic structures involved in antigen-specific human T cell function. *J. Exp. Med.* **157**:705.
29. Reinherz, E.L., S. Meuer, K.A. Fitzgerald, R.E. Hussey, H. Levine, and S.F. Schlossmann. 1982. Antigen recognition by human T lymphocytes is linked to surface expression of the T3 molecular complex. *Cell* **30**:735.
30. LeBien, T.W., D.R. Boue, J. Bradley, and J.M. Kersey. 1982. Antibody affinity may influence antigenic modulation of the common acute lymphoblastic leukemia antigen *in vitro*. *J. Immunol.* **129**:2287.
31. Reinherz, E.L., P.C. Kung, G. Goldstein, and S.F. Schlossman. 1979. A monoclonal antibody with selective reactivity with functionally mature thymocytes and all peripheral human T cells. *J. Immunol.* **123**:1312.
32. Van Wauwe, J., J. De Mey, and J. Goossens. 1980. OKT3: a monoclonal antihuman T lymphocyte antibody with potent mitogenic properties. *J. Immunol.* **124**:2708.

CHAPTER 43

Specific Membrane Lectin of Human T Suppressor Cells

Claudine Kieda and Michel Monsigny

Introduction

Membrane lectins on murine lymphocytes have previously been described (1,2). They are sugar-specific receptors distributed on subpopulations of cells. Their presence has also been investigated on human peripheral blood leukocytes (3,4), where they are also distributed on distinct subpopulations. Furthermore, it could be shown that a suppressive effect on B cell immunoglobulin production can be inhibited by α-L-rhamnosyl derivatives (4–6).

In this communication, we report that α-L-rhamnosyl derivatives are recognized by and bind to a subset of T cells. This binding can be shown by the use of a synthetic neoglycoprotein: α-L-rhamnosylated bovine serum albumin (7). On the basis of this property, a separation of the α-L-rhamnose-specific subset of T cells was set up and the immunological and biological properties of this subset were investigated. Cytological and functional characterizations of the separated subpopulations showed that the specific recognition of sugar residues by lymphoid cells is a property determining subpopulations with defined immunological behavior. The α-L-rhamnose specific cells have the properties of T suppressor cells.

Materials and Methods

Leukocytes were obtained by Ficoll–Hypaque density gradient centrifugation (8) from heparinized venous blood given by normal healthy donors. T cells were identified by sheep erythrocyte rosetting (9). Monocytes and macrophages were detected by nonspecific esterase staining (10). B cells were identified with fluorescein-labeled F(ab')$_2$ fragments of anti–human immunoglobulins (11). Pokeweed mitogen was purchased from IBF Réactifs (Pointet-Girard, Villeneuve la Garenne, France).

Separation and Characterization of α-L-Rhamnose-Specific T Cells

The separation procedure is described in detail elsewhere (12). Briefly, the T cell-enriched fraction (9) was incubated in the presence of α-L-rhamnosylated BSA for 1 hr at 4°C, washed, and incubated in petri dishes coated with rabbit anti-BSA antibodies for 1 hr at 4°C. Nonadherent cells (Rha$^-$–TCE) were collected and then adherent cells (Rha$^+$–TCE) were released upon adding BSA-containing buffer. The two subpopulations were characterized by flow cytofluorimetry using a FACS analyzer (Becton-Dickinson, Sunnyvale, CA, USA) and fluorescein-labeled α-L-rhamnosylated serum albumin, and by their reactivity with monoclonal antibodies binding monocytes (Leu-M$_3$), T cells (Leu-1), helper/inducer T cells (Leu-3), and cytoxic/suppressor T cells (Leu-2) from Becton-Dickinson; monoclonal antibodies binding B cells (B$_2$) from Coultronics, Margency (France); and fluorescein-labeled goat anti–mouse IgG (H + L) from Becton-Dickinson.

Immunological Function of Rha$^+$–TCE and Rha$^-$–TCE Cells

Cells obtained as described were tested for their ability to modulate the secretion of immunoglobulins by pokeweed mitogen-stimulated B cells (13). Leukocytes or B cell-enriched populations were cultured for 9 days in the presence of an optimal dose of pokeweed mitogen and either T cell subpopulations or culture supernatants of T cell subpopulations.

Results

α-L-Rhamnosylated-BSA Fractionation of Human Peripheral T Cells

The T cell-enriched fraction (TCE) obtained by double E-rosetting with sheep erythrocytes containing less than 1% esterase-positive cells was split into two subfractions: the Rha$^-$–TCE cells which do not bind a significant amount of α-L-rhamnosylated BSA and thus do not adhere to rabbit anti-BSA antibody-coated petri dishes (60 ± 5% of the TCE population) and the Rha$^+$–TCE cells which, under the conditions used, do adhere to precoated petri dishes and are released in the presence of BSA-containing buffer (30 ± 5% of the TCE population).

The cell recovery was higher than 90% and cell viability of Rha$^+$–TCE and Rha$^-$–TCE cells was always higher than 95%, showing that the procedure is quite suitable. Rha$^-$–TCE cells do not bind α-L-rhamnosylated BSA, anti-Leu-M$_3$, or B$_4$ monoclonal antibodies. A large proportion of Rha$^-$–TCE cells strongly bind anti-Leu-1 (80%) and anti-Leu-3 ($\approx$60%)

monoclonal antibodies, while a minor proportion (15%) binds anti-Leu-2 monoclonal antibody.

Rha$^+$–TCE cells do not bind anti-Leu-M$_3$ or B$_4$ monoclonal antibodies but do bind α-L-rhamnosylated BSA. A large proportion of Rha$^+$–TCE cells strongly binds anti-Leu-1 (80%) and anti-Leu-2 (60%) while a small proportion ($\approx$7%) binds anti-Leu-3 monoclonal antibody.

Immunological Function of Rha$^+$–TCE and Rha$^-$–TCE Cells

These two subpopulations were shown to be almost inefficient in modulating the blastic transformation of pokeweed mitogen-activated B cells. Conversely, Rha$^+$–TCE cells as well as culture supernatant of Rha$^+$–TCE cells strongly inhibit the production of antibodies by pokeweed mitogen-activated B cells as shown by plaque-forming cell experiments (14) (Table 43.1). Rha$^-$–TCE cells and culture supernatants of Rha$^-$–TCE cells slightly enhance the production of antibodies by pokeweed mitogen-activated B cells. So, it appears that Rha$^+$–TCE cells release a soluble suppressor factor of B cell immunoglobulin production similar to the suppressor factor elaborated by concanavalin A-activated human mononuclear cells (5).

Conclusion

The presence of sugar-binding receptors at the surface of human lymphocytes is for the first time shown to be related to the immunological function of specific lymphocyte subsets. The reported cytological character-

Table 43.1. Modulation of the antibody production of pokeweed mitogen-stimulated B cells by Rha$^+$–TCE and Rha$^-$–TCE cells or their culture supernatants.

Adducts	Cells Δ PFC%	Supernatants Δ PFC%
Rha$^+$–TCE	−60 ± 4	−65 ± 4
Rha$^-$–TCE	+12 ± 2	+20 ± 2

Δ PFC%: percent inhibition (−) or enhancement (+) of the number of plaque-forming cells relative to the number of plaque-forming cells obtained with pokeweed mitogen-stimulated unfractionated human leukocytes in the absence of Rha$^+$–TCE, Rha$^-$–TCE cells, or their culture supernatants. The ratio of added T cells/unfractionated leukocytes was 1/10. Supernatants isolated from 2×10^6 T cells cultured for 48 hr in 2.5-ml complete medium were diluted fourfold before being added to the leukocyte culture wells.

izations and functional studies of two subsets of T cells isolated on the basis of their specific binding to a given neoglycoprotein show that:

1. A subpopulation of T cells does bind α-L-rhamnosylated bovine serum albumin.
2. The binding is strong and specific enough to allow the isolation of the subset.
3. The Rha$^+$–TCE cell subset predominantly contains cytotoxic/suppressor T cells.
4. The suppressor effect of Rha$^+$–TCE cells on immunoglobulin production is quite potent.
5. This suppressor effect is mediated by a soluble factor released in the culture supernatant of Rha$^+$–TCE cells.

Acknowledgments. This work was supported by Institut National de la Santé et de la Recherche Médical, grant CRL 84.0041, and by Association pour la Recherche sur le Cancer (ARC), grant allowing the purchase of a flow cytofluorimeter.

References

1. Kieda, C.M., D.J. Bowles, A. Ravid, and N. Sharon. 1978. Lectins in lymphocytes membranes. *FEBS Lett.* **94**:391.
2. Kieda, C.M., A.C. Roche, F. Delmotte, and M. Monsigny. 1979. Lymphocytes membrane lectins: Direct visualization by the use of fluorescent glycosylated cytochemical markers. *FEBS Lett.* **99**:329.
3. Barzilay, M., M. Monsigny, and N. Sharon. 1982. Interaction of soybean agglutinin with human peripheral blood lymphocytes subpopulations: evidence for the existence of a lectin-like substance on the lymphocyte surface. In: *Lectins: Biology, biochemistry and clinical biochemistry,* Vol. 2, T.C. Bog-Hansen, ed. W. de Gruyter, Berlin, New York, pp. 67–81.
4. Kieda, C.M., M. Monsigny, and M.J. Waxdal. 1982. Endogenous lectins on human peripheral blood lymphocytes. In: *Lectins: Biology, biochemistry and clinical biochemistry,* Vol. 3, T.C. Bog-Hansen and G.A. Spengler, eds. W. de Gruyter, Berlin, pp. 427–433.
5. Fleisher, T.A., W.C. Greene, R.M. Blaese, and T.A. Waldmann. 1981. Soluble suppressor supernatants elaborated by Concanavalin A activated human mononuclear cells. 1. Characterization of a soluble suppressor of T cells proliferation. *J. Immunol.* **126**:1192.
6. Greene, W.C., T.A. Fleisher, and T.A. Waldmann. 1981. Soluble suppressor supernatants elaborated by Concanavalin A activated human mononuclear cells. 2. Characterization of a soluble suppressor of B cells immunoglobulin production. *J. Immunol.* **126**:1158.
7. Monsigny, M., C.M. Kieda, and A.C. Roche. 1983. Membrane glycoproteins, glycolipids and membrane lectins as recognition signals in normal and malignant cells. *Biol. Cell.* **47**:95.
8. Boyum, A. 1968. Isolation of mononuclear cells and granulocytes from human blood. *Scand. J. Clin. Lab. Invest.* **21**:1.

9. Bentwich, Z., S.D. Douglas, F.D. Siegal, and H.G. Kunkel. 1973. The formation of stable E rosettes after neuraminidase treatment of either human peripheral blood lymphocytes or sheep red blood cells. *Clin. Immunol. Immunopathol.* **1**:511.
10. Koski, I.R., D.G. Poplack, and R.M. Blaese. 1976. A non specific esterase stain for the identification of monocytes and macrophages. In: *In vitro methods in cell mediated and tumor immunity*, B.R. Bloom and J.R. David, eds. Academic Press, New York, pp. 359–362.
11. Johnson, G.D., E.J. Holborow, and J. Dorling. 1978. Immunofluorescence and immunoenzyme techniques. In: *Handbook of experimental immunology*, D.M. Weir ed. Blackwell Scientific, Oxford, pp. 15.1–15.30.
12. Kieda, C.M., M.J. Waxdal, and M. Monsigny. Involvement of membrane glycoconjugates and membrane lectins in lymphocytes homing. *J. Immunol.* (submitted).
13. Gronowicz, E., A. Coutinho and F. Melchers. 1976. A plaque assay for all cells secreting immunoglobulin of a given type or class. *Eur. J. Immunol.* **6**:588.
14. Ginsburg, W.W., F.D. Finkelman, and P.E. Lipsky. 1978. Circulating and mitogen-induced immunoglobulin secreting cells in human peripheral blood: evaluation by a reverse hemolytic plaque assay. *J. Immunol.* **120**:33.

Index